Host Interactions in HIV Infection

Host Interactions in HIV Infection

Edited by **Chris Stinson**

FOSTER
ACADEMICS

New Jersey

Published by Foster Academics,
61 Van Reypen Street,
Jersey City, NJ 07306, USA
www.fosteracademics.com

Host Interactions in HIV Infection
Edited by Chris Stinson

International Standard Book Number: 978-1-63242-234-7 (Hardback)

Printed in China.

Contents

Preface

Every book is initially just a concept; it takes months of research and hard work to give it the final shape in which the readers receive it. In its early stages, this book also went through rigorous reviewing. The notable contributions made by experts from across the globe were first molded into patterned chapters and then arranged in a sensibly sequential manner to bring out the best results.

There is no vaccine or cure available for HIV; hence it is a prominent global health threat. To beat the challenges of HIV/AIDS, one must have sufficient knowledge of HIV infection. This book discusses various forms of HIV-host interactions in vitro and in vivo, like the interrelation between cellular components and HIV proteins, Integrase, Tat, and Nef, as well as the clinical pertinence of HIV superinfection. The book also examines the function of innate immunity along with dendritic cells and defensins in HIV infections and the effects of host factors on HIV pathogenesis. Topics like co-infection are also included that talk about the influence of Human herpesvirus 6 and Trichomonas vaginalis on HIV infection. The book also includes a discussion on the generations of HIV molecular clones that can be applied in macaques and the potential usage of cotton rats for HIV studies.

It has been my immense pleasure to be a part of this project and to contribute my years of learning in such a meaningful form. I would like to take this opportunity to thank all the people who have been associated with the completion of this book at any step.

Editor

Part 1

Viral Components and Host Interactions

1

Molecular Crosstalk between HIV-1 Integration and Host Proteins – Implications for Therapeutics

Youichi Suzuki[1], Yasutsugu Suzuki[1,2] and Naoki Yamamoto[1]
[1]*Yong Loo Lin School of Medicine, National University of Singapore*
[2]*Graduate School of Biostudies, Kyoto University*
[1]*Singapore*
[2]*Japan*

1. Introduction

The human immunodeficiency virus (HIV) is the causative agent of acquired immunodeficiency syndrome (AIDS), which is one of the leading causes of infectious disease-related mortality worldwide (UNAIDS, 2010). An HIV infection is a chronic disease. While there is no regimen to eradicate the HIV from an infected person, there are more than 20 drugs approved for the treatment of HIV infection, the majority of which target viral reverse transcriptase (RT) and protease (PR). In addition to the development of chemotherapeutic agents such as RT and PR inhibitors (RTI and PI), the advent of the combination therapy of different classes of antiviral drugs, the highly active antiretroviral therapy (HAART), has brought a significant decrease in the morbidity and mortality associated with HIV infections for over a decade. Nowadays, HAART is a standard treatment for HIV infection and AIDS (Palella et al., 1998). However, despite the successful suppression of HIV RNA detected in plasma over prolonged periods of time and a dramatic decrease in patient mortality, HAART is still facing problems, including the emergence of drug resistant viruses and serious side effects in treated individuals. In addition, current treatments only suppress the HIV replication, and eradication of virus from the body cannot be achieved. Therefore, considerable efforts have been made to develop novel anti-HIV drugs that exhibit entirely distinct mechanisms of action. To date, three additional classes of inhibitors have been approved by the US Food and Drug Administration (FDA) as oral anti-HIV agents: a fusion inhibitor blocking the fusion step of the viral and cellular membranes, an entry inhibitor targeting coreceptor binding by the virus, and an integrase (IN) inhibitor blocking the integration step of viral DNA.

Although many promising inhibitors against HIV replication have arisen over recent years, the current approach in anti-HIV chemotherapy is mostly based on competitive agents targeting the active sites of viral enzymes or the binding pockets of cellular receptors. One of the drawbacks of existing drugs, particularly the antivirals exhibiting allosteric effects, is the rapid emergence of mutant HIV strains resistant to the drugs due to the innately high mutational rate in of viral enzymes. On the other hand, it is becoming increasingly clear that protein-protein interactions (PPIs) could also serve as attractive targets of drugs for human therapeutics (Cochran, 2001; Arkin & Wells, 2004; Pagliaro et al., 2004; Ryan & Matthews, 2005). PPIs are central to most biological processes including virus infection and many human diseases are attributed to aberrant PPIs in cells. Not surprisingly, there are a number of interactions between viral and cellular proteins involved in all stages of HIV replication (Goff, 2007; Arhel & Kirchhoff, 2010) and recent evidence demonstrates that these PPIs can be potential targets for the development of a novel class of anti-HIV drugs termed small molecule protein-protein interaction inhibitors (SMPPIIs) (Busschots et al., 2009; Christ et al., 2010). Although a challenging approach, an advantage of SMPPIIs in HIV chemotherapy is that the mutation rate in the PPI interface is considerably low compared to the mutation rate in the active sites of viral enzymes, particularly for the host proteins. Therefore, SMPPIIs targeting HIV and cellular proteins hold great promise with regards to preventing the emergence of drug resistant viruses in administrated persons. Thus, understanding the molecular basis of virus-host interactions should provide new insights into alternative strategies for the treatment of HIV infection and AIDS. In this chapter, we focus our attention on integration, an essential step in the HIV replication cycle catalyzed by IN, and review the current knowledge of molecular interactions between IN and cellular cofactors.

2. HIV infection - from cell entry to integration

HIV belongs to lentivirus, a separate genus of the *Retroviridae* family, and it can be further divided into antigenically distinct members, HIV-1 and HIV-2 (Levy, 2009). In the case of HIV-1, the enveloped viral particle contains two copies of positive sense RNA of 9.7-kb in length which encode two regulatory (*tat* and *rev*) and four accessory (*vpr*, *vif*, *vpu*, and *nef*) genes in addition to the characteristic retroviral *gag*, *pol*, and *env* genes. These protein-coding regions are flanked by the 5′ and 3′ long terminal repeat (LTR) sequences that are required for reverse transcription, integration, and gene expression steps.

HIV-1 infection begins with the specific binding of the viral envelope (Env) glycoprotein gp120 to the CD4 receptor molecule on the surface of target cells. This interaction triggers a conformational change in the gp120 that facilitates subsequent binding to a coreceptor. As for the coreceptor, most of HIV-1 strains use either the α-chemokine receptor CXCR4 or the β-chemokine receptor CCR5. The formation of the gp120, CD4, and coreceptor complex then induces refolding of the gp41 subunit of Env, allowing the fusion of the HIV-1 and cell membranes.

After penetrating the cell membrane, the HIV-1 core particle, which contains genomic RNA and the proteins needed to establish an infection, is first released into the cytoplasm where it then undergoes the uncoating process. Although this uncoating is defined as the loss of HIV-1 capsid (CA) protein after the entry step, the nature and timing of the uncoating process is poorly understood (Arhel, 2010). The formation of the reverse transcription complex (RTC), in which reverse transcription from viral RNA to DNA takes place, accompanies the uncoating of infecting virion core (Warrilow et al., 2009; Arhel, 2010). Currently, little is known about the components of the RTC, although several studies have shown that matrix (MA), Vpr, RT, and IN are contained in the HIV-1 RTC (Fassati & Goff, 2001; McDonald et al., 2002; Iordanskiy et al., 2006). CA is only found in the HIV-1 RTC very early after cell entry but it becomes barely detectable at later times (Fassati & Goff, 2001). Interestingly, in the case of the Moloney murine leukemia virus (MoMLV), CA has shown to be stably associated with the RTC even at the later stages (Fassati & Goff, 1999). These pieces of evidence suggest that dissociation of CA from the HIV-1 core proceeds rapidly as compared to other retroviruses.

The newly synthesized full-length viral DNA remains associated with viral and cellular proteins in a high molecular weight nucleoprotein complex. This integration-competent nucleoprotein complex is called the preintegration complex (PIC) (Goff, 2001; Suzuki & Craigie, 2007). Although the structure of the PIC is also poorly understood, a number of studies using immunoprecipitation assays have revealed that HIV-1 PICs retain many components of the RTC (Farnet & Haseltine, 1990, 1991; Bukrinsky et al., 1993; Gallay et al., 1995; Farnet & Bushman, 1997; Miller et al., 1997; Iordanskiy et al., 2006). Additionally, several cellular proteins have been shown to associate with the HIV-1 PIC (Farnet & Bushman, 1997; Li et al., 2001; Lin & Engelman, 2003; Llano et al., 2004). A defining characteristic of the PIC is its full fidelity to the authentic integration reaction. When purified IN alone is used for an *in vitro* integration reaction, most of the products are the result of the integration of only a single viral DNA end into one strand of target DNA (Bushman & Craigie, 1991; Turlure et al., 2004). In contrast, a PIC isolated from virus-infected cells is able to efficiently insert both viral DNA ends into the target DNA in a pairwise manner *in vitro*, and this is a hallmark of the integration reaction *in vivo* (Farnet & Haseltine, 1990; Chen & Engelman, 2001). Another striking feature of PICs is that suicidal intramolecular integration into its own viral DNA, a reaction termed autointegration, is precluded and it has been reported that cellular proteins are implicated in this barrier to autointegration in HIV-1 PICs (Yan et al., 2009).

The PIC formed in the cytoplasm also serves as the vehicle for the translocation of its genetic cargo (i.e. viral DNA) into the nucleus. Once the PIC reaches the nuclear periphery it must gain entry into the nucleus for integration. In non-dividing cells such as macrophages, the PIC must permeate the barrier of an intact nuclear envelope. This is particularly important as macrophages are a major target of HIV-1 infection. How is the PIC to cross the nuclear envelope? Passive diffusion cannot explain the translocation because the size of the HIV-1 PIC exceeds the allowances of a nuclear pore. Molecules up to 9 nm in diameter can pass through the nuclear pore complex by diffusion (Mattaj & Englmeier, 1998), but the HIV-1 PIC is estimated to be more than 50 nm in diameter (Miller et al., 1997; McDonald et al., 2002; Nermut & Fassati, 2003). Thus, active transport mechanisms are necessary for this task; one widely accepted model is that the HIV-1 PIC possesses karyophilic signals and many viral and cellular proteins have been proposed as the karyophilic proteins that cause the nucleoprotein complex to be imported into the nucleus (Fouchier & Malim, 1999; Fassati, 2006; Luban, 2008). Although the actual participation of these proteins in the nuclear import of HIV-1 PICs is a matter of debate (Fassati, 2006; Suzuki & Craigie, 2007), this property is important in the pathogenesis of HIV-1 (Blankson et al., 2002). Additionally, the ability of HIV-1 to infect non-dividing cells makes the virus an attractive candidate for a gene transfer vector (Verma & Somia, 1997).

In the nucleus, chromosomal DNA serves as the target for integration. Integration is essential in the replication of all retroviruses including HIV-1, and this step as well as reverse transcription are hallmarks of retroviral infection. The integration process occurs in three well-characterized reactions referred to as 3′-end processing, DNA strand transfer and gap repair (described below). IN catalyzes the first two reactions whereas the last reaction is likely carried out by yet-to-be identified cellular enzymes (Turlure et al., 2004). Once integrated, the viral DNA, called the provirus, is acted upon by cellular transcription factors to express viral genes and can persist indefinitely in the host cell genome (Fig. 1).

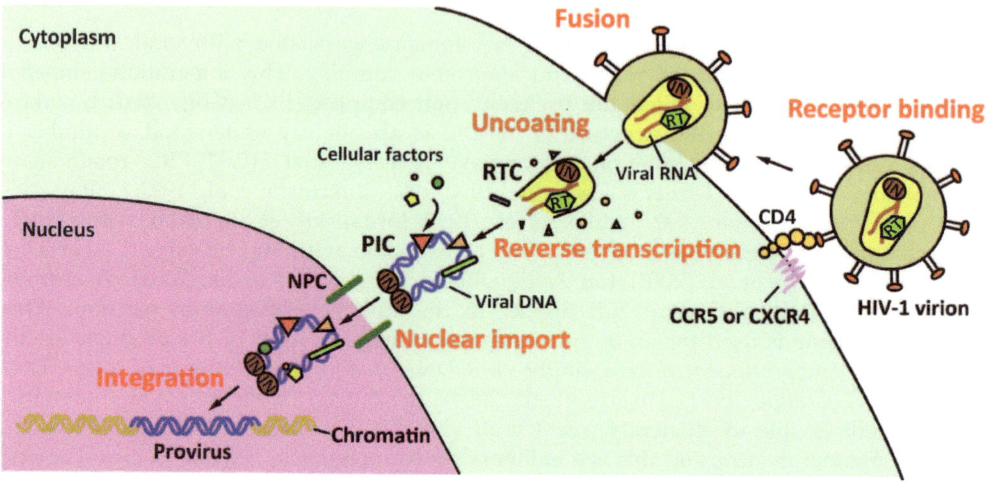

Fig. 1. Early stages of HIV-1 replication. HIV-1 infection begins with the binding of Env to the CD4 receptor and a coreceptor (CCR5 or CXCR4), allowing fusion between the cellular and viral membranes. After entry, the viral nucleoprotein core containing the genomic RNA is released into cytoplasm and reverse transcription takes place in a nucleoprotein complex called the RTC. The resulting full-length viral DNA remains associated with viral and cellular proteins in an integration-competent nucleoprotein complex termed the PIC. This PIC mediates integration of viral DNA into chromatin. Integrated viral DNA, called the provirus, then acts as a transcription template for the synthesis of viral RNAs.

3. HIV-1 IN and the mechanism of integration

3.1 IN structure

During HIV-1 replication, IN is expressed from the provirus as the C-terminal part of a 160-kDa Gag-Pol polyprotein and it is incorporated into nascent virions. Following the budding and release of viral particles from infected cells, viral PR cleaves the Gag-Pol precursor protein to generate the mature form of IN (Swanstrom & Wills, 1997). In the HIV-1 genome, Gag (a precursor for structural proteins such as MA, CA and nucleocapsid [NC]) and Pol (a precursor for enzymes such as PR, RT and IN) are encoded by overlapping open reading frames (ORFs), and the Gag-Pol precursor is generated by ribosomal frameshifting during translation of the *gag* gene. This translation mechanism results in the synthesis of Gag-Pol at a 20-fold lower level than Gag's in HIV-1 infected cells (Jacks et al., 1988). Consequently, only 50 to 100 molecules of IN are contained in a viral particle. Although the production of Gag protein has been reported to suffice for generation of virus-like particles (VLP) (Mergener et al., 1992), incorporation and processing of the Gag-Pol protein is required for the formation of infectious HIV-1 virions (Swanstrom & Wills, 1997; Wu et al., 1997).

HIV-1 IN is a 32-kDa protein that consists of three structurally and functionally distinct domains called the N-terminal domain (NTD), the catalytic core domain (CCD), and the C-terminal domain (CTD) (Fig. 2A) (Lewinski & Bushman, 2005). The structures of these individual domains have been determined by X-ray crystallography or NMR (Craigie, 2001; Vandegraaff & Engelman, 2007). The CCD is highly conserved amongst retroviral INs and contains a triad of conserved amino acids comprising of Asp64, Asp116, and Glu152and this is termed the D,D-35-E motif. By coordinating divalent metal ions such as Mg^{2+} to this motif, the CCD domain plays a key role during the integration reaction (Lewinski & Bushman, 2005). This domain is dimeric in solution and the crystal structure of the dimer shows that the CCD domain consists of a five-stranded β-sheet and six α-helices. This structure is also found in many nucleotidyl transferases including RNase H, bacterial Mu, and the Argonaute protein of the RNA-induced silencing complex (RISC). Hence, IN belongs to the superfamily of polynucleotidyltransferases (Vandegraaff & Engelman, 2007).

A well-conserved motif is also found in the NTD, which comprises two His and two Cys residues (HHCC motif). This domain contains a bundle of three α-helices, and the HHCC motif stabilizes the helices by coordinating Zn^{2+}. Mutation studies of the NTD have indicated that the HHCC motif contributes to the multimerization and catalytic function of HIV-1 IN (Lewinski & Bushman, 2005).

In contrast to the NTD and CCD, the CTD is the least conserved domain of retroviral INs. Although the functional role of the CTD for catalysis is less clear, this domain exhibits strong and non-specific DNA-binding activity *in vitro*. The isolated CTD forms dimers in solution, and its monomer has an all β-strand SH3-type fold (Lewinski & Bushman, 2005).

3.2 Integration reaction

The chemical mechanism of the integration catalyzed by HIV-1 IN has been elucidated by *in vitro* biochemical studies using recombinant IN protein and oligonucleotide DNA substrates (Craigie, 2001; Lewinski & Bushman, 2005; Vandegraaff & Engelman, 2007). This reaction proceeds with well-defined 3′ processing and strand transfer steps (Fig. 2B). In the 3′ processing step, IN specifically recognizes the viral attachment (*att*) sites on the 5′ and 3′ LTRs where it removes two nucleotides from each of the 3′ ends of the viral DNA to expose a recessed hydroxyl immediately following a CA dinucleotide that is conserved among retroviruses and many transposons. Water serves as the nucleophile this cleavage of viral DNA. Next, in the strand transfer step, the exposed hydroxyl groups attack a pair of phosphodiester bonds on opposite strands of the target DNA, causing the viral DNA termini to be covalently linked to the protruding 5′ phosphoryl ends of the target DNA. Since the cleavage sites on the opposite strands of target DNA are separated by 5 bp, HIV-1 integration generates a five-base duplication flanking the provirus. Stereochemical analysis has revealed that these reactions occur by single-step transesterification mechanism (Engelman et al., 1991).

The 3′ processing and strand transfer steps are reproducible *in vitro* using recombinant IN and DNA substrates, indicating that IN alone is sufficient to carry out the DNA breakage and joining reactions. However, these events yield short staggered DNA breaks at the points of joining, and so in virus-infected cells the mispaired 5′ viral DNA ends must be excised and the resulting nicks filled in order to produce the provirus (gap repair step). However, this final step is likely carried out by yet-to-be identified cellular enzymes and the molecular mechanisms involved in this reaction have not yet been elucidated (Smith & Daniel, 2006; Yoder et al., 2006; Turlure et al., 2004).

4. Cellular proteins interacting with HIV-1 IN

Although the enzymatic activities of HIV-1 IN in the integration reaction have been clearly defined by *in vitro* biochemical studies, numerous genetic analysis of HIV-1 DNA have demonstrated that mutations in the *IN* gene, including deletion mutants, influence many other stages of viral replication in addition to integration. This pleiotropic effect of IN is characterized by defects in uncoating, reverse transcription, nuclear import, viral gene expression, virion precursor protein processing, and virion morphology (Shin et al., 1994; Engelman et al., 1995; Masuda et al., 1995; Bukovsky & Gottlinger, 1996; Leavitt et al., 1996; Nakamura et al., 1997; Engelman, 1999; Tsurutani et al., 2000; Lu et al., 2004; Dar et al., 2009; Briones et al., 2010). However, the mechanisms for these pleiotropic effects of the *IN* gene are still poorly understood.

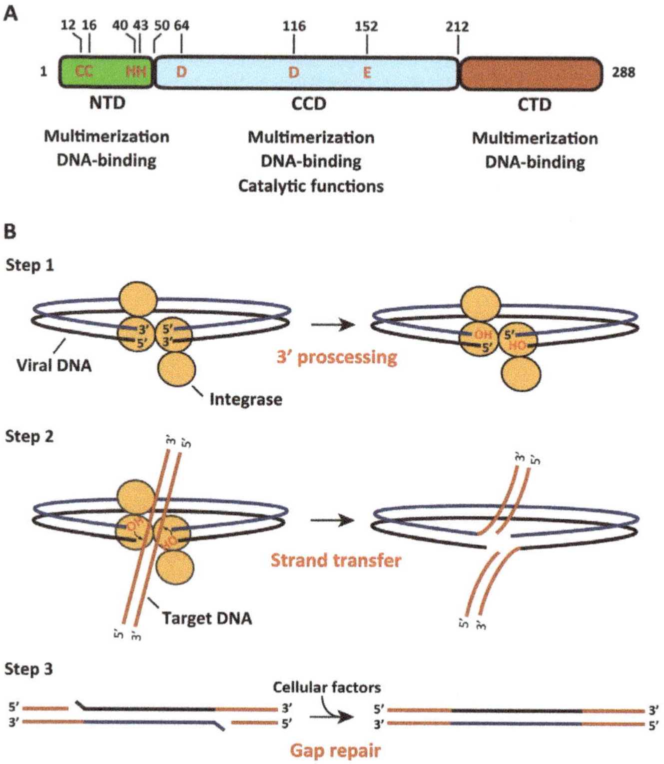

Fig. 2. HIV-1 integration reaction. (A) Domain organization of HIV-1 IN. Retroviral IN , including HIV-1 IN, consists of the N-terminal domain (NTD), catalytic core domain (CCD), and C-terminal domain (CTD). Highly concerved aspartic (D) and glutamic acid (E) residues are found in the CCD, forming the catalytic centre in IN (D,D-35-E motif). Likewise, the NTD contains a well-conserved motif that is formed from two histidine and two cystein residues (HHCC motif) while the CTD is the least conserved of the retroviral INs domains. (B) Mechanism of DNA integration. IN recognizes both ends of the viral DNA and removes two nucleotides from each of the ends (3′ processing). This reaction takes place in the cytoplasm. After entering the nucleus and binding to chromosomal DNA, IN cleaves the target DNA in a staggered fashion via the exposed hydroxyl groups (OH) on the viral DNA ends, the viral DNA termini are then joined to the cuts (strand transfer step). Finally, the resulting nicks at the viral-target DNA junction are repaired by cellular enzymes to complete the integration process (gap repair step).

Meanwhile, a number of cellular proteins have been identified as binding partners for HIV-1 IN (Turlure et al., 2004; Al-Mawsawi & Neamati, 2007; Ao et al., 2007; Christ et al., 2008; Woodward et al., 2009; Ao et al., 2010). Some of these cellular interactors have been reported to assist in HIV-1 integration in infected cells (Turlure et al., 2004). However, other cellular partners for HIV-1 IN appear to have functional roles in steps other than the integration process including reverse transcription, nuclear import, and infectious particle production (Yung et al., 2001; Hamamoto et al., 2006; Al-Mawsawi & Ao et al., 2007; Mousnier et al., 2007; Neamati, 2007; Christ et al., 2008; Ao et al., 2010). These pieces of evidence suggests that PPIs between IN and its cellular partner could be the molecular basis for the pleiotropic effects that have been observed in genetic studies using HIV-1 with mutant IN.
Below, we summarize the current knowledge of the HIV-1 IN-binding cellular proteins and their possible roles in virus replication.

4.1 Cellular interactors affecting on integration step

So far, identification of HIV-1 IN cofactors has mostly been conducted by using yeast two-hybrid screenings or co-immunoprecipitation assays (Turlure et al., 2004). Integrase interactor 1 (INI1) was the first IN-binding protein identified by the yeast two-hybrid screening (Kalpana et al., 1994). INI1 is the human homologue of yeast SNF5, a core subunit of the ATP-dependent SWI/SNF chromatin-remodeling complex (Wang et al., 1996). Thus, INI1 is also known as hSNF5. By exposing transcriptionally active regions of chromatin, SNF5 regulates the expression of numerous genes in eukaryotic cells (Carlson & Laurent, 1994). INI1/hSNF5 is a 385 amino acid protein that is composed of three conserved domains including two direct imperfect repeat (Rpt) regions (Rpt1 and Rpt2) and a C-terminal coiled-coil domain referred to as the homology region III (HRIII) (Morozov et al., 1998). A yeast two-hybrid assay has revealed that the Rpt1 is necessary for binding to HIV-1 IN (Morozov et al., 1998).

In an early study using recombinant HIV-1 IN, INI1/hSNF5 was found to stimulate the integration reaction *in vitro* (Kalpana et al., 1994). However, when the minimal IN-binding domain of INI1/hSNF5, including the Rpt1 region (residues 183-294) termed S6, was co-transfected with HIV-1 proviral DNA in HEK293 cells, a 10,000-fold reduction in virus production from the transfected cells was observed (Yung et al., 2001). Moreover, expression of the S6 fragment in Jurkat T cells protected the cells against HIV-1 replication (Yung et al., 2001). Although this inhibitory effect was not detected in full-length INI1/hSNF5, the WT INI1/hSNF5 has been shown to be incorporated into virions during virus production (Yung et al., 2001; Yung et al., 2004). Given the recent report that depletion of endogenous INI1/hSNF5 did not affect the transduction efficiency of an HIV-1-based vector, this suggests that INI1/hSNF5 is likely implicated in post-integration steps, rather than the integration step as we shall see below, particularly in HIV-1 production (Ariumi et al., 2006).
In terms of integration cofactors, lens epithelium-derived growth factor (LEDGF) is the first host protein whose role has been most clearly elucidated (Engelman & Cherepanov, 2008). LEDGF, a transcriptional regulator that belongs to the hepatoma-derived growth factor (HDGF) related protein (HRP) family, was identified as an IN-binding protein as a result of co-immunoprecipitation analysis using FLAG-tagged HIV-1 IN (Cherepanov et al., 2003). LEDGF is a 530 amino acid protein that consists of several functional domains (Fig. 3A) (Engelman & Cherepanov, 2008). The N-terminal 92 amino acid region is termed the PWWP (Pro-Trp-Trp-Pro) domain. The PWWP domain is conserved amongst the HRP family

proteins and is thought to function as a protein-protein interaction domain and/or DNA-binding domain (Stec et al., 2000; Qiu et al., 2002). LEDGF also includes three segments of polar amino acids called CR (charged region) domains, and a putative nuclear localization signal (NLS) and dual copies of the AT-hook DNA-binding motif can be identified in the N-terminal half of the protein. In addition, a limited proteolysis analysis of recombinant LEGFP has revealed an evolutionarily conserved domain at the C terminus, which mediates the interaction with HIV-1 IN (integrase-binding domain: IBD) (Cherepanov et al., 2004). The IBD is a compact right-handed bundle composed of five α helices (Cherepanov et al., 2005b). As for HIV-1 IN, CCD has been identified as the main determinant for interactions with LEDGF (Fig. 3A) (Maertens et al., 2003; Cherepanov et al., 2005a).

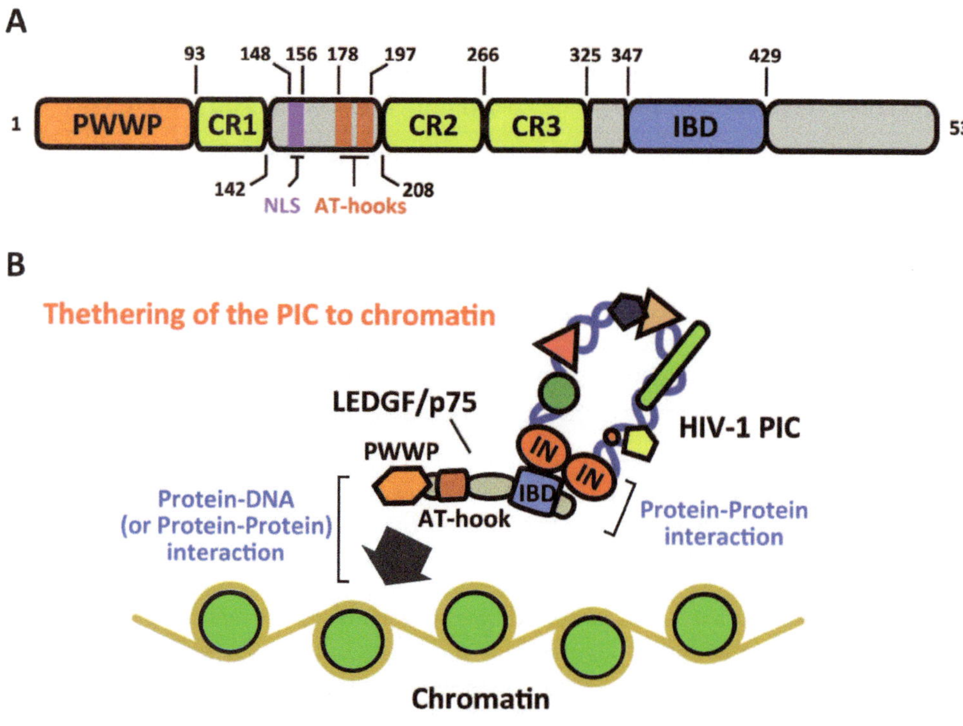

Fig. 3. Function of LEDGF in HIV-1 integration. (A) Domain structure of LEDGF. LEDGF is a 530 amino acid protein containing the PWWP domain, CR domains, a putative NLS, and dual copies of the AT-hook DNA-binding motif. Interaction of HIV-1 IN and LEDGF occurs between the CCD of IN and the C-terminal IBD of LEDGF, and this has been demonstrated to be critical for enhancement of the intgration reaction *in vitro* and *in vivo*. (B) LEDGF-mediated tethering of the HIV-1 PIC to chromain. The most widely accepted model of LEDGF function in HIV-1 infection is that LEDGF serves as an adaptor molecule to anchor the PIC to chromain via i) protein-protein interaction between IN and LEDGF and ii) subsequent protein-DNA interaction between LEDGF and chromatin. This thethering function may also regulate integraton-site selection of the HIV-1 PICs in virus-infected cells.

Early works using recombinant proteins have shown that LEDGF is able to stimulate the integration activity of the HIV-1 IN *in vitro* (Cherepanov et al., 2003, 2004). Furthermore, LEDGF associates with HIV-1 PICs (Llano et al., 2004). While these studies have raised the possibility that LEDGF might be implicated in the integration reaction of HIV-1 infection, subsequent *in vivo* studies using RNA interference reported that depletion of endogenous LEDGF resulted in only a modest effect or none at all on the replication efficiency of HIV-1 (Llano et al., 2004; Vandegraaff et al., 2006; Zielske & Stevenson, 2006). However, if residual expression of LEDGF is sufficient to complement the activity of HIV-1 IN in virus-infected cells, the results obtained by experiments using RNA interference-based knockdown assays might downplay the contribution of LEDGF to HIV-1 replication. Indeed, a significant reduction of HIV-1 infection was observed in human $CD4^+$ T cells in which there was a more complete knockdown of endogenous LEDGF (Llano et al., 2006a), and in mouse embryo fibroblasts (MEFs) derived from LEDGF knockout mice (Marshall et al., 2007; Shun et al., 2007), indicating a crucial role of LEDGF in virus replication. These genetic knockdown and knockout studies have revealed that the defect in HIV-1 replication in the absence of LEDGF clearly occurred at the DNA integration step (Llano et al., 2006a; Marshall et al., 2007; Shun et al., 2007). How is LEDGF involved in the integration process of HIV-1? Several lines of evidence have demonstrated that although *in vitro* integration by recombinant IN or PIC derived from HIV-1-infected cells occurs almost randomly, *in vivo* integration sites of HIV-1 are enriched with active transcription units (TUs) (Bushman et al., 2005). Considering the fact that the N-terminal PWWP domain/AT-hook motifs mediate chromatin-binding of LEDGF (Llano et al., 2006b; Turlure et al., 2006) and are also required for HIV-1 infection as much as the IBD (Llano et al., 2006a; Shun et al., 2007), the simplest model would be that LEDGF functions as a molecular adaptor for tethering HIV-1 IN within the PIC to chromatin, thereby promoting the integration process (Fig. 3B). Since LEDGF is a transcriptional coactivator, it would be plausible that the distribution of LEDGF on certain regions of chromatin is a primary determinant for the integration site specificity of HIV-1 (De Rijck et al., 2010). Indeed, genome-wide studies analyzing integration sites in HIV-1-infected cells have shown that a significant reduction in the frequency of integration into TUs was observed in LEDGF knockdown and knockout cells (Ciuffi et al., 2005; Marshall et al., 2007; Shun et al., 2007).

Posttranslational modifications of HIV-1 IN by cellular enzymes have also been reported to be implicated in integration. p300, a histone acetyltransferase (HAT), was first identified as a cellular protein that directly binds to HIV-1 IN *in vitro* and in human cells (Cereseto et al., 2005). HATs are known as enzymes that catalyze the transfer of acetyl groups from acetyl coenzyme A (acetyl-CoA) to specific lysine residues within the N-terminal tails of nucleosomal histones. This histone acetylation leads to chromatin decondensation and transcriptional activation (Roth et al., 2001). In addition to histones, HATs are able to acetylate other proteins including transcription factors. *In vitro* analysis using recombinant proteins showed that p300 can also acetylate three specific lysines (Lys264, Lys266, and Lys273) in the C-terminus of HIV-1 IN (Cereseto et al., 2005). Interestingly, the acetylation increased IN binding to LTR DNA its catalysis of the strand transfer reaction *in vitro* (Cereseto et al., 2005). Because HIV-1 harbouring mutations in the Lys264, Lys266, and Lys273 of IN exhibited replication defect at the integration step, these results suggest that acetylation of IN is important for efficient integration during HIV-1 infection (Cereseto et al., 2005). A recent study from the same group showed that another HAT, GCN5, was also able to mediate the acetylation of HIV-1 IN, and provirus formation was inefficient in GCN5-

depleted cells (Terreni et al., 2010). However, it should be noted that the role of acetylation of IN in HIV-1 replication remains controversial (Topper et al., 2007; Vandegraaff & Engelman, 2007).

Another type of posttranslational modification of IN that regulates HIV-1 infection has also been demonstrated. The c-Jun NH_2-terminal kinase (JNK), a member of mitogen-activated protein kinase (MAPK) family, is reported to phosphorylate a highly conserved serine residue (Ser57) in the CCD of HIV-1 IN. This phosphorylated IN is, in turn, recognized by the cellular peptidyl-prolyl *cis-trans* isomerase Pin1, and this association with Pin1 induces a conformational change in HIV-1 IN, eventually resulting in an increase in IN stability (Manganaro et al., 2010). Intriguingly, expression of JNK is very low in resting $CD4^+$ T cells, which are resistant to the establishment of productive infection by HIV-1, but not in activated cells permissive to HIV-1 infection. Hence, JNK and Pin1 may collaborate to increase the permissivity of T lymphocytes to HIV-1 via the phosphorylation and subsequent stabilization of IN (Manganaro et al., 2010).

Several other cellular proteins including uracil DNA glycosylase (UDG), heat-shock protein (HSP) 60, Rad18, and *Polycomb* group protein EED (embryonic ectoderm development) have also been found to interact with HIV-1 IN (Willetts et al., 1999; Parissi et al., 2001; Mulder et al., 2002; Violot et al., 2003), and some of them have been shown to stimulate *in vitro* integration activity of recombinant IN (Parissi et al., 2001; Violot et al., 2003). Yet, the contributions of these cellular interactors in HIV-1 integration and infection remain unclear (Turlure et al., 2004).

4.2 Cellular interactor affecting on reverse transcription step

It has been demonstrated that a specific interaction occurs between the HIV-1 IN and RT (Wu et al., 1999; Zhu et al., 2004), and that IN stimulates RT-catalyzed early synthesis of viral DNA *in vitro* (Dobard et al., 2007). This suggests that interaction between IN and RT has a functional consequence during the reverse transcription step of HIV-1 infection. Supporting the role of IN in viral DNA synthesis, a cellular binding protein for IN has been implicated in the reverse transcription of HIV-1. Gemin2 is a component of the survival of motor neurons (SMN) complex that is essential for the biogenesis of spliceosomal small nuclear ribonucleoproteins (snRNPs). The SMN complex, which is composed of an SMN protein and 7 additional proteins (Gemin2-8), recognizes specific sequences and structures of small nuclear RNAs and serves as an assembly complex for snRNP formation (Paushkin et al., 2002). A yeast two-hybrid screening identified Gemin2 as a novel interactor of HIV-1 IN (Hamamoto et al., 2006). This interaction involves the CTD alongside partial contribution from the CCD of HIV-1 IN (Hamamoto et al., 2006). Although Gemin2 was found in the HIV-1 PIC, knockdown experiments using small interfering RNA (siRNA) revealed that depletion of endogenous Gemin2 significantly reduced HIV-1 infectivity in human primary monocyte-derived macrophage (MDM), and importantly, the replication defect was observed at the early reverse transcription step during virus replication (Hamamoto et al., 2006). Moreover, a recent study shows that viral DNA synthesis by RT is augmented by IN in a Gemin2-dependent manner *in vitro* (Nishitsuji et al., 2009). These results suggest that the concerted action of IN and Gemin2 enhances the RT-catalyzed reverse transcription step in HIV-1 infection.

4.3 Cellular interactors affecting on nuclear import step

As mentioned above, a striking feature of HIV-1 is its ability to infect non-dividing cells. The nuclear envelope is intact in the non-dividing cells, and the HIV-1 PIC must cross this nuclear envelope to integrate viral DNA into chromosomal DNA. Therefore, it is believed that the HIV-1 PIC carries karyophilic signals that cause it to be transported into the nucleus through nuclear pore complexes (NPCs) (Suzuki & Craigie, 2007). HIV-1 IN has been implicated as a karyophilic protein that facilitates the nuclear import of the PICs (Ikeda et al., 2004). Although many studies using reporter proteins have shown that HIV-1 IN accumulates in the nucleus (Petit et al., 1999; Pluymers et al., 1999; Ikeda et al., 2004), recent evidences suggest that IN may lack a transferable NLS and that the accumulation of HIV-1 IN may be attributed to its interactions with the cellular karyophilic protein(s) (Devroe et al., 2003; Llano et al., 2004).

Shortly after its identification as an interactor of HIV-1 IN, LEDGF was proposed as the karyophilic factor (Maertens et al., 2003). A siRNA-mediated knockdown experiment showed that depletion of endogenous LEDGF abolished nuclear accumulation of HIV-1 IN in HeLa cells (Maertens et al., 2003). Because the LEDGF is the cellular component of HIV-1 PICs (Llano et al., 2004), this suggests that LEDGF is the nuclear import factor directing IN and viral DNA into the nucleus (Maertens et al., 2003). However, this overplays the role of LEDGF in HIV-1 replication; replication defect of HIV-1 in LEDGF knockdown and knockout cells was not observed at the step of nuclear import of the PIC, as measured by the formation of a circular ligation product of viral DNA in the nucleus (Llano et al., 2006a; Shun et al., 2007). Thus, LEDGF should contribute to the stable tethering of IN and viral DNA (i.e. the PIC) to chromatin, thereby regulating integration efficiency and integration-site selection of HIV-1 (Fig. 3B) (Engelman & Cherepanov, 2008).

Translocation of proteins (cargo molecule) across the NPC requires specific transport receptors. Importin is one of the best-studied receptors for nuclear translocation. Importin contains two subunits, importin α and importin β. The NLS of a cargo molecule is first recognized by importin α, and after binding to importin β, the cargo-receptor complex is targeted to the NPC via direct association of importin β with components of the NPC called nucleoporin (NUP) (Mattaj & Englmeier, 1998). To date, several importins have been reported to interact with HIV-1 IN (Krishnan et al., 2010). By employing the *in vitro* nuclear import assay, importin 7, a member of importin β family acting as an import receptor for ribosomal proteins and histone H1, was shown to mediate nuclear import of the HIV-1 PICs (Fassati et al., 2003). Although HIV-1 IN was found to interact with importin 7 through the CTD (Ao et al., 2007), the functional role of this cellular protein in the nuclear entry of the PIC remains a matter of debate (Zielske & Stevenson, 2005).

Another member of the importin β family, transportin 3 (TNPO3/transportin-SR2), has also been identified by yeast two-hybrid screening as an HIV-1 IN-binding protein that directs the PICs to the nucleus (Christ et al., 2008). The requirement of TNPO3 in HIV-1 replication was confirmed by studies using siRNA-mediated knockdown (Brass et al., 2008; Konig et al., 2008; Krishnan et al., 2010). However, a recent study reveals that CA, but not IN, determines the TNPO3 dependency during HIV-1 replication (Krishnan et al., 2010). Additionally, later studies disclosed that the different cellular proteins regulating nucleocytoplasmic trafficking, importin α3 and NUP153, also interact with HIV-1 IN (Woodward et al., 2009; Ao et al., 2010). Understanding how the HIV-1 PIC crosses the intact nuclear envelope in non-dividing cells is one of the most fascinating areas in retroviral research. Further experiments will be therefore required to unveil the role of IN and its cellular cofactors in the active transport of the HIV-1 PIC into the nucleus (Suzuki & Craigie 2007).

4.4 Cellular interactors affecting on postintegration steps

Following integration, the provirus serves as a template for viral gene expression. During this postintegration process, disassembly of IN from the integrated viral DNA is a prerequisite for efficient transcription (Yoder & Bushman, 2000). It is well known that when HIV-1 IN is solely expressed in mammalian cells it undergoes proteasome-mediated degradation via ubiquitination (Mulder & Muesing, 2000). Although the function of this ubiquitin-mediated degradation of IN in HIV-1 replication remains unclear, one ubiquitination pathway has been suggested to participate in the gene expression step of HIV-1 replication through the degradation of IN (Mousnier et al., 2007). von Hippel-Lindau-binding protein 1 (VBP1) was identified as a cellular partner for HIV-1 IN by yeast two-hybrid screening. VBP1, also known as a subunit of the prefoldin chaperone, associates with the substrate recognition component of the cullin2-based von Hippel-Lindau (Cul2/VHL) ubiquitin ligase complex. Co-immunoprecipitation assays showed that HIV-1 IN bound both VBP1 and pVHL, and this IN-pVHL interaction was reduced by siRNA-mediated knockdown of endogenous VBP1 expression (Mousnier et al., 2007). Intriguingly, the depletion of VBP1 by siRNA had a negative impact on the transcriptional activity of integrated HIV-1 DNA without affecting provirus formation. Additionally, the specific knockdown of components of the Cul2/VHL ubiquitin ligase complex, including VBP1, resulted in a slower degradation and a decreased ubiquitination of HIV-1 IN as observed in pVHL deficient cells, indicating that Cul2/VHL ubiquitin ligase is responsible for the proteasomal degradation of IN (Mousnier et al., 2007). This study suggests that the recruitment of Cul2/VHL ubiquitin ligation complex by VBP1-IN interaction may play a pivotal role in degradation of IN, leading to efficient transition from integration to viral gene expression during HIV-1 infection.

Recently, a different class of ubiquitin ligase was found to interact with HIV-1 IN (Yamamoto et al., 2011). By employing a tandem affinity purification (TAP) procedure combined with mass spectrometry (MS) analysis, we have identified Huwe1 (HECT, UBA, and WWE domain containing 1), a HECT (homologous to E6-AP carboxyl terminus)-type E3 ubiquitin ligase, as a novel cellular interactor of MoMLV IN. Interestingly, Huwe1 also interacts with HIV-1 IN, and the binding was mediated through the CCD of IN and a wide-segment of Huwe1 (Fig. 4A). Because Huwe1 was associated with the PICs in immunoprecipitation assays, this ubiquitin ligase was expected to have a role in the integration process. However, when endogenous Huwe1 was depleted from a human T cell line by RNA interference technique, comparable levels of reverse transcription, integration, and gene expression were observed in HIV-1-infected knockdown and control cells. On the other hand, the knockdown experiment revealed that the infectivity of HIV-1 virions released from Huwe1-depleted T cells was significantly augmented compared to the virions produced from control cells, suggesting that Huwe1 has a negative impact on the production of infectious virions during HIV-1 replication (Yamamoto et al., 2011).

One question to be pondered is how the IN-binding protein Huwe1 modulates HIV-1 infectivity. IN is expressed as the C-terminal part of the Gag-Pol protein that is required for the formation of infectious virions during retroviral replication (Swanstrom & Wills, 1997). Further analysis showed that Huwe1 also associates with the HIV-1 Gag-Pol polyprotein in a C-terminal IN domain dependent manner (Yamamoto et al., 2011). Given that incorporation of Huwe1 into HIV-1 virions was not detected, one possibility would be that Huwe1 blocks the proper intracellular localization of the Gag-Pol precursor. It has been well demonstrated that during HIV-1 particle assembly, viral structural proteins, including Gag-

Pol, are taken up by the detergent-resistant membrane (DRM) fraction, the so called lipid raft, which is characterized by its insolubility against non-ionic detergents such as NP-40 (Halwani et al., 2003; Ono, 2010). In contrast, Huwe1 was distributed in a NP-40-soluble (non-DRM) fraction (Yamamoto et al., 2011). Thus, Gag-Pol precursor protein may be sequestered by Huwe1 present in the non-DRM domains of the cytoplasm through the IN region, resulting in interference of proper localization of Gag-Pol to the lipid raft where assembly of infectious virions is meant to take place (Fig. 4B, left).

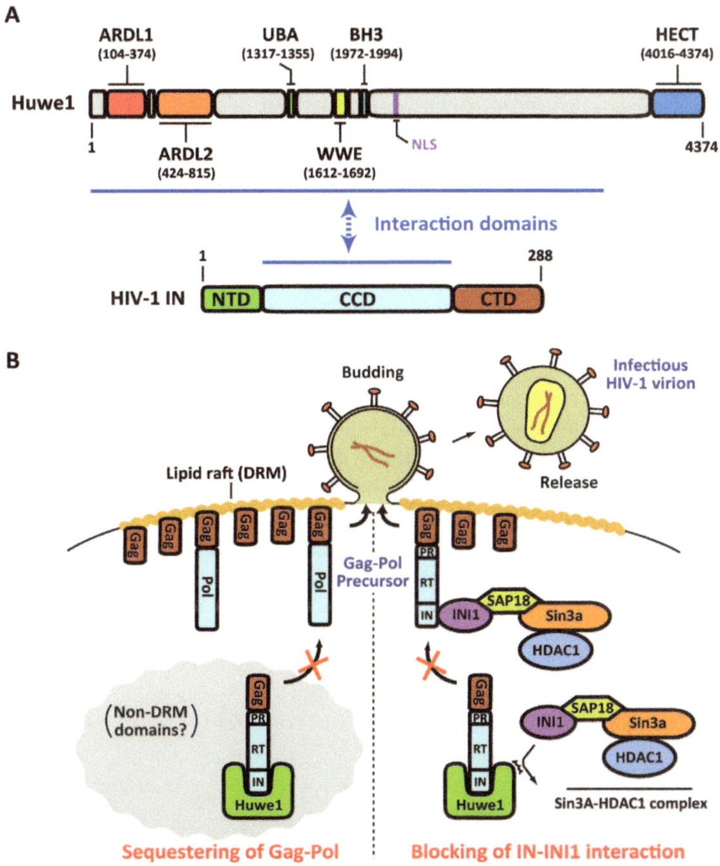

Fig. 4. A novel HIV-1 IN-binding protein, Huwe1. (A) Interacting domains between Huwe1 and HIV-1 IN. Huwe1 is a HECT-type E3 ubiquitin ligase which possesses several recognizable domains; ARLD (Armadillo [ARM] repeat like domain) 1 and 2 in the N-terminus, UBA (ubiquitin-associated), WWE, and the well-conserved BH3 domain in the middle, and a HECT domain in the C-terminus. Our study shows that Huwe1 interacts with the CCD of HIV-1 IN through a broad region spanning 3,500 amino acids (Yamamoto et al., 2011). (B) Possible mechanisms by which Huwe1 hampers the formation of infectious HIV-1. In virus producing cells, Huwe1 may act as a scaffolding modulator that reduces infectivity of virions by interfering with the proper localization (left) or function (right) of HIV-1 Gag-Pol precursor through interactions with IN.

Another possible mechanism for the Huwe1-mediated negative modulation of HIV-1 infectivity is that Huwe1 could mask the IN region of Gag-Pol, thereby blocking the incorporation of INI1/hSNF5 and its associated cellular factors into HIV-1 virions (Fig. 4B, right). As described above, INI1/hSNF5 has been shown to be specifically encapsidated into HIV-1 virions, probably through the IN region of Gag-Pol (Yung et al., 2001, 2004). In addition, a recent study demonstrates that the IN-INI1/hSNF1 interaction selectively recruits SAP18 and HDAC1, components of the Sin3a-HDAC complex, into the HIV-1 virion, increasing the infectivity of the virions (Sorin et al., 2009). Although Huwe1 is an E3 ubiquitin ligase, our study suggests that enzymatic activity of Huwe1 is not involved in the ubiquitination and subsequent proteasomal-degradation of IN and Gag-Pol (Yamamoto et al., 2011). Therefore, in HIV-1 producer cells, Huwe1 may function as a scaffolding modulator that hampers proper localization or function of the Gag-Pol precursor protein via interaction with IN region (Fig. 4B).

5. Conclusion and implications for future treatment of HIV infection

This chapter highlights the functional role of PPIs between HIV-1 IN and its cellular cofactors for virus replication. Although the indispensability of these IN interactors in the HIV-1 infection cycle requires further validation, research into intracellular binding proteins of IN provide an important insight for the development of novel classes of anti-HIV drugs: inhibitors blocking IN-cellular protein interactions that can act synergistically with existing drugs. The design of this class of inhibitors (i.e. SMPPIIs) is an emerging field in retroviral research, but the rationale for their availability in blocking HIV-1 replication has been demonstrated in SMPPIIs against IN-LEDGF interaction (Christ et al., 2010). One impact on the pharmacological aspect is that, because cellular interactors for IN appear to be implicated in steps other than the integration process, SMPPIIs targeting IN could block HIV-1 replication at multiple steps. Therefore, further analysis of the mechanism by which the IN interactors regulate virus infection can be the basis of a promising new strategy for the treatment of HIV-1 infection and AIDS.

6. Acknowledgment

We are grateful Wei Xin Chin for proofreading and comments on the manuscript.

7. References

Al-Mawsawi, L.Q.; Neamati, N. (2007). Blocking interactions between HIV-1 integrase and cellular cofactors: an emerging anti-retroviral strategy. *Trends Pharmacol. Sci.*, Vol. 28, No. 10, pp. 526-535

Ao, Z.; Danappa Jayappa, K.; Wang, B.; Zheng, Y.; Kung, S.; Rassart, E.; Depping, R.; Kohler, M.; Cohen, E.A.; Yao, X. (2010). Importin α3 interacts with HIV-1 integrase and contributes to HIV-1 nuclear import and replication. *J. Virol.*, Vol. 84, No. 17, pp. 8650-8663

Ao, Z.; Huang, G.; Yao, H.; Xu, Z.; Labine, M.; Cochrane, A.W.; Yao, X. (2007). Interaction of human immunodeficiency virus type 1 integrase with cellular nuclear import receptor importin 7 and its impact on viral replication. *J. Biol. Chem.*, Vol. 282, No. 18, pp. 13456-13467

Arhel, N. (2010). Revisiting HIV-1 uncoating. *Retrovirology,* Vol. 7, pp. 96

Arhel, N.; Kirchhoff, F. (2010). Host proteins involved in HIV infection: new therapeutic targets. *Biochim. Biophys. Acta,* Vol. 1802, No. 3, pp. 313-321

Ariumi, Y.; Serhan, F.; Turelli, P.; Telenti, A.; Trono, D. (2006). The integrase interactor 1 (INI1) proteins facilitate Tat-mediated human immunodeficiency virus type 1 transcription. *Retrovirology,* Vol. 3, pp. 47

Arkin, M.R.; Wells, J.A. (2004). Small-molecule inhibitors of protein-protein interactions: progressing towards the dream. *Nat. Rev. Drug. Discov.,* Vol. 3, No. 4, pp. 301-317

Blankson, J.N.; Persaud, D.; Siliciano, R.F. (2002). The challenge of viral reservoirs in HIV-1 infection. *Annu. Rev. Med.,* Vol. 53, pp. 557-593

Brass, A.L.; Dykxhoorn, D.M.; Benita, Y.; Yan, N.; Engelman, A.; Xavier, R.J.; Lieberman, J.; Elledge, S.J. (2008). Identification of host proteins required for HIV infection through a functional genomic screen. *Science,* Vol. 319, No. 5865, pp. 921-926

Briones, M.S.; Dobard, C.W.; Chow, S.A. (2010). Role of human immunodeficiency virus type 1 integrase in uncoating of the viral core. *J. Virol.,* Vol. 84, No. 10, pp. 5181-5190

Bukovsky, A.; Gottlinger, H. (1996). Lack of integrase can markedly affect human immunodeficiency virus type 1 particle production in the presence of an active viral protease. *J. Virol.,* Vol. 70, No. 10, pp. 6820-6825

Bukrinsky, M.I.; Sharova, N.; McDonald, T.L.; Pushkarskaya, T.; Tarpley, W.G.; Stevenson, M. (1993). Association of integrase, matrix, and reverse transcriptase antigens of human immunodeficiency virus type 1 with viral nucleic acids following acute infection. *Proc. Natl. Acad. Sci. USA,* Vol. 90, No. 13, pp. 6125-6129

Bushman, F.; Lewinski, M.; Ciuffi, A.; Barr, S.; Leipzig, J.; Hannenhalli, S.; Hoffmann, C. (2005). Genome-wide analysis of retroviral DNA integration. *Nat. Rev. Microbiol.,* Vol. 3, No. 11, pp. 848-858

Bushman, F.D.; Craigie, R. (1991). Activities of human immunodeficiency virus (HIV) integration protein in vitro: specific cleavage and integration of HIV DNA. *Proc. Natl. Acad. Sci. USA,* Vol. 88, No. 4, pp. 1339-1343

Busschots, K.; De Rijck, J.; Christ, F.; Debyser, Z. (2009). In search of small molecules blocking interactions between HIV proteins and intracellular cofactors. *Mol. Biosyst.,* Vol. 5, No. 1, pp. 21-31

Carlson, M.; Laurent, B.C. (1994). The SNF/SWI family of global transcriptional activators. *Curr. Opin. Cell Biol.,* Vol. 6, No. 3, pp. 396-402

Cereseto, A.; Manganaro, L.; Gutierrez, M.I.; Terreni, M.; Fittipaldi, A.; Lusic, M.; Marcello, A.; Giacca, M. (2005). Acetylation of HIV-1 integrase by p300 regulates viral integration. *EMBO J.,* Vol. 24, No. 17, pp. 3070-3081

Chen, H.; Engelman, A. (2001). Asymmetric processing of human immunodeficiency virus type 1 cDNA in vivo: implications for functional end coupling during the chemical steps of DNA transposition. *Mol. Cell. Biol.,* Vol. 21, No. 20, pp. 6758-6767

Cherepanov, P.; Maertens, G.; Proost, P.; Devreese, B.; Van Beeumen, J.; Engelborghs, Y.; De Clercq, E.; Debyser, Z. (2003). HIV-1 integrase forms stable tetramers and associates with LEDGF/p75 protein in human cells. *J. Biol. Chem.,* Vol. 278, No. 1, pp. 372-381

Cherepanov, P.; Devroe, E.; Silver, P.A.; Engelman, A. (2004). Identification of an evolutionarily conserved domain in human lens epithelium-derived growth factor/transcriptional co-activator p75 (LEDGF/p75) that binds HIV-1 integrase. *J. Biol. Chem.*, Vol. 279, No. 47, pp. 48883-48892

Cherepanov, P.; Ambrosio, A.L.; Rahman, S.; Ellenberger, T.; Engelman, A. (2005a). Structural basis for the recognition between HIV-1 integrase and transcriptional coactivator p75. *Proc. Natl. Acad. Sci. USA*, Vol. 102, No. 48, pp. 17308-17313

Cherepanov, P.; Sun, Z.Y.; Rahman, S.; Maertens, G.; Wagner, G.; Engelman, A. (2005b). Solution structure of the HIV-1 integrase-binding domain in LEDGF/p75. *Nat. Struct. Mol. Biol.*, Vol. 12, No. 6, pp. 526-532

Christ, F.; Thys, W.; De Rijck, J.; Gijsbers, R.; Albanese, A.; Arosio, D.; Emiliani, S.; Rain, J.C.; Benarous, R.; Cereseto, A.; Debyser, Z. (2008). Transportin-SR2 imports HIV into the nucleus. *Curr. Biol.*, Vol. 18, No. 16, pp. 1192-1202

Christ, F.; Voet, A.; Marchand, A.; Nicolet, S.; Desimmie, B.A.; Marchand, D.; Bardiot, D.; Van der Veken, N.J.; Van Remoortel, B.; Strelkov, S.V.; De Maeyer, M.; Chaltin, P.; Debyser, Z. (2010). Rational design of small-molecule inhibitors of the LEDGF/p75-integrase interaction and HIV replication. *Nat. Chem. Biol.*, Vol. 6, No. 6, pp. 442-448

Ciuffi, A.; Llano, M.; Poeschla, E.; Hoffmann, C.; Leipzig, J.; Shinn, P.; Ecker, J.R.; Bushman, F. (2005). A role for LEDGF/p75 in targeting HIV DNA integration. *Nat. Med.*, Vol. 11, No. 12, pp. 1287-1289

Cochran, A.G. (2001). Protein-protein interfaces: mimics and inhibitors. *Curr. Opin. Chem. Biol.*, Vol. 5, No. 6, pp. 654-659

Graigie, R. (2001). HIV integrase, a brief overview from chemistry to therapeutics. *J. Biol.Chem.*, Vol. 276, No. 26, pp. 23213-23216

Dar, M.J.; Monel, B.; Krishnan, L.; Shun, M.C.; Di Nunzio, F.; Helland, D.E.; Engelman, A. (2009). Biochemical and virological analysis of the 18-residue C-terminal tail of HIV-1 integrase. *Retrovirology*, Vol. 6, pp. 94

De Rijck, J.; Bartholomeeusen, K.; Ceulemans, H.; Debyser, Z.; Gijsbers, R. (2010). High-resolution profiling of the LEDGF/p75 chromatin interaction in the ENCODE region. *Nucleic Acids Res.*, Vol. 38, No. 18, pp. 6135-6147

Devroe, E.; Engelman, A.; Silver, P.A. (2003). Intracellular transport of human immunodeficiency virus type 1 integrase. *J. Cell Sci.*, Vol. 116, Pt 21, pp. 4401-4408

Dobard, C.W.; Briones, M.S.; Chow, S.A. (2007). Molecular mechanisms by which human immunodeficiency virus type 1 integrase stimulates the early steps of reverse transcription. *J. Virol.*, Vol. 81, No. 18, pp. 10037-10046

Engelman, A.; Mizuuchi, K.; Craigie, R. (1991). HIV-1 DNA integration: mechanism of viral DNA cleavage and DNA strand transfer. *Cell*, Vol. 67, No. 6, pp. 1211-1221

Engelman, A.; Englund, G.; Orenstein, J.M.; Martin, M.A.; Craigie, R. (1995). Multiple effects of mutations in human immunodeficiency virus type 1 integrase on viral replication. *J. Virol.*, Vol. 69, No. 5, pp. 2729-2736

Engelman, A. (1999). *In vivo* analysis of retroviral integrase structure and function. *Adv. Virus Res.*, Vol. 52, No. pp. 411-426

Engelman, A.; Cherepanov, P. (2008). The lentiviral integrase binding protein LEDGF/p75 and HIV-1 replication. *PLoS Pathog.*, Vol. 4, No. 3, pp. e1000046

Farnet, C.M.; Haseltine, W.A. (1990). Integration of human immunodeficiency virus type 1 DNA in vitro. *Proc. Natl. Acad. Sci. USA*, Vol. 87, No. 11, pp. 4164-4168

Farnet, C.M.; Haseltine, W.A. (1991). Determination of viral proteins present in the human immunodeficiency virus type 1 preintegration complex. *J. Virol.*, Vol. 65, No. 4, pp. 1910-1915

Farnet, C.M.; Bushman, F.D. (1997). HIV-1 cDNA integration: requirement of HMG I(Y) protein for function of preintegration complexes in vitro. *Cell*, Vol. 88, No. 4, pp. 483-492

Fassati, A.; Goff, S.P. (1999). Characterization of intracellular reverse transcription complexes of Moloney murine leukemia virus. *J. Virol.*, Vol. 73, No. 11, pp. 8919-8925

Fassati, A.; Goff, S.P. (2001). Characterization of intracellular reverse transcription complexes of human immunodeficiency virus type 1. *J. Virol.*, Vol. 75, No. 8, pp. 3626-3635

Fassati, A.; Gorlich, D.; Harrison, I.; Zaytseva, L.; Mingot, J.M. (2003). Nuclear import of HIV-1 intracellular reverse transcription complexes is mediated by importin 7. *EMBO J.*, Vol. 22, No. 14, pp. 3675-3685

Fassati, A. (2006). HIV infection of non-dividing cells: a divisive problem. *Retrovirology*, Vol. 3, pp. 74

Fouchier, R.A.; Malim, M.H. (1999). Nuclear import of human immunodeficiency virus type-1 preintegration complexes. *Adv. Virus Res.*, Vol. 52, pp. 275-299

Gallay, P.; Swingler, S.; Song, J.; Bushman, F.; Trono, D. (1995). HIV nuclear import is governed by the phosphotyrosine-mediated binding of matrix to the core domain of integrase. *Cell*, Vol. 83, No. 4, pp. 569-576

Goff, S.P. (2001). Intracellular trafficking of retroviral genomes during the early phase of infection: viral exploitation of cellular pathways. *J. Gene Med.*, Vol. 3, No. 6, pp. 517-528

Goff, S.P. (2007). Host factors exploited by retroviruses. *Nat. Rev. Microbiol.*, Vol. 5, No. 4, pp. 253-263

Halwani, R.; Khorchid, A.; Cen, S.; Kleiman, L. (2003). Rapid localization of Gag/GagPol complexes to detergent-resistant membrane during the assembly of human immunodeficiency virus type 1. *J. Virol.*, Vol. 77, No. 7, pp. 3973-3984

Hamamoto, S.; Nishitsuji, H.; Amagasa, T.; Kannagi, M.; Masuda, T. (2006). Identification of a novel human immunodeficiency virus type 1 integrase interactor, Gemin2, that facilitates efficient viral cDNA synthesis in vivo. *J. Virol.*, Vol. 80, No. 12, pp. 5670-5677

Ikeda, T.; Nishitsuji, H.; Zhou, X.; Nara, N.; Ohashi, T.; Kannagi, M.; Masuda, T. (2004). Evaluation of the functional involvement of human immunodeficiency virus type 1 integrase in nuclear import of viral cDNA during acute infection. *J. Virol.*, Vol. 78, No. 21, pp. 11563-11573

Iordanskiy, S.; Berro, R.; Altieri, M.; Kashanchi, F.; Bukrinsky, M. (2006). Intracytoplasmic maturation of the human immunodeficiency virus type 1 reverse transcription complexes determines their capacity to integrate into chromatin. *Retrovirology*, Vol. 3, pp. 4

Jacks, T.; Power, M.D.; Masiarz, F.R.; Luciw, P.A.; Barr, P.J.; Varmus, H.E. (1988). Characterization of ribosomal frameshifting in HIV-1 gag-pol expression. *Nature*, Vol. 331, No. 6153, pp. 280-283

Kalpana, G.V.; Marmon, S.; Wang, W.; Crabtree, G.R.; Goff, S.P. (1994). Binding and stimulation of HIV-1 integrase by a human homolog of yeast transcription factor SNF5. *Science,* Vol. 266, No. 5193, pp. 2002-2006

Konig, R.; Zhou, Y.; Elleder, D.; Diamond, T.L.; Bonamy, G.M.; Irelan, J.T.; Chiang, C.Y.; Tu, B.P.; De Jesus, P.D.; Lilley, C.E.; Seidel, S.; Opaluch, A.M.; Caldwell, J.S.; Weitzman, M.D.; Kuhen, K.L.; Bandyopadhyay, S.; Ideker, T.; Orth, A.P.; Miraglia, L.J.; Bushman, F.D.; Young, J.A.; Chanda, S.K. (2008). Global analysis of host-pathogen interactions that regulate early-stage HIV-1 replication. *Cell,* Vol. 135, No. 1, pp. 49-60

Krishnan, L.; Matreyek, K.A.; Oztop, I.; Lee, K.; Tipper, C.H.; Li, X.; Dar, M.J.; Kewalramani, V.N.; Engelman, A. (2010). The requirement for cellular transportin 3 (TNPO3 or TRN-SR2) during infection maps to human immunodeficiency virus type 1 capsid and not integrase. *J. Virol.,* Vol. 84, No. 1, pp. 397-406

Leavitt, A.D.; Robles, G.; Alesandro, N.; Varmus, H.E. (1996). Human immunodeficiency virus type 1 integrase mutants retain in vitro integrase activity yet fail to integrate viral DNA efficiently during infection. *J. Virol.,* Vol. 70, No. 2, pp. 721-728

Levy, J.A. (2009). HIV pathogenesis: 25 years of progress and persistent challenges. *AIDS,* Vol. 23, No. 2, pp. 147-160

Lewinski, M.K.; Bushman, F.D. (2005). Retroviral DNA integration--mechanism and consequences. *Adv. Genet.,* Vol. 55, pp. 147-181

Li, L.; Olvera, J.M.; Yoder, K.E.; Mitchell, R.S.; Butler, S.L.; Lieber, M.; Martin, S.L.; Bushman, F.D. (2001). Role of the non-homologous DNA end joining pathway in the early steps of retroviral infection. *EMBO J.,* Vol. 20, No. 12, pp. 3272-3281

Lin, C.W.; Engelman, A. (2003). The barrier-to-autointegration factor is a component of functional human immunodeficiency virus type 1 preintegration complexes. *J. Virol.,* Vol. 77, No. 8, pp. 5030-5036

Llano, M.; Vanegas, M.; Fregoso, O.; Saenz, D.; Chung, S.; Peretz, M.; Poeschla, E.M. (2004). LEDGF/p75 determines cellular trafficking of diverse lentiviral but not murine oncoretroviral integrase proteins and is a component of functional lentiviral preintegration complexes. *J. Virol.,* Vol. 78, No. 17, pp. 9524-9537

Llano, M.; Saenz, D.T.; Meehan, A.; Wongthida, P.; Peretz, M.; Walker, W.H.; Teo, W.; Poeschla, E.M. (2006a). An essential role for LEDGF/p75 in HIV integration. *Science,* Vol. 314, No. 5798, pp. 461-464

Llano, M.; Vanegas, M.; Hutchins, N.; Thompson, D.; Delgado, S.; Poeschla, E.M. (2006b). Identification and characterization of the chromatin-binding domains of the HIV-1 integrase interactor LEDGF/p75. *J. Mol. Biol.,* Vol. 360, No. 4, pp. 760-773

Lu, R.; Limon, A.; Devroe, E.; Silver, P.A.; Cherepanov, P.; Engelman, A. (2004). Class II integrase mutants with changes in putative nuclear localization signals are primarily blocked at a postnuclear entry step of human immunodeficiency virus type 1 replication. *J. Virol.,* Vol. 78, No. 23, pp. 12735-12746

Luban, J. (2008). HIV-1 infection: going nuclear with TNPO3/Transportin-SR2 and integrase. *Curr. Biol.,* Vol. 18, No. 16, pp. R710-713

Maertens, G.; Cherepanov, P.; Pluymers, W.; Busschots, K.; De Clercq, E.; Debyser, Z.; Engelborghs, Y. (2003). LEDGF/p75 is essential for nuclear and chromosomal targeting of HIV-1 integrase in human cells. *J. Biol. Chem.,* Vol. 278, No. 35, pp. 33528-33539

Manganaro, L.; Lusic, M.; Gutierrez, M.I.; Cereseto, A.; Del Sal, G.; Giacca, M. (2010). Concerted action of cellular JNK and Pin1 restricts HIV-1 genome integration to activated CD4+ T lymphocytes. *Nat. Med.*, Vol. 16, No. 3, pp. 329-333

Marshall, H.M.; Ronen, K.; Berry, C.; Llano, M.; Sutherland, H.; Saenz, D.; Bickmore, W.; Poeschla, E.; Bushman, F.D. (2007). Role of PSIP1/LEDGF/p75 in lentiviral infectivity and integration targeting. *PLoS One,* Vol. 2, No. 12, pp. e1340

Masuda, T.; Planelles, V.; Krogstad, P.; Chen, I.S. (1995). Genetic analysis of human immunodeficiency virus type 1 integrase and the U3 att site: unusual phenotype of mutants in the zinc finger-like domain. *J. Virol.*, Vol. 69, No. 11, pp. 6687-6696

Mattaj, I.W.; Englmeier, L. (1998). Nucleocytoplasmic transport: the soluble phase. *Annu. Rev. Biochem.*, Vol. 67, No. pp. 265-306

McDonald, D.; Vodicka, M.A.; Lucero, G.; Svitkina, T.M.; Borisy, G.G.; Emerman, M.; Hope, T.J. (2002). Visualization of the intracellular behavior of HIV in living cells. *J. Cell Biol.*, Vol. 159, No. 3, pp. 441-452

Mergener, K.; Facke, M.; Welker, R.; Brinkmann, V.; Gelderblom, H.R.; Krausslich, H.G. (1992). Analysis of HIV particle formation using transient expression of subviral constructs in mammalian cells. *Virology,* Vol. 186, No. 1, pp. 25-39

Miller, M.D.; Farnet, C.M.; Bushman, F.D. (1997). Human immunodeficiency virus type 1 preintegration complexes: studies of organization and composition. *J. Virol.*, Vol. 71, No. 7, pp. 5382-5390

Morozov, A.; Yung, E.; Kalpana, G.V. (1998). Structure-function analysis of integrase interactor 1/hSNF5L1 reveals differential properties of two repeat motifs present in the highly conserved region. *Proc. Natl. Acad. Sci. USA,* Vol. 95, No. 3, pp. 1120-1125

Mousnier, A.; Kubat, N.; Massias-Simon, A.; Segeral, E.; Rain, J.C.; Benarous, R.; Emiliani, S.; Dargemont, C. (2007). von Hippel Lindau binding protein 1-mediated degradation of integrase affects HIV-1 gene expression at a postintegration step. *Proc. Natl. Acad. Sci. USA,* Vol. 104, No. 34, pp. 13615-13620

Mulder, L.C.; Chakrabarti, L.A.; Muesing, M.A. (2002). Interaction of HIV-1 integrase with DNA repair protein hRad18. *J. Biol. Chem.*, Vol. 277, No. 30, pp. 27489-27493

Mulder, L.C.; Muesing, M.A. (2000). Degradation of HIV-1 integrase by the N-end rule pathway. *J. Biol. Chem.*, Vol. 275, No. 38, pp. 29749-29753

Nakamura, T.; Masuda, T.; Goto, T.; Sano, K.; Nakai, M.; Harada, S. (1997). Lack of infectivity of HIV-1 integrase zinc finger-like domain mutant with morphologically normal maturation. *Biochem. Biophys. Res. Commun.*, Vol. 239, No. 3, pp. 715-722

Nermut, M.V.; Fassati, A. (2003). Structural analyses of purified human immunodeficiency virus type 1 intracellular reverse transcription complexes. *J. Virol.*, Vol. 77, No. 15, pp. 8196-8206

Nishitsuji, H.; Hayashi, T.; Takahashi, T.; Miyano, M.; Kannagi, M.; Masuda, T. (2009). Augmentation of reverse transcription by integrase through an interaction with host factor, SIP1/Gemin2 Is critical for HIV-1 infection. *PLoS One,* Vol. 4, No. 11, pp. e7825

Ono, A. (2010). Relationships between plasma membrane microdomains and HIV-1 assembly. *Biol. Cell,* Vol. 102, No. 6, pp. 335-350

Pagliaro, L.; Felding, J.; Audouze, K.; Nielsen, S.J.; Terry, R.B.; Krog-Jensen, C.; Butcher, S. (2004). Emerging classes of protein-protein interaction inhibitors and new tools for their development. *Curr. Opin. Chem. Biol.*, Vol. 8, No. 4, pp. 442-449

Palella, F.J., Jr.; Delaney, K.M.; Moorman, A.C.; Loveless, M.O.; Fuhrer, J.; Satten, G.A.; Aschman, D.J.; Holmberg, S.D. (1998). Declining morbidity and mortality among patients with advanced human immunodeficiency virus infection. HIV Outpatient Study Investigators. *N. Engl. J. Med.*, Vol. 338, No. 13, pp. 853-860

Parissi, V.; Calmels, C.; De Soultrait, V.R.; Caumont, A.; Fournier, M.; Chaignepain, S.; Litvak, S. (2001). Functional interactions of human immunodeficiency virus type 1 integrase with human and yeast HSP60. *J. Virol.*, Vol. 75, No. 23, pp. 11344-11353

Paushkin, S.; Gubitz, A.K.; Massenet, S.; Dreyfuss, G. (2002). The SMN complex, an assemblyosome of ribonucleoproteins. *Curr. Opin. Cell Biol.*, Vol. 14, No. 3, pp. 305-312

Petit, C.; Schwartz, O.; Mammano, F. (1999). Oligomerization within virions and subcellular localization of human immunodeficiency virus type 1 integrase. *J. Virol.*, Vol. 73, No. 6, pp. 5079-5088

Pluymers, W.; Cherepanov, P.; Schols, D.; De Clercq, E.; Debyser, Z. (1999). Nuclear localization of human immunodeficiency virus type 1 integrase expressed as a fusion protein with green fluorescent protein. *Virology*, Vol. 258, No. 2, pp. 327-332

Qiu, C.; Sawada, K.; Zhang, X.; Cheng, X. (2002). The PWWP domain of mammalian DNA methyltransferase Dnmt3b defines a new family of DNA-binding folds. *Nat. Struct. Biol.*, Vol. 9, No. 3, pp. 217-224

Roth, S.Y.; Denu, J.M.; Allis, C.D. (2001). Histone acetyltransferases. *Annu. Rev. Biochem.*, Vol. 70, No. pp. 81-120

Ryan, D.P.; Matthews, J.M. (2005). Protein-protein interactions in human disease. *Curr. Opin. Struct. Biol.*, Vol. 15, No. 4, pp. 441-446

Shin, C.G.; Taddeo, B.; Haseltine, W.A.; Farnet, C.M. (1994). Genetic analysis of the human immunodeficiency virus type 1 integrase protein. *J. Virol.*, Vol. 68, No. 3, pp. 1633-1642

Shun, M.C.; Raghavendra, N.K.; Vandegraaff, N.; Daigle, J.E.; Hughes, S.; Kellam, P.; Cherepanov, P.; Engelman, A. (2007). LEDGF/p75 functions downstream from preintegration complex formation to effect gene-specific HIV-1 integration. *Genes Dev.*, Vol. 21, No. 14, pp. 1767-1778

Smith, J.A.; Daniel, R. (2006). Following the path of the virus: the exploitation of host DNA repair mechanisms by retroviruses. *ACS Chem. Biol.*, Vol. 1, No. 4, pp. 217-226

Sorin, M.; Cano, J.; Das, S.; Mathew, S.; Wu, X.; Davies, K.P.; Shi, X.; Cheng, S.W.; Ott, D.; Kalpana, G.V. (2009). Recruitment of a SAP18-HDAC1 complex into HIV-1 virions and its requirement for viral replication. *PLoS Pathog.*, Vol. 5, No. 6, pp. e1000463

Stec, I.; Nagl, S.B.; van Ommen, G.J.; den Dunnen, J.T. (2000). The PWWP domain: a potential protein-protein interaction domain in nuclear proteins influencing differentiation? *FEBS Lett.*, Vol. 473, No. 1, pp. 1-5

Suzuki, Y; Craigie, R. (2007). The road to chromatin - nuclear entry of retroviruses. *Nat. Rev. Microbiol.*, Vol. 5, No. 3, pp. 187-196

Swanstrom, R.; Wills, J.W. (1997). Synthesis, assembly, and processing of viral proteins, In: *Retroviruses*, Coffin, J.; Hughes, S.; Varmus, H., pp. 263, Cold Spring Harbor Laboratory Press, Cold Spring Harbor Laboratory

Terreni, M.; Valentini, P.; Liverani, V.; Gutierrez, M.I.; Di Primio, C.; Di Fenza, A.; Tozzini, V.; Allouch, A.; Albanese, A.; Giacca, M.; Cereseto, A. (2010). GCN5-dependent acetylation of HIV-1 integrase enhances viral integration. *Retrovirology* Vol. 7, pp. 18

Topper, M.; Luo, Y.; Zhadina, M.; Mohammed, K.; Smith, L.; Muesing, M.A. (2007). Posttranslational acetylation of the human immunodeficiency virus type 1 integrase carboxyl-terminal domain is dispensable for viral replication. *J. Virol.*, Vol. 81, No. 6, pp. 3012-3017

Tsurutani, N.; Kubo, M.; Maeda, Y.; Ohashi, T.; Yamamoto, N.; Kannagi, M.; Masuda, T. (2000). Identification of critical amino acid residues in human immunodeficiency virus type 1 IN required for efficient proviral DNA formation at steps prior to integration in dividing and nondividing cells. *J. Virol.*, Vol. 74, No. 10, pp. 4795-4806

Turlure, F.; Devroe, E.; Silver, P.A.; Engelman, A. (2004). Human cell proteins and human immunodeficiency virus DNA integration. *Front. Biosci.*, Vol. 9, No. pp. 3187-3208

Turlure, F.; Maertens, G.; Rahman, S.; Cherepanov, P.; Engelman, A. (2006). A tripartite DNA-binding element, comprised of the nuclear localization signal and two AT-hook motifs, mediates the association of LEDGF/p75 with chromatin *in vivo*. *Nucleic Acids Res.*, Vol. 34, No. 5, pp. 1653-1665

UNAIDS (2010). In: *UNAIDS Report on the Global AIDS Epidemic*. Available from : <http://www.unaids.org/globalreport/Global_report.htm>

Vandegraaff, N.; Devroe, E.; Turlure, F.; Silver, P.A.; Engelman, A. (2006). Biochemical and genetic analyses of integrase-interacting proteins lens epithelium-derived growth factor (LEDGF)/p75 and hepatoma-derived growth factor related protein 2 (HRP2) in preintegration complex function and HIV-1 replication. *Virology*, Vol. 346, No. 2, pp. 415-426

Vandegraaff, N.; Engelman, A. (2007). Molecular mechanisms of HIV integration and therapeutic intervention. *Expert Rev. Mol. Med.*, Vol. 9, No. 6, pp. 1-19

Verma, I.M.; Somia, N. (1997). Gene therapy -- promises, problems and prospects. *Nature*, Vol. 389, No. 6648, pp. 239-242

Violot, S.; Hong, S.S.; Rakotobe, D.; Petit, C.; Gay, B.; Moreau, K.; Billaud, G.; Priet, S.; Sire, J.; Schwartz, O.; Mouscadet, J.F.; Boulanger, P. (2003). The human polycomb group EED protein interacts with the integrase of human immunodeficiency virus type 1. *J. Virol.*, Vol. 77, No. 23, pp. 12507-12522

Wang, W.; Cote, J.; Xue, Y.; Zhou, S.; Khavari, P.A.; Biggar, S.R.; Muchardt, C.; Kalpana, G.V.; Goff, S.P.; Yaniv, M.; Workman, J.L.; Crabtree, G.R. (1996). Purification and biochemical heterogeneity of the mammalian SWI-SNF complex. *EMBO J.*, Vol. 15, No. 19, pp. 5370-5382

Warrilow, D.; Tachedjian, G.; Harrich, D. (2009). Maturation of the HIV reverse transcription complex: putting the jigsaw together. *Rev. Med. Virol.*, Vol. 19, No. 6, pp. 324-337

Willetts, K.E.; Rey, F.; Agostini, I.; Navarro, J.M.; Baudat, Y.; Vigne, R.; Sire, J. (1999). DNA repair enzyme uracil DNA glycosylase is specifically incorporated into human immunodeficiency virus type 1 viral particles through a Vpr-independent mechanism. *J. Virol.*, Vol. 73, No. 2, pp. 1682-1688

Woodward, C.L.; Prakobwanakit, S.; Mosessian, S.; Chow, S.A. (2009). Integrase interacts with nucleoporin NUP153 to mediate the nuclear import of human immunodeficiency virus type 1. *J. Virol.*, Vol. 83, No. 13, pp. 6522-6533

Wu, X.; Liu, H.; Xiao, H.; Conway, J.A.; Hunter, E.; Kappes, J.C. (1997). Functional RT and IN incorporated into HIV-1 particles independently of the Gag/Pol precursor protein. *EMBO J.*, Vol. 16, No. 16, pp. 5113-5122

Wu, X.; Liu, H.; Xiao, H.; Conway, J.A.; Hehl, E.; Kalpana, G.V.; Prasad, V.; Kappes, J.C. (1999). Human immunodeficiency virus type 1 integrase protein promotes reverse transcription through specific interactions with the nucleoprotein reverse transcription complex. *J. Virol.*, Vol. 73, No. 3, pp. 2126-2135

Yamamoto, S.P.; Okawa, K.; Nakano, T.; Sano, K.; Ogawa, K.; Masuda, T.; Morikawa, Y.; Koyanagi, Y.; Suzuki, Y. (2011). Huwe1, a novel cellular interactor of Gag-Pol through integrase binding, negatively influences HIV-1 infectivity. *Microbes Infect.* Vol. 13, No. 4, pp. 339-349

Yan, N.; Cherepanov, P.; Daigle, J.E.; Engelman, A.; Lieberman, J. (2009). The SET complex acts as a barrier to autointegration of HIV-1. *PLoS Pathog.*, Vol. 5, No. 3, pp. e1000327

Yoder, K.; Sarasin, A.; Kraemer, K.; McIlhatton, M.; Bushman, F.; Fishel, R. (2006). The DNA repair genes XPB and XPD defend cells from retroviral infection. *Proc. Natl. Acad. Sci. USA*, Vol. 103, No. 12, pp. 4622-4627

Yoder, K.E.; Bushman, F.D. (2000). Repair of gaps in retroviral DNA integration intermediates. *J. Virol.*, Vol. 74, No. 23, pp. 11191-11200

Yung, E.; Sorin, M.; Pal, A.; Craig, E.; Morozov, A.; Delattre, O.; Kappes, J.; Ott, D.; Kalpana, G.V. (2001). Inhibition of HIV-1 virion production by a transdominant mutant of integrase interactor 1. *Nat. Med.*, Vol. 7, No. 8, pp. 920-926

Yung, E.; Sorin, M.; Wang, E.J.; Perumal, S.; Ott, D.; Kalpana, G.V. (2004). Specificity of interaction of INI1/hSNF5 with retroviral integrases and its functional significance. *J. Virol.*, Vol. 78, No. 5, pp. 2222-2231

Zhu, K.; Dobard, C.; Chow, S.A. (2004). Requirement for integrase during reverse transcription of human immunodeficiency virus type 1 and the effect of cysteine mutations of integrase on its interactions with reverse transcriptase. *J. Virol.*, Vol. 78, No. 10, pp. 5045-5055

Zielske, S.P.; Stevenson, M. (2005). Importin 7 may be dispensable for human immunodeficiency virus type 1 and simian immunodeficiency virus infection of primary macrophages. *J. Virol.*, Vol. 79, No. 17, pp. 11541-11546

Zielske, S.P.; Stevenson, M. (2006). Modest but reproducible inhibition of human immunodeficiency virus type 1 infection in macrophages following LEDGFp75 silencing. *J. Virol.*, Vol. 80, No. 14, pp. 7275-7280

2

HIV Infection «HIV Tat Protein, a Key Factor in Pathogenesis and Immune System Dysregulation: Implication of IL-10»

Ben Haij N., Planès R., Mzoughi O. and Bahraoui E.
Université Paul Sabatier, Unité mixte INSERM/CNRS/UPS 1043, Toulouse France

1. Introduction

Human Immunodeficiency Virus (HIV) is the causative agent of AIDS (Acquired Immune Deficiency Syndrome). Currently, the infection by HIV is considered as one of the major problem of public health and social stability. The scale of HIV/AIDS epidemic has exceeded all expectations since its identification 30 years ago. Currently, according to the report on HIV/AIDS by UNAIDS and World Health Organization (WHO) in 2009, we estimated approximately 33 million people are currently living with HIV-1 and about 25 millions have already died (Piot, Feachem et al. 2004). HIV infection leads to a decline in the number of T helper CD4 cells leading to a progressive dysfunction of the immune system. This weakening of the immune system results in the development of opportunistic infections leading to death of the patient. Despite prevention policies and anti-retroviral therapies, AIDS still remains one of the most serious humanitarian crises that we have never known.

1.1 HIV taxonomy, structure and genome organization

Identified in 1983, HIV belongs to lentivirus genus of Retroviridaea (Barre-Sinoussi, Chermann et al. 1983). Lentiviruses are host-specific viruses which cause slowly progressive diseases in their hosts and are characterized by selective T CD4 depletion (Fauci 1988) associated with a severe immunological and neurological disorders. These disorders are amplified by the fact that the virus infects the key cells of the immune system. As consequences, immunological disorders in HIV infected patients are observed since the asymptomatic stage. Two major subtypes of HIV have been identified: HIV-1 and HIV-2 (Clavel, Guetard et al. 1986). The first, HIV-1, is world wide, virulent and responsible of HIV infection globally. However, the second, HIV-2, is less pathogenic and is largely confined to West Africa. These two types of virus share a 40% homology in their sequences. HIV-1 strain is subdivided into three genetically groups: M (Major), N (New or non M non O) and O (Outlier) (Clavel, Guetard et al. 1986). The M strain is the most spread worldwide, it represents more than 95% of the global virus isolates. The variability within the sequence of *env* gene of HIV-1, allowed it to be subdivided into 10 clades A to L (McCutchan 2000). At least 15 additional circulating recombinant forms (CRF) has been identified in HIV-1 patients living in different geographic regions of the world (Peeters and Sharp 2000). However, the presence of these CRF seems to be more present in Africa, Asia and South of America. Despite the high sequence homology between HIV-1 and HIV-2 and the existence of co-infection *in vivo* with the two viruses, no recombination between HIV-1 and -2 have been reported. About the question of the origin of HIV-1 and HIV-2 transmission to human, it is admitted that it comes respectively from a cross-species of SIVcpz (Simian Immunodeficiency Virus which infects chimpanzees) in Central Africa and SIVsm (Simian Immunodeficiency Virus which infects sooty mangabey) in West Africa (Hirsch, Olmsted et al. 1989; Gao, Gorelick et al. 2003).

HIV-1 is an enveloped virus. The viral particles are produced as immature virions by budding from infected cells. After maturation by the viral protease, mature particles adopt spherical forms with a diameter of 90-100 nm (figure 1).

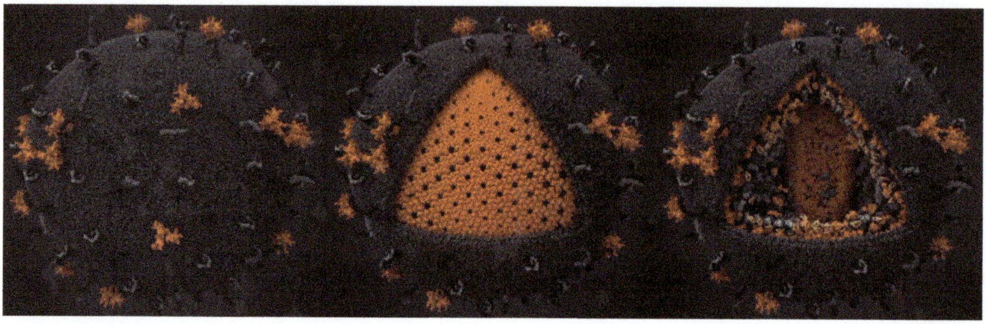

This spatial representation takes into account and summarizes the results from more than 100 latest scientific publications in the fields of virology, X-ray analysis and NMR spectroscopy. The depicted spatial configurations of 17 different viral and cellular proteins found in HIV particle are in strict accordance with known 3D-structures. This model of HIV virion is put on the cover of the special issue of Nature Medicine (September 8, 2010) prepared by the Global HIV Vaccine Enterprise.

Fig. 1. Model reconstitution of spatial structure of HIV-1.

Those mature particles have a cone shaped core composed of the p24 viral protein. It was estimated that each viral particle contains 1500-2000 Gag and 100-200 Pol molecules. The envelope glycoproteins are present as trimers of gp120/gp41 and were estimated to ten trimers per particle. The HIV capsid contains the viral genome composed of two identical single stranded RNA molecules allowing the establishment of frequent genetic changes by recombination. The RNA viral genome is capped at its 5′-end and polyadenylated at its 3′-end. The viral reverse transcriptase, integrase and nucleoproteins were found associated with the viral genome. The HIV genome of approximately 10kb encodes for 16 distinct proteins (Sodroski, Rosen et al. 1985). A schematic representation of HIV genome and proteins is illustrated in figure 2. As in all retroviruses, those proteins are derived from three essential genes *gag, pol* and *env*. The first gene *gag* encodes for Gag precursor p55, which is cleaved by viral protease to give capside, matrice and nucleocapside proteins : p24, p17, p7 and p6. Enzymatic proteins are encoded by *pol* gene and give three viral enzymes : protease p11, transcriptase reverse p65/51 and integrase p32. The *env* gene encodes for the precursor gp160 which is later proteotically cleaved by a cellular protease into the two envelope proteins gp120 and gp41. These steps of maturation by the viral or the cellular proteases are crucial for the production of infectious viral particles. In addition to these structural and enzymatic gene products, HIV genome encodes for two regulatory proteins Tat (transcriptional transactivator) and Rev (regulator of virion gene expression) and also for four accessory proteins : Vif (viral infectivity factor), Vpr (viral protein r), Vpu (viral protein

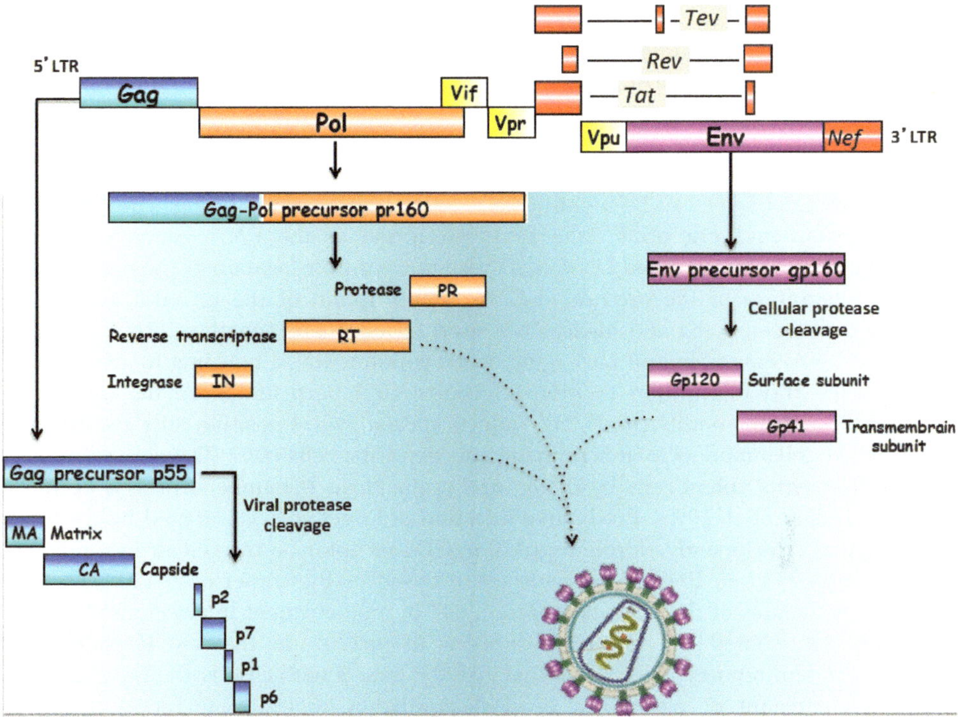

Gag (group specific antigen) and Gag-Pol (polymerase) are polyprotein precursors that are processed by viral protease. The 9 mature subunits are protease (PR), reverse transcriptase (RT), integrase (IN), matrix (MA), capsid (CA), p2, nucleocapside (NC), p1 and p6. Envelope is also cleaved, however by a host cellular protease into surface (SU) gp120 and transmembrane gp41 moieties. HIV genome encodes also for accessory and regulatory proteins: transcriptional transactivator (Tat), regulator of virion gene expression (Said, Dupuy et al.), viral infectivity factor (Vif), viral proteins u (Vpu), viral proteins r (Vpr) and negative factor (Nef). Tev contains Tat, Env and Rev sequences and functions like Tat and Rev.

Fig. 2. HIV genome organization and proteins.

u) and Nef (negatif factor) (Emerman and Malim 1998). The gene products of *rev* and *tat* are produced early in the viral cycle and their expression is essential for the viral replication. Deletion of one of them leads to an abortive viral cycle. The Tat protein is implicated in the initiation and elongation/stabilisation of transcribed viral mRNA. Tat binds to a specific site called TAR (Tat responsive region) located in the LTR. Tat is the major protein involved in the upregulation of HIV-1 replication. In parallel, the Rev protein interacts with a structure called RRE (Rev responsive element) located in the *env* gene (Emerman and Malim 1998). This interaction permits mono and unspliced mRNA to cross the nuclear membrane in order to enter in the cytoplasm, where, they will be translated to proteins or encapsidated in the nascent viral particles. As Tat and Rev, Nef is also an early produced protein. This protein has at least three distinct activities including down regulation of cell surface CD4 and MHC class I molecules and enhancement of virion infectivity. It has been reported that this protein is essential for proviral DNA synthesis. It is also important for cell-cell transmission of the virus. In fact, the Vif protein seems to be involved in the final stages of the nucleoprotein core packaging (Peterlin and Trono 2003). The Vpr protein affects the nuclear localization of viral nucleic acids in non dividing cells and induces cell differentiation (Peterlin and Trono 2003), while the Vpu protein enhances virion release and degrades CD4 in the endoplasmic reticulum (Hoglund, Ohagen et al. 1994). Many studies have put forward that Vpr, Vif, Nef and perhaps Tat are found associated in the viral particles.

1.2 HIV-1 tropism and replication cycle

At least 11 distinct steps can be identified in HIV-1 viral cycle including: viral attachment, entry by fusion and uncoating, reverse transcription of the RNA genome by reverse transcriptase to double stranded DNA (dsDNA), nuclear translocation of the pre-integration complex, integration of the proviral dsDNA, transcription of the proviral genome after cellular activation, splicing and nuclear transport of mono and unspliced RNA, translation of the viral RNA, assembly and packaging of the genomic RNA, budding to give immature viral particles and maturation to give infectious viral particles. Since the infection are mediated through the bodily fluids, HIV infects specially CD4 positive cells and essentially T-CD4 helper cells, monocyte/macrophage and dendritic cells (DC) (Dalgleish, Beverley et al. 1984). The virus enters cells by fusion and endocytosis (Chambers, Pringle et al. 1990; Bernstein, Tucker et al. 1995). Productive infection of target cells is initiated by the binding of the external envelope glycoprotein gp120 to CD4 receptor on the cell surface membrane (Bour, Geleziunas et al. 1995). At the surface of the virus the trimer of gp120 is associated with three molecules of the transmembrane gp41 by non-covalent interactions. CD4-gp120 interaction is mediated by conserved domains of gp120 and the first domain of CD4 receptor. Different reports have shown that gp120 interacts with CD4 with high affinity with dissociation constant of nanomolar level (Fenouillet, Clerget-Raslain et al. 1989). It is interesting to note that the conserved domains of gp120 appear to be few or non-immunogenic in HIV-1 infected patients. Generation antibodies against the conserved domains of gp120 are of great interest. In fact, despite the great variability observed in HIV-1 sequence, all viruses recognize the same receptor CD4. Thus, the production of such antibodies will probably exhibit a large spectrum of HIV neutralization by blocking gp120-CD4 interaction with all HIV-1 subtypes despite their variability. A great number of studies are working to design potential vaccine candidates based on these conserved domains of HIV-1 envelope glycoproteins. Entry of HIV requires also an interaction of gp120 with a coreceptor: CCR5 (R5 tropic virus) and/or CXCR4 (X4 tropic virus) (Maddon, Dalgleish et al. 1986; Kozak, Platt et al. 1997; Platt, Wehrly et al. 1998). At the time of primo-infection, HIV recognizes and infects principally cells that express CCR5 proteins (monocytes/macrophages) (Dragic, Litwin et al. 1996). With time the virus switch from R5 to X4 tropic to infects T cells (Grivel and Margolis 1999; Shankarappa, Margolick et al. 1999). This tropic evolution correlates with late stage of HIV infection : AIDS stage. Thus, interaction of gp120 to CD4 receptor and coreceptors induces HIV entry by allowing viral and host cell membranes fusion. This mechanism continues to be largely investigated at a molecular level, by different groups. We will briefly summarize here the key steps.

Subsequently to gp120-CD4 interaction, conformational changes occurs firstly in the viral gp120 and then, in the transmembrane gp41. Modifications in gp120 structure contribute to the exposure of V3 region, which contains the binding site of the viral chemokine receptors CCR5 or CXCR4. This latter interaction mediates further modifications in the gp41 structure leading to the exposition of the hydrophobic N-terminal gp41 fusion domain. Then the insertion of this fusion domain into the membrane of the host cell allows its fusion with the viral membrane (Chan, Fass et al. 1997) (figure 3).

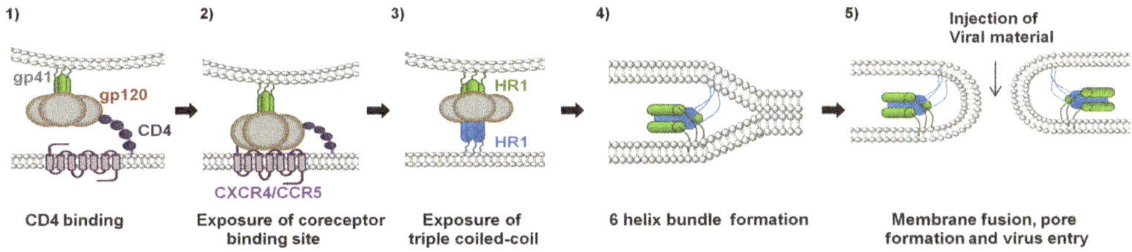

The mechanism of HIV-1 entry can be summarized in the following model. After binding of gp120 to receptor and coreceptor (step 1-2), gp41 undergoes conformational changes leading to the exposure of the fusion peptide and the accessibility of trimeric HR1 and the hydrophobic N-terminal domain, which contains the fusogenic region, and the trimeric HR2 domains (step 3). Then, HR1 and HR2 interacts together forming a 6-helix bundle leading to the membrane fusion and virus entry (step 4-5). The triple stranded coiled-coil structure (step 3), which probably explains its low immunogenicity in human patients infected with HIV-1.

Fig. 3. Representation of the different steps from the viral-host interaction and the viral entry after membranes fusion.

The chemokine coreceptors CCR5 and CXCR4 of HIV are preferentially found in lipid rafts (Kozak, Heard et al. 2002). These cholesterol and sphingolipid-enriched microdomains in the plasma membrane mirror the optimal lipid bilayer of the virus and provide likely a better environment for membrane fusion (Chambers, Pringle et al. 1990; Chazal and Gerlier 2003). Several inhibitors including T20 (enfuvirtide) have been developed. T20 is a synthetic peptide of 36 amino acids which blocks HIV-1 entry by interfering with the formation of the six helix bundle formed following the interaction between the trimeric HR1 and HR2 domains of the transmembrane envelope glycoprotein gp41 (Kilby, Hopkins et al. 1998). More recently a selective CCR5 antagonist, named maraviroc or vicriviroc has been developed. By blocking gp120-CCR5 interaction this antagonist present a potent anti-HIV-1 activity (Kromdijk, Huitema et al.; Perry). As T20, maraviroc is also active at nanomolar concentrations. It is postulated that CCR5 antagonists may be of great interest, if we consider that HIV-1 infection is essentially mediated by CCR5 tropic viruses (Kromdijk, Huitema et al.). The use of these type of entry inhibitors has been found to effectively inhibit infection of cells *in vitro* and *in vivo* by R5 strains tropic HIV-1 that have developed resistance to the other major classes of anti-retroviral drugs (anti reverse transcriptase and anti protease inhibitors). It is interesting to note that this is the first anti-HIV drug that targets the host cells rather than the virus directly. However, one potential limitation of such inhibitors is the possible selection and rapid emergence of CXCR4 tropic viruses. In fact, the isolation of HIV-1 from patients, who have never received an anti-retroviral therapy, naïve for HAART, showed the presence, of R5 tropic viruses in 85% of the cases. These results are in agreement with the natural resistance of persons harbouring CCR5delta32 deletion (Dean, Carrington et al. 1996; Huang, Paxton et al. 1996; Liu, Paxton et al. 1996; Samson, Libert et al. 1996). While the early stage of infection was characterized by the predominance of R5 tropic viruses, the emergence of viruses with CXCR4 tropism were associated with the late stage of infection (Scarlatti, Tresoldi et al. 1997). The molecular basis of this R5 to CXCR4 switch remains to be clarified. CXCR4 strains seem to emerge only in 50% patients who develop AIDS (Connor, Sheridan et al. 1997; Scarlatti, Tresoldi et al. 1997). In addition to these two selective HIV-1 strains, an intermediate strain named dual tropic HIV-1 strain which use indifferently R5 and CXCR4 was also reported in some HIV-1 infected patients.

The external envelope gp120 is a highly glycosylated protein. Carbohydrates represent about 50% of its molecular weight (Fenouillet, Clerget-Raslain et al. 1989). The majority of these carbohydrates are of N-type glycosylation. O-glycosylation seems to be rarely present in HIV-1 envelope glycoproteins. Viruses use glycosylation as tool to escape immune responses, resist to protease degradation, and adopt structural native conformation or to bind cellular receptors. By its carbohydrate parts, envelope glycoprotein gp120 recognizes and interacts with high affinity (Kd of nM level) with DC-SIGN (Dendritic Cell-Specific Intercellular adhesion molecule-3-Grabbing Non integrin) receptor. DC-SIGN is a C-type lectin present on the surface of membranes of dendritic and monocyte/macrophage cells (Geijtenbeek, Kwon et al. 2000; Geijtenbeek, Torensma et al. 2000).

Submucosal DC, which normally process and present antigens to immune cells, bind HIV-1 using C-type lectin essentially at the vaginal mucosa. However this interaction does not trigger the conformational changes necessary for the fusion of the virus and DC membranes. But virus bound on DC, or internalized by endocytosis, can migrate to regional lymph nodes where its target T-helper cells are found. Thus, dendritic cells expressing DC-SIGN appear to act as a "Trojan horse" facilitating the spread of the infection from mucosal surfaces to lymphatic organs (Geijtenbeek, Kwon et al. 2000; Geijtenbeek, Torensma et al. 2000; Kwon, Gregorio et al. 2002).

After entry and uncoating, the viral genome is released into the cytoplasm. This step is concomitant with the start of reverse transcription. The resulted dsDNA migrates into the nucleus where it is integrated by the viral integrase into host genome. The integration site is preferentially located into active genes locus because HIV like many other viruses cannot replicate into quiescent/latent cells. This DNA is flanked by two repeated sequence named LTRs (Long Terminal Repeats). Following cell activation, the viral DNA is transcribed by cellular RNA polymerase II (RNA pol II). Viral transcription is initiated when cellular RNA pol II is recruited at the 5'end of LTR provirus. For efficient transcription elongation a 5'end TAR-hairpin structure named TAR (Tat associated region) element have to be present and bind HIV Tat protein. When Tat protein is absent, the initiation can begin but elongation is abrogated and/or inefficient. After translation, of viral protein and assembly in cholesterol rich lipid rafts, immature virions are released by budding from plasma membrane infected cells.

1.3 HIV-1 genome transactivation: an essential role of HIV-1 Tat protein

Once integrated, HIV genome behaves like the host genes and can be transcribed using the cellular RNA pol II and host cell machineries in addition to the viral Tat protein. The HIV LTR contains proximal core sequence and a distal promoter. The core element is composed by the initiator (Inr) and TATA box (TATA). The distal promoter carries enhancer sequences that contain two NF-κB and three SP1 binding sites that position RNA pol II at the correct site for transcription initiation (Peterlin and Trono 2003; Peterlin and Price 2006). Downstream the core element, HIV LTR contains a short nascent stem bulged loop leader RNA named TAR (Transcription associated Region) (Berkhout, Silverman et al. 1989; Jeang, Xiao et al. 1999). HIV Tat protein is known to be the transcriptional activator that binds to this TAR RNA structure and HIV transcription mediated by Tat is illustrated in figure 4.

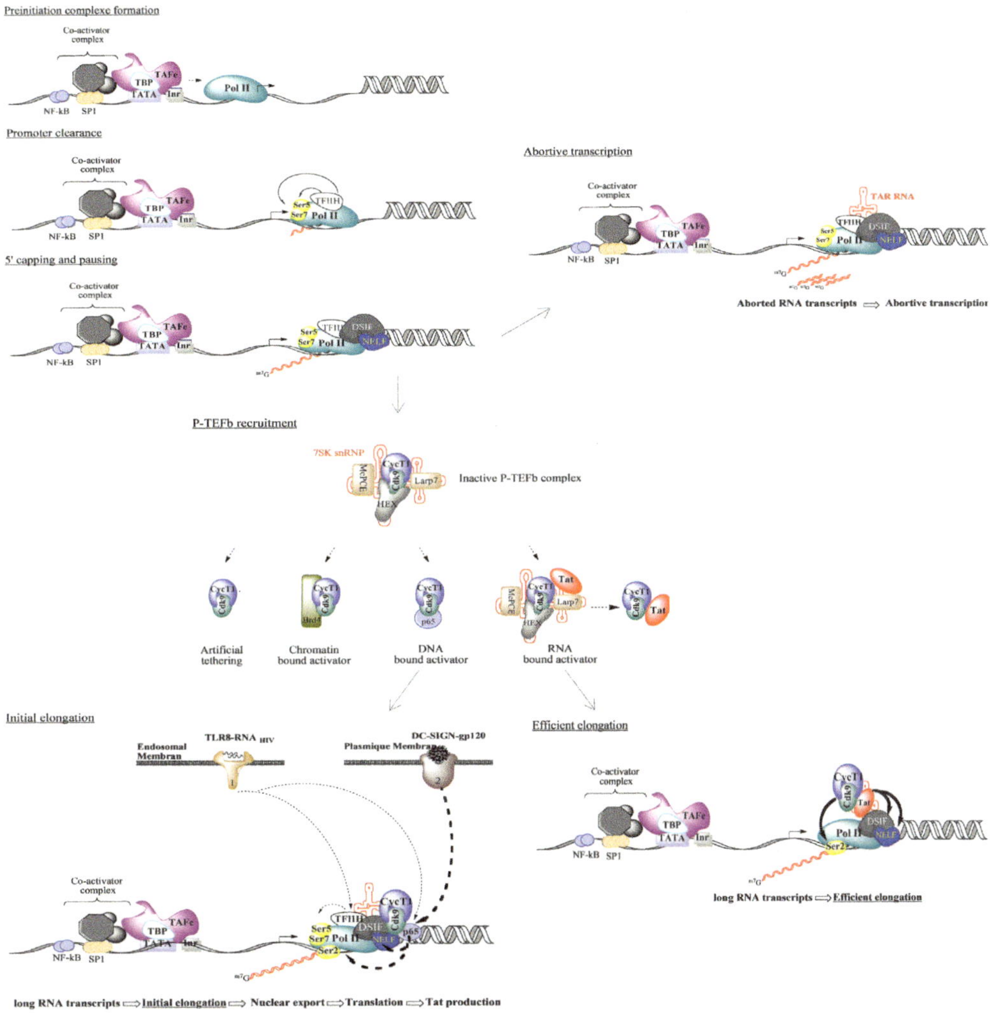

The first step of HIV transcription consists of the formation of the pre-initiation complex by RNA pol II recruitment to the promoter. The second step consists to clear the promoter by phosphorylation of the RNA pol II at serine position 5 of the CTD by cyclin dependent kinase : CDK7 of the TFIIH protein. This phosphorylation increases the binding and affinity of human enzyme capping (Brenchley, Price et al. 2006) that leads to the 5′end capping of nascent RNA transcripts. At this step a pausing of RNA pol II occurs by the recruitment of two negatives elongation factors named: DSIF (DRB sensitivity inducing factor) and NELF. Finally, productive elongation occurs by the recruitment of P-TEFb. P-TEFb activity is tightly regulated by its association with a complex composed by 7SK snRNA and heterodimer HEXIM1/2. Tat recruitment of P-TEFb leads to efficient elongation and the obtaining of totally RNA transcripts production.

Fig. 4. Transcription of the HIV genome and implication of its Tat protein.

For summary, after PIC formation and clearance of the promoter a pause of RNA pol II occurs. Without recruitment of P-TEFb (positive transcription elongation factor b), only short RNA transcripts are formed and subsequently aborted. In fact, in absence of Tat, transcription is initiated but elongation do not occurs and only short RNA abortive transcripts are produced (Peterlin and Price 2006). At a molecular level, P-TEFb can be recruited by several mechanisms (figure 4) and notably by HIV Tat protein. Indeed, transcription from the HIV-1 LTR is several hundred folds higher in presence of Tat than in its absence. So, the question that follows is how can HIV initiate the synthesis of the first viral proteins, including Tat protein, in the absence of the latter viral factor essential for an efficient elongation ? Or how the first Tat molecules are synthetized ?

Several studies have demonstrated that, in HIV, LTR transcription can be separated in two steps, the first is Tat independent whereas the second is Tat dependent. Recent studies from Greijtenbeek et al. and Gringhuis, van der Vlist et al.(Greijtenbeek et al. 2000; Gringhuis, Van der vlist et al. 2010) have shown that HIV can activate initiation and elongation by two separate mechanisms. The first, transcription initiation, is activated in endosomal structure following the HIV RNA-Toll Like Receptor 8 (TLR8) interaction. More precisely, HIV ssRNA-TLR8 interaction induces activation of NF-κB p65 and RNA pol II phosphorylation at serine 5 residue leading to the recruitment of CDK7 to the transcription units. In parallel, they have also shown that elongation depends upon gp120-DC-SIGN interaction. This membrane interaction activates elongation by phosphorylation of serine 276 and serine 5 of NF-κB p65 and RNA pol II respectively and their recruitments with CDK9 to the HIV LTR. This mechanism can explain how the HIV initiates the production of the first HIV-Tat protein. Then, Tat proteins take over and amplify viral transcription by its capacity to bind the 7SK small nuclear RNA (7SK nRNA) complex and recruits P-TEFb to the paused RNA pol II, by interacting cooperatively with TAR element. This interaction is mediated by Tat arginine rich motif. Once recruited to the transcription units, P-TEFb phosphorylates NELF (negative elongation factor) and the CTD of RNA pol II at serine 2 residue. Tat has also been reported to interact with many factor/co-factor implicated in transcription as: Sp1, TATA box binding protein, CDK2, CBP/p300, TFIIH and RNA pol II. Overall, Tat permits an efficient elongation and co-transcriptional processing by splicing and polyadenylation machineries. When levels of the regulatory Tat protein fall to below threshold levels, HIV becomes latent.

1.4 HIV-1 infection and its effects on immune and the central nervous system

1.4.1 Natural history of HIV-1 infection

The course of HIV infection could be divided into three distinct clinical phases: acute infection, asymptomatic stage or chronic infection and symptomatic stage characterized by AIDS development (Furrer, Opravil et al. 2001) (figure 5).

The first step called acute phase corresponds to the contamination, the primary viral replication and the beginning of immune sensitization. The most common routes of HIV infection are mediated by sexual transmission of the virus, transfusion by contaminated blood products, the use of unsafe needles by drug users, and perinatal transmission from infected mother to infant. This latter case of HIV transmission can occur either in utero or during breast-feeding (Coovadia, Rollins et al. 2007). Cases of contamination during delivery are also reported. Early after exposure, the virus reaches some strategic organs such as the secondary lymphoid organs (mucosa-associated lymphoid tissue and gut-associated lymphoid tissues), which content most of the cells targeted by HIV. At this stage, the virus replicates actively during a period of 6 to 12 weeks called the acute phase. Viral load reaches several millions copies of viral RNA per millilitre (ml) of plasma. T cells are depleted in blood and the gastro-intestinal tract, but the pool of T cells present in the blood compartment was restored by the central lymphoid organs. In general this step remains asymptomatic, but some patients could develop signs of of routine infection including, fever, lymphadenopathy and rash (Quinn 1997). These symptoms may last in general two to three weeks. At this stage of infection, the innate and adaptive immune systems react strongly to control HIV replication to lower the viral load to a set point often below 20000 RNA copies per ml of plasma (figure 5).

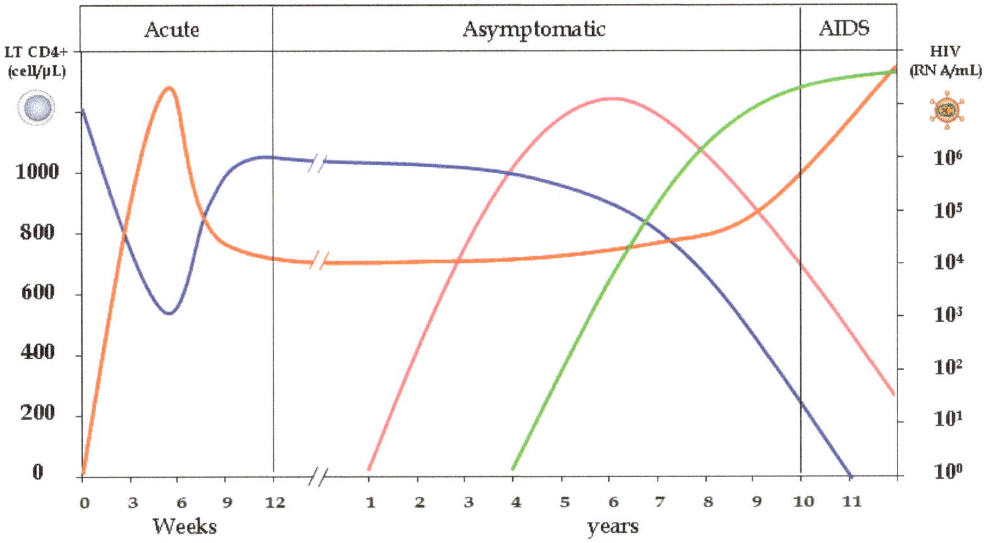

A generalized graph that represent the relationship between T cells number by blood microliter (blue line) and HIV viral RNA copies by blood ml (red line) over the time course of untreated HIV infection. Two major mechanisms involved in T cells dysfunction and progression toward AIDS are represented (arbitrary units) such as increase in pro-inflammatory factors TNF-α, IL-6, IFN-α (pink line), and upregulation of immunosuppressive factors including IL-10, PD-1, PD-L1 and IDO (green line).

Fig. 5. Evolution of T cell count and viral load over the different stages of untreated HIV infection.

The second stage is an asymptomatic phase where the virus persists and the infection becomes chronic. During this period, that varies from 6 months to several decades depending on the patients, the virus replicates continuously mainly in the reservoir cell such as macrophages, the nervous system and regulatory T cells (Treg) (Tran, de Goer de Herve et al. 2008). During this phase, most of the patients maintain a normal CD4 T cell count with apparent normal health. The immune system is still continuously activated against viral replication but HIV will escape to this immune pressure by different mechanisms including the emergence of new variants. One of the most dramatic viral emergence is the appearance of X4 and dual tropic R5/X4 viruses, which replicate more rapidly, produces high amount of viruses progeny and are more cytopathic (Schuitemaker,

Koot et al. 1992; Connor, Sheridan et al. 1997; Singh and Collman 2000). In fact, a loss of $CD4^+$ cells of about 30 to 60 cells per microlitre and per year was observed in HIV-1 infected patients (figure 5). This asymptomatic phase has duration of 6 to 10 years and may be greatly modulated by highly anti-retroviral therapy (HAART). However in less than 1% of HIV-1 infected patients this asymptomatic phase is highly reduced (1 to 2 years), and can last longer, more than 25 years, in patients under HAART (Markowitz, Mohri et al. 2005). In addition to the direct lyses of infected cells this phase is accompanied with several immune disorders leading to immune exhaustion.

One hallmark of this immune disorder is chronic immune activation characterized by increase production of pro-inflammatory cytokines such as TNF-α and IL-6. TNF-α, thus, lead to the activation of HIV replication, loss of CD4 and CD8 through apoptosis (Said, Dupuy et al. 2010) and to neuronal disorders including HIV associated dementia (Nixon and Landay 2010). Increase of IL-6 production has been associated with immunological disorders including B cell lymphoma and hypergammaglobulinemie. It is interesting to note that Tat protein is able to induce TNF-α and IL-6. Production of these two cytokines has also been correlated with a systemic increase of bacterial products such as LPS. Indeed Brencley et al., (Brenchley, Price et al. 2006) have shown that chronic phase of HIV infection is characterized by an increase in circulating bacterial products related to the damage of the intestinal epithelium by the HIV-1 cytopathic effect. Released viral antigens and bacterial products contribute to the constant persistence of a chronic immune activation and T cells death. Other mechanism involved in immune activation is mediated by IFN-α produced by plasmacytoïd DC (pDC), a particular DC population specialized in antiviral immunity. It was reported that HIV induce IFN-α production by pDC through the activation of TLR7 by viral ssRNA. This cytokine acts on CD4+ and CD8+ lymphocytes to induce an activated phenotype (CD69+, CD38+) and will in turn lead to T cell apoptosis (Martinson, Montoya et al. 2010). This great and continual immune activation fails, however, to contain HIV infection. This phenomenon could be explained by the upregulation of several immunosuppressive factors that impaired T cell responses. Among those, it has been reported an a) increase in the production of the immunosuppressive cytokine IL-10, principally by monocytes cells; b) increase expression of programmed death 1 (PD-1) on monocytes (Said, Dupuy et al. 2010), LT CD4+ and LT CD8+, and its ligand PD-L1 on monocytes, macrophages, mDC and pDC. Subsequently, PD-1/PD-L1 interaction stimulates IL-10 production, induces negative signals for TCR activation and leads to T cell death; c) enhancement in the activation of the immunosuppressive enzyme indoleamine 2,3-dioxygenase (IDO) in mDC and pDC which acts by depleting the essential amino acid tryptophan and inhibits T cell proliferation and d) increase in the generation and activation of T reg, a subset of T lymphocytes with immunosuppressive activity. All of these immunosuppressive factors will contribute to immune inactivation and have been associated with disease progression to AIDS. As the CD4+ cell count drops below 200 cells/mm3 the risk of developing opportunistic infections including *pneumocystis carini, CMV, JC* or malignancies increases Kaposi's sarcoma (Clifford and Demierre 2005; Bonnet, Balestre et al. 2006). Advanced HIV-disease is characterized by a strong T CD4 depletion to less than 50 cell/mm^3, high viral load and multiple opportunistic infections and malignancies.

AIDS represents the final stage of HIV-1 infection and is characterized by a profound depletion of CD4 positive T cells. In fact, after several years of unresolved chronic infection, the rate of CD4+ T cells drops dramatically in the blood to a critical rate of 200 T CD4 cells microliter. This phase is characterized by the occurrence of several rare opportunistic infections. The first opportunists that are taking advantage of immunocompromised patients are oral candidiasis, pneumococcal infections, mycobacterial infections and reactivation of herpes simplex and varicella virus. AIDS is also associated with tumor proliferations such as Kaposi's sarcoma, due to Human Herpes Virus 8 (HHV8), lymphoma associated with Epstein-Barr virus and cervical and anal carcinoma associated with human papilloma virus. In fact, this stage results in an extreme immunosuppression with diverse clinical features including opportunistic infections, malignancies and neurological disorders (So, Holtzman et al. 1988; Coopman, Johnson et al. 1993; Simpson and Tagliati 1994) and without treatment will irremediably lead to death of the patient within a few months.

1.4.2 Neuropathogenesis of HIV-1 infection

In addition to its tropism for the cells of the immune system, HIV is also known for its neurotropism. The virus is early found in the CNS carried by infected cells essentially macrophages. The virus can be directly isolated and cultured from the cerebrospinal fluids (CSF) from HIV-1 infected patients. In the CNS the virus replicates strongly in macrophages and microglia and moderately in astrocytes. Although HIV-1 is qualified as a neurotropic virus, it does not infect neurons. Consequently to CNS infection, about 60% of HIV-1 infected patients showed HIV associated neurological, which includes dementia and neuropsychiatric and cognitive motor impairments (Ozdener 2005; Giunta, Obregon et al. 2006). Infiltration of the virus in the brain is concomitant with the development of astrocytosis and microgliosis. While HIV-1 productively replicates in macrophages and microglia, infection of astrocytes allow only, the expression of early proteins Rev, Tat and Nef (Tornatore, Nath et al. 1991; Lipton and Gendelman 1995; Kutsch, Oh et al. 2000). It is interesting to note that astrocytes function also as an reservoir for HIV-1. Neuronal injury observed in the CNS of HIV-1 infected patients results from the activation direct by the virus or indirectly by inflammatory neurotoxins. For example it has been shown that the infection of astrocytes allowed to the impairment of the uptake and secretion of glutamate and to the modulation of glutamate receptor expression (Bezzi, Carmignoto et al. 1998). It was also demonstrated that, by its Tat protein, HIV stimulates the production of various chemokines including MCP-1, IL-8 and IP-10 which participate in the recruitment of macrophages and various type of leukocytes (Conant, Garzino-Demo et al. 1998; Kutsch, Oh et al. 2000). Production by HIV-1 infected macrophages of neurotoxins including quinolate, glutamate and L-cysteine, and inflammatory mediators including, IFN-α, IFN-β, IL-6, IL-1α, IL-1β, TNF-α, and TNF-β play an essential role in HAND. The loss of neurons in HAND by apoptosis and other mechanisms is directly related to these release of toxic mediators by activated and infected cells (Zink, Zheng et al. 1999). Tat, Nef, Vpr, gp120 and gp41 have been described as directly implicated as neuropathogenic factors. By acting with CXCR4, gp120 induces apoptosis of neurons. Also by acting on voltage gated calcium channels and N-methyl-D-aspartate receptor (NMDAR) gp120 induces calcium mobilization which mediates the production of reactive oxygen species (ROS), apoptosis and various neurotoxin mediators (Medina, Ghose et al. 1999). As gp120, HIV-1 Tat protein has been reported to be implicated in neuron injury directly via apoptosis (Sabatier, Clerget-Raslain et al. 1989; Shi, Raina et al. 1998; Nath, Haughey et al. 2000) and indirectly via the induction of inflammatory cytokines including TNF-α and IL-1β.

1.4.3 HIV and Kaposi's sarcoma: Effect of Tat protein

The high incidence of Kaposi's sarcoma (KS) in patients with HIV-1 infection has been related to the co-infection with HHV-8 also named KSHV (Kaposi sarcoma-associated herpes virus) (Schulz, Arbusow et al. 1998; Sirianni, Vincenzi et al. 1998; Aoki and Tosato 2004). It was shown that the presence of KSHV alone is not sufficient for KS development. The presence of HIV-1 seems to be essential for the development of KS lesions. This observation is in agreement with the drastic decrease of KS in patients under HAART. The analysis of the HIV-1 viral factor implicated underlined the essential role of Tat protein which acts as a transactivator factor for KSHV lytic cycle and activates proliferation, MAP-kinase activation, angiogenesis and tumoregenesis. It was shown that Tat promotes the tumorogenesis of endothelial cells both by acting at different ways by: stimulating the production of β-FGF, recruiting VEGF-2 receptor, both on KS and on endothelial cells, whose stimulation is essential for VEGF angiogenic effects (Albini, Benelli et al. 1996; Albini, Soldi et al. 1996; Ganju, Munshi et al. 1998), blocking apoptosis, and stimulating KSHV replication (Pyakurel, Pak et al. 2007). In addition Tat is able to stimulate the production of inflammatory cytokines following its interaction with chemokine receptors.

1.4.4 HIV and immunological disorders

From the asymptomatic stage and before T CD4 lymphocyte depletion, a generalized immune depression is observed in HIV-1 infected patients including disorders of both in the specific/acquired and innate immunities. This immunodepression in HIV-1 infected patients is associated with a profound alteration of the cytokine production (McMichael, Borrow et al. 2010; Clerici and Shearer 1993; Fauci 1996). These alterations have effects on target cells and influence also the virus replication. Increased production of pro-inflammatory cytokines stimulates HIV-1 replication *via* the activation of NF-κB pathway. In fact the LTR promoter of HIV-1 contains NF-κB binding sites. HIV-1 infection is associated, since the asymptomatic stage with a chronic immune activation and dysfunctional cytokine production. The acute host response to primary HIV-1 infection is characterized by Th0 cytokine profile, including the pro-inflammatory cytokines IL-1, IL-2, IL-6, TNF-α, IFN–α/β and IFN-γ as well as the anti-inflammatory cytokines IL-4, IL-10 and IL-13 (Harrich, Garcia et al. 1989; Hatada, Saito et al. 1999). At later stages of infection with disease progression, the pattern of cytokine production shifts toward a strongly based Th2 response mediated by IL-4, IL-6 and IL-10 (Rinaldo, Armstrong et al. 1990; Graziosi, Gantt et al. 1996; Takizawa, Ohashi et al. 1996). This profile was revealed inefficient to eradicate the virus. The mechanism of HIV induced cytokine production has been largely studied. There are many HIV-1 proteins that are capable of inducing the production of several cytokines. These proteins include HIV-1 glycoprotein gp120 that induce the secretion of many pro-inflammatory cytokines including IL-1, IL-6, IL-8, TNF-α, and IFN-γ (Francis and Meltzer 1993; Ameglio, Capobianchi et al. 1994; Ankel, Capobianchi et al. 1994; Capobianchi, Barresi et al. 1997). Interestingly, gp120 is also able to induce the secretion of IL-4 and IL-13 in basophils and IL-10 in mononuclear cells. Nef protein is able to induce the production of IL-1β, IL-6, IL-10, IL-15, TNF-α and IFN-γ in various human leukocyte populations (Schols and De Clercq 1996; Patella, Florio et al. 2000). There is also evidence that Vpr induces the expression of IL-6, IL-8, IL-10, TNF-α and IFN-γ in a variety of cell types (Brigino, Haraguchi et al. 1997).

Another HIV-1 protein, Tat, is known to stimulate the production of many cytokines and chemokines including IL-1β, IL-2, IL-6, IL-8, IL-10, TNF-α and MCP-1 (Clerici and Shearer 1993; Moore, O'Garra et al. 1993; Badou, Bennasser et al. 2000; Nath, Haughey et al. 2000;

Bennasser, Badou et al. 2002; Bennasser and Bahraoui 2002; Contreras, Bennasser et al. 2005). Our laboratory has shown that HIV-1 Tat protein induces the production of IL-10, a highly immunosuppressive cytokine by human peripheral blood monocytes. Since IL-10 levels have been shown to progressively increase as the disease progresses toward AIDS, one can hypothesize that this event can play a crucial role in the immune deregulation observed during HIV-1 infection. In line with this hypothesis, Shearer's group in a study including more than 1000 patients identified four patient classes depending on the capacity of their CD4 T lymphocytes to respond to different stimuli (mitogen, alloantigen, influenza virus, and HIV antigens). The progressive loss of the response of the immune system to these stimuli was found to be associated with a course leading to AIDS. Considerable production of IL-10 by peripheral blood mononuclear cells was observed in these patients and paralleled the alteration in CD4 T cell proliferative function. In addition, the immunosuppressive effect of IL-10 also correlated with the restoration of the capacity of isolated mononuclear cells of patients infected by HIV and immunodepressed to proliferate *in vitro* after stimulation by peptide antigens of HIV-1 envelope glycoprotein in the presence of a neutralizing anti-IL-10 antibody (Clerici, Wynn et al. 1994). In another study, Stylianou et al. evaluated the level of IL-10 in the sera of HIV-1 infected patients at different stages of infection. In agreement with Shearer's conclusion, they showed an increase in IL-10 level with disease progression. They also showed a decrease in IL-10 level in patients under highly active retroviral therapy (HAART). Inversely, it was reported an increase of IL-10 levels in patients with failure in tri-therapy treatment. Similarly low level of IL-10 was observed in HIV-1 long term non progressors or elite controllers (Clerici, Wynn et al. 1994). Inversely, it was showed that the persistence of a great level of IL-10 in the sera correlates with the failure in HAART (Stylianou, Aukrust et al. 1999).

HIV-1 infection affects cellular signaling. The two most important signaling pathways involved in cytokine production include the PKC and calcium pathway (figure 6). These pathways are activated after ligand-receptor interaction. Subsequently, this interaction activates phospholipase C which then cleaves its substrate PIP2 (phosphoinositol biphosphate) in IP3 (inositol 1,4,5-triphospate), responsible of the mobilization of intracellular calcium and to DAG (diacylglycerol), which initiates PKC activation. These two pathways lead to the phosphorylation and activation of cellular proteins mitogen-activated protein (MAP) kinase and of transcriptional factors including NF-AT, NF-κB, CREB and AP-1 responsible for the induction of cytokine genes (Spitaler et Cantrell 2004). In our laboratory we have accumulated several data showing the mechanism recruited by Tat protein to stimulate the production of the highly immunosuppressive cytokine IL-10. In the following part we will describe the role of Tat protein at different levels including its structure, secretion and uptake, mode of action for the transactivation of HIV-1 transcription, activation of signaling pathways and in the conclusion we will discuss Tat as potential target for drug or vaccine development.

2. HIV Tat protein

2.1 Background

HIV Tat protein is one of HIV conserved protein. It is early produced after HIV infection. Tat is a 9-14 kDa protein encoded by two exons separated by a non coding region. The first exon encodes the 72 first amino acids (figure 7). The length of HIV-1 Tat protein ranges from 86 to 101 amino acids and consists of 130 amino acids for HIV-2 (Johri, Mishra et al. 2011).

The 101 amino acids form of Tat is predominant in clinical isolates. Another form that comprises 86 amino acids is also found in some subtype B isolates and in the laboratory strain HXB2. The Tat sequence can be subdivided into six functional domains including N-terminal a proline and cysteine rich region, an hydrophobic core, a basic region followed by a glutamine rich region and a C terminal domain that contain a tripeptide RGD (Arginine, glycine, aspartatic acid) (figure 7). In addition, a domain containing the basic region is also called protein transduction domain (PTD), which renders Tat to have the ability to cross cell membranes and to be used as vector for gene transfer. Thus, viral Tat protein can be either intracellular or extracellular. The main function of HIV Tat protein is to transactivate the HIV long term repeat for retroviral transcription.

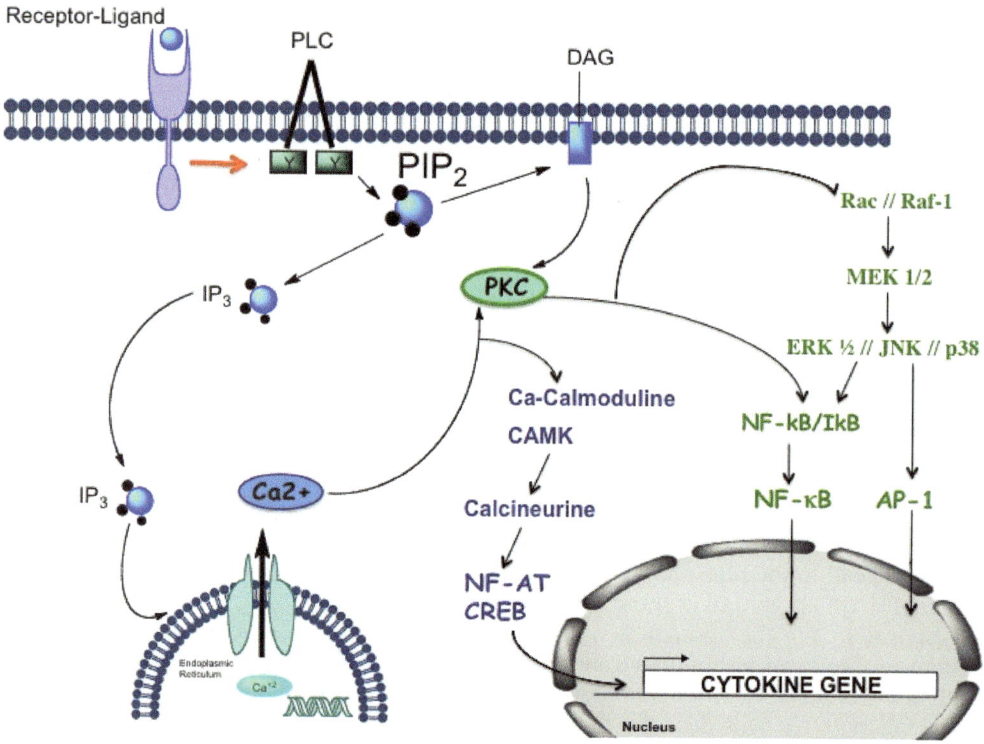

External stimulus activates a G protein coupled receptor, which activates a stimulating G protein. This G protein activates phospholipase C (PLC), which cleaves phosphoinositol-4,5-biphosphate (PIP2) into 1,2 diacylglycerol (DAG) and inositol-1, 4, 5-triphosphate (IP3). The IP3 interacts with calcium channel in the endoplasmic reticulum (ER), releasing calcium (Ca2+) into the cytoplasm. Intracytosolic calcium can interact with calmoduline proteins. This, leads to the activation of CAM kinases and calcineurine. Activation of CAMK and calcineurine induce activation and nuclear translocation of CREB and NF-AT respectively. In other hand, the increase in calcium levels activates PKC, which translocates to the membrane, anchoring to DAG and phosphatidylserine. Active catalytic PKC then, phosphorylate targets such as Rac, Raf that lead to downstream activation of MAP kinases and NF-□B and AP-1 transcription factor.

Fig. 6. The Protein Kinase C and calcium pathways.

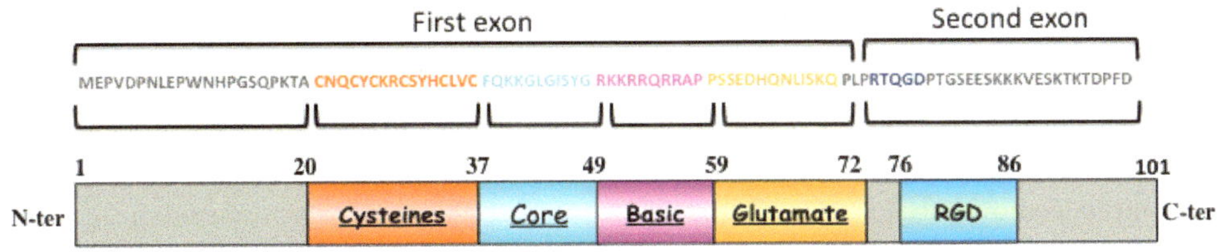

Tat is encoded by 2 exons in the HIV genome and it is composed by several regions. N-ter region 1-21 is a rich proline region. A region implicated in HIV transactivation is the 21-37 amino acids cysteine rich region and the core region 38-48 implicated in the Tat binding of HIV RNA. The basic rich region 49-59 is involved in Tat internalization whereas the glutamine rich region 60-72 in HIV replication. Finally the last region with the RGD sequence is encoded by the second exon.

Fig. 7. Organization of HIV-1 Tat protein: primary amino acids sequence and different domain of Tat.

2.1.1 HIV-1 Tat structure

Few studies have been devoted to studying secondary and tertiary structure of Tat protein. It seems clear that Tat belongs to the family of intrinsically unstructured proteins (Foucault, Mayol et al. 2010; Bayer, Kraft et al. 1995). Circular dichroïsme studies of Tat (analyze of secondary structure) showed a majority of β-turns structure and the absence of α-helical and β-sheets structures when the spectra were performed in aqueous solutions. However about 20 to 50% of alpha helical structures were detected when the protein was analyzed in organic solvant. Tertiary studies with using NMR confirmed that HIV Tat was generally an unfolded protein (Bayer, Kraft et al. 1995; Shojania and O'Neil 2006). They also demonstrated that the cysteine and basic regions are highly flexible and the N-terminal region is localized between the hydrophobic core and the glutamic rich domains (Watkins, Campbell et al. 2008). The X-ray cristallographic determination of Tat structure is not available. In summury all the available data indicated that Tat contains no ordered α-helical or β-sheet structures. Thus the biological active Tat protein seems to be conformation independent and perhaps only a limited gain of structure is necessary for its function. All these studies suggest that Tat protein does not have a defined secondary or tertiary structures and that biological active Tat protein is natively unfolded and only a limited gain of structure is necessary for its function.

2.1.2 HIV-1 Tat secretion and internalization

Despite the importance of extracellular Tat, few studies have focused on its mechanism of secretion from infected cells and its entry into uninfected cells (Rayne and Debaisieux et al. 2010; Vendeville and Rayne et al. 2004) (Westendorp, Frank et al. 1995). In fact, HIV Tat protein does not have a signal sequence and seems to be secreted by infected cells by an non conventionnal pathway. It is found present in the sera of HIV-1 infected patients at the nanomolar level (Ensoli, Buonaguro et al. 1993; Xiao, Neuveut et al. 2000) a value which may be underestimated since Tat may be trapped by its potential receptors, and particularly the heparan sulfates which are largely expressed on cell surfaces. Thus, the concentration of Tat, *in vivo*, is probably higher in the vicinity of the active HIV replication sites. After its secretion, Tat protein is taken up by neighboring cells infected or not. Despite the previous data reporting a particular mechanism for Tat uptake, it is clear now, that Tat protein enter viable cells essentially by endocytosis. This entry is mediated by the basic domain of Tat, also named PTD (protein transduction domain) and used for the development of peptidic vectors (Futaki and Suzuki 2001).

2.2 Tat activates the production of IL-10 in human monocytes

Our group has shown that HIV-1 Tat protein, by acting at cell membrane level, induces the production of IL-10, by non infected human monocytes (Badou and Bennasser 2000; Bennasser and Bahraoui 2002). To this end monocytes from healthy donors were purified and stimulated during 24 hours with increasing concentrations of recombinant Tat protein. Results showed that Tat protein induced strong and dose dependent IL-10 production. In contrast in the absence of Tat no IL-10 production was observed. This Tat induced IL-10 production persists after 48 and 72 hours of Tat stimulation. The amount of IL-10 produced by monocytes in response to Tat is dose and stimulation time dependent. Specifity of Tat effect was demonstrated by showing that chemically modified Tat, after H_2O_2 oxidation, becomes unable to stimulate IL-10 production. The specificity of Tat effect was further demonstrated by showing that when the stimulation of monocytes was performed in the presence of anti-Tat antibodies, IL-10 production by monocyte was totally inhibited (figure 8).

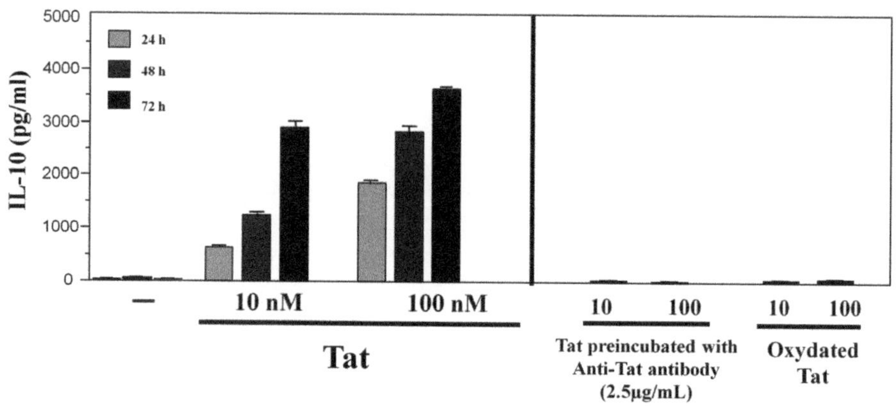

Tat 1-86 at 10 and 100 nM were incubated with or without anti-Tat antibody 2.5 □g/mL or were oxidated by H2O2 treatment. After 1 hour treatment, Tat treated or not, was incubated with human primary monocytes for 24h. IL-10 production was measured by ELISA.

Fig. 8. HIV-1 Tat induces specifically IL-10 production by human monocytes.

To determine the active domain of Tat that is responsible for the activity of Tat, monocytes were stimulated with GST-Tat deleted mutants including GST-Tat 1-72 (deleted form RGD domain), GST-Tat 1-55 (deleted from RGD and glutamate domains), GST-Tat 1-54 (deleted from RGD and basic domains), GST-Tat 20-72 (deleted from the N-Terminal domain), and GST-Tat 30-72 (deleted from de N-Terminal domain). Only GST-Tat deleted mutants but containing the N-terminal domain continues to stimulate IL-10 production. While the deleted mutants GST-Tat 20-72 and GST-Tat 30-72 as GST alone were unable to stimulate IL-10 production (figure 9). These data underlined the importance of the N-Terminal domain in IL-10 Tat induced activity.

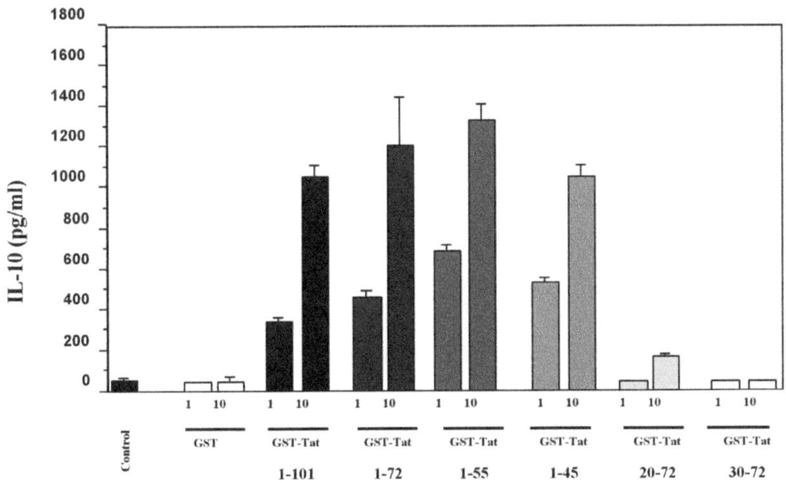

Monocytes were treated with 1 and 10 nM of wild type GST-Tat 1-101 or deleted mutant of Tat or GST alone as negative control. After 24 h of stimulation IL-10 production was measured by ELISA.

Fig. 9. The N-terminal domain of Tat : 1-45 is sufficient to induce IL-10 production by human monocytes.

As previously demonstrated in different report Tat protein is able to enter cells and to localize in the nucleus. So Tat protein is able to activate IL-10 production by acting at the cell membrane level or inside the cell. To understand its mechanism of action during the first steps of the activation, Tat protein was immobilized by coating in wells before adding purified human monocytes. In this condition, immobilized Tat leads to a dose dependent production of IL-10 indicating that Tat mediates its action by acting at the cell membrane. These results are in line with the capacity of the Tat deleted mutant, GST-Tat 1-45, to stimulate IL-10 production. In contrast to native Tat protein, the deleted mutant GST-Tat 1-45 is unable to penetrate into cells because it lacks the basic domain, responsible for penetration and nuclear localization of Tat.

The specific receptor implicated in this interaction remains to be characterized, despite the fact that different regions of Tat have been implicated in interaction with various receptors: the N-terminal region with CD26 receptor (Gutheil, Subramanyam et al. 1994), the tripeptide RGD with integrins $\alpha_v\beta_3$ and $\alpha_5\beta_1$ of DC, and the basic region with membrane lipids and the VEGFR of endothelial cells (Rubartelli, Poggi et al. 1998). Other reports, demonstrated the interaction of the cysteine rich region of Tat 24-51 with CCR2, CCR3 and CCR5 chemokine receptors and the heparan sulfate proteoglycans (Johri, Mishra et al. 2010; Ensoli, Buonaguro et al. 1993). It has been proposed that Tat could interact with the coreceptor CXCR4 and thus competitively inhibit infection by X4-tropic HIV-1 strains (Xiao, Neuveut et al. 2000). In this way, Tat contributes to immune system disorders as it induces apoptosis of T-lymphocytes, inhibits MHC class I expression, alters cell activity by blocking L-type channels (Li, Li et al. 2009).

Using chemical inhibitors and molecular analysis, we showed that Tat-cell interaction lead to activation of different signaling pathways including PKC. In fact, the PKC pathway, one of the major pathway involved in the production of cytokines, plays an essential role in this induction. Downstream PKC, activation of MAP kinases and NF-κB pathways by Tat is crucial for Tat induced IL-10 (Bennasser and Bahraoui 2002; Leghmari and Bennasser 2008; Leghmari and Bennasser 2008; Contreras 2008).

2.3 Analysis of the activated signaling pathways

Calcium and PKC pathways are activated following the action of the phospholipase C (PLC). Implication of PLC signaling in the production of IL-10 following Tat activation was evaluated by using U73122, an inhibitor of PLC. In the presence of this inhibitor a strong inhibition, more than 50% of the production of IL-10 by Tat was observed. Thus, the activation of PKC signaling pathways known to induce the expression of cytokine genes was further investigated.

2.3.1 Tat activates PKC pathway

2.3.1.1 The PKC pathway

The PKC belongs to the serine/threonine kinase family. It represents a key element recruited to regulate cell responses to external stimuli. Eleven PKC isoforms have been identified and classified into three groups based on their ability to be activated by Ca^{2+} and DAG (Spitaler and Cantrell 2004). The classical PKC-α,–βI,–βII and -γ, isoforms are activated by Ca^{2+} and DAG, the novel PKC-θ, -η, -δ and -ε, are Ca^{2+} independent but DAG dependent, finally the atypical PKC–ζ, –μ and -λ (also named -α in murine cells) are Ca^{2+} and DAG independent (Lee, Duan et al. 2008) (figure 10). PKC are single polypeptide chains of heterogeneous size, ranging from 67.2 kDa for PKC–τ to 83.5 kDa for, PKC–ε. Each PKC isoform is the product of a separate gene, except for PKC-βI and PKC-βII which are alternative spliced variants of the same gene. At the structural level, PKC contained four conserved domains (C1 to C4) (figure 10) and five variable regions (V1 to V5) that encode isoform-specific properties. The conserved region mediates binding to the activating cofactors: C1 for DAG or to PMA when used as pharmacological tool, and C2 for Ca^{2+}.

2.3.1.2 Effects of HIV-1 Tat on PKC pathway

The implication of PKC pathway in the control of IL-10 production mediated by Tat was analyzed by complementary approaches. Pre-treatment of cells with Ro31-8220, an inhibitor of all PKC isozymes inhibits totally Tat induced IL-10, thus demonstrating the crucial role of PKC pathway. In agreement with the essential role of PKC pathway, Tat becomes unable to stimulate IL-10 production in monocyte previously treated during 48h with PMA. In order to understand the nature of PKC isoforms activated by Tat and essential for IL-10 production, monocytes isolated from healthy donors were cultured in the presence of Tat at 10 or 100nM and cytoplasmic and membrane proteins were isolated after 30 min or after 1 or 2 hours. Whereas PKC is localized in the cytoplasm in unstimulated human monocytes, Tat stimulation induces in a dose dependent manner, PKC translocation to the membrane indicating PKC activation. This activation observed after 30min of Tat stimulation reaches a peak in 1h and decreases after 2 hours of stimulation. Thus HIV-1 Tat induces PKC activation in a dose and time dependent manner in human monocytes. To investigate the involvement of PKC activation in Tat-induced IL-10 production, monocytes were incubated with different PKC inhibitors. Ro318220 as well as Gö6983 which inhibits several PKC isoforms including PKC–α, –β (IC50= 7 nM), PKC-γ (IC50 = 6 nM), PKC-δ (IC50 = 10 nM), PKC-ζ (IC50= 60 nM) and PKC-μ (IC50 = 20 μM) totally inhibit IL-10 production (Bennasser and Bahraoui 2002; Leghmari and Bennasser 2008; Contreras 2008). Gö6976 which inhibits classical PKC isoforms -α and -βI has no effect on the capacity of Tat to induce IL-10 production by monocytes. Altogether, these results suggest that PKC isoforms -α, -βI and –μ are not primarily involved in the signaling pathways implicated in IL-10 production. To evaluate the implication of PKC-βII and δ two other inhibitors were used. Hispidin, PKC-βI and βII inhibitor (IC50 = 20 μM), and rottlerin, an inhibitor of PKC-δ (IC50 = 3-6 μM). Hispidin used at 2-20 μM inhibits IL-10 production by Tat in a dose dependent manner, an inhibition of 60% is reached in the presence of 20 μM of Hispidin. The implication of PKC-δ in IL-10 production was further evaluated by using rottlerin 5-30 μM. In these conditions an inhibition reaching 90% was observed. Interestingly, PKC-βII and PKC–δ inhibitors used separately at 2 and 5 μM inhibited IL-10 production induced by Tat by 15 and 45% respectively, but when used in combination, they inhibited IL-10 production by 85% thus suggesting a possible synergistic effect between these two PKC isoforms (Bennasser and Bahraoui 2002).

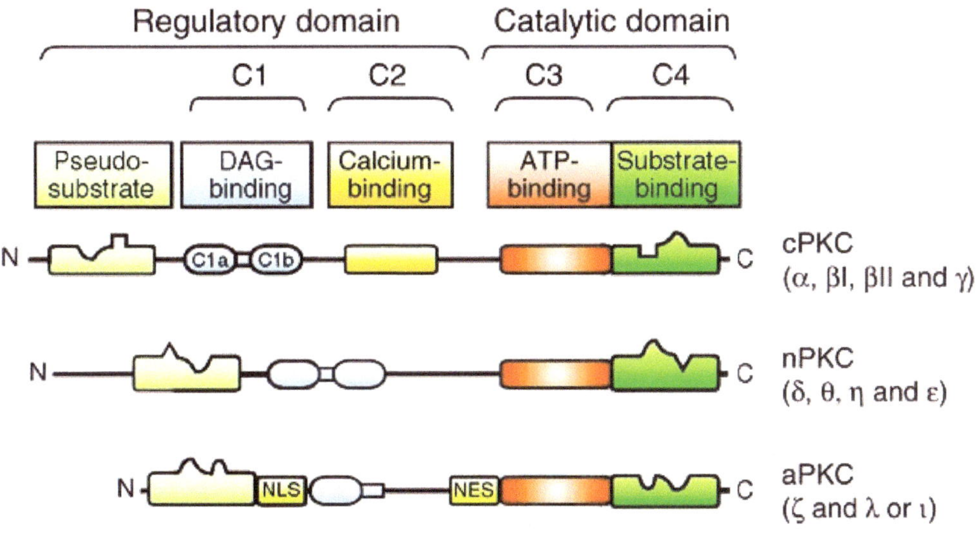

The three subgroups of PKC have been identified and their regulatory domains identified. The classical PKC isoforms (cPKC) share all typical regulatory features: the autoinhibitory pseudosubstrate motif, two DAG-binding C1 domains (C1a and C1b) and the calcium-binding C2 domain. Novel PKC isoforms (nPKC) lack a calcium-binding motif but contain an extended N-ter domain that can receive regulatory signals. They are regulated by DAG. The catalytic activity of atypical PKC isoforms (aPKC) is independent of DAG and calcium, and they seem to be regulated by regulatory proteins in association with the nuclear localization signal (NLS) and nuclear export signal (NES) in their regulatory domain

Fig. 10. Primary structure and identification of the different PKC family and their functional domains adapted from Spitaler et Cantrell 2004.

After ligand-receptor interaction on the cell surface, phospolipids are hydrolyzed by PLC, producing DAG and IP3 both acting as second messengers. Subsequently, DAG activates PKC, which in turn phosphorylates a range of cellular proteins. More precisely activation of PKC is mediated by phospatidylserine (PS) binding domain that includes C2, the basic pseudosubstrate peptide, and the cysteine rich region that contributes to the increased affinity of PKC to PS by interacting with DAG. These PS binding domains have also been reported to be involved in affinity, PKC localization, membrane translocation and binding to potential receptors. In resting cells, PKC is localized in the cytoplasm in an inactive form where the pseudosubstrate sequence upstream from C1 binds to the catalytic domain, but cannot be phosphorylated since it lacks a phospho-receptor amino acid. Upon activation, Ca^{2+} and or phosphoinositides induce a conformational change leading to the release of the pseudosubstrate. Thus the catalytic site becomes accessible to anchoring proteins called RACK (receptor for activated kinase) or substrates STICK (substrate that interacts with C-kinase). This PKC activation is accompanied by a translocation from the cytoplasm to the membrane. Subsequent to membrane translocation and PKC activation, a second messenger seems to be stimulated and leads to the phosphorylation of PKC binding proteins thus, reducing their affinity for PKC and PS.

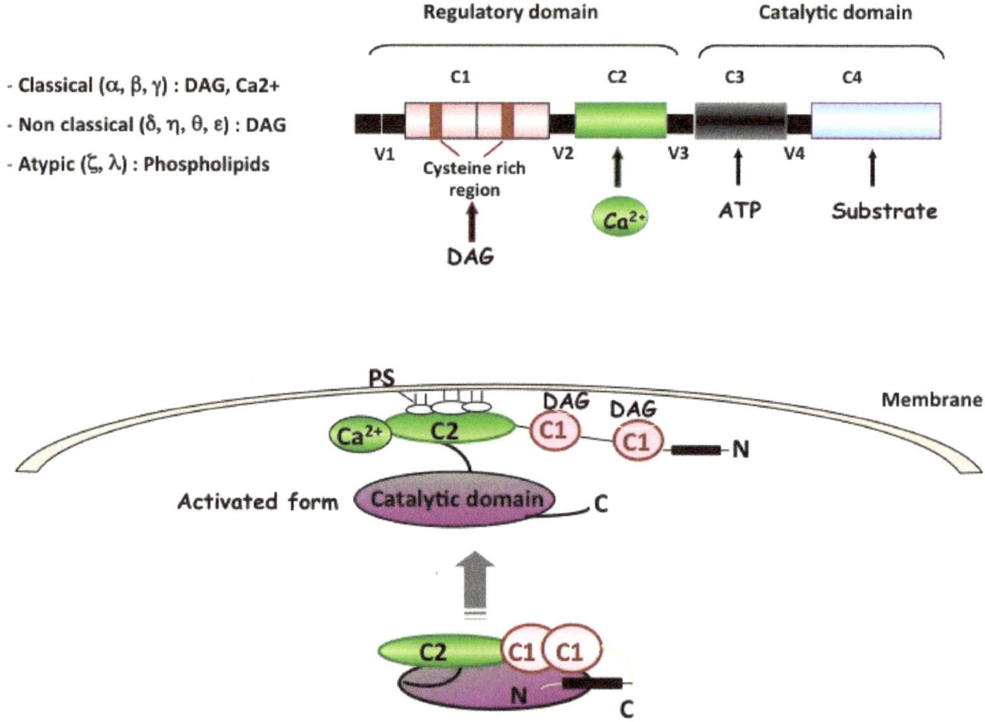

In the cytoplasm, PKC is present as an inactive form. After its activation by phosphorylation, it undergoes conformational modifications leading to its translocation from the cytoplasmic to the membrane compartment. In membrane compartment, PKC associates with a second messenger DAG (and in the case of classical PKC isoforms, calcium) produced after receptor stimulation. Binding to the second messengers is also required for the release of the pseudosubstrate motif from the active site to give an active enzyme.

Fig. 11. Activation of PKC pathway

We next investigated which isoforms of PKC are activated by Tat protein. Monocytes were incubated with Tat at 10 nM for 15, 30 min or 1 hour and PKC localization was analyzed by western blot using specific antibodies. Results showed that as soon as 15 min Tat induces translocation to the membrane of four PKC isoforms: PKC-α, PKC-βII, PKC-δ, and PKC-ε. To further analyze the implicated PKC isoforms in Tat induced IL-10 production, these PKC isoforms activated by Tat were targeted with isoform specific antisense oligonucleotides. Monocytes were pre-incubated during 24 hours with PKC-α, PKC-βII, PKC-δ, and PKC-ε or with the corresponding sense sequences as negative controls. After 24h monocytes were stimulated during 1h by Tat at 10 nM and then the level of each isoform in the cytoplasmic and membrane compartments were determined by western blot (Bennasser and Bahraoui 2002). Treatment with 5 μM of PKC-α antisense oligonucleotide down regulates PKC-α expression and the use of 15 μM oligonucleotide totally inhibits PKC-α expression. The use of antisense PKC-α inhibits specifically PKC-α, since PKC-βII is still detected in the same monocytes and is activated by Tat at 10 nM (figure 12). The same specificity of inhibition

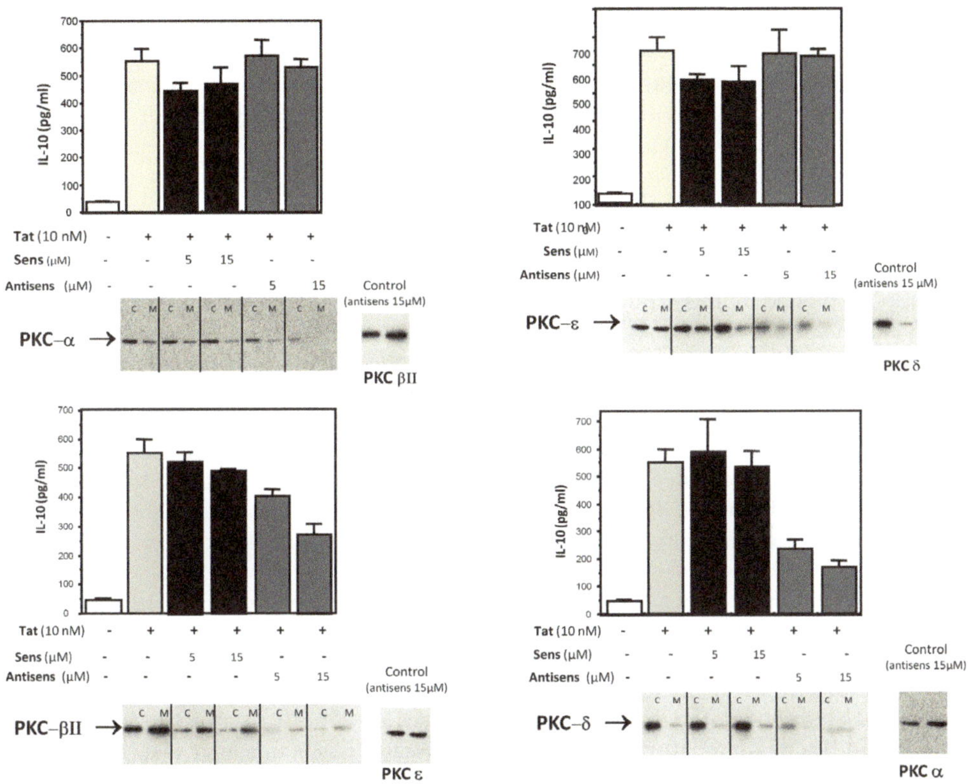

Monocytes were treated with sense or antisense oligonucleotides (5, 15 μM) specific for PKC-α, PKC-βII, PKC-δ, PKC-ε. After washing, cells were stimulated with HIV-1 Tat protein at 10 nM for 1 hour. Isoform specific PKC inhibition was assessed by western blot (bottom). IL-10 production was measured by ELISA 24h later (Sirianni, Vincenzi et al. 1998). In each case, specific inhibition of each isoform was verified by visualizing in the same cell extracts another PKC isoform activation by Tat.

Fig. 12. Effects of isoform specific PKC inhibition with antisense oligonucleotides on Tat induced IL-10 production.

was observed with the other isoforms: PKC-βII, δ, and ε antisense oligonucleotides caused a specific down regulation in the level of their corresponding isoforms (figure 12). In agreement with the data obtained with chemical inhibitors, an inhibition of Tat induced IL-10 was observed in the presence of antisense oligonucleotides directed against PKC-βII and δ. In contrast no significant inhibition was observed with antisense oligonucleotides directed against PKC-α and -ε (figure 12) (Bennasser and Bahraoui 2002).
Overall, it was shown that HIV-1 Tat, activates four PKC isoforms in human monocytes: PKC-α, PKC-βII, PKC-δ, and PKC-ε. These data introduce a way to explore the role of PKC in signaling pathways in Tat activated monocytes and on search for the partners of PKC-βII and δ involved in the production of IL-10, an immunosuppressive cytokine that participates in the deregulation of the immune system as early as the asymptomatic stage of HIV-1 infection.
Monocytes were treated with sense or antisense oligonucleotides (5, 15 μM) specific for PKC-α, PKC-βII, PKC-δ, PKC-ε. After washing, cells were stimulated with HIV-1 Tat protein at 10 nM for 1 hour. Isoform specific PKC inhibition was assessed by western blot (bottom). IL-10 production was measured by ELISA 24h later (Sirianni, Vincenzi et al. 1998). In each case, specific inhibition of each isoform was verified by visualizing in the same cell extracts another PKC isoform activation by Tat.

2.3.2 Tat activate NF-κB pathway

In this part, we will describe the NF-κB signaling pathways implicated in the IL-10 production induced by Tat protein in the human monocytes, and the mechanism of NF-κB regulation exploited by this viral protein.
NF-κB is a major transcriptional regulator for the expression of cytokines that are involved in the control of the immune and inflammatory response (Baeuerle and Baltimore 1996; Baldwin 1996). NF-κB is a dimeric transcription factor that consists of REL family members, including RelA/p65, c-Rel, RelB, p50 and p52 (Li and Verma 2002). p50 and p52 are derived from the larger precursors p105 and p100, respectively, through proteolytic processing by the proteasome. All NF-κB proteins contain a highly conserved REL-homology domain (RHD) that is responsible for DNA binding, dimerization, nuclear translocation and interaction with the inhibitory proteins IκB within the cytoplasm. The IκB proteins, bind to NF-κB and block its nuclear import and, thereby, its transcriptional activity. The p105 and p100 precursors also contain the IκB-like repeats that must be degraded to generate the mature p50 and p52 subunits, respectively. In contrast to the other NF-κB family members, p50 lacks a transactivation domain and therefore, usually forms heterodimers with p65 to bind to NF-κB sites in the nucleus. Homodimers p50:p50 can also be formed but they act as a suppressor of inflammatory cytokine gene expression (Ghosh, May et al. 1998). Three distinct NF-κB activating pathways have emerged (Viatour, Merville et al. 2005) (figure 13).
Most of our knowledge concerns the "canonical" pathway, which mostly targets ubiquitous heterodimers p65:p50 and p50:c-Rel. The critical event in initiating this pathway is activation of an IκB-phosphorylating protein kinase, IKKβ/IKK2, which occurs within the "IKK signalosome", in association with a structurally homologous kinase, IKKα/IKK1, and an adaptor protein, IKKγ/NEMO (Yamaoka, Courtois et al. 1998). IKKβ-mediated phosphorylation of IκBα and leads to its proteasomal degradation and, hence, activation of its associated NF-κB dimers that translocate in the nucleus. This pathway is normally triggered in response to microbial and viral infections or exposure to pro-inflammatory

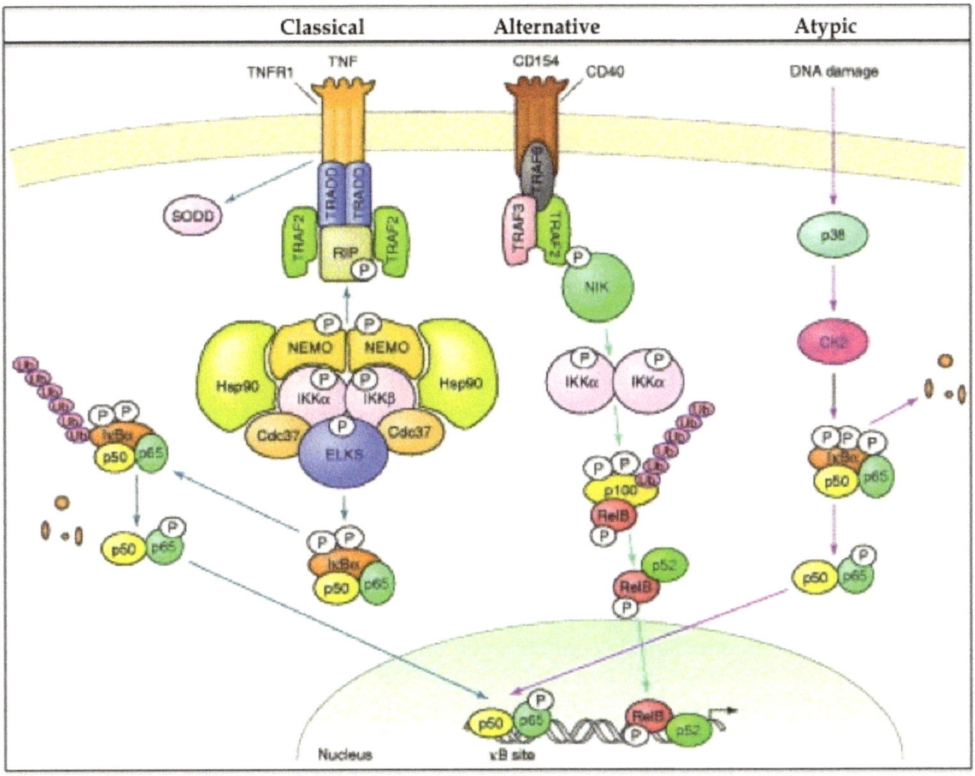

The classical, alternative and atypical NF-κB-activating pathways as illustrated by the TNF-α-mediated, CD40-mediated and DNA-damage-mediated NF-κB activation pathways, respectively. In the classical NF-κB-activating pathway, upon binding of TNF-α to TNFR1, SODD is released from the receptor and triggers the sequential recruitment of the adaptors TRADD, RIP and TRAF2 to the membrane. Then, TRAF2 mediates the recruitment of the IKK complex composed of IKKα, IKKβ and NEMO. Hsp90 and Cdc37 are also part of the IKK complex and are required for- IKK activation. Activation of the IKK complex leads to the phosphorylation of IκBα at specific residues, ubiquitination and its degradation via the proteasome pathway. Then, the heterodimer p50–p65 is released and migrates to the nucleus where it binds to specific κB sites and activates a variety of NF-κB target genes. The alternative pathway is triggered by binding of the CD40 ligand to its receptor, leading to recruitment of TRAF proteins and the sequential activation of NIK and IKKα, which induces the processing of the inhibitory protein p100. p100 proteolysis releases p52 which forms heterodimers with RelB. This pathway is NEMO-independent and relies on IKKα homodimers. The atypical pathway, which is triggered by DNA damage relies on sequential p38 and CK2 activations, and involves phosphorylation and degradation of subsequent IκBα via an IKK-independent pathway. Abbreviations: CK2, casein kinase 2; ELKS, Glu-Leu-Lys-Ser; Hsp90, heat shock protein 90; IκB, inhibitor of NF-κB; IKK, IκB kinase; NEMO, NF-κB essential modulator; NF-κB, nuclear factor-κB; NIK, NF-κB-inducing kinase; RIP, receptor-interacting protein; RSK1, ribosomal S6 kinase 1; SODD, silencer of death domains; TNF-α, tumour necrosis factor α; TNFR1, TNF receptor 1; TRADD, TNF-receptor-associated death domain protein; TRAF, TNF-receptor-associated factor; Ub, ubiquitin.

Fig. 13. Three pathways of NF-κB modified by Viatour & al. 2005.

cytokines such as tumour necrosis factor TNF–α. By contrast, the "alternative" pathway, occurs independently of IKKβ or NEMO, but is dependent on NF-κB -inducing kinase and IKKα. Activation of this pathway leads to a limited proteasomal processing of the NF-κB precursor protein, allowing the resulting p52 fragment to translocate to the nucleus in association with some NF-κB proteins (mainly RelB) (Xiao, Harhaj et al. 2001). This pathway is triggered by cytokines such as lymphotoxin B (Dejardin, Droin et al. 2002), or CD40 ligand (Coope, Atkinson et al. 2002), and by viruses such as the Epstein-Barr virus (Eliopoulos, Caamano et al. 2003). The third signaling pathway is classified as "atypical" because it is independent of IKK proteins but it still requires the proteasome and is triggered by DNA damage such as UV oxidative stress (Imbert, Rupec et al. 1996; Tergaonkar, Bottero et al. 2003). However, recent data suggest another role for IKKα in NF-κB dependent gene expression in response to cytokine treatment (Anest, Hanson et al. 2003; Yamamoto, Verma et al. 2003). Independently of its previously described cytoplasmic role, IKKα functions in the nucleus by activating the expression of NF-κB-responsive genes after TNF-α stimulation. IKKα recruited to NF-κB-responsive promoters, interacts with the histone acetyltransferase CBP/p300 (CREB-binding protein). Then it mediates phosphorylation and subsequent acetylation of specific residues of histone H3 leading to the NF-κB binding sites accessibility. In inactivated cells, NF-κB is sequestreted in the cytoplasm by the inhibitory protein IκB, which masks its nuclear localization sequence. In order to be active, NF-κB. The involvement of NF-κB was first tested by the capacity of Tat to activate the nuclear translocation of this factor by using the mobility shift technic assay. These experiments were performed with an oligonucleotide containing an NF-κB site and showed the formation of a complex with nuclear extracts of monocytes stimulated with Tat (figure 14). The observed interaction between NF-κB and the probe seems to be specific, since no complex was observed when the protein extract was incubated in the same conditions with the mutated NF-κB site (Badou and Bennasser 2000).

In agreement with the inability of this mutant to stimulate the production of IL-10, no complex was detected in these conditions. These results showed that Tat induces NF-κB activation specifically in monocytes. Then the region of Tat involved in NF-κB activation was investigated by stimulating monocytes with different GST-Tat deleted mutants. EMSA analysis showed that only, the C-terminally deleted mutants GST-Tat 1-72 and GST-Tat 1-45 activate NF-κB as the wild type GST-Tat 1-101. In contrast, no activation was observed with GST-Tat 30-72 or GST alone (figure 14). These results showed that NF-κB activation correlates with the ability of Tat and Tat mutant to mediate IL-10 production. In addition the role of NF-κB activation in the production of IL-10 was evaluated. Monocytes were treated with non toxic doses of TLCK (an inhibitor of NF-κB pathways), and then stimulated with Tat at 10 nM. Then, NF-κB activation and IL-10 production were analyzed by EMSA and ELISA respectively. In this conditions no NF-κB activation nor IL-10 production were obtained. Thus, Tat activates transcriptional factor NF-κB, one of the substrates of PKC, thereby causing induction of IL-10 gene.

Three distinct NF-κB activating pathways have emerged. Interestingly by using the same approache we showed that Tat protein is also able to stimulate the nuclear translocation of p52 in addition of p65 (figure 15). This results suggest that Tat protein activates both classical and alternative NF-κB pathways, while TNF-α activates only the classical pathway.

The critical event in initiating this pathway is activation of an IκB-phosphorylating protein kinase, IKKβ/IKK2, which occurs within the "IKK signalosome", in association with a structurally homologous kinase, IKKα/IKK1, and an adaptor protein, IKKγ/NEMO (Yamaoka, Courtois et al. 1998). IKKβ-mediated phosphorylation of IκBα leads to its proteasomal degradation and, hence, activation of its associated NF-κB dimers that translocate in the nucleus. This pathway is normally triggered in response to microbial and viral infections or exposure to pro-inflammatory cytokines such as tumour necrosis factor TNF-α. By contrast, the "alternative" pathway, occurs independently of IKKβ or NEMO, but is dependent on NF-κB inducing kinase and IKKα. Activation of this pathway leads to a limited proteasomal processing of the NF-κB 2/p100 precursor protein, allowing the resulting p52 fragment to translocate to the nucleus in association with some NF-κB proteins (mainly RelB).

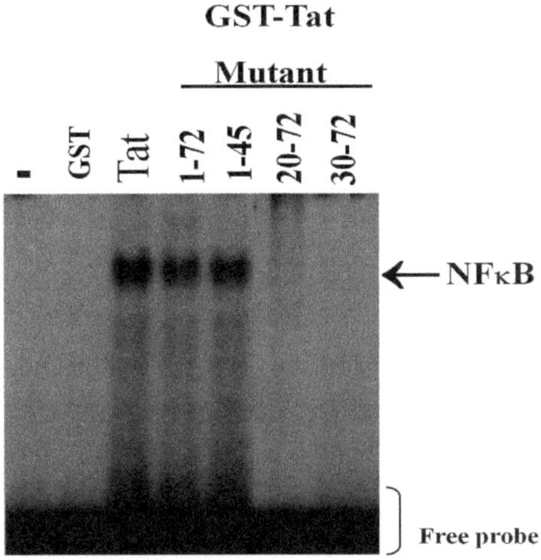

Nuclear protein extracts of human monocytes treated with wild type GST-Tat 1-101 or Tat deleted mutants or negatif control GST at 10 nM for 16 h were incubated with a 32P-labeled NF-κB probe sequence containing the wild type NF-□B site. To verify that NF-κB activation was specifically mediated by Tat, monocytes were treated with chemically mutated Tat (oxidized Tat), and nuclear extracts were analyzed by EMSA.

Fig. 14. Activation of NF-κB by HIV-1 Tat 1-45 in human monocytes.

The analysis of signaling pathways allowed to demonstarte the crucial role of NF-κB transctivation factor as showed by the capacity of Tat to activate the nuclear translocation of the transcription factor NF-κB which is shown to be required for the IL-10 production (Badou and Bennasser 2000). At the light of the known mechanisms of NF-κB activation pathways, the molecular mechanisms recruited by Tat to activate NF-κB was further investigated. To this end, and in order to use transfection approach, we have developed and validated the U937 promonocytic cells as model, in addition to primary human monocytes.
Treated in the same conditions as primary human monocytes, U937 monocytic cells produced IL-10 (Leghmari and Bennasser 2008; Contreras 2008). U937 promonocytic cells previously cotransfected with a NF-κB reporter plasmid, pNF-κBLuc, expressing the luciferase gene under the control of four NF-κB sites and the pCMV-βGal, expressing the β-galactosidase gene under the control of the CMV promoter were treated by different concentrations of Tat.The obtained results showed that Tat protein is able to activate NF-κB

in a dose dependent manner. In agreement with the data obtained in primary human monocytic cells, only, the totally Tat protein or its N-terminal fragment Tat 1-45 are able to activate NF-κB. In contrast no activation was observed with Tat 30-72 or with GST alone (Figure 13, 14).

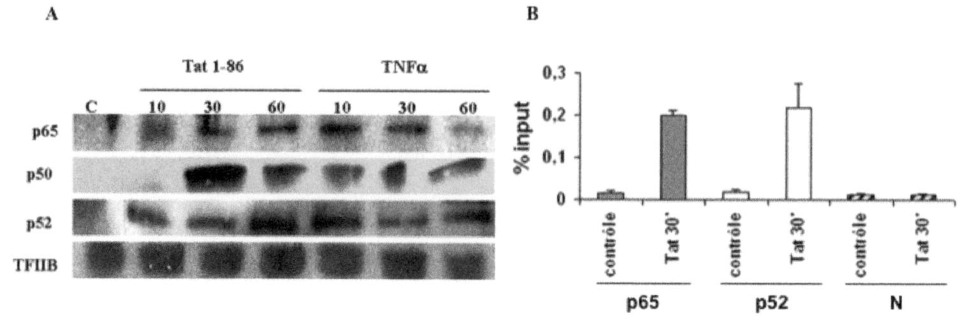

Tat induces recruitment of p65 and p52 to the IL-10 promoter. (A) Primary monocytes (107 cells) were stimulated or not with Tat 1-86 (10 nM) or TNF-α (20 ng/ml). Nuclear extracts were prepared and analyzed by Western blot. Anti-TFIIB was used as a loading control. (B) Monocytes were treated or not with 10nM Tat 1-86 for 30 min, and ChIP assays were performed with anti-p65, anti-p52 or without (N) antibodies. The proportion of co-immunoprecipitated IL-10 promoter was analyzed by quantitative realtime PCR.

Fig. 15. Tat activates classical and alternative NF-κB pathways.

Using negative transdominant mutants of NIK, IKKα and IKKβ, we showed that their expression inhibit strongly NF-κB activation induced by Tat. Interestingly when both IKKα and IKKβ are inhibited simultaneously by their corresponding negative transdominants, NF-κB activation was totally inhibited. In summury our data indicate that Tat induced NF-κB activation requires NIK, IKKα and IKKβ kinases.

To adress the question whether Tat was also able to induce nuclear translocation of IKKα, nuclear extracts from Tat treated cells was analysed by SDS-PAGE and western blot using antibodies specific to IKKα. This analysis clearly showed that Tat protein is able to stimulate IKKα translocation from the cytoplasm to the nucleus. This activation is also obtained with wild type Tat protein and its N-terminal fragment but not with Tat 30-72. However, recent data suggest another role for IKKα in NF-κB dependent gene expression in response to cytokine treatment. Independently of its previously described cytoplasmic role, IKKα functions in the nucleus by activating the expression of NF-kB-responsive genes after TNF-α stimulation. IKKα recruited to NF-κB-responsive promoters, interacts with the histone acetyltransferase CBP/p300 (CREB-binding protein). Then it mediates phosphorylation and subsequent acetylation of specific residues of histone H3 leading to the NF-κB binding sites accessibility.

In summury, Tat protein secreted by infected cells will be taken up by neighboring cells to activate HIV-1 replication in HIV-1 infected latent cells, and also to activate non infected cells to produce different chemokines and cytokines including IL-10 a highly immunosuppressive cytokine greatly implicated in the dysregulation of the immune system in HIV-1 infected patients. The analysis of the signaling pathway activated by Tat underlined the crucial role of PKC and NF-κB pathways.

3. Conclusion

HIV-1 infection hijacks the cellular machinery and uses cellular signaling pathways to its own advantage. Early secreted Tat protein, as gp120 via its interaction with CD4 receptor and CCR5 coreceptor, trigger a signaling cascade which activates calcium and protein kinase C pathways (Contreras 2008; Sieczkarski S et al. 2003). All these signaling pathways regulate cell activation by acting on the state of cell differentiation, transcription activation, cell survival or cytoskeleton dynamics which are required for viral replication (Lamph et al 1988; Burnette et al 1993; Llewellyn et al 2006).

Among the activated pathways, PKC pathway plays a critical role for HIV-1 replication. Indeed, PKCs stimulate NF-κB (Meichle et al 1990; Junttila et al. 2003; Taunton et al. 2001) via the phosphorylation of IκB. NF-κB binds to the HIV promoter and is involved in initiation and elongation of transcription. In addition, PKCs activate other transcription factors like AP-1 and NF-AT, which have specific binding sites on the HIV-1 promoter. Thus, activation of PKCs can reverse HIV-1 latency in infected T cells and in cell lines (Guy et al. 1987). Moreover, PKCs have been suggested to phosphorylate a number of viral proteins such as p17 Gag (Yang et al. 1999), Nef (Popik et al. 1998; Ghosh et al. 1990; Hamamoto et al. 1990) and Rev (Fantuzzi et al. 2000). The PKC pathway is also critical for the step of entry of a number of enveloped viruses like rhabdoviruses, alphaviruses and herpesviruses (Yang et al 1999) and for type 2 adenovirus (Owen et al. 1996). Thus, the understanding of the signaling pathways implicated in the stimulation of virus replication or in the production of immunopathogenic cytokines may suggest possible targeted therapeutic approaches to neutralize such key steps.

Taking into account the role of Tat protein in viral replication and induction of immunological and neurological disorders, this Tat protein represents a potential vaccine candidate (Caputo, Gavioli et al. 2009). Tat protein appears to be an effective candidate to include for an HIV vaccine, since its gene product is produced early during the viral life cycle. Targeting the immune responses against Tat which plays an important role in viral infectivity and pathogenicity could aid in lowering the viral load through the destruction of HIV-1 replicating cells by CTL or antibody dependent cell-cytotoxicity. It is important to underline the critical role of HIV-1 Tat in the dysregulation of the immune system by the the induction of the higly immunosuprressive cytokine: IL-10 (Badou and Bennasser 2000). Interestingly several reports showed that humoral or cellular responses against Tat are associated with the control of HIV-1 infection as showed by the low viral load and the protection against AIDS progression (Wieland et al 1990; Krone et al. 1988; Reiss 1990; Re 1996; Rezza et al. 2005; Zagury et al. 1998). In agreement with these observations the group of Ensoli showed that vaccination of macaque with native Tat protein allowed protection against viral infection and disease development (Cafaro et al. 1999; Maggiorella et al. 2004). However, experiments performed by other groups showed no protection, or only a partial protection in rhesus macaques immunized with native or denatured Tat protein (Allen et al. 2002; Silvera et al. 2002; Goldstein et al. 2000; Pauza et al. 2000). This apparent discrepancy may be related to the nature of animal used cynomolgus versus rhesus and the nature of the virus used for the challenge, SHIV89.6P, SIVmac239 or SHIV33.

It is interesting to note that a therapeutic phase I clinical trial in human, using recombinant Tat protein as vaccine candidate is under investigation by the group of Ensoli.

4. References

Albini, A., R. Benelli, et al. (1996). "HIV-tat protein is a heparin-binding angiogenic growth factor." Oncogene 12(2): 289-97.

Albini, A., R. Soldi, et al. (1996). "The angiogenesis induced by HIV-1 tat protein is mediated by the Flk-1/KDR receptor on vascular endothelial cells." Nat Med 2(12): 1371-5.

Ameglio, F., M. R. Capobianchi, et al. (1994). "Recombinant gp120 induces IL-10 in resting peripheral blood mononuclear cells; correlation with the induction of other cytokines." Clin Exp Immunol 95(3): 455-8.

Anest, V., J. L. Hanson, et al. (2003). "A nucleosomal function for IkappaB kinase-alpha in NF-kappaB-dependent gene expression." Nature 423(6940): 659-63.

Ankel, H., M. R. Capobianchi, et al. (1994). "Interferon induction by HIV glycoprotein 120: role of the V3 loop." Virology 205(1): 34-43.

Aoki, Y. and G. Tosato (2004). "HIV-1 Tat enhances Kaposi sarcoma-associated herpesvirus (KSHV) infectivity." Blood 104(3): 810-4.

Badou, A., Y. Bennasser, et al. (2000). "Tat protein of human immunodeficiency virus type 1 induces interleukin-10 in human peripheral blood monocytes: implication of protein kinase C-dependent pathway." J Virol 74(22): 10551-62.

Baeuerle, P. A. and D. Baltimore (1996). "NF-kappa B: ten years after." Cell 87(1): 13-20.

Baldwin, A. S., Jr. (1996). "The NF-kappa B and I kappa B proteins: new discoveries and insights." Annu Rev Immunol 14: 649-83.

Barre-Sinoussi, F., J. C. Chermann, et al. (1983). "Isolation of a T-lymphotropic retrovirus from a patient at risk for acquired immune deficiency syndrome (AIDS)." Science 220(4599): 868-71.

Bayer, P., M. Kraft, et al. (1995). "Structural studies of HIV-1 Tat protein." J Mol Biol 247(4): 529-35.

Bennasser, Y., A. Badou, et al. (2002). "Signaling pathways triggered by HIV-1 Tat in human monocytes to induce TNF-alpha." Virology 303(1): 174-80.

Bennasser, Y. and E. Bahraoui (2002). "HIV-1 Tat protein induces interleukin-10 in human peripheral blood monocytes: involvement of protein kinase C-betaII and -delta." Faseb J 16(6): 546-54.

Berkhout, B., R. H. Silverman, et al. (1989). "Tat trans-activates the human immunodeficiency virus through a nascent RNA target." Cell 59(2): 273-82.

Bernstein, H. B., S. P. Tucker, et al. (1995). "Oligomerization of the hydrophobic heptad repeat of gp41." J Virol 69(5): 2745-50.

Bezzi, P., G. Carmignoto, et al. (1998). "Prostaglandins stimulate calcium-dependent glutamate release in astrocytes." Nature 391(6664): 281-5.

Bonnet, F., E. Balestre, et al. (2006). "Factors associated with the occurrence of AIDS-related non-Hodgkin lymphoma in the era of highly active antiretroviral therapy: Aquitaine Cohort, France." Clin Infect Dis 42(3): 411-7.

Bour, S., R. Geleziunas, et al. (1995). "The human immunodeficiency virus type 1 (HIV-1) CD4 receptor and its central role in promotion of HIV-1 infection." Microbiol Rev 59(1): 63-93.

Brenchley, J. M., D. A. Price, et al. (2006). "Microbial translocation is a cause of systemic immune activation in chronic HIV infection." Nat Med 12(12): 1365-71.

Brigino, E., S. Haraguchi, et al. (1997). "Interleukin 10 is induced by recombinant HIV-1 Nef protein involving the calcium/calmodulin-dependent phosphodiesterase signal transduction pathway." Proc Natl Acad Sci U S A 94(7): 3178-82.

Burke, B., N. R. Derby, et al. (2006). "Viral evolution in macaques coinfected with CCR5- and CXCR4-tropic SHIVs in the presence or absence of vaccine-elicited anti-CCR5 SHIV neutralizing antibodies." Virology 355(2): 138-151.

Burnette, B., G. Yu, et al. (1993). "Phosphorylation of HIV-1 gag proteins by protein kinase C." J Biol Chem 268(12): 8698-8703.

Cafaro, A., A. Caputo, et al. (1999). "Control of SHIV-89.6P-infection of cynomolgus monkeys by HIV-1 Tat protein vaccine." Nat Med 5(6): 643-650.

Cannell, L. J., J. E. Taunton, et al. (2001). "A randomised clinical trial of the efficacy of drop squats or leg extension/leg curl exercises to treat clinically diagnosed jumper's knee in athletes: pilot study." Br J Sports Med 35(1): 60-64.

Capobianchi, M. R., C. Barresi, et al. (1997). "Human immunodeficiency virus type 1 gp120 stimulates cytomegalovirus replication in monocytes: possible role of endogenous interleukin-8." J Virol 71(2): 1591-7.

Caputo, A., R. Gavioli, et al. (2009). "HIV-1 Tat-based vaccines: an overview and perspectives in the field of HIV/AIDS vaccine development." Int Rev Immunol 28(5): 285-334.

Chambers, P., C. R. Pringle, et al. (1990). "Heptad repeat sequences are located adjacent to hydrophobic regions in several types of virus fusion glycoproteins." J Gen Virol 71 (Pt 12): 3075-80.

Chan, D. C., D. Fass, et al. (1997). "Core structure of gp41 from the HIV envelope glycoprotein." Cell 89(2): 263-73.

Chazal, N. and D. Gerlier (2003). "Virus entry, assembly, budding, and membrane rafts." Microbiol Mol Biol Rev 67(2): 226-37, table of contents.

Clavel, F., D. Guetard, et al. (1986). "Isolation of a new human retrovirus from West African patients with AIDS." Science 233(4761): 343-6.

Clerici, M. and G. M. Shearer (1993). "A TH1-->TH2 switch is a critical step in the etiology of HIV infection." Immunol Today 14(3): 107-11.

Clerici, M., T. A. Wynn, et al. (1994). "Role of interleukin-10 in T helper cell dysfunction in asymptomatic individuals infected with the human immunodeficiency virus." J Clin Invest 93(2): 768-75.

Clifford, K. S. and M. F. Demierre (2005). "Progression of classic Kaposi's sarcoma with rituximab." J Am Acad Dermatol 53(1): 155-7.

Conant, K., A. Garzino-Demo, et al. (1998). "Induction of monocyte chemoattractant protein-1 in HIV-1 Tat-stimulated astrocytes and elevation in AIDS dementia." Proc Natl Acad Sci U S A 95(6): 3117-21.

Connor, R. I., K. E. Sheridan, et al. (1997). "Change in coreceptor use correlates with disease progression in HIV-1--infected individuals." J Exp Med 185(4): 621-8.

Contreras, X., Y. Bennasser, et al. (2005). "Human immunodeficiency virus type 1 Tat protein induces an intracellular calcium increase in human monocytes that requires DHP receptors: involvement in TNF-alpha production." Virology 332(1): 316-28.

Coope, H. J., P. G. Atkinson, et al. (2002). "CD40 regulates the processing of NF-kappaB2 p100 to p52." Embo J 21(20): 5375-85.

Coopman, S. A., R. A. Johnson, et al. (1993). "Cutaneous disease and drug reactions in HIV infection." N Engl J Med 328(23): 1670-4.

Coovadia, H. M., N. C. Rollins, et al. (2007). "Mother-to-child transmission of HIV-1 infection during exclusive breastfeeding in the first 6 months of life: an intervention cohort study." Lancet 369(9567): 1107-16.

Dalgleish, A. G., P. C. Beverley, et al. (1984). "The CD4 (T4) antigen is an essential component of the receptor for the AIDS retrovirus." Nature 312(5996): 763-7.

Dean, M., M. Carrington, et al. (1996). "Genetic restriction of HIV-1 infection and progression to AIDS by a deletion allele of the CKR5 structural gene. Hemophilia Growth and Development Study, Multicenter AIDS Cohort Study, Multicenter Hemophilia Cohort Study, San Francisco City Cohort, ALIVE Study." Science 273(5283): 1856-62.

Dejardin, E., N. M. Droin, et al. (2002). "The lymphotoxin-beta receptor induces different patterns of gene expression via two NF-kappaB pathways." Immunity 17(4): 525-35.

Dragic, T., V. Litwin, et al. (1996). "HIV-1 entry into CD4+ cells is mediated by the chemokine receptor CC-CKR-5." Nature 381(6584): 667-73.

Eliopoulos, A. G., J. H. Caamano, et al. (2003). "Epstein-Barr virus-encoded latent infection membrane protein 1 regulates the processing of p100 NF-kappaB2 to p52 via an IKKgamma/NEMO-independent signaling pathway." Oncogene 22(48): 7557-69.

Emerman, M. and M. H. Malim (1998). "HIV-1 regulatory/accessory genes: keys to unraveling viral and host cell biology." Science 280(5371): 1880-4.

Ensoli, B., L. Buonaguro, et al. (1993). "Release, uptake, and effects of extracellular human immunodeficiency virus type 1 Tat protein on cell growth and viral transactivation." J Virol 67(1): 277-87.

Fantuzzi, L., L. Conti, et al. (2000). "Regulation of chemokine/cytokine network during in vitro differentiation and HIV-1 infection of human monocytes: possible importance in the pathogenesis of AIDS." J Leukoc Biol 68(3): 391-399.

Fauci, A. S. (1988). "The human immunodeficiency virus: infectivity and mechanisms of pathogenesis." Science 239(4840): 617-22.

Fauci, A. S. (1996). "Host factors and the pathogenesis of HIV-induced disease." Nature 384(6609): 529-34.

Fenouillet, E., B. Clerget-Raslain, et al. (1989). "Role of N-linked glycans in the interaction between the envelope glycoprotein of human immunodeficiency virus and its CD4 cellular receptor. Structural enzymatic analysis." J Exp Med 169(3): 807-22.

Foucault, M., K. Mayol, et al. (2010). "UV and X-ray structural studies of a 101-residue long Tat protein from a HIV-1 primary isolate and of its mutated, detoxified, vaccine candidate." Proteins 78(6): 1441-56.

Francis, M. L. and M. S. Meltzer (1993). "Induction of IFN-alpha by HIV-1 in monocyte-enriched PBMC requires gp120-CD4 interaction but not virus replication." J Immunol 151(4): 2208-16.

Furrer, H., M. Opravil, et al. (2001). "Discontinuation of primary prophylaxis in HIV-infected patients at high risk of Pneumocystis carinii pneumonia: prospective multicentre study." Aids 15(4): 501-7.

Futaki, S., T. Suzuki, et al. (2001). "Arginine-rich peptides. An abundant source of membrane-permeable peptides having potential as carriers for intracellular protein delivery." J Biol Chem 276(8): 5836-40.

Ganju, R. K., N. Munshi, et al. (1998). "Human immunodeficiency virus tat modulates the Flk-1/KDR receptor, mitogen-activated protein kinases, and components of focal adhesion in Kaposi's sarcoma cells." J Virol 72(7): 6131-7.

Gao, K., R. J. Gorelick, et al. (2003). "Cofactors for human immunodeficiency virus type 1 cDNA integration in vitro." J Virol 77(2): 1598-603.

Geijtenbeek, T. B., D. S. Kwon, et al. (2000). "DC-SIGN, a dendritic cell-specific HIV-1-binding protein that enhances trans-infection of T cells." Cell 100(5): 587-97.

Geijtenbeek, T. B., R. Torensma, et al. (2000). "Identification of DC-SIGN, a novel dendritic cell-specific ICAM-3 receptor that supports primary immune responses." Cell 100(5): 575-85.

Ghosh, S., M. J. May, et al. (1998). "NF-kappa B and Rel proteins: evolutionarily conserved mediators of immune responses." Annu Rev Immunol 16: 225-60.

Giunta, B., D. Obregon, et al. (2006). "EGCG mitigates neurotoxicity mediated by HIV-1 proteins gp120 and Tat in the presence of IFN-gamma: role of JAK/STAT1 signaling and implications for HIV-associated dementia." Brain Res 1123(1): 216-25.

Graziosi, C., K. R. Gantt, et al. (1996). "Kinetics of cytokine expression during primary human immunodeficiency virus type 1 infection." Proc Natl Acad Sci U S A 93(9): 4386-91.

Gringhuis, S. I., M. van der Vlist, et al. (2010). "HIV-1 exploits innate signaling by TLR8 and DC-SIGN for productive infection of dendritic cells." Nat Immunol 11(5): 419-26.

Grivel, J. C. and L. B. Margolis (1999). "CCR5- and CXCR4-tropic HIV-1 are equally cytopathic for their T-cell targets in human lymphoid tissue." Nat Med 5(3): 344-6.

Gutheil, W. G., M. Subramanyam, et al. (1994). "Human immunodeficiency virus 1 Tat binds to dipeptidyl aminopeptidase IV (CD26): a possible mechanism for Tat's immunosuppressive activity." Proc Natl Acad Sci U S A 91(14): 6594-8.

Guy, B., M. P. Kieny, et al. (1987). "HIV F/3' orf encodes a phosphorylated GTP-binding protein resembling an oncogene product." Nature 330(6145): 266-269.

Hamamoto, Y., T. Matsuyama, et al. (1990). "Augmentation of cytotoxic effect of tumor necrosis factor on human immunodeficiency virus-infected cells by staurosporine, a potent protein kinase C inhibitor." Cancer Res

Harrich, D., J. Garcia, et al. (1989). "Role of SP1-binding domains in in vivo transcriptional regulation of the human immunodeficiency virus type 1 long terminal repeat." J Virol 63(6): 2585-91.

Hatada, E., S. Saito, et al. (1999). "Mutant influenza viruses with a defective NS1 protein cannot block the activation of PKR in infected cells." J Virol 73(3): 2425-33.

Hirsch, V. M., R. A. Olmsted, et al. (1989). "An African primate lentivirus (SIVsm) closely related to HIV-2." Nature 339(6223): 389-92.

Hoglund, S., A. Ohagen, et al. (1994). "Role of vif during packing of the core of HIV-1." Virology 201(2): 349-55.

Huang, Y., W. A. Paxton, et al. (1996). "The role of a mutant CCR5 allele in HIV-1 transmission and disease progression." Nat Med 2(11): 1240-3.

Imbert, V., R. A. Rupec, et al. (1996). "Tyrosine phosphorylation of I kappa B-alpha activates NF-kappa B without proteolytic degradation of I kappa B-alpha." Cell 86(5): 787-98.

Jeang, K. T., H. Xiao, et al. (1999). "Multifaceted activities of the HIV-1 transactivator of transcription, Tat." J Biol Chem 274(41): 28837-40.

Johri, M. K., R. Mishra, et al. (2011). "Tits and bits of HIV Tat protein." Expert Opin Biol Ther 11(3): 269-83.

Junttila, I., R. P. Bourette, et al. (2003). "M-CSF induced differentiation of myeloid precursor cells involves activation of PKC-delta and expression of Pkare." J Leukoc Biol 73(2): 281-288.

Kilby, J. M., S. Hopkins, et al. (1998). "Potent suppression of HIV-1 replication in humans by T-20, a peptide inhibitor of gp41-mediated virus entry." Nat Med 4(11): 1302-7.

Kozak, S. L., J. M. Heard, et al. (2002). "Segregation of CD4 and CXCR4 into distinct lipid microdomains in T lymphocytes suggests a mechanism for membrane destabilization by human immunodeficiency virus." J Virol 76(4): 1802-15.

Kozak, S. L., E. J. Platt, et al. (1997). "CD4, CXCR-4, and CCR-5 dependencies for infections by primary patient and laboratory-adapted isolates of human immunodeficiency virus type 1." J Virol 71(2): 873-82.

Kromdijk, W., A. D. Huitema, et al. (2010) "Treatment of HIV infection with the CCR5 antagonist maraviroc." Expert Opin Pharmacother 11(7): 1215-23.

Krone, W. J., C. Debouck, et al. (1988). "Natural antibodies to HIV-tat epitopes and expression of HIV-1 genes in vivo." J Med Virol 26(3): 261-270.

Kronke, M., S. Schutze, et al. (1990). "Tumour necrosis factor signal transduction." Cell Signal 2(1): 1-8.

Kutsch, O., J. Oh, et al. (2000). "Induction of the chemokines interleukin-8 and IP-10 by human immunodeficiency virus type 1 tat in astrocytes." J Virol 74(19): 9214-21.

Kwon, D. S., G. Gregorio, et al. (2002). "DC-SIGN-mediated internalization of HIV is required for trans-enhancement of T cell infection." Immunity 16(1): 135-44.

Lee, M. R., W. Duan, et al. (2008). "Protein kinase C isozymes as potential therapeutic targets in immune disorders." Expert Opin Ther Targets 12(5): 535-52.

Lamph, W. W., P. Wamsley, et al. (1988). "Induction of proto-oncogene JUN/AP-1 by serum and TPA." Nature 334(6183): 629-631.

Leghmari, K., Y. Bennasser, et al. (2008). "HIV-1 Tat protein induces IL-10 production in monocytes by classical and alternative NF-kappaB pathways." Eur J Cell Biol 87(12): 947-62.

Leghmari, K., Y. Bennasser, et al. (2008). "HIV-1 Tat protein induces IL-10 production by an alternative TNF-alpha-independent pathway in monocytes: role of PKC-delta and p38 MAP kinase." Cell Immunol 253(1-2): 45-53.

Leghmari, K., X. Contreras, et al. (2008). "HIV-1 Tat protein induces TNF-alpha and IL-10 production by human macrophages: differential implication of PKC-betaII and -delta isozymes and MAP kinases ERK1/2 and p38." Cell Immunol 254(1): 46-55.

Li, Q. and I. M. Verma (2002). "NF-kappaB regulation in the immune system." Nat Rev Immunol 2(10): 725-34.

Li, W., G. Li, et al. (2009). "Role of Tat protein in HIV neuropathogenesis." Neurotox Res 16(3): 205-20.

Lipton, S. A. and H. E. Gendelman (1995). "Seminars in medicine of the Beth Israel Hospital, Boston. Dementia associated with the acquired immunodeficiency syndrome." N Engl J Med 332(14): 934-40.

Liu, R., W. A. Paxton, et al. (1996). "Homozygous defect in HIV-1 coreceptor accounts for resistance of some multiply-exposed individuals to HIV-1 infection." Cell 86(3): 367-77.

Llewellyn, N., R. Zioni, et al. (2006). "Continued evolution of HIV-1 circulating in blood monocytes with antiretroviral therapy: genetic analysis of HIV-1 in monocytes and CD4+ T cells of patients with discontinued therapy." J Leukoc Biol 80(5): 1118-1126.

Maddon, P. J., A. G. Dalgleish, et al. (1986). "The T4 gene encodes the AIDS virus receptor and is expressed in the immune system and the brain." Cell 47(3): 333-48.

Maggiorella, M. T., S. Baroncelli, et al. (2004). "Long-term protection against SHIV89.6P replication in HIV-1 Tat vaccinated cynomolgus monkeys." Vaccine 22(25-26): 3258-3269.

Markowitz, M., H. Mohri, et al. (2005). "Infection with multidrug resistant, dual-tropic HIV-1 and rapid progression to AIDS: a case report." Lancet 365(9464): 1031-8.

Martinson, J. A., C. J. Montoya, et al. (2010) "Chloroquine modulates HIV-1-induced plasmacytoid dendritic cell alpha interferon: implication for T-cell activation." Antimicrob Agents Chemother 54(2): 871-81.

McCutchan, F. E. (2000). "Understanding the genetic diversity of HIV-1." Aids 14 Suppl 3: S31-44.

McMichael, A. J., P. Borrow, et al. "The immune response during acute HIV-1 infection: clues for vaccine development." Nat Rev Immunol 10(1): 11-23.

Medina, I., S. Ghose, et al. (1999). "Mobilization of intracellular calcium stores participates in the rise of [Ca2+]i and the toxic actions of the HIV coat protein GP120." Eur J Neurosci 11(4): 1167-78.

Meichle, A., S. Schutze, et al. (1990). "Protein kinase C-independent activation of nuclear factor kappa B by tumor necrosis factor." J Biol Chem 265(14): 8339-8343.

Moore, K. W., A. O'Garra, et al. (1993). "Interleukin-10." Annu Rev Immunol 11: 165-90.

Nath, A., N. J. Haughey, et al. (2000). "Synergistic neurotoxicity by human immunodeficiency virus proteins Tat and gp120: protection by memantine." Ann Neurol 47(2): 186-94.

Nixon, D. E. and A. L. Landay (2010). "Biomarkers of immune dysfunction in HIV." Curr Opin HIV AIDS 5(6): 498-503.

Owen, P. J., G. D. Johnson, et al. (1996). "Protein kinase C-delta associates with vimentin intermediate filaments in differentiated HL60 cells." Exp Cell Res 225(2): 366-373.

Ozdener, H. (2005). "Molecular mechanisms of HIV-1 associated neurodegeneration." J Biosci 30(3): 391-405.

Patella, V., G. Florio, et al. (2000). "HIV-1 gp120 induces IL-4 and IL-13 release from human Fc epsilon RI+ cells through interaction with the VH3 region of IgE." J Immunol 164(2): 589-95.

Pauza, C. D., P. Trivedi, et al. (2000). "Vaccination with tat toxoid attenuates disease in simian/HIV-challenged macaques." Proc Natl Acad Sci U S A 97(7): 3515-3519.

Peeters, M. and P. M. Sharp (2000). "Genetic diversity of HIV-1: the moving target." Aids 14 Suppl 3: S129-40.

Perry, C. M. "Maraviroc: a review of its use in the management of CCR5-tropic HIV-1 infection." Drugs 70(9): 1189-213.

Peterlin, B. M. and D. H. Price (2006). "Controlling the elongation phase of transcription with P-TEFb." Mol Cell 23(3): 297-305.

Peterlin, B. M. and D. Trono (2003). "Hide, shield and strike back: how HIV-infected cells avoid immune eradication." Nat Rev Immunol 3(2): 97-107.

Piot, P., R. G. Feachem, et al. (2004). "Public health. A global response to AIDS: lessons learned, next steps." Science 304(5679): 1909-10.

Platt, E. J., K. Wehrly, et al. (1998). "Effects of CCR5 and CD4 cell surface concentrations on infections by macrophagetropic isolates of human immunodeficiency virus type 1." J Virol 72(4): 2855-64.

Popik, W., J. E. Hesselgesser, et al. (1998). "Binding of human immunodeficiency virus type 1 to CD4 and CXCR4 receptors differentially regulates expression of inflammatory genes and activates the MEK/ERK signaling pathway." J Virol 72(8): 6406-6413.

Pyakurel, P., F. Pak, et al. (2007). "KSHV/HHV-8 and HIV infection in Kaposi's sarcoma development." Infect Agent Cancer 2: 4.

Quinn, T. C. (1997). "Acute primary HIV infection." Jama 278(1): 58-62.

Rayne, F., S. Debaisieux, et al. (2010). "Phosphatidylinositol-(4,5)-bisphosphate enables efficient secretion of HIV-1 Tat by infected T-cells." Embo J 29(8): 1348-62.

Re, M. C., G. Furlini, et al. (1996). "Antibody against human immunodeficiency virus type 1 (HIV-1) Tat protein may have influenced the progression of AIDS in HIV-1-infected hemophiliac patients." Clin Diagn Lab Immunol 3(2): 230-232.

Reiss, P., J. M. Lange, et al. (1990). "Speed of progression to AIDS and degree of antibody response to accessory gene products of HIV-1." J Med Virol 30(3): 163-168.

Rezza, G., V. Fiorelli, et al. (2005). "The presence of anti-Tat antibodies is predictive of long-term nonprogression to AIDS or severe immunodeficiency: findings in a cohort of HIV-1 seroconverters." J Infect Dis 191(8): 1321-1324.

Rhodes, R. E., A. D. Martin, et al. (2001). "Temporal relationships of self-efficacy and social support as predictors of adherence in a 6-month strength-training program for older women." Percept Mot Skills 93(3): 693-703.

Rinaldo, C. R., Jr., J. A. Armstrong, et al. (1990). "Relation of alpha and gamma interferon levels to development of AIDS in homosexual men." J Exp Pathol 5(3): 127-32.

Robinson, J. M., J. L. Cook, et al. (2001). "The VISA-A questionnaire: a valid and reliable index of the clinical severity of Achilles tendinopathy." Br J Sports Med 35(5): 335-341.

Rubartelli, A., A. Poggi, et al. (1998). "HIV-I Tat: a polypeptide for all seasons." Immunol Today 19(12): 543-5.

Sabatier, J. M., B. Clerget-Raslain, et al. (1989). "Use of synthetic peptides for the detection of antibodies against the nef regulating protein in sera of HIV-infected patients." Aids 3(4): 215-20.

Said, E. A., F. P. Dupuy, et al. (2010). "Programmed death-1-induced interleukin-10 production by monocytes impairs CD4+ T cell activation during HIV infection." Nat Med 16(4): 452-9.

Samson, M., F. Libert, et al. (1996). "Resistance to HIV-1 infection in caucasian individuals bearing mutant alleles of the CCR-5 chemokine receptor gene." Nature 382(6593): 722-5.

Sassone-Corsi, P., L. J. Ransone, et al. (1988). "Direct interaction between fos and jun nuclear oncoproteins: role of the 'leucine zipper' domain." Nature 336(6200): 692-695.

Scarlatti, G., E. Tresoldi, et al. (1997). "In vivo evolution of HIV-1 co-receptor usage and sensitivity to chemokine-mediated suppression." Nat Med 3(11): 1259-65.

Schols, D. and E. De Clercq (1996). "Human immunodeficiency virus type 1 gp120 induces anergy in human peripheral blood lymphocytes by inducing interleukin-10 production." J Virol 70(8): 4953-60.

Schuitemaker, H., M. Koot, et al. (1992). "Biological phenotype of human immunodeficiency virus type 1 clones at different stages of infection: progression of disease is associated with a shift from monocytotropic to T-cell-tropic virus population." J Virol 66(3): 1354-60.

Schulz, P., V. Arbusow, et al. (1998). "Highly variable distribution of HSV-1-specific DNA in human geniculate, vestibular and spiral ganglia." Neurosci Lett 252(2): 139-42.

Shankarappa, R., J. B. Margolick, et al. (1999). "Consistent viral evolutionary changes associated with the progression of human immunodeficiency virus type 1 infection." J Virol 73(12): 10489-502.

Shi, B., J. Raina, et al. (1998). "Neuronal apoptosis induced by HIV-1 Tat protein and TNF-alpha: potentiation of neurotoxicity mediated by oxidative stress and implications for HIV-1 dementia." J Neurovirol 4(3): 281-90.

Shojania, S. and J. D. O'Neil (2006). "HIV-1 Tat is a natively unfolded protein: the solution conformation and dynamics of reduced HIV-1 Tat-(1-72) by NMR spectroscopy." J Biol Chem 281(13): 8347-56.

Sieczkarski, S. B., H. A. Brown, et al. (2003). "Role of protein kinase C betaII in influenza virus entry via late endosomes." J Virol 77(1): 460-469.

Silvera, P., M. W. Richardson, et al. (2002). "Outcome of simian-human immunodeficiency virus strain 89.6p challenge following vaccination of rhesus macaques with human immunodeficiency virus Tat protein." J Virol 76(8): 3800-3809.

Simpson, D. M. and M. Tagliati (1994). "Neurologic manifestations of HIV infection." Ann Intern Med 121(10): 769-85.

Singh, A. and R. G. Collman (2000). "Heterogeneous spectrum of coreceptor usage among variants within a dualtropic human immunodeficiency virus type 1 primary-isolate quasispecies." J Virol 74(21): 10229-35.

Sirianni, M. C., L. Vincenzi, et al. (1998). "gamma-Interferon production in peripheral blood mononuclear cells and tumor infiltrating lymphocytes from Kaposi's sarcoma patients: correlation with the presence of human herpesvirus-8 in peripheral blood mononuclear cells and lesional macrophages." Blood 91(3): 968-76.

So, Y. T., D. M. Holtzman, et al. (1988). "Peripheral neuropathy associated with acquired immunodeficiency syndrome. Prevalence and clinical features from a population-based survey." Arch Neurol 45(9): 945-8.

Sodroski, J., C. Rosen, et al. (1985). "Trans-acting transcriptional regulation of human T-cell leukemia virus type III long terminal repeat." Science 227(4683): 171-3.

Spitaler, M et D. A. Cantrell (2004). " Protein kinase C and beyond." Nature Rev. Immunology 5, 785 - 790.

Stylianou, E., P. Aukrust, et al. (1999). "IL-10 in HIV infection: increasing serum IL-10 levels with disease progression--down-regulatory effect of potent anti-retroviral therapy." Clin Exp Immunol 116(1): 115-20.

Takizawa, T., K. Ohashi, et al. (1996). "Possible involvement of double-stranded RNA-activated protein kinase in cell death by influenza virus infection." J Virol 70(11): 8128-32.

Tergaonkar, V., V. Bottero, et al. (2003). "IkappaB kinase-independent IkappaBalpha degradation pathway: functional NF-kappaB activity and implications for cancer therapy." Mol Cell Biol 23(22): 8070-83.

Tornatore, C., A. Nath, et al. (1991). "Persistent human immunodeficiency virus type 1 infection in human fetal glial cells reactivated by T-cell factor(s) or by the cytokines tumor necrosis factor alpha and interleukin-1 beta." J Virol 65(11): 6094-100.

Tran, T. A., M. G. de Goer de Herve, et al. (2008). "Resting regulatory CD4 T cells: a site of HIV persistence in patients on long-term effective antiretroviral therapy." PLoS One 3(10): e3305.

Vendeville, A., F. Rayne, et al. (2004). "HIV-1 Tat enters T cells using coated pits before translocating from acidified endosomes and eliciting biological responses." Mol Biol Cell 15(5): 2347-60.

Viatour, P., M. P. Merville, et al. (2005). "Phosphorylation of NF-kappaB and IkappaB proteins: implications in cancer and inflammation." Trends Biochem Sci 30(1): 43-52.

Watkins, J. D., G. R. Campbell, et al. (2008). "Homonuclear 1H NMR and circular dichroism study of the HIV-1 Tat Eli variant." Retrovirology 5: 83.

Westendorp, M. O., R. Frank, et al. (1995). "Sensitization of T cells to CD95-mediated apoptosis by HIV-1 Tat and gp120." Nature 375(6531): 497-500.

Wieland, U., J. E. Kuhn, et al. (1990). "Antibodies to recombinant HIV-1 vif, tat, and nef proteins in human sera." Med Microbiol Immunol 179(1): 1-11.

Xiao, G., E. W. Harhaj, et al. (2001). "NF-kappaB-inducing kinase regulates the processing of NF-kappaB2 p100." Mol Cell 7(2): 401-9.

Xiao, H., C. Neuveut, et al. (2000). "Selective CXCR4 antagonism by Tat: implications for in vivo expansion of coreceptor use by HIV-1." Proc Natl Acad Sci U S A 97(21): 11466-71.

Yamamoto, Y., U. N. Verma, et al. (2003). "Histone H3 phosphorylation by IKK-alpha is critical for cytokine-induced gene expression." Nature 423(6940): 655-9.

Yamaoka, S., G. Courtois, et al. (1998). "Complementation cloning of NEMO, a component of the IkappaB kinase complex essential for NF-kappaB activation." Cell 93(7): 1231-40.

Yang, X., Y. Chen, et al. (1999). "ERK MAP kinase links cytokine signals to activation of latent HIV-1 infection by stimulating a cooperative interaction of AP-1 and NF-kappaB." J Biol Chem 274(39): 27981-27988.

Yang, X. and D. Gabuzda (1999). "Regulation of human immunodeficiency virus type 1 infectivity by the ERK mitogen-activated protein kinase signaling pathway." J Virol 73(4): 3460-3466.

Zagury, J. F., A. Sill, et al. (1998). "Antibodies to the HIV-1 Tat protein correlated with nonprogression to AIDS: a rationale for the use of Tat toxoid as an HIV-1 vaccine." J Hum Virol 1(4): 282-292. Zink, W. E., J. Zheng, et al. (1999). "The neuropathogenesis of HIV-1 infection." FEMS Immunol Med Microbiol 26(3-4): 233-41.

3

Clinical Relevance of HIV-1 Superinfection

Daniëlle Hoogmoed, Marion Cornelissen and Antoinette van der Kuyl
University of Amsterdam
The Netherlands

1. Introduction

Over time a single patient can be infected by multiple intra- or intersubtype human immunodeficiency viruses type 1 (HIV-1) strains. These so-called dual infections are divided into co-infections and superinfections. HIV-1 co-infection is described as a second infection taking place before measurable HIV-1 antibody production by the immune system (seroconversion) and HIV-1 superinfection is defined as a second infection occurring after seroconversion. Here the focus lays on superinfections, which have implications for HIV-1 transmission, treatment and vaccine development (Gottlieb et al., 2004). Moreover superinfections can give rise to HIV-1 circulating recombinant forms (CRF); this significantly increases the global epidemiology (Gottlieb et al., 2007). Also due to these recombination events, two different drug resistant HIV-1 viruses could lead to multi drug resistance or even to more pathogenic viruses (Gottlieb et al., 2004, Blackard et al., 2004, Fernandez Larrosa et al., 2006).

Another important issue that is not extensively surveyed in literature is the clinical relevance of HIV-1 superinfection, as most descriptions rely on case reports and not on controlled cohort studies. The individual cases differ in severity, as several superinfected patients with rapidly progressive HIV-1 disease have been described since 2002, but superinfection cases were also found by coincidence in long-term non-progressors (LTNPs). These patients were able to control HIV-1 disease before and sometimes also after the superinfection event. So it is not resolved yet how superinfection affects disease progression in general and, if any, specific host or viral factors are involved. In this chapter, first an overview will be given of HIV-1 superinfected patients from several studies, with regard to HIV-1 disease progression. Disease progression is indicated by an increase in the HIV-1 plasma viral load, a decrease in the CD4+ T-cell count, acquired immunodeficiency syndrome (AIDS) related events and/or the start of antiretroviral treatment. These outcomes are compared to values of disease progression for single HIV-1 infected patients, resulting in an indication of the clinical relevance of HIV-1 superinfection.

2. Experimental studies with multiple lentivirus strains

An in vitro HIV-1 superinfection system for the analysis of viral dynamics and production of pseudotypes was used by Fernandez Larrosa et al. (2006). In vitro superinfected cells showed higher cell mortality, favoured viral spread and enhanced viral replication compared to non-superinfected cells. The results suggest that HIV-1 superinfection could result in progressive disease, as viral replication, a marker of pathogenicity, is enhanced after superinfection. A second study also showed that superinfection of cells infected with a defective HIV-1 virus, with a second replication-competent strain, results in the production of highly cytopathogenic HIV-1 particles (Iwabu et al., 2006).

In an in vivo cat model, both co- and superinfection compared to monoinfection with the related lentivirus feline immunodeficiency virus (FIV) increases neuroinflammation and subsequent neurodegeneration in the cat brain, also indicating enhanced pathogenicity (Afkhami-Goli et al., 2009).

A mathematical model of the within-host dynamics of HIV superinfection suggested that only superinfection with a fitter strain will lead to faster progression to AIDS (Fung et al., 2010). Probably, the HIV-1 superinfections in patients that are clinically detected are productive superinfections that indeed largely occur with fitter strains (Kozaczynska et al., 2010). Superinfections with less-fit strains may go unnoticed in vivo due to a low or localized replication of the less-fit strain. Another computer simulation study suggested that regulated superinfection of single cells might increase HIV-1 fitness through recombination (Leontiev and Hadany, 2010). Enhanced viral fitness is often associated with increased replication and pathogenicity. If different strains superinfect single cells, adaptation of HIV-1 could be more optimal than if only a single strain is present. Superinfection should be regulated so that competition for host resources does not result in less virions produced per cell as compared to single infected cells. If that happens, superinfection will not increase viral fitness. However, the authors speculate that HIV-1 is able to regulate superinfections by multiple virions. Indeed, this phenomenon is called superinfection resistance (SIR), and has been observed for many retrovirus infections (for a review, see: Nethe et al., 2005). SIR can be induced by simply down-regulating the virus receptor on the cell surface, but more complex retroviruses, such as HIV, often carry accessory genes specifically involved in resistance to superinfection of an already infected cell.

Thus, the few in vivo (FIV), in vitro (HIV-1) or in silico (HIV-1) studies that have been performed with lentiviruses with emphasis on growth characteristics, suggest that infection with multiple strains results in enhanced replication capacity, fitness and pathogenicity.

3. Disease progression in HIV-1 single infected patients

3.1 Markers of disease progression

Accepted indicators for HIV disease progression, especially in the post-ART (antiretroviral therapy) era, are increases in the plasma viral load and/or decreases in the CD4+ T-cell count below a certain limit (Mellors et al., 1997), although these markers are not clearly correlated (Rodríguez et al., 2006), and should preferentially be combined (Mellors et al., 1997). Korenromp et al. (2009) collected and analysed longitudinal viral load and CD4+ T-cell count data from untreated HIV-1 infected patients included in 30 studies and 16 cohorts, from the moment of seroconversion. The plasma viral loads of these patients ranged between 3.7 $\log_{10}$ and 5.6 $\log_{10}$ copies/ml, with an overall median of 4.4 $\log_{10}$ copies/ml. No significant change was seen in this median viral load for over 8 years. Mean CD4+ T-cell counts decreased from 600 to 360 cells/µl in 8 years. This is in agreement with the typical progression to AIDS in untreated HIV-1 infected patients within 8-10 years after infection (Gottlieb et al., 2004). However, the course of infection is variable; with approximately 5% of HIV-1 infected patients developing AIDS within 3 years, whereas up to 12% of the infected patients remain free of AIDS for over 20 years (Mellors et al., 1997).

The viral setpoint, e.g. the plasma viral load level stabilization after the acute infection period, has been found to be highly predictive of the rate of disease progression (Geskus et al., 2007). However, another study found that setpoint and disease progression are only linked in patients of European descent, and not in Africans (Müller et al., 2009).

Nowadays, HIV-1 disease progression until the occurrence of an AIDS-defining event or death from AIDS as a clinical end-point is replaced with CD4+ T-cell count decline to a certain level (mostly the level that indicates start of ART) or the start of antiretroviral treatment. Treatment is currently initiated in most western countries when CD4+ T-cell levels are below 350 cells/µl.

3.2 Disease progression profiles among risk groups

HIV-1 incidence varies among risk groups. Some risk groups in the western world, for example men having sex with men (MSM) and intravenous drug users (IDUs), have a high risk of acquiring HIV-1. The route of infection could be related to the type of initial immune response, which could theoretically influence the pattern of disease progression.

Pehrson et al. (1997) compared the disease progression parameters for HIV-1 infected MSM and IDUs, using the criteria of AIDS defining events and death from AIDS as endpoint markers. They observed a significant lower HIV-1 disease progression for IDUs. A similar outcome was found in an Italian study of 1078 HIV-1 seroconverters, were IDUs began antiretroviral therapy significantly later than homo- or heterosexual patients, even when corrected for CD4+ T-cell counts (Dorrucci et al., 1997). Such a difference in disease progression between MSM and IDUs was not seen in 12 European cohorts, where only a higher pre-AIDS mortality was obvious for IDUs (Prins and Veugelers, 1997). A similar outcome was seen in the Swiss Cohort Studies, where a uniform mortality risk was found among the sexes and risk groups, with only an increased risk of death for IDU without CD4+ cell depletion at entry, also probably not attributable to HIV-1 infection (van Overbeck et al., 1994). In homosexual men from different continents, no differences were found in time to development of AIDS, and also year of infection (before or after 1985) did not affect disease progression (Biggar, 1990). Adults with haemophilia infected through blood transfusion progressed slower towards AIDS than homosexual men before the introduction of ART due to the highly increased risk of Kaposi's sarcoma in the latter group (Biggar, 1990).

Overall, an age-related effect was seen whereby younger age at seroconversion was mostly beneficial (Biggar, 1990; Rosenberg et al., 1994; Collaborative Group on AIDS Incubation, 2000). However, perinatally infected children were found to have a much lower survival in the pre-ART era than children infected post-natally from breastfeeding (Marston et al., 2011).

Gender differences between men and women have also been reported, with women generally having lower initial HIV-1 plasma viral loads independent of exposure group, e.g. heterosexual or IDU (Rezza et al., 2000) or within an IDU cohort (Sterling et al., 2001), but this difference was not associated with lower disease progression rates (Sterling et al., 2001).

Concluding, disease progression profiles after HIV infection do generally not differ within and between risk groups. HIV-1 infected individuals do show variation in progression over time depending on the specific host characteristics, which includes age at seroconversion. For a review on this topic with similar conclusions, see: Hessol and Palacio (1996).

3.3 Disease progression in relation to HIV-1 subtype

HIV-1 group M is a highly variable virus. By now 9 subtypes (named A-D, F-G, J-K) are circulating worldwide accompanied by at least 48 described CRF's (circulating recombinant forms) and numerous URF's (unique recombinant forms) (Hemelaar et al., 2011). Distribution of these virus strains is variable, with all strains being present in Africa, but specific strains dominating epidemics on other continents. For an overview of the geographical distribution of HIV-1 strains in 2000-2007, see: Hemelaar et al. (2011).

It is reasonable to assume that HIV-1 isolates differ in their pathogenicity. Indeed, attenuated circulating virus strains that promote long-term disease free survival have been described, e.g. a nef-deleted strain found in Australia among blood-product recipients (Deacon et al., 1995). It is less clear if subtypes in general also differ in their capacity to induce AIDS, irrespective of host genetics. Most studies, mainly in African women, that describe a difference indicate that subtype D induces faster disease progression, especially when compared with subtype A (Kanki et al., 1999; Kaleebu et al., 2001; Vasan et al., 2006; Baeten et al., 2007; Kiwanuka et al., 2008). One Swedish/African study found similar rates of disease progression among persons infected with either subtypes A, B, C or D (Alaeus et al., 1999), in line with an Israeli study that showed no differences in progression between Ethiopian immigrants infected with subtype C and Israeli homosexual men infected with subtype B (Galai et al., 1997). In contrast, Singaporese seroconverters infected with CRF01_AE had an increased rate of CD4+ T-cell decline and a shorter time to initiation of ART than their non-CRF01_AE infected counterparts (Ng et al., 2011).

Env-V3 loop variation within a subtype can also affect disease progression, as Brazilians infected with a variant subtype B strain (B′-GWGR motif) had a lower progression towards AIDS and a lower chance of experiencing AIDS-defining events than Brazilian patients infected with the US/European subtype B strain (B-GPGR motif) (Casseb et al., 2002; de Brito et al., 2006).

Concluding, it is not unlikely that some subtypes, primarily subtype D and possibly CRF01_AE are more pathogenic than other HIV-1 subtypes, but generally subtypes do not differ appreciably in disease-inducing potential. However, when comparing disease progression in cohorts, it would be advisable to mainly evaluate patients infected with a certain subtype or recombinant form.

3.4 Disease progression in relation to host genetics

Infection of a host species by a pathogen is counteracted first by the innate and secondly by the adaptive immune system. The immune system of vertebrates has evolved into a highly variable gene complex, so that immune responses between individuals can differ depending upon the specifically inherited alleles.

Genome-wide association studies have suggested that the major genetic variation associated with control of HIV infection in humans is found in the Major Histocompatibility Complex (MHC) located on chromosome 6 (Fellay et al., 2007; International HIV Controllers Study, 2010). Decreased disease progression and lower plasma viral load at setpoint have been associated with carrying MHC class I alleles HLA-B*2705, HLA-B*5701/02/03 and HLA-B*5801 (reviewed by Goulder and Watkins, 2008, for a specific study, see: Altfeld et al., 2003). Rapid disease progression and high plasma viral load at setpoint is found in individuals carrying HLA-B*1801, HLA-B*3502/03, or HLA-B*5802 alleles. However, it has been observed that HIV-1 strains are escaping from HLA-B pressure (Goulder et al., 2001;

Cornelissen et al., 2009). Immune escape had already been described for individual patients, but more importantly, it is now also visible in the general epidemic.

Specific HLA alleles differ in their distribution worldwide, so that HIV disease progression related to HLA variation can differ not only between individuals, but also between populations. In a Swiss cohort study, a lower average CD4+ T-cell decline was seen for patients from African descent compared with Europeans (Müller et al., 2009). Earlier in a UK cohort, it was already observed that African descent was associated with lower plasma viral load after correction for CD4+ T-cell counts, compared with European ancestry (Smith et al., 2003). However, an earlier in-depth analysis of published studies did not reveal obvious differences in progression towards AIDS-defining events in correlation with race or ethnicity (Hessol and Palacio, 1996). Probably, in a certain population advantageous and disadvantageous alleles are generally more or less balanced, and other cofactors are also of importance. Therefore, although the inherited HLA type is important for the individual patient with regard to disease progression, ethnicity itself is no indicator for (loss of) control of HIV replication.

Variation in other genes is also implicated in disease progression rates, be it delayed or accelerated (reviewed by Fellay, 2009). Especially polymorphisms in the chemokine receptors CCR2 and CCR5 promoter regions have been found to be influential, as is the CCR5-Δ32 variant that is only present in Caucasians. In a large study on HIV controllers, the only variation outside the MHC-I regions that was significantly associated with control of infection, were polymorphisms in CCR2/CCR5, albeit only in European samples (International HIV Controllers Study, 2010).

Concluding, host genetic variation is important in HIV-1 disease progression, but it is not practically possible to compare only individuals with a similar genetic make-up. Also, viral factors are important, making disease outcome in the individual patient a trade-off between host and viral genetics. Besides, HIV might be in the process of circumventing adverse host factors, as is ongoing for some HLA-B alleles. Another important issue is the level of expression of a certain trait, e.g. how well functions the adaptive immune system, and the balance between traits is of importance. Consequently, one has to recognize that host (and viral) genetics influence disease progression, but is complicated in practice to draw firm conclusions, even when genetic information would be entirely available.

4. Clinical progression and HIV-1 superinfection

4.1 HIV-1 superinfection: Introduction

In the earlier days of the epidemic, many were sceptic about the existence of HIV-1 superinfections, e.g. a re-infection with an unrelated HIV-1 strain after seroconversion. For some time, it was assumed that infection with HIV would protect against such a second infection. Recombinant strains observed already early in the epidemic were explained as having been generated by HIV co-infection during the acute, early phase of the infection when the adaptive immunity is not fully developed, or be the ultimate result of long-term evolution (Gonzalez et al., 2003).

The first reported HIV-1 superinfection was detected in an MSM who experienced an acute retroviral syndrome in 1998 after infection with a CRF01_AE strain, and who was superinfected with a HIV-1 subtype B strain in 2001 (Jost et al., 2002). In the same year a second HIV-1 superinfected patient was described, another MSM who controlled initial HIV-1 infection after supervised ART interruption (Altfeld et al., 2002). Although many researchers did not find HIV-1 superinfections when examining their diverse cohorts (Tsui et al., 2004; Diaz et al., 2005), many others did, so that the concept of HIV-1 superinfection being a regular event was gradually accepted. For example, Hu et al. (2005) identified two superinfected individuals amongst 80 HIV-1 infected Thai IDUs with a sample available 12 months after seroconversion, and concluded that superinfection is not an uncommon event. In several cohorts, especially in Africa, sometimes high incidences of HIV-1 dual infections were found (Manigart et al., 2004; Chohan et al., 2005; Piantadosi et al., 2007), so that the authors reached conclusions similar to Hu et al. However, most studies do not report on clinical progression of the superinfected individuals, leaving the question whether or not HIV-1 superinfection is harmful to the individual patient.

4.2 Superinfection cases with rapid clinical progression

Gottlieb et al. (2004) found amongst 34 HIV-1 positive patients, 4 patients who were co-infected with HIV-1 (3 MSM and one African female sex worker) and one MSM who was intrasubtype superinfected with HIV-1 subtype B. He had a rapid CD4+ T-cell decrease after initial infection and became superinfected approximately 1 year after seroconversion (Gottlieb et al., 2007). Antiretroviral treatment was initiated half a year after superinfection. In these five patients, a CD4+ T-cell count of <200 cells/µl was reached <3.1 years after seroconversion and AIDS-defining events occurred <3.4 years after seroconversion. Due to the rapid disease progression in HIV-1 dually infected patients, including a superinfected patient, compared with single infected patients; the authors suggested a general association between dual infection and HIV-1 disease progression.

A fast progressing MSM, reaching an AIDS diagnosis within 1.5 years from primary infection and infected with two unrelated HIV-1 populations early in infection, had already been reported in 1997 (Liu et al., 1997). It was, however, in this study unclear whether the source partner had a dual infection or whether the second HIV-1 population in this patient originated from a second source.

Published reports on rapid disease progression after HIV-1 superinfection are rare, and only one of them concerns an actually confirmed superinfection (Gottlieb et al., 2004). In single HIV-1 infection cases, rapid progression to AIDS is also infrequent, and estimated to occur in only 5% of patients.

4.3 Superinfection cases with markers of increased clinical progression

The first case of superinfection to be described involved an MSM with initial CRF01_AE infection who acquired a subtype B superinfection when interrupting his ART regimen (Jost et al., 2002). The superinfection was accompanied by transient fatigue and fever, a rebound in the plasma viral load remaining at 200,000-400,000 copies/ml and a steady decline of the CD4+ T-cell count. ART was resumed four months after the rebound in plasma viral load.

In a Swiss IDU cohort, two CRF11_cpx superinfections after initial subtype B infection were found in chronically infected patients that had low viral loads without antiretroviral treatment for years (Yerly et al., 2004). In both patients, a Caucasian female and an African male patient, HIV-1 superinfection was associated with an acute retroviral syndrome, stably increased viral loads and a significant decrease of the CD4+ T-cell counts.

Three HIV-1 superinfection cases were reported from a North American Acute Infection and Early Disease cohort of HIV infected patients (Smith et al., 2004). The superinfections occurred within 6-12 months from primary infection, and were associated with a unfavourable change in disease markers. Within 6 months of superinfection, the plasma viral loads of these 3 patients increased with a mean of 1.6 $\log_{10}$ copies/ml and the CD4+ T-cell count decreased with a mean of 132 cells/µl. Two of the three individuals were initially infected with a drug resistant HIV-1 strain and became superinfected with a wild-type strain. The third individual was initially infected with a wild-type strain and became superinfected with a drug resistant strain (see also: Smith et al., 2005). In all individuals the superinfecting strain was fitter than the initial infecting strain, so that a change in antiretroviral susceptibility was seen. In two individuals the wild-type superinfecting strain masked the initial drug resistant strain.

A similar observation was published by Koelsch et al. (2003), were a male patient initially infected with a subtype B drug-resistant strain was superinfected with a wild-type subtype B strain four months later. After primary infection, the patient had a low viral load of around 6000 viral RNA copies/ml at setpoint, in line with the finding that drug-resistance mutations often decrease viral fitness (see: De Luca, 2006). After superinfection, the viral load increased sharply to 200,000 copies/ml and CD4+ T-cells declined steadily from 792 cells/µl at enrolment to ± 500 cells/µl four months post-infection (immediately before superinfection) till 283 cells/µl eleven months post-infection (approximately 7 months after superinfection), suggestive of increased disease progression.

Drug-resistant virus strains have also been identified in further superinfection cases. An MSM first infected with a multidrug resistant HIV-1 subtype B strain was superinfected 10 months later with another multidrug resistant subtype B strain from a new partner (Brenner et al., 2004). The first infection was associated with low viremia: 1305 copies/ml decreasing to undetectable levels without antiretroviral treatment four months after infection. Superinfection was associated with a rise in the plasma viral load from undetectable levels to 13,888 copies/ml. CD4+ T-cell counts were not documented during that time, although they were very high after the acute infection phase (1200 cells/µl).

In a cohort of female South African sexworkers infected with HIV-1 subtype C, many intrasubtype dual infections were observed during primary infection (Grobler et al., 2004). It was unclear how many of these dual infections could be attributed to early superinfections. Dual infection was significantly associated with an elevated viral setpoint compared to the single infected patients. No superinfections were detected in any patient during follow-up.

A triple HIV-1 infection in a Dutch MSM was reported by van der Kuyl et al. (2005). In March 2001 the patient was diagnosed with an HIV-1 subtype B infection. His plasma viral load was then approximately 3.4 $\log_{10}$ copies/ml and his CD4+ T-cell count was around 850 cells/µl. Retrospective analysis showed that he became superinfected with another subtype B strain in October 2002. His plasma viral load was then 4.5 $\log_{10}$ copies/ml with a CD4+ T-cell count of 550 cells/µl. No medical symptoms were reported by the patient around the time of the first superinfection. However, in July 2003, the patient presented with acute fever and an increased plasma viral load of 6 $\log_{10}$ copies/ml and a decreased CD4+ T-cell count of 300 cells/µl. Analysis of the viral genotype indicated that he was again superinfected, this time with a CRF01_AE strain. After the second superinfection, the plasma viral load stabilized at an increased level while the CD4+ T-cell counts continued to decrease. Therefore, ART was initiated in June 2005, two years after the second superinfection.

An African female barworker, who was initially infected with a HIV-1 ACD recombinant strain, became superinfected 6 till 9 months after seroconversion with an AC recombinant strain. At that time, the plasma viral load was 5.6 $\log_{10}$ copies/ml (McCutchan et al., 2005), while CD4+ T-cell counts were unavailable. Six months after seroconversion, the patient

showed recurring short episodes of malaise, fever, cough, diarrhoea and had moderate weight loss, symptoms indicative of an acute HIV infection. Genotyping indeed indicated that a superinfection with an AC recombinant strain had occurred around that time. Three months after superinfection a setpoint value of 4.8 $\log_{10}$ copies/ml was maintained, while CD4+ T-cell count declined from 482 cells/µl to 377 cells/µl 24 to 30 months after primary infection, suggestive of increased disease progression.
An Asian-American MSM presenting with an acute HIV-1 infection syndrome was found to be infected with a multi-drug resistant HIV-1 subtype B strain, of which he controlled viremia after the acute infection period (Yang et al., 2005). His viral load was 1000 copies/ml, and his CD4+ T-cell count rose above 600 cells/µl after an initial decline to 396 cells/µl). However, before he could reach long-term non-progressor status, he was superinfected 4 months later with a distinct, drug-sensitive subtype B strain. Viremia immediately rose to 30,000-40,000 copies/ml with a concomitant decline in CD4+ T-cell counts to 450 cells/µl. Ten months after the first infection CD4+ T-cell counts decreased further to <400 cells/µl.
Smith et al. (2006) described 3 superinfected homosexual male patients from the USA and compared them to 11 control patients primarily to analyse (neutralizing) antibody profiles. Over the study period (6 months after first antibody measurement), viral loads (ΔHIV RNA) showed a significant increase ($p=0.02$) in the superinfected patients compared to the control group, but there was no statistically significant difference ($p = 0.29$) in the CD4+ T-cell count reductions (ΔCD4) between the groups.
Reports describing increased disease progression, mainly inferred from rising plasma viral load or decreasing CD4+ T-cell counts, but not always in combination, are more common. In some cases, increasing plasma viral load can be attributed to re-infection with a virus that has higher replication capacity, e.g. in the case of infection with a drug-sensitive virus after primary infection with a drug-resistant strain. Also, in other cases with enhanced progression, superinfection could have occurred with a fitter strain. Possibly, cases with increased disease progression are more easily detected, as patients suddenly presenting with adverse clinical characteristics are more likely to be scrutinized.

4.4 Superinfection cases with low or normal clinical progression

HIV-1 superinfection events in IDU's which did obviously not result in enhanced disease progression were reported from Thailand (Ramos et al., 2002). In October 1996, a female patient was found to be infected with the recombinant strain CRF01_AE. She became superinfected with HIV-1 subtype B, probably 3-6 weeks after initial infection. Her plasma viral load varied within 2 logs (mean 4 $\log_{10}$ copies/ml), while the CD4+ T-cell counts remained around 500 cells/µl, only dropping below this number once. A second, male patient was identified with an initial HIV-1 subtype B infection in August 1996. He became superinfected 5-9 months later with strain CRF01_AE and experienced fluctuating viral loads between 3.7 $\log_{10}$ and 4.9 $\log_{10}$ copies/ml for 3 years. His CD4+ T-cell counts remained >500 cells/µl. Both patients showed at the time before superinfection limited or absent specific T-cell and antibody immune responses (see also: Promadej-Lanier et al., 2009).
Analysis of a Swiss IDU cohort revealed three subtype B/CRF11_cpx co-infected patients and a transient subtype B superinfection in an initially CRF11_cpx infected female individual in a cohort with recent HIV infection (Yerly et al., 2004). No symptoms were associated with the transient superinfection, and both the plasma viral load and CD4+ T-cell counts were stable in this patient.

Manigart et al. (2004) reported 2 superinfected women out of 147 HIV-1 infected commercial sex workers in a cohort from Burkina Faso. In November 1999 the first woman was found to be single infected with CRF02_AG. In samples from January 2001 onwards, a second virus strain, CRF06_cpx, was always present. Plasma viral load levels increased till July 2001, with a steady decline thereafter. A second woman was found to be HIV-1 seropositive with a CRF02_AG infection in March 2000 and a plasma viral load of around 55,000 copies/ml. A subsequent superinfection with CRF06_cpx occurred before November 2000 with a tripling of the plasma viral load in the November 2000 sample. Thereafter, her plasma viral load decreased to 11,000 copies/ml. Unfortunately, she was lost to follow-up after she died in 2001 from obstetric complications.

A superinfected Kenyan female sex worker from the pre-antiretroviral therapy period was presented by Fang et al. (2004). In February 1985, this patient from Nairobi tested HIV-1 seropositive and was, retrospectively, found to be infected with a subtype A strain. In April 1992, at least 7 years after primary infection, she presented an acute febrile illness with chills and had a greatly decreased CD4+ T-cell count (<100 cells/µl) compared with a measurement in March 1991 (794 cells/µl). A superinfection with a subtype C strain was suspected but due to a lack of samples, only in later samples from 1995 and 1997 subtype C sequences could be detected from subtype A/C recombinant strains that had already been formed then. The patient never received antiretroviral treatment. From 1994, symptoms indicating the onset of the AIDS phase, e.g. weight loss, tuberculosis and cryptococcal infection appeared and she died in 1998, e.g. over 14 years after her primary HIV-1 infection (Fang et al., 2004). In this cohort of sex-workers, mean survival was 4.4 years, and surviving over 10 years was rare, suggesting that this woman had a remarkably slow disease progression despite an HIV-1 superinfection in the chronic phase of the infection.

Also from Kenya, but now from its second-largest city Mombasa, three additional superinfection cases in a cohort of intermediate risk heterosexual women were described during the 1993-2000 period (Chohan et al., 2005). During follow-up, none of these women received antiretroviral therapy. All three women were inter-subtype superinfected with HIV-1; two women were infected with a subtype D strain and became superinfected with an subtype A strain, while the third women was infected with a subtype C strain and was superinfected with an A/C recombinant strain. The first patient experienced a superinfection 264-385 days after primary HIV infection. Follow-up was done for 2282 days (> 6 years), and during this time her plasma viral load was high ($\approx$ 6 $\log_{10}$ copies/ml), but stable, with no obvious increase at the estimated time of superinfection. The second woman experienced an HIV-1 superinfection 303-591 days after primary HIV infection. She was followed for 2069 days (> 5.5 years), during which her plasma viral load was stable at 5 $\log_{10}$ copies/ml. The third woman became superinfected between 101-485 days after primary HIV infection. During follow-up (1262 days $\approx$ 3.5 years), her plasma viral load rose from a very low level of 1.7 $\log_{10}$ copies/ml at day 485 to the modest level of 4.1 $\log_{10}$ copies/ml at end-point. It is possible, however, that in this patient, viraemia continues to rise after the 3.5 years of follow-up. But even then, this patient cannot be classified as a fast progressor.

From the same Kenyan cohort, 7 additional HIV-1 superinfection cases were reported two years later (Piantadosi et al., 2007). Four of these women were inter-subtype superinfected, while the other 3 were superinfected with a second strain of the same subtype. The women were superinfected as early as around 2 months after primary HIV infection to as late as 5 years after seroconversion. Plasma viral load changes were measured before and after the superinfection moment, and were either similar or modestly increased in the subjects. Only one of the intra- and one of the inter-subtype infected women showed a 1.5 $\log_{10}$ increase in her plasma viral load. CD4+ T-cell counts measured at the first moment after superinfection ranged between 553-628 cells/µl for 3 patients, between 296-309 cells/µl for 2 other patients, and were not available for the two remaining women. Unfortunately, no CD4+ T-cell counts were available from earlier moments. The two patients with the lowest available CD4+ T-cell counts had both been superinfected around 2.5 years from their primary HIV infection moment, suggesting that the relatively low CD4+ T-cell counts were not necessarily due to an already advanced disease stage. Four patients had viral load data for more than 2 years after superinfection (range 2.1-5 years). In all four, including a patient with 309 CD4+ cells/µl, the plasma viral load was stable at around 5 $\log_{10}$ copies/ml. The other patient with <300 CD4+ T-cells/µl after superinfection also had a stable viral load after approximately one year of follow-up. So, in this female African cohort, HIV-1 superinfection was not correlated with plasma viral load increases. In 2008, two more superinfected women from this cohort were described (Piantadosi et al., 2008). One woman was intrasubtype superinfected with two subtype A strains, and also showed no significant plasma viral load increases after more than 3.5 years of follow-up, although her viral load had increased from 4.3 $\log_{10}$ copies/ml to 4.9 $\log_{10}$ copies/ml directly after superinfection. The other patient, infected with a subtype D strain, did however show continuous plasma viral load increases in the three years after superinfection with a subtype A strain. On the other hand, the plasma viral load of this patient was already increasing during the mono-infection period.

Pernas et al. (2006) described a Spanish HIV-1 triple infected patient who was an IDU but also had unprotected heterosexual contacts. In 1987 this patient became infected with a subtype A HIV-1 strain. Antiretroviral treatment was started in 1996 due to strongly declining CD4+ T-cell counts. Plasma viral load data were only available from 1998 onward. The patient was poorly compliant, and treatment was interrupted several times voluntarily. In 1999, twelve years after primoinfection, the patient was found to have been superinfected, probably at the same moment, with both a subtype B and a subtype C strain. The superinfecting strain B had several drug resistance mutations in the pol gene. After the superinfection moment, the patient's viral load increased steadily from 4.2 $\log_{10}$ copies/ml directly after superinfection till 5.3 $\log_{10}$ copies/ml in 2001. His CD4+ T-cell count decreasing accordingly; from approx. 280 cells/µl directly after superinfection till 55 cells/µl in February 2003.

Patients with no obvious increased disease progression after HIV-1 superinfection have been mainly reported from cohort studies examining viral diversity in general. It is remarkable that most non-progressors described above are women (15 women versus 2 males in the mentioned studies). However, this probably has to do with the time-frame of the studies. Female sex-workers in Africa have probably been exposed to repeated HIV-1 infections from the start of the epidemic due to their risk behaviour. The male cohorts examined mainly consist of MSM from Europe and the USA. In this risk group, risk behaviour, and thus risk exposure sharply diminished after HIV-1 diagnosis before the availability of ART (Rachinger et al., 2010). In line with this reduced risk behaviour, no HIV-1 superinfections were reported from MSM cohorts before the year 2000 (Gonzalez et al., 2003; Rachinger et al., 2010).

4.5 Superinfection cases in long-term non progressors

Long-term non progressors (LTNPs) are HIV-1 infected patients who control viral replication without anti-retroviral therapy to low levels and have stable CD4+ T-cell counts in the normal range for over 10 years. Only a minor group of HIV-1 infected patients are LTNPs (Deeks et al., 2007; Canducci et al., 2009). An even smaller LTNP subgroup is constituted of the so-called elite HIV controllers. Elite HIV controllers are atypical HIV-1 infected patients who have continuous undetectable viral loads of <50 copies/ml, and no decline in CD4+ T-cell count for at least 10 years, also without the help of antiretroviral therapy (Deeks et al., 2007; Clerc et al., 2009).

Casado et al. (2007) reported two HIV-1 infected LTNP patients, who remained in control of their HIV-1 infection even after a potential superinfection. The patients were an IDU who was HIV-1 infected for at least 18 years and an MSM who was infected for at least 20 years. Both had CD4+ T-cell counts of >500 cells/ml, remained asymptomatic and antiretroviral therapy naïve. In time, the IDU had multiple peaks in the viral load and a slow decrease in CD4+ T-cell count whereas the MSM had undetectable viral loads and a steady CD4+ T-cell count. The time of HIV-1 infection for both patients was estimated based on the genetic distance to a reconstructed most recent common ancestor. These calculations suggested that the IDU was most likely co-infected with two HIV-1 subtype B strains, but a superinfection could not be ruled out, and that the MSM became HIV-1 subtype B superinfected 9 years after initial infection. Both patients did not show any indications for faster disease progression after long-term follow-up, suggesting that here a putative superinfection is not associated with progressive HIV-1 disease. However, the presumed superinfection event is based on nucleotide distance estimation, and not on actual sampling, so that the superinfection could in reality be a co-infection and vice versa. Still, no increased disease progression is seen in these two LTNP's, whether or not they have been co- or superinfected.

A haemophiliac harbouring two separate clusters of replication-competent HIV-1 subtype B strains was controlling his HIV-1 infection without antiretroviral treatment and with > 90% of plasma viral load measurements being below 400 copies/ml (Lamine et al., 2007). The patient received contaminated blood products, most likely on distinct occasions. He was thus possibly superinfected, but did not experience disease progression after more than 10 years of follow-up.

An HIV-1 elite controller who showed HIV-1 viremic control before and after superinfection was described from The Netherlands (Rachinger et al., 2008). The patient, an MSM, was diagnosed HIV-1 positive in 1991. His viral load was under the detection limit of the assays used then, and the CD4+ T-cell counts were > 600 cells/µl from 1996 onwards. In May 2005, the plasma viral load of the elite controller increased. In April 2006, the viral load peaked at 25,000 copies/ml. Sequence analysis of the 2006 sample showed that a superinfection with another subtype B strain had occurred. Indeed, the patient reported unprotected sexual intercourse with a new partner at that time. HIV-1 RNA levels continued to decline again till around 1000-2000 copies/ml during November 2006 - March 2008, suggesting that the former elite controller was regaining control of his HIV-1 viremia. CD4+ T-cell counts, however, were slowly declining to 480 cells/µl in March 2008 (approximately 2 years after superinfection), suggestive of disease progression. Two other patients, the source partner and a second partner that had been infected with the same virus strain, showed rapidly decreasing CD4+ T-cell counts and high viral loads. Therefore, this specific virus strain is not attenuated. Host factors are important in controlling infection, and indeed, the index patient was shown to carry the protective HLA class I B*5701 allele.

However, not all (initial) controllers of HIV viral replication are able to control a second HIV infection. Streeck et al. (2008) described a HIV–controller who rapidly lost control due to an HIV-1 superinfection. The patient, expressing the protective HLA-B27 allele, had at initial infection a peak viral load of 5.7 $\log_{10}$ copies/ml and a CD4+ T-cell count of approximately 900 cells/µl. He controlled viral replication as early as 22 days after infection with a plasma viral load well below 10,000 copies/ml, most likely due to his rapidly increasing CD8+ T-cell immune responses. However after 1.4 years, the viral load increased to 5.6 $\log_{10}$ copies/ml followed by a steady decrease in CD4+ T-cell count. Three years after initial infection (1.5 years after superinfection) the CD4+ T-cell count was below 300 cells/µl. Phylogenetic analysis of viral sequences showed that the patient was superinfected with a distinct subtype B HIV strain. The superinfecting strain dominated the blood plasma for the following 3 years with no control of viral replication.

Clerc et al. (2010) also showed that elite controllers are not exempt from HIV-1 superinfection and risk of disease progression. Two HIV-1 infected IDU elite controllers contracted an HIV-1 superinfection and subsequently experienced progressive disease. In 1996, a Swiss woman was tested positive for HIV-1 infection with a subtype B strain. For over 6 years, she had undetectable plasma viral loads and CD4+ T-cell counts >800 cells/µl. However in July 2002, she presented with a syndrome of high fever, general weakness and multiple adenopathies. A viral load of 5.9 $\log_{10}$ copies/ml was measured with a decreased CD4+ T-cell count (600 cells/µl). A diagnosis of acute retroviral syndrome was made due to superinfection with a CRF11_cpx strain. In August 2007 she started with antiretroviral therapy, as her CD4+ T-cell count was then as low as 240 cells/µl, and had already been around the 400 cells/µl level from January 2005 onwards. After the superinfection moment, the plasma viral load had always been high.

An African male IDU patient with the protective HLA B*81 allele was tested HIV-1 subtype B positive in March 1999. His viral load was undetectable and he had normal CD4+ T-cell counts. In October 2002, he showed fatigue, general weakness and multiple new adenopathies. His plasma viral load was then 5 $\log_{10}$ copies/ml and the CD4+ T-cell count decreased from 1225 to 674 cells/µl. Also this patient was superinfected with a CRF11_cpx strain and showed HIV-1 disease progression. After superinfection, the plasma viral load remained high at around 5 $\log_{10}$ copies/ml, while CD4+ T-cell counts dropped below 400 cells/µl. Nineteen months after the HIV-1 superinfection event the patient died from a drug overdose and was lost to follow-up.

A homosexual male patient infected with an attenuated HIV-1 subtype B strain that lacked the *nef* gene lost control of HIV-1 replication when he was subsequently superinfected with a wild-type subtype B strain (Braibant et al., 2010). The patient had been included in a French long-term nonprogressors cohort after 10 years of seropositivity with 5 years of stable CD4+T-cell counts >600 cells/µl. However, in March 1999, almost 4 years after inclusion in the cohort, plasma viral load increased progressively to 10,350 copies/ml and CD4+ T-cell counts declined <600 cells/µl, necessitating the start of antiretroviral therapy. Retrospective analysis showed that the patient had been superinfected with a wild-type subtype B strain around the time of inclusion in the controller cohort. Although control of HIV-1 replication was lost by this patient after superinfection, disease progression was relatively slow, e.g. 4 years after superinfection, CD4+ T-cell counts were still around 500 cells/µl, and plasma viral load was only slowly increasing till ±10,000 copies/ml.

LTNPs and elite controllers are not free from HIV-1 superinfection. This should come as no surprise, because although these atypical patients are able to control replication of HIV, they are fully susceptible to infection with the virus. How viral control is achieved is not completely clear. Favourable HLA-B types are associated with control, as are infections with low-replicating virus variants. In the latter case, re-infection with a more competent strain could easily result in loss-of-control. If the adaptive immune system is controlling the virus, there is a possibility that control will not be lost or can be regained after superinfection. From the above described patient cases, it is clear that all hypothetical situations exist in real life, but that control is more often lost than recovered.

5. Conclusion

The course of an HIV-1 infection in humans varies greatly. From rapid progression to AIDS within a few years to control of viral replication for more than 20 years: it all exists. The studies presented above indicate that patients who get infected with a second HIV-1 strain follow similar divergent tracks of disease progression: from rapid to no obvious progression. Assigning HIV-1 superinfection cases (leaving out the questionable cases) into progression or non-progression categories results in 20 cases immediately exhibiting markers of disease progression versus 21 cases that do not, e.g. in 50% of cases HIV-1 superinfection results in an accelerated loss of viral control. However, larger studies, e.g. case-control studies, are needed to assess the effect of HIV-1 superinfection upon disease progression in a controlled way, as most reports published have low numbers of superinfected patients.

6. References

Afkhami-Goli, A., Liu, S-H., Zhu, Y., Antony, J.M., Arab, H. & Power, C. (2009). Dual lentivirus infection potentiates neuroinflammation and neurodegeneration: viral copassage enhances neurovirulence. *Journal of NeuroVirology*, Vol. 15, No. 2, pp. 139-152.

Altfeld, M., Allen, T., Yu, X.G., Johnston, M.N., Agrawal, D., Korber, B.T. , Montefiori, D. C., O'Connor, D.H. Davis, B.T. Lee, P.K. Maier, E.L. Harlow, J. Goulder, P.J. Brander, C. Rosenberg, E.S. & Walker, B.D. (2002). HIV-1 superinfection despite broad CD8+ T-cell responses containing replication of the primary virus. *Nature*, Vol. 420, No. 28, pp. 434-439.

Altfeld, M., Addo, M.M., Rosenberg, E.S., Hecht, F.M., Lee, P.K., Vogel, M., Xu, X.G., Draenert, R., Johnston, M.N., Strick, D., Allen, T.M., Feeney, M.E., Kahn, J.O., Sekaly, R.P., Levy, J.A., Rockstroh, J.K., Goulder, P.J., & Walker, B.D. (2003). Influence of HLA-B57 on clinical presentation and viral control during acute HIV-1 infection. *AIDS*, Vol. 17, No. 18, pp. 2581-2591.

Anderson, R.M., & Medley, G.F. (1988). Epidemiology of HIV infection and AIDS: incubation and infectious periods, survival and vertical transmission. *AIDS*, Vol. 2 Suppl 1, pp. S57-63.

Biggar, R.J. (1990) AIDS incubation in 1891 HIV seroconverters from different exposure groups. International Registry of Seroconverters. *AIDS*, Vol. 4, No. 11, pp. 1059-1066.

Blackard, J.T. & Mayer, K.H. (2004). HIV superinfection in the era of increased sexual risk-taking. *Sexually Transmitted Diseases*, Vol. 31, No. 4, pp. 201–204.

Braibant, M., Xie, J., Samri, A., Agut H., Autran, B., & Barin F. (2010). Disease progression due to dual infection in an HLA-B57-positive asymptomatic long-term nonprogressor infected with a *nef*-deleted HIV-1 strain. *Virology*, Vol. 405, No. 1, pp. 81-92.

Brenner, B., Routy, J-P., Quan, Y., Moisi D., Oliveira, M., Turner, D., Wainberg, W.A., & co-investigators of the Quebec Primary Infection Study. (2004). Persistence of multidrug-resistant HIV-1 in primary infection leading to superinfection. *AIDS*, Vol. 18, No. 12, pp. 1653-1660.

Canducci, F., Marinozzi, M.C., Sampaolo, M., Berrè, S., Bagnarelli, P., Degano, M., Gallotta, G., Mazzi, B., Lemey, P., Burioni R., & Clementi, M. (2009). Dynamic features of the selective pressure on the human immunodeficiency virus type 1 (HIV-1) gp120 CD4-binding site in a group of long term non progressor (LTNP) subjects. *Retrovirology*, Vol. 6, No. 4.

Casado, C., Pernas, M., Alvaro, T., Sandonis, V., García, S., Rodríguez, C., Romero, J.D., Grau, E., Ruiz, L., & Lopez-Galindez, C. (2007). Coinfection and superinfection in patients with long-term, nonprogressive HIV-1 disease. *The Journal of Infectious Diseases*, Vol. 196, No. 6, pp. 895–899.

Chohan, B., Lavreys, L., Rainwater, S.M. J., & Overbaugh, J. (2005). Evidence for frequent reinfection with Human Immunodeficiency Virus Type 1 of a different subtype. *Journal of Virology*, Vol. 79, No. 16, pp. 10701–10708.

Clerc, O., Cavassini, M., Böni, J., Schüpbach, J., & Bürgisser, P. (2009). Prolonged seroconversion in an elite controller of HIV-1 infection. *Journal of Clinical Virology*, Vol. 46, No. 4, pp. 371–373.

Clerc, O., Colombo, S., Yerly, S., Telenti, A., & Cavassini, M. (2010). HIV-1 elite controllers: Beware of super-infections. *Journal of Clinical Virology*, Vol. 47, No. 4, pp.376–378.

Collaborative Group on AIDS Incubation and HIV Survival including the CASCADE EU Concerted Action. Concerted Action on SeroConversion to AIDS and Death in Europe. (2000). Time from HIV-1 seroconversion to AIDS and death before widespread use of highly-active antiretroviral therapy: a collaborative re-analysis. *Lancet*, Vol. 355, No. 9210, pp. 1131-1137.

Cornelissen, M., Hoogland, F.M., Back, N.K.T., Jurriaans, S., Zorgdrager, F., Bakker, M., Brinkman, K., Prins, M., & van der Kuyl, A.C. (2009). Multiple transmissions of a stable human leucocyte antigen-B27 cytotoxic T-cell-escape strain of HIV-1 in The Netherlands. *AIDS*, Vol. 23, No. 12, pp. 1495-1500.

Deacon, N.J., Tsykin, A., Solomon, A., Smith, K., Ludford-Menting, M., Hooker, D.J., McPhee, D.A., Greenway, A.L., Ellett, A., Chatfield, C., Lawson, V.A., Crowe, S., Maerz, A., Sonza, S., Learmont, J., Sullivan, J.S., Cunningham, A., Dwyer, D., Dowton, D., & Mills, J. (1995). Genomic structure of an attenuated quasi species of HIV-1 from a blood transfusion donor and recipients. *Science*, Vol. 270, No. 5238, pp. 988-91.

Deeks, S.G., & Walker, B.D. (2007). Human immunodeficiency virus controllers: mechanisms of durable virus control in the absence of antiretroviral therapy. *Immunity*, Vol. 27, No. 3, pp. 406- 416.

Diaz, R.S., Pardini, R., Catroxo, M., Operskalski, E.A., Mosley, J.W., & Busch, M.P. (2005). HIV-1 superinfection is not a common event. *Journal of Clinical Virology*, Vol. 33, No. 4, pp. 328–330.

Dorrucci, M., Pezzotti, P., Phillips, A.N., Alliegro, M.B., Rezza, G. (1997). Antiretroviral treatment and progression to AIDS in HIV seroconverters from different risk groups. HIV Italian Seroconversion Study. *AIDS* Vol. 11, No. 4, pp. 461-467.

Fang, G., Weiser, B., Kuiken, C., Philpott, S.M., Rowland-Jones S, Plummer, F., Kimani, J., Shi, B., Kaul, R., Bwayo, J., Anzala, O., & Burger, H. (2004). Recombination following superinfection by HIV-1. *AIDS*, Vol. 18, No. 2, pp. 153-159.

Fellay, J., Shianna, K.V., Ge, D., Colombo, S., Ledergerber, B., Weale, M., Zhang, K., Gumbs, C., Castagna, A., Cossarizza, A., Cozzi-Lepri, A., De Luca, A., Easterbrook, P., Francioli, P., Mallal, S., Martinez-Picado, J., Miro, J.M., Obel, N., Smith, J.P., Wyniger, J., Descombes, P., Antonarakis, S.E., Letvin, N.L., McMichael ,A.J., Haynes, B.F., Telenti, A., & Goldstein, D.B. (2007). A whole-genome association study of major determinants for host control of HIV-1. *Science*, Vol. 317, No. 5840, pp. 944-947.

Fellay, J. (2009). Host genetics influences on HIV type-1 disease. *Antiviral Therapy*, Vol. 14, No. 6, pp. 731-738.

Fernandez Larrosa, P.N., Ceballos, A., Andreani, G., Marquina, S., Martinez Peralta, L. & Rabinovich, R.D. (2006). Viral reactivation and pseudotype production in an in vitro superinfection system with two different strains of HIV-1. *Archives of Virology*, Vol. 151, No. 4, pp. 651-662.

Fung, I. C-H., Gambhir, M., van Sighem, A., de Wolf, F., & Garnett, G.P. (2010). Superinfection with a heterologous HIV strain per se does not lead to faster progression. *Mathematical Biosciences*, No. 224, pp 1–9.

Geskus, R.B., Prins, M., Hubert, J.B., Miedema, F., Berkhout, B., Delfraissy, J.F., & Meyer, L. (2007). The HIV RNA setpoint theory revisited. (2007). *Retrovirology*, Vol. 4, No. 65.

Gonzales, M.J., Delwart, E., Rhee, S-Y., Tsui, R., Zolopa, A.R., Taylor, J. & Shafer, R.W. (2003). Lack of detectable human immunodeficiency virus type 1 superinfection during 1072 person-years of observation. *Journal of Infectious Diseases*, Vol. 188, No. 3, pp. 397–405.

Gottlieb, G.S., Nickle, D.C., Jensen, M.A., Wong, K.G., Grobler, J., Li, F. Liu, S.L., Rademeyer, C., Learn, G.H., Karim, S.S., Williamson, C., Corey, L., Margolick, J.B., & Mullins, J.I. (2004). Dual HIV-1 infection associated with rapid disease progression. *Lancet*, Vol. 363, No. 9415, pp. 619–22.

Gottlieb, G.S., Nickle, D.C., Jensen, M.A., Wong, K.G., Kaslow, R.A., Shepherd, J.C., Margolick, J.B., & Mullins, J.I. (2007). HIV type 1 superinfection with a dual-tropic virus and rapid progression to AIDS: A case report. *Clinical Infectious Diseases*, Vol. 45, No. 4, pp. 501–509.

Goulder, P.J., Brander, C., Tang, Y, Tremblay, C., Colbert, R.A., Addo, M.M., Rosenberg, E.S., Nguyen, T., Allen, R., Trocha, A., Altfeld, M., Bunce, M., Funkhouser, R., Pelton, S.I., Burchett, S.K., McIntosh, K., Korber, B.T., & Walker, B.D. (2001). Evolution and transmission of stable CTL escape mutations in HIV infection. *Nature*, Vol. 412, No. 6844, pp. 334-338.

Goulder, P.J.R., & Watkins, D.I. (2008). Impact of MHC class I diversity on immune control of immunodeficiency virus replication. *Nature Reviews Immunology*, Vol. 8, No. 8, pp. 619-630.

Grobler, J., Gray, C.M., Rademeyer, C., Seoighe, C., Ramjee, G., Karim, S.A., Morris, L., & Williamson, C. (2004). Incidence of HIV-1 dual infection and its association with increased viral load setpoint in a cohort of HIV-1 subtype C-infected female sex workers. *Journal of Infectious Diseases*, Vol. 190, No. 7, pp. 1355-1359.

Hemelaar, J., Gouws, E., Ghys, P.D., Osmanov, S. & WHO-UNAIDS Network for HIV Isolation and Characterisation. (2011). Global trends in molecular epidemiology of HIV-1 during 2000-2007. *AIDS*, Vol. 25, No. 5, pp. 679-689.

Hessol, N.A., & Palacio, P. (1996). Gender, ethnicity and transmission category variation in HIV disease progression. *AIDS*, Vol. 10, Suppl. A, pp. S69-74.

Hu, D.J., Subbarao, S., Vanichseni, S., Mock, P.A., Ramos, A., Nguyen, L., Chaowanachan, T., Griensven, F., Choopanya, K., Mastro, T.D., & Tappero, J.W. (2005). Frequency of HIV-1 dual subtype infections, including intersubtype superinfections, among injection drug users in Bangkok, Thailand. *AIDS*, Vol. 19, No. 3, pp. 303–308.

International HIV Controllers Study. (2010). The major genetic determinants of HIV-1 control affect HLA class I peptide presentation. *Science*, Vol. 330, No. 601, pp. 1551-1557.

Iwabu, Y., Goto, T., Tsuji, S., Warachit, J., Li, G.M., Shoji S., Kameoka, M., & Ikuta, K (2006). Superinfection of human immunodeficiency virus type 1 (HIV-1) to cell clone persistently infected with defective virus induces production of highly cytopathogenic HIV-1. *Microbes and Infection*, Vol. 8, No. 7, pp. 1773-1782.

Jost, S., Bernard. M-C., Kaiser, L., Yerly, S., Hirschel, B., Samri, A., Autran, B., Goh, L.E., & Perrin, L. (2002). A patient with HIV-1 superinfection. *New England Journal of Medicine*, Vol. 347, No. 10, pp. 731-736.

Koelsch, K.K., Smith, D.M., Little, S.J., Ignacio, C.C., Macaranas, T.R. Leigh Brown, A.J., Petropoulos, C.J., Richman, D.D., & Wong, J.K. (2003). Clade B HIV-1 superinfection with wild-type virus after primary infection with drug-resistant clade B virus. *AIDS*, Vol. 17, No. 7, pp. F11-F16.

Korenromp, E.L., Williams, B.G., Schmid, G.P. & Dye C. (2009) Clinical prognostic value of RNA viral load and CD4 cell counts during untreated HIV-1 infection—A quantitative review. *PLoS ONE*, Vol. 4, No. 6, pp 1-12.

Lamine, A., Caumont-Sarcos, A., Chaix, M-L., Saez-Cirion, A., Rouzioux, C., Delfraissy, J-F. Pancino, G., & Lambotte, O. (2007). Replication-competent HIV strains infect HIV controllers despite undetectable viremia (ANRS EP36 study). *AIDS*, Vol. 21, No. 8, pp. 1043–1058.

Leontiev, V., & Hadany, L. (2010). Regulated superinfection may help HIV adaptation on rugged landscape. *Infection, Genetics and Evolution*, Vol. 10, No. 4. , pp. 505-510.

Liu, S-H., Schacker, T., Musey, L., Shriner D., McElrath M.J., Corey, L., and Mullins, J.I. (1997). Divergent patterns of progression to AIDS after infection from the same source: human immunodeficiency virus type 1 evolution and antiviral responses. *Journal of Virology*, Vol. 71, No. 6, pp. 4284-4295.

De Luca, A. (2006). The impact of resistance on viral fitness and its clinical implications. In: *Antiretroviral resistance in clinical practice*, A.M. Geretti, (Ed.), chapter 12, Mediscript, ISBN-13: 978-0-955-16690-7, London, UK.

Manigart, O., Courgnaud, V., Sanou, O., Valéa, D., Nagot, N., Meda, N., Delaporte, E., Peters, M., & Van de Perre, P. (2004). HIV-1 superinfections in a cohort of commercial sex workers in Burkina Faso as assessed by an autologous heteroduplex mobility procedure. *AIDS*, Vol. 18, No. 12, pp. 1645–1651.

Marston, M., Becquet, R., Zaba, B., Moulton, L.H., Gray, G., Coovadia, H., Essex, M., Ekouevi, D.K., Jackson, D., Coutsoudis, A., Kilewo, C., Leroy, V., Wiktor, S., Nduati, R., Msellati, P., Dabis, F., Newell, M.L., & Ghys, P.D. (2011). Net survival of perinatally and postnatally HIV-infected children: a pooled analysis of individual data from sub-Saharan Africa. *International Journal of Epidemiology*, Vol. 40, No. 2, pp. 385-396.

McCutchan, F.E., Hoelscher, M., Tovanabutra, S., Piyasirisilp, S, Sanders-Buell, E., Ramos, G., Jagodzinski, L., Polonis, V., Maboko, L., Mmbando, D., Hoffmann, O., Riedner, G., von Sonnenberg, F., Robb, M., & Birx, D.L. (2005). In-depth analysis of a heterosexually acquired human immunodeficiency virus type 1 superinfection: evolution, temporal fluctuation, and intercompartment dynamics from the seronegative window period through 30 months postinfection. *Journal of Virology*, Vol. 79, No. 18, pp. 11693–11704.

Mellors, J.W., Muñoz, A., Giorgi, J.V., Margolick, J.B., Tassoni, C.J., Gupta, P., Kingsley, L. A., Todd, J.A., Saah, A.J., Detels, R., Phair, J.P., & Rinaldo, C.R. jr. (1997). Plasma viral load and CD4+ lymphocytes as prognostic markers of HIV-1 infection. *Annals of Internal Medicine*, Vol. 126, No. 12, pp. 946-954.

Müller, V., von Wyl., V., Yerly, S., Böni, J., Klimkait, T., Bürgisser, P., Ledergerber, B., Günthard, H.F., Bonhoeffer, S., & Swiss HIV Cohort Study. (2009). African descent is associated with slower CD4 cell count decline in treatment-naïve patients of the Swiss HIV Cohort Study. *AIDS*, Vol. 23, No. 10, pp. 1269-1276.

Nethe, M., Berkhout, B., & van der Kuyl, A.C. (2005). Retroviral superinfection resistance. Review. *Retrovirology*, Vol. 2, No. 52.

von Overbeck, J., Egger, M., Smith, G.D., Schoep, M., Ledergerber, B., Furrer, H., Malinverni, R. (1994). Survival in HIV infection: do sex and category of transmission matter? Swiss HIV Cohort Study. *AIDS*, Vol. 8, No. 9, pp. 1307-1313.

Pehrson, P., Lindbäck, S., Lidman, C., Gaines, H. & Giesecke, J. (1997). Longer survival after HIV infection for injecting drug users than for homosexual men: implications for immunology. *AIDS*, Vol. 11, No. 8, pp. 1007–1012.

Pernas, M., Casado, C., Fuentes, R., Pérez-Elías, M.J. & López-Galíndez, C. (2006). A dual superinfection and recombination within HIV-1 subtype B 12 years after primoinfection. *JAIDS*, Vol. 42, No. 1, pp. 12-18.

Piantadosi, A., Chohan, B., Chohan, V., McClelland, R.S. & Overbaugh, J. (2007). Chronic HIV-1 infection frequently fails to protect against superinfection. *PLoS Pathogens*, Vol. 3, No. 11, pp. 1745-1760.

Piantadosi, A., Ngayo, M.O., Chohan, B., & Overbaugh, J. (2008) Examination of a second region of the HIV type 1 genome reveals additional cases of superinfection. *AIDS Research and Human Retroviruses*, Vol. 24, No. 9, pp. 1221-1224.

Prins, M., & Veugelers, P.J. (1997). Comparison of progression and non-progression in injecting drug users and homosexual men with documented dates of HIV-1 seroconversion. *AIDS*, Vol. 11, No. 5, pp. 621–631.

Promadej-Lanier, N., Thielen, C., Hu, D. J., Chaowanachan, T., Gvetadze, R., Choopanya, K., Vanichseni, S., & McNicholl, J.M. (2009). Cross-reactive T-cell responses in HIV CRF01_AE and B'-Infected intravenous drug users: implications for superinfection and vaccines. *AIDS Research and Human Retroviruses*, Vol. 25, No. 1, pp. 73-81.

Rachinger, A., Navis, M., van Assen, S., Groeneveld, P.H.P., & Schuitemaker, H. (2008). Recovery of viremic control after superinfection with pathogenic HIV type 1 in a long-term elite controller of HIV type 1 infection. *Clinical Infectious Diseases*, Vol. 47, No. 11, pp. 86–89.

Rachinger, A., Stolte, I.G., Derks van de Ven, T., Burger, J.A., Prins, M., Schuitemaker, H., & van 't Wout, A. (2010). Absence of HIV-1 superinfection 1 year after infection between 1985-1997 coincides with a reduction in sexual risk behavior in the seroincident Amsterdam Cohort of homosexual men. *Clinical Infectious Diseases*, Vol. 50, No. 9, pp. 1309-1315.

Ramos, A., Hu, D.J., Nguyen, L., Phan, K-O., Vanichseni, S., Promadej, N., Choopanya, K., Callahan, M., Young, N.L., McNicholl, J., Mastro, T.D., Folks, T.M., & Subbarao, S. (2002). Intersubtype human immunodeficiency virus type 1 superinfection following seroconversion to primary infection in two injection drug users. *Journal of Virology*, Vol. 76, No. 15, pp. 7444–7452.

Rezza, G., Lepri, A.C., d'Arminio Monforte, A., Pezzotti, P., Castelli, F., Dianzani, F., Lazzarin, A., De Luca, A., Arlotti, M., Leoncini, F., Manconi, P.E., Rizzardini, G., Minoli, L., Poggio, A., Philips, A.N., & Moroni, M. (2000). Plasma viral load concentrations in women and men from different exposure categories and with known duration of HIV infection. I.CO.N.A. Study Group. *JAIDS*, Vol. 25, No. 1, pp. 56-62.

Rodríguez, B., Sethi, A.K., Cheruvu, V.K., Mackay, W., Bosch, R.J., Kitahata, M., Boswell, S. L., Mathews, W.C., Bangsberg, D.R., Martin, J., Whalen, C.C., Sieg, S., Yadavalli, S., Deeks, S.G., & Lederman, M.M. (2006). Predictive value of plasma HIV RNA level on rate of CD4 T-cell decline in untreated HIV infection. *JAMA*, Vol. 296, No. 12, pp. 1498-506.

Rosenberg, P.S., Goedert, J.J., & Biggar, R.J. (1994) Effect of age at seroconversion on the natural AIDS incubation distribution. Multicenter Hemophilia Cohort Study and the International Registry of Seroconverters. *AIDS*, Vol. 8, No. 6, pp. 803-810.

Smith, D.M., Wong, J.K., Hightower, G.K., Ignacio, C.C., Koelsch, K.K., Daar, E.S., Richman, D.D., & Little, S.J. (2004). Incidence of HIV superinfection following primary infection. *JAMA*, Vol. 292, No. 10, pp. 1177-1178.

Smith, D.M., Wong, J.K., Hightower, G.K., Ignacio, C.C., Koelsch, K.K., Petropoulos, C.J. Richman, D. D., & Little, S. J. (2005). HIV drug resistance acquired through superinfection. *AIDS*, Vol. 19, No. 12, pp. 1251-1256.

Smith, D.M., Strain, M.C., Frost, S.D., Pillai, S.K., Wong, J.K., Wrin, T., Liu, Y., Petropolous, C.J., Daar, E.S., Little, S.J., & Richman, D.D. (2006). Lack of neutralizing antibody response to HIV-1 predisposes to superinfection. *Virology*, Vol. 355, No. 1, pp. 1–5.

Smith, P.R., Sarner, L., Murphy, M., James, B., Thomas, J.M., Skinner, C.J., & Aitken, C. (2003). Ethnicity and discordance in plasma HIV-1 RNA viral load and CD4+ lymphocyte count in a cohort of HIV-1 infected individuals. *Journal of Clinical Virology*, Vol. 26, No. 1, pp. 101-107.

Sterling, T.R., Vlahov, D., Astemborski, J., Hoover, D.R., Margolick, J.B., & Quinn, T.C. (2001). Initial plasma HIV-1 RNA levels and progression to AIDS in women and men. *New England Journal of Medicine*, Vol. 344, No. 10, pp. 720-725.

Streeck, H., Li, B., Poon, A.F.Y., Schneidewind, A., Gladden, A.D., Power, K.A., Daskalakis, D., Bazner, S., Zuniga, R., Brander, C., Rosenberg, E.S., Frost, S.D., Altfeld, M., & Allen, T.M. (2008). Immune-driven recombination and loss of control after HIV superinfection. *The Journal of Experimental Medicine*, Vol. 205, No. 8, pp. 1789-1796.

Tsui, R., Herring, B.L., Barbour, J.D., Grant, R.M., Bacchetti, P., Kral, A., Edlin, B.R., & Delwart, E.L. (2004). Human immunodeficiency virus type 1 superinfection was not detected following 215 years of injection drug user exposure. *Journal of Virology*, Vol. 78, No. 1, pp. 94–103.

van der Kuyl, A.C., Kozaczynska, K., van den Burg, R., Zorgdrager, F., Back, N., Jurriaans, S., Berkhout, B., Reiss, P., & Cornelissen, M. (2005). Triple HIV-1 Infection. *New England Journal of Medicine*, Vol. 352, No. 24, pp. 2557-2559.

Yang, O.O., Daar, E.S., Jamieson, B.D., Balamurugan, A., Smith, D.M., Pitt, J.A., Petropoulos, C.J., Richman, D.D., Little, S.J., & Leigh Brown, A.J. (2005). Human Immunodeficiency Virus Type I clade B superinfection: evidence for differential immune containment of distinct clade B strains. *Journal of Virology*, Vol. 79, No. 2, pp. 860-868.

Yerly, S., Jost, S., Monnat, M., Telenti, A., Cavassini, M., Chave, J-P., Kaiser, L., Burgisser, P., Perrin, L., & Swiss HIV Cohort Study. (2004). HIV-1 co/super-infection in intravenous drug users. *AIDS*, Vol. 18, No. 10, pp. 1413–1421.

4

HIV-1 Nef Transfer and Intracellular Signalling in Uninfected Cells

Zulema A. Percario[1], Giorgio Mangino[1,4], Valentina Gallo[1], Maria Vincenza Chiantore[2], Gianna Fiorucci[2,3], Giovanna Romeo[2,4] and Elisabetta Affabris[1]

[1]*Department of Biology, University Roma Tre, Rome*
[2]*Department of Infectious, Parasitic and Immune-Mediated Diseases, Istituto Superiore di Sanità, Rome*
[3]*Institute of Molecular Biology and Pathology, Consiglio Nazionale delle Ricerche, Rome,*
[4]*Department of Medical-Surgical Sciences and Biotechnologies, Sapienza University of Rome, Rome*
Italy

1. Introduction

Several lymphotropic viruses manipulate host innate immune response to escape immune recognition and improve viral replication and spreading. From this point of view HIV (Human Immunodeficiency Virus-1) represents a paradigmatic example (for review see Peterlin & Trono, 2003). HIV-1 encodes the classical structural and enzymatic factors of all retroviruses codified from the *gag* (group-specific antigen), *pol* (polymerase) and *env* (envelope) genes. In addition it codes two regulatory proteins that are essential for viral replication (i.e., the transcriptional transactivator Tat and the regulator of virion gene expression Rev) and four accessory proteins (i.e., the ill-named 'negative effector' Nef, the viral infectivity factor Vif, the viral protein r Vpr and the viral protein u Vpu). With time has become increasingly clear that the so-called accessory proteins carry out several critical functions for both viral replication and pathogenesis (Malim & Emerman, 2008). In particular, the Nef protein was demonstrated to be an important virulence factor of primate lentiviruses. In fact Nef-defective HIV leads to an attenuated clinical phenotype with reduced viral loads in mouse models, monkeys, and in human disease (Daniel et al., 1992; Deacon et al., 1995; Gulizia et al., 1997; Kestler et al., 1991; Kirchhoff et al., 1995) and *nef* transgenic mice develop an AIDS-like disease (Hanna et al., 1998) confirming that this viral protein is a major determinant of pathogenicity.

Studies on structure and mechanism of action of the protein highlighted its multifunctional properties at cellular and molecular level. The open reading frame encoding Nef is located 3′ of the *env* gene, overlaps the untranslated sequences of the 3′ viral long terminal repeat and is translated from multiply spliced transcripts. Nef is expressed early and most abundantly during the infection cycle together with Tat and Rev and evidences have been reported of possible expression also before integration of the proviral genome (Wu & Marsh, 2001). It acts as a molecular adaptor inside the cell inducing genetically distinguishable, yet highly conserved, effects via specific protein-protein interaction motifs (Arold & Baur, 2001; Doms & Trono, 2000; Geyer et al., 2001, Foster et al., 2011). In general, Nefs from all primate lentiviruses (*i.e.* HIV-1, HIV-2, and SIV) share multiple activities *in vitro*, but differences between the ability of human and simian immunodeficiency viruses to induce Nef-mediated internalization of the CD3 component of the T-cell receptor complex have been observed and have been correlated with the greater pathogenicity of HIV and the reduction of T-cell activation in simian immunodeficiency virus (SIV) (Schindler et al., 2006). It has been also observed that HIV-1 Nef treatment of uninfected cells in culture causes internalization of the protein in some cell types and/or activates specific intracellular signalling pathways. Interestingly, Nef has been found inside uninfected B cells of lymphoid follicles from infected individuals (Qiao et al., 2006) and recently it has been provided experimental evidencies that it can be transferred to uninfected cells from the infected ones via cellular protrusions and/or exosomes (Lenassi et al., 2010; Muratori et al., 2009; Xu et al., 2009) opening a new road to deepen our insight on the roles of this multifunctional protein. This review will focus on those recent observations trying to provide a unifying reading.

2. Nef: A multifunctional viral adaptor

Nef is a protein of about 200 aminoacids and the different alleles may vary slightly in length. Sequence analysis has identified a number of conserved motifs that are responsible for protein–protein interactions and for specific biological functions. The protein is co-translationally modified by N-terminal myristoylation and is phosphorylated on specific aminoacid residues. Its membrane binding is critical for Nef function on cell signalling and membrane trafficking and requires both the covalently attached myristic acid moiety and a cluster of N-terminal basic residues (Bentham et al., 2006; Gerlach et al., 2010; Szilluweit et al., 2009). Myristoylation appears only a weak membrane-targeting signal, but the N-terminal basic residues, especially the arginine-rich cluster (R^{17} to R^{22}), are needed for the stable association of the viral protein with cellular membranes. Nef appears to be a cytoplasmic protein partially associated with cell membrane and often accumulated in perinuclear regions. Cellular-fractionation assays from transient transfection experiments showed that less than 60% of the protein is localized at membranes, while the remaining portion was found to be cytosolic (Kaminchik et al., 1994). Structurally the 24-29 kDa HIV-1 Nef protein adopts a two-domain structure encompassing a flexible membrane anchor domain (residues 2-61 in Nef_{SF2}) and a folded core domain (residues 62-210). The core domain, again, contains a C-terminal flexible loop of 33 residues (152-184) that is thought to mediate trafficking interactions (Geyer et al., 2001). Arold and Baur speculated that after translation the protein adopts a close conformation where the myristoyl moiety interacts with a hydrophobic region on the core domain, which could explain why the majority of the protein is localized in the cytosol and not attached to membranes (Arold & Baur, 2001). Biochemical indication for myristoylation-dependent conformational changes in HIV-1 Nef has been obtained (Breuer et al., 2006; Dennis et al., 2005). Indeed, Nef is readily soluble in aqueous solution, suggesting the shielding of the lipid moiety within the protein. Protein structures of Nef have been determined for the core domain by NMR spectroscopy and X-ray crystallography (Arold et al., 1997; Grzesiek et al., 1997; Lee et al., 1996) and for the flexible anchor domain by NMR (Geyer et al., 1999), but not yet for the full-length protein due to the low stability and solubility and the high degree of intrinsic flexibility. The protein mediates a multitude of functions, increasing the production and infectivity of viral particles and inducing alteration of specific cellular signalling and trafficking pathways. It has been also demonstrated that the protein is able to induce the transient translocation to the cell membrane of the Polycomb Group protein Eed, a nuclear transcriptional repressor, leading to a potent stimulation of Tat-dependent HIV transcription (Witte et al., 2004). The cytoplasmic translocation of Eed seems to result in the removal of a block on Tat-mediated HIV transcription essential to promote viral transcription at low concentrations of the transactivator protein found at the very early phase of the infection or reactivation from latency. It has been proposed that Nef adopts different structural conformations inside the cell that allows different localizations and interaction with different partners, realizing the so called "Nef interaction cycle" (Arold & Baur, 2001). In particular, Nef, after translation, could adopt the closed conformation in which its binding sites are mainly hidden (closed conformation). Contact with the cell membrane could then trigger a conformational change via the interaction of the negative charges of the membrane lipid heads with the positive charges in the N-terminus of Nef, thus relieving the interaction between the N-terminus and the core. This conformational change could also expose several motifs capable of binding signalling molecules (signalling conformation), many of which are present in lipid rafts. The association of Nef molecules with the membrane might persist for only a short period of time because of the exposure of the core loop, which would then bind molecules of the cellular endocytotic machinery mediating internalization of Nef together with specific interaction partners.

The best characterized Nef functions are: (a) acceleration of endocytosis and lysosomal degradation of CD4, thereby avoiding both super-infection of infected cells and the interaction of budding virions with CD4 of the infected cells; (b) down-regulation of HLA-A and -B MHC-I molecules thereby protecting infected cells from recognition and lysis by cytotoxic T lymphocytes (CTL); (c) induction of a pre-activation state in CD4+ T cells favouring viral gene expression (Simmons et al., 2001); (d) regulation of apoptosis, promoting apoptosis in bystander uninfected cells meanwhile protecting the infected cells by apoptotic stimuli through more than one mechanism (Das & Jameel, 2005). Nef perturbs the trafficking of many different plasma membrane-associated proteins but how Nef traffics within the endosomal system to reach the perinuclear endosomal region where it is concentrated at steady state is not yet understood (Burtey et al., 2007; Roeth & Collins, 2006). The list of cellular proteins whose transport is affected has continued to grow over the past several years. To date it has been reported to decrease the cell surface expression of MHC-I, MHC-II, CD4, CD28, transferrin and mannose receptors, CD80, CD86, CD8, and CCR5 and to increase the expression of TNF, LIGHT, DC-SIGN, and the invariant chain (Anderson et al., 1993; Chaudhry et al., 2005; Lama & Ware, 2000; Madrid et al., 2005; Schindler et al., 2003; Schwartz et al., 1996; Sol-Foulon et al., 2002; Stove et al., 2005; Stumptner-Cuvelette et al., 2001). The acceleration of endocytosis and lysosomal degradation of the transmembrane glycoprotein CD4 was one of the first discovered actions. To recruit CD4 into the endocytotic pathway, Nef acts as an adaptor between CD4 and components of the clathrin coated pits. In T cells this involves disruption of the CD4-Lck tyrosine kinase complex by Nef and its interaction with adaptor protein (AP) complexes and the regulatory subunit of the vacuolar proton pump v-ATPase. Nef binds also to the beta subunit of COPI coatomers (β-COP) to direct CD4 to a degradation pathway. Surprisingly, Nef uses different domains and mechanism to downregulate MHC-I molecules (Blagoveshchenskaya et al., 2002; Doms & Trono, 2000). Regarding the Nef ability to induce a state of pre-activation in T cells several publications have reported its direct interaction with T Cell Receptor (TCR) ζ chain,

glycolipid enriched membrane microdomains (i.e., GEMs also called lipid "rafts") and proteins of the submembrane TCR environment including the adaptor proteins Vav and LAT, and the kinases Lck, PAK and PKC (Renkema & Saksela, 2000). Mutational analysis suggests that most of the signaling molecules that bind to Nef interact with its core domain, often via the Pro-rich sequence that binds the SH3 domain of Src kinases. Nef displays high (*i.e.* nanomolar) affinity for the SH3 domain of Hck and Lyn, and rather modest (*i.e.* micromolar) affinity for those of Lck, Fyn and Src. *In vivo,* the individual tissue distribution of Src kinases become relevant because Hck is restricted to macrophages, therefore in T cells Nef might interact with lower-affinity targets such as Fyn or Lck. As far as regulation of apoptosis concerns, it appears that Nef causes bystander cell apoptosis in uninfected cells through its induction of FasL expression on the infected $CD4^+$ T cell (Xu et al., 1999; Xu et al., 1997). Conversely, it inhibits apoptosis in virally infected host T cells both through its concomitant suppressive effects on ASK1, a key intermediate in the Fas and TNFα death signaling cascade, and via Akt-indipendent phosphorylation of Bad (Geleziunas et al., 1996; Geleziunas et al., 2001; Wolf et al., 2001). In addition it has been described to inhibit p53-mediated apoptosis binding the tumor suppressor (Greenway et al., 2002).
As a consequence of Nef ability to bind multiple targets it is plausible that depending on Nef subcellular localization and the availability of particular subset of targets (for example Hck versus Lck tyrosine kinase), certain Nef effects dominate over others in a time- and cell type-dependent manner thus differing in infected monocyte/macrophages versus T lymphocytes, DC, astrocytes or microglial cells (see Quaranta et al., 2009 for the different regulatory effects of Nef in immune cells). In macrophages, that are important target of HIV infection and reservoir of the virus, Nef expression induces the release of a set of paracrine factors including a marked increase of CCL2/MIP-1α and CCL4/MIP-1β chemokines. These factors are able to recruit T cells and make them susceptible to HIV replication (Swingler et al., 2003; Swingler et al., 1999). In particular, Nef expression in macrophages induces also the production of the soluble forms of the intercellular adhesion molecule ICAM-1 (sICAM) and of the coactivation molecule CD23 (sCD23). sICAM and sCD23 act on B cells that cooperate with macrophages in inducing T cell recruitment and their permissivity to productive infection *in vitro.* The effects of Nef expression in macrophages mimics those of CD40 Ligand (CD40L) in activating the CD40 signalling cascades suggesting that Nef intersects a macrophages pathway that is regulated by the CD40 receptor and requires nuclear factor kappa B (NF-κB) activation (Swingler et al., 2003; Swingler et al., 1999).

3. Effects induced by extracellular Nef in uninfected cells

Evidences that Nef produced by recombinant DNA technology can induce cell signalling effects when added to cell cultures has been provided (Alessandrini et al., 2000; Brigino et al., 1997; Fujii et al., 1996c; Fujinaga et al., 1995; Huang et al., 2004; James et al., 2004; Lehmann et al., 2006; Okada et al., 1998; Okada et al., 1997; Qiao et al., 2006; Quaranta et al., 1999; Quaranta et al., 2003; Tobiume et al., 2002; Varin et al., 2003). Different Nef alleles have been expressed in *E. coli* and both myristoylated (myr^+) or not myristoylated (myr^-) proteins have been produced (Breuer et al., 2006; Dennis et al., 2005). Myr^+ Nef was obtained via co-trasformation of *E. coli* with expression vectors coding the viral protein and the human N-myristoyl-transferase and supplementing the culture medium with myristic acid. Purified myr^+ and myr^- wild type (wt) Nef proteins showed different oligomerisation properties *in vitro.* Indeed, myristoylated Nef prevails in a monomeric state in solution whereas the nonlipidated protein forms dimers, trimers, or even oligomers of greater magnitude. When cell signalling effects induced by myr+ and myr- wtNef were compared in cultures of human monocyte-derived macrophages (MDMs), myr+ wt Nef was found to be much more active than the myr- protein (Mangino et al., 2007; Olivetta et al., 2003). Table 1 briefly summarizes the effects induced by cell treatment with Nef. In particular, negative effects on $CD4^+$ T cell survival has been described (Fujii et al., 1996a; b; Fujii et al., 1996c), *e.g.* Nef treatment of $CD4^+$ T lymphocytes in culture induced apoptosis via the interaction with the CXCR4 receptor (Huang et al., 2004; James et al., 2004). On immature dendritic cells (iDCs) exogenous Nef enhances CXCR4 expression and up-regulates MHC-II molecules, possibly favouring their migration and nonspecific $CD4^+$ T cell activation (Quaranta et al., 2002). Exogenous Nef enters iDCs, promoting their functional and morphological differentiation. Specifically, Nef promotes interleukin (IL)-12 release, which closely fits with nuclear factor NF-κB activation, and targets Vav promoting its tyrosine phosphorylation associated with its nucleus-to-cytoplasm redistribution. Nef induces also the rearrangement of actin microfilaments, leading to uropod and ruffle formation and increases the capacity of DCs to form clusters with allogeneic $CD4^+$ T cells, improving immunological synapse formation (Quaranta et al., 2003). In addition to iDCs, Nef is internalized by primary human MDMs and IgD^+ B cells in culture (Alessandrini et al., 2000; Qiao et al., 2006). Myr+ Nef treatment of primary human IgD^+ B cells induced to differentiate in culture by the addition of CD40L, IL-4 and IL-10 inhibits switching to IgG, IgA, and IgE by inducing the negative regulators I-κB-α and SOCS proteins, which block CD40L and cytokine signalling rendering Nef-containing B cell less responsive to $CD4^+$ T cell help (Qiao et al., 2006). Nef treatment of primary human MDMs down-regulated CD4 surface expression, thus reproducing an effect widely observed in cells endogenously expressing the viral protein. In addition, myr+ Nef treatment of MDMs induces the rapid (15-30′) activation of IKK/NF-κB, MAPKs (i.e., ERK1/2, JNK and p38) and IRF-3, the main transcriptional regulator of the IFNβ gene expression, thereafter regulating the expression of many cellular transcripts (Federico et al., 2001; Mangino et al., 2007; Olivetta et al., 2003; Percario et al., 2003). The prompt transcriptional reprogramming leads in 2 hours to the synthesis and release of a set of proinflammatory cytokines/chemokines, including TNFα, IL-1β, IL-6, CCL2/MIP-1α and CCL4/MIP-1β, and of IFNβ that, in turn, immediately activate the signal transducers and activators of transcription STAT1, -2 and -3 in autocrine and paracrine manner. A transient STAT1, -2 and -3 tyrosine phosporylation was also observed early after (*i.e.* 8-16 hrs later) *in vitro* infection of 7-day old human MDMs with *nef*-expressing Δ*env*, but not Δ*nef*/Δ*env*, HIV-1 pseudotypes suggesting that intracellular signalling induced in Nef-treated MDMs might also be activated via Nef intracellular expression soon after MDMs infection with HIV-1 or viral reactivation from latency. In an attempt to identify the Nef structural motifs required for the activation of those signaling pathways, MDMs were treated with different myr^+ $recNef_{SF2}$ proteins lacking specific conserved aminoacid residues (Mangino et al., 2007). In particular, the viral protein was modified in the consensus sequence required for myristoylation (mutant $G^2 \rightarrow A$), in the polyproline-rich region (mutant $P^{76}XXP^{79}XR^{81} \rightarrow AXXAXA$), in the domain required for the interaction with CD4 (mutant $C^{59}AWL^{62} \rightarrow AAAA$) or with elements of the endocytic machinery, such as the V1H subunit of the vacuolar-membrane ATPase (mutant $E^{178}D^{179} \rightarrow AA$) or the adaptor protein complex (mutant $L^{168}L^{169} \rightarrow AA$) Finally a Nef protein with a deletion of the first 44 amino acids (ΔN-term) was also used. Overall the experimental results indicated that myristoylation of the protein was required for the activation of the signaling cascades, because $G^2 \rightarrow A$ and ΔN-term Nef were the only two Nef mutants unable to induce signalling. These data were in agreement with lack of induction of STAT1, STAT2 and STAT3 tyrosine phosphorylation in MDMs 8 to 16 h after infection with VSV-G Δ*env* HIV-1 pseudotypes expressing the $G^2 \rightarrow A$ Nef mutant (Mangino et al., 2007; Percario et al., 2003). As previously mentioned myristoylation of Nef is a weak membrane-targeting signal and N-terminal basic residues, especially an arginine-rich cluster (R^{17} to R^{22}), are needed for the stable association of the viral protein with cellular membranes. Presently, it is not possible to exclude the hypothesis that also these residues are important together with myristoylation for the activation of NF-κB and IRF-3 in MDMs.

Regarding the production of IFNβ we propose that Nef, abundantly expressed early after HIV infection together with Tat and Rev, induces IFNβ at a very early stage of viral infection or soon after reactivation of viral gene expression in latently infected cells, before the appearance of other viral proteins that can inhibit type I IFN production or mechanisms of action to allow the viral release from infected cells. In fact, even if type I IFNs inhibit the release of retroviral particles and their infectivity in cells chronically infected by the simplest retroviruses without inducing relevant reduction of viral proteins synthesis (Peng et al., 2006; Pitha-Rowe & Pitha, 2007), the lentivirus HIV has evolved specific strategies to inhibit IFN-mediated antiretroviral effects at least via Vif and Vpu accessory protein functions. Both these viral proteins are produced later than the early HIV regulatory protein Nef and inhibit the function of APOBEC3 and tetherin, two cellular antiretroviral proteins specifically increased by type I IFN via positive transcriptional regulation (Malim & Emerman, 2008). In addition a recent analysis of antiviral defences in $CD4^+$ cells during HIV-1 infection indicates that viral expression can also direct a global disruption of innate immune signalling through suppression of IRF-3 (Doehle et al., 2009). In particular, a marked depletion of IRF-3, but not IRF-7, was observed in HIV-1-infected cells which supported robust viral replication. Indeed, IRF-3 depletion was dependent on a productive HIV-1 replication cycle and caused the specific disruption of Toll-like and RIG-I-like receptors innate immune signalling. In agreement with these *in vitro* results, IRF-3 levels were found reduced *in vivo* within $CD4^+$ T cells from patients with acute HIV-1 infection, but not from long-term non-progressors (Doehle et al., 2009). A decrease of IRF-3 expression after HIV-1 infection was observed also in THP-1 cells, a human monocyte/macrophage-like cell line, as HIV-1 infection progressed over a 48-h period. The ability of Nef to induce transient IFNβ production in HIV-1 infected cells *in vivo* needs to be investigated. Nef might induce IFNβ production in cells neighbouring the infected ones if the protein is secreted or released after cell lysis or when transferred via cell-to-cell contact to uninfected cells (Peterlin, 2006). This cytokine could exert its effects on bystander cells, such as the plasmacytoid dendritic cells, priming them to IFNα production. Other HIV products (*i.e.*, gp120) induce the production of type I IFNs in MDMs, as well as in PBMCs (Ankel et al., 1994; Capobianchi et al., 1993; Capobianchi et al., 1992; Gessani et al., 1994). Induction of both IFNα and -β as a consequence of *in vitro* infection of MDMs cultures has been reported (Gessani et al., 1994; Szebeni et al., 1991) and a rapid and transient elevations in IFNα has been observed during the cytokine storms that accompany the increase in plasma viremia in acute HIV-1 infection (Stacey et al., 2009). It is interesting to note that in early 1980's one of the first clear-cut HIV isolate was obtained using cultured T lymphocytes, derived from a lymphonode biopsy specimen of a patient with lymphadenopathy, with the help of IL-2 and anti-IFNα serum (Barre-Sinoussi et al., 1983).

Ref.	recNef Alleles	Cell type	Induced Effects
Alessandrini et al., 2000	NL4-3	primary hu MDMs	- CD4 downmodulation - Inhibition of M- and Dual-tropic strains replication
Brigino et al., 1997	LAV	PBMC H9 U937	- IL-10 induction in a calcium/calmodulin dependent manner
Creery et al., 2002		PBMC primary hu monocytes	- CD14 upregulation
Federico et al., 2001 Mangino et al., 2007 Olivetta et al., 2003 Percario et al., 2003	NL4-3 BH10 SF2	primary hu MDMs	-- Activation of NF-kB, MAPKs and IRF-3 signalling pathways - Synthesis of pro-inflammatory cyto- and chemokines including CCL2/MIP-1α, CCL4/MIP-1β, TNFα, IL-1β, IL-6 and IFNβ that induce STAT1, STAT2 and STAT3 phosphorylation in autocrine and paracrine manner - Induction of IRF-1
Fujii et al., 1996 a,b,c	NL4-3	$CD4^+$ T lymphocytes	- Cytotoxic effects on T cells - Inhibition of proliferaton
Fujinaga et al., 1995		MOLT-20-2	- HIV reactivation from latency
Huang et al., 2004	NL4-3	PBMC Jurkat	- Apoptosis induction through Nef-CXCR4 interaction
James et al., 2004	NL4-3	Jurkat H9	- Apoptosis induction
Okada et al., 1997 Okada et al., 1998	ELI III B	JA-4, Balb3T3 EL-4, WEHI	- Fas-independent apoptosis induction
Qiao et al., 2006	BaL	primary B cells	- Suppression of CD40-dependent Ig class switching
Quaranta et al., 1999	ELI	hu monocyte /macrophages	IL-15 synthesis induction
Quaranta et al., 2002 Quaranta et al., 2003	ELI	primary hu Dendritic Cells	- DC maturation - Cytoskeleton rearrangements through Vav/Rac-1 dependent signaling
Tobiume et al., 2002			- HIV activation from latency through Ras/MAPKs signaling
Varin et al.,2003	SIVmac SF2 BH10	U937 U1	- Stimulation of HIV transcription through NF-κB, AP-1 and c-JNK signaling

Table 1. Effects induced by cell treatment with recombinant Nef

Regarding the response of astrocytes to extracellular Nef, treatment of uninfected cells (*i.e.* human glioblastoma/astrocytoma cell line U373MG) with the purified viral proteins Nef induces the synthesis of C3 (Speth et al., 2002). A significant difference in the C3 synthesis in Nef-treated cells was visible after 3 days and maximal effect was reached after 9 days. Besides Nef, also whole HIV virions and gp41 were biologically active in upregulating C3, whereas Tat, gp120, and gp160 were not (Speth et al., 2002). The complement system is of special importance in the brain because the elements of adaptive immunity have only limited access due to the blood-brain barrier. The complement factor C3 is a central protein of the cascade, and its fragments (C3b, iC3b, C3d, and C3a) affect many cellular processes in the brain, such as activation of signalling pathways and modulation of cytokine synthesis. In general, all complement proteins can be synthesized by various brain cells, including astrocytes, neurons, microglia, and oligodendrocytes, with astrocytes being the most potent complement producers. Although normal synthesis in the brain is low, inflammatory cytokines such as IFNγ and TNFα considerably increase complement production, especially of complement factor C3. Increased levels of C3 and C4 were found in the cerebrospinal fluid of HIV-infected patients with neurological symptoms and signs of central nervous system dysfunction, supporting the hypothesis of an association between complement and HIV-induced neurodegeneration. HIV-induced upregulation of C3 expression in astrocytes may be an important reason for increased complement levels in the cerebrospinal fluid of HIV-infected patients. HIV-1 increased the C3 levels in astrocyte culture supernatants from 30 to up to 400 ng/ml. Signal transduction studies revealed that adenylate cyclase activation with upregulation of cyclic AMP is the central signalling pathway to mediate that increase. Furthermore, activity of protein kinase C was necessary for HIV induction of C3, since inhibition of protein kinase C by prolonged exposure to the phorbol ester tetradecanoyl phorbol acetate partly abolished the HIV effect.

Confocal microscopy analysis of human MDMs treated with myr- and myr+ Nef–FITC indicated that both proteins are internalized and localize in an intracytoplasmic punctate pattern and at the cell margin (Alessandrini et al., 2000; Olivetta et al., 2003) as described for cells that endogenously express the protein (Greenberg et al., 1997). The protein lacking the acceptor signal for myristoylation ($G^2 \rightarrow A$ Nef) is internalized, but loose at least in part the co-localization signal with the cell membrane (Alessandrini et al., 2000). The wt protein does not bind MDMs at 4 °C suggesting that it does not recognize specific receptor on the cell membrane, but it might be internalized exploiting the endocytic/pinocytotic MDMs machinery. Indeed Nef was shown to perturb model membranes opening an avenue for its translocation through cell membranes (Gerlach et al., 2010; Szilluweit et al., 2009).

All these experimental evidences suggest that extracellular Nef if present *in vivo* could induce specific cellular response in uninfected cells that might contribute directly and indirectly to the onset of AIDS. Indeed the presence of extracellular Nef in infected individuals has not been extensively evaluated. The viral protein has been found in the serum of some HIV-1 infected patients at concentration ranging from 1 to 10 ng/ml (Fujii et al., 1996c). This concentration might be even higher in the lymphonodal germinal centers, where virion-trapping dendritic cells, virion-infected $CD4^+$ T cells and macrophages are densely packed (Pantaleo et al., 1991). In addition antibodies directed against this viral protein have been found in HIV-1 infected seronegative individuals supporting the possible detection of extracellular molecule (Ameisen et al., 1989). Nef can be released in culture supernatant of 293, Jurkat and THP-1 cells transfected with HIV-$1_{NL4\text{-}3}$-, HIV-2- or SIV-Nef expressing vectors indicating that it can be secreted (James et al., 2004). The genetic characterization of Nef-induced secretion has identified that the N-terminal 70 amino acids were sufficient for induction of secretion of Nef- containing vescicles in several cell lines and identified critical aminoacid residues: (1) a basic cluster of four arginine residues (aa 17, 19, 21, 22), (2) the phosphofurin acidic cluster sequence (PACS; Glu62–65), and (3) a previously uncharacterized domain spanning amino acid residues 66–70 (VGFPV), which has been named the secretion modification region (SMR). Interestingly, *in vivo* analysis performed on infected follicles of lymphoid tissue showed the presence of Nef positive IgD^+ B cells at the edge of the germinal center and in the interfollicular area even if these cells were unlikely to be infected by HIV-1 (Qiao et al., 2006). This observation suggested that Nef, produced inside the HIV infected cells via the transcription of the proviral genome, can be transferred *in vivo* to bystander non infected cells.

4. Nef transfer from infected to uninfected cells

The transfer of HIV viral proteins by nanotubes (Sowinski et al., 2008) and the transfer of Nef by vesicles (Campbell et al., 2008) has been recently documented. Interestingly in September 2009, Xu and collaborators (Xu et al., 2009) reported that HIV-1 infected macrophages form B cell–targeting conduits in response to Nef expression. These conduits translocate membrane-bound Nef and Nef-containing endosomes from macrophages to follicular B cells via a mechanism propelled by actin, mediated by Vav and dependent on GTPases. These results provided the evidence that infected cells can transfer the viral protein via cell to cell contact to uninfected cells. It appears that Nef-mediated activation of membrane trafficking is bidirectional, connecting endocytosis with exocytosis as occurs in activated T cells. Interestingly Nef expression induced an extensive secretory activity also in infected and, surprisingly, in non infected T cells, leading to the massive release of microvesicle clusters, a phenotype observed in vitro and in 36%–87% of primary $CD4^+$ T cells from HIV-infected individuals. Consistent with exocytosis in noninfected cells, Nef is transferred to bystander cells upon cell-to-cell contact and subsequently induces secretion in an Erk1/2-dependent manner. Thus, Nef alters membrane dynamics mimicking those of activated T cells and causing a transfer of infected cell signalling to bystander cells (Muratori et al., 2009). Based on these findings, it was hypothesized that Nef transfer could potentially explain the effects observed in bystander cells *in vivo*. In agreement with this hypothesis conduits-mediated shuttling of Nef from infected macrophages to B cells attenuated IgG2 and IgA class switching in systemic and intestinal lymphoid follicles suggesting that HIV-1 exploits intercellular 'highways' as a 'Trojan horse' to deliver Nef to B cells and evade specific humoral immunity systemically and at mucosal sites of entry. The stronger virus-specific IgG2 and IgA responses observed in Long Term Non Progressor infected by Nef-deficient HIV-1 further supports this possibility (Xu et al., 2009). In addition Lenassi et al. (Lenassi et al., 2010) demonstrated that the expression of Nef not only augmented the production of the exosomes from T cells (Jurkat, SupT1 and primary T cells) but also resulted in the packaging of Nef into these vesicles which, upon contact, leads to an activation-induced cell death in the resting CD4+ T lymphocytes (bystander cells). It is known that subsets of cellular proteins are specifically targeted to exosomes reflecting the site of their formation. Proteomic profiling of Nef exosomes originating from Jurkat and SupT1 cells indicates that Nef exosomes form at the plasma membrane in Jurkat and in Multivescicular Bodies in SupT cells. Instead Nef exosomes from PBLs represent a mixture of secreted vesicles of plasma membrane and late endosomal origin. Therefore, Nef increases the production of exosomes from several distinct cellular compartments. Nef release through exosomes was conserved also during HIV-1 infection of peripheral blood lymphocytes (PBLs). Thus, HIV-infected cells export Nef in bioactive vesicles that might facilitate the depletion of CD4+ T cells *in vivo*.

Figure 1 schematically summarizes Nef-induced effects and transfer in uninfected cells.

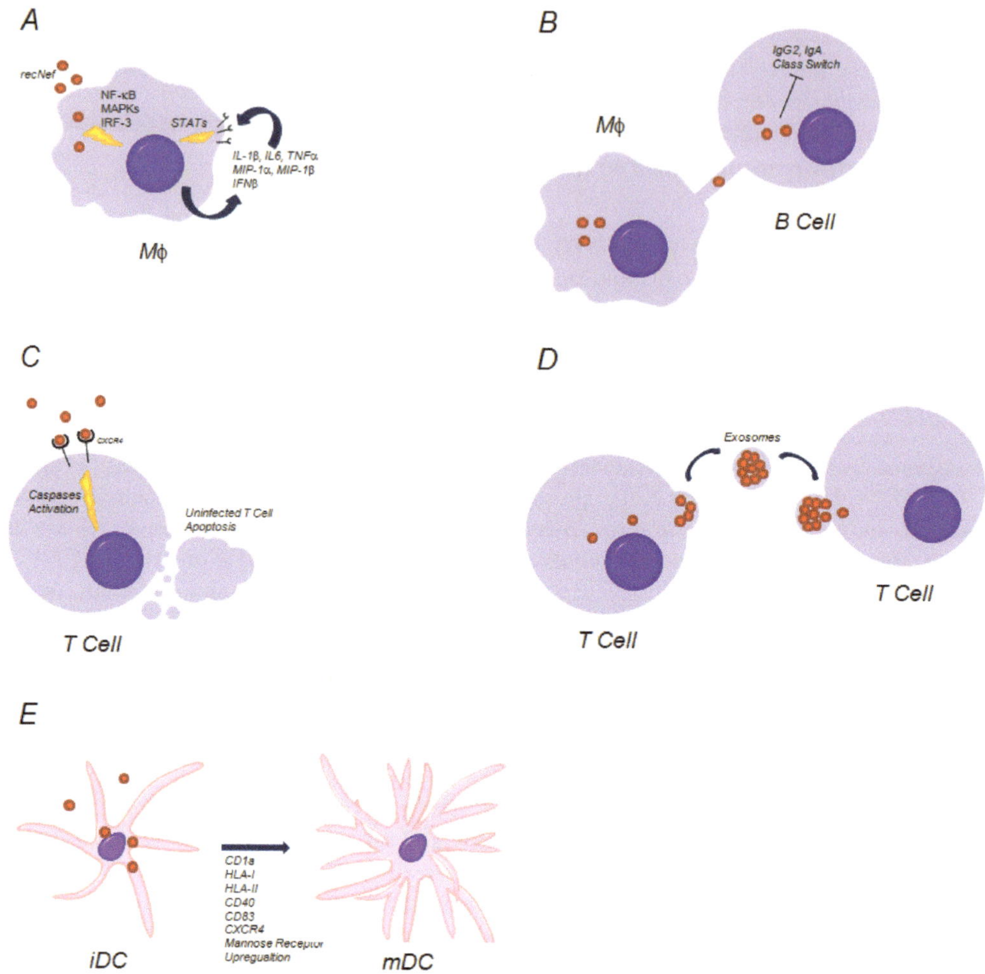

Fig. 1. Schematic representation of Nef-induced signalling and transfer in uninfected cells. A: Nef treatment of MDMs induces signal transduction events followed by production of inflammatory chemo/cytokines and IFNβ; B: infected MDMs transfer Nef via cellular protusions; C: exogenous Nef induces apoptosis in T cells via interaction with CXCR4; D: T cells expressing Nef release Nef-containing - exosomes that are transferred to bystander cells; E: extracellular Nef induces up regulation of specific maturation markers in immature DC.

5. Perspectives and future directions

In recent years, it has become apparent that many viruses induce signal transduction events in concert with virus entry and/or as a consequence of the intracellular expression and release of viral proteins. These events can trigger a variety of changes in the cell, including induction of apoptosis, cytoskeleton rearrangements and global reprogramming of cellular transcription to favour viral replication or persistence. At the same time the innate sensing of some viral components by cells triggers signal transduction pathways to induce antiviral responses. At present, we are only beginning to decipher the mechanism and the consequences of these events to viral replication and pathogenesis in the host. As far as Nef concerns, its ability to induce exosome formation and cell to cell connection mediating its transfer and the transfer of signalling molecules between cells open new road to understand its complex role in HIV-1-host interaction and highlights the complexity of functions of biological molecules. How Nef is able to switch on signalling events in uninfected cells and the patho-physiological relevance of this phenomenon requires further investigations and might disclosure new therapeutic targets for treatment of seropositive patients.

6. References

Alessandrini, L., Santarcangelo, A. C., Olivetta, E., Ferrantelli, F., d'Aloja, P., Pugliese, K., Pelosi, E., Chelucci, C., Mattia, G., Peschle, C., Verani, P. & Federico, M. (2000). T-tropic human immunodeficiency virus (HIV) type 1 Nef protein enters human monocyte-macrophages and induces resistance to HIV replication: a possible mechanism of HIV T-tropic emergence in AIDS. *Journal of General Virology*, Vol.81, No.12, (December 2000), pp. 2905-2917, ISSN 0022-1317

Ameisen, J., Guy, B., Chamaret, S., Loche, M., Mouton, Y., Neyrinck, J., Khalife, J., Leprevost, C., Beaucaire, G. & Boutillon, C. (1989). Antibodies to the nef protein and to nef peptides in HIV-1-infected seronegative individuals. *AIDS Research and Human Retroviruses*, Vol.5, No.3, (June 1989), pp. 279-291, ISSN 0889-2229

Anderson, S., Shugars, D. C., Swanstrom, R. & Garcia, J. V. (1993). Nef from primary isolates of human immunodeficiency virus type 1 suppresses surface CD4 expression in human and mouse T cells. *Journal of Virology*, Vol.67, No.8, (August 1993), pp. 4923-4931, ISSN 0022-538X

Ankel, H., Capobianchi, M. R., Castilletti, C. & Dianzani, F. (1994). Interferon induction by HIV glycoprotein 120: role of the V3 loop. *Virology*, Vol.205, No.1, (November 1994), pp. 34-43, ISSN 0042-6822

Arold, S., Franken, P., Strub, M. P., Hoh, F., Benichou, S., Benarous, R. & Dumas, C. (1997). The crystal structure of HIV-1 Nef protein bound to the Fyn kinase SH3 domain suggests a role for this complex in altered T cell receptor signaling. *Structure*, Vol.5, No.10, (October 1997), pp. 1361-1372 ISSN 0910-8270

Arold, S. T. & Baur, A. S. (2001). Dynamic Nef and Nef dynamics: how structure could explain the complex activities of this small HIV protein. *Trends in Biochemical Sciences*, Vol.26, No.6, (June2001), pp. 356-363, ISSN 0968-0004

Barre-Sinoussi, F., Chermann, J. C., Rey, F., Nugeyre, M. T., Chamaret, S., Gruest, J., Dauguet, C., Axler-Blin, C., Vezinet-Brun, F., Rouzioux, C., Rozenbaum, W. & Montagnier, L. (1983). Isolation of a T-lymphotropic retrovirus from a patient at risk for acquired immune deficiency syndrome (AIDS). *Science*, Vol.220, No.4599, (May 1983), pp. 868-871, ISSN 0193-4511

Bentham, M., Mazaleyrat, S. & Harris, M. (2006). Role of myristoylation and N-terminal basic residues in membrane association of the human immunodeficiency virus type 1 Nef protein. *Journal of General Virology*, Vol.87, No.3, (May 2006), pp. 563-571, ISSN 0022-1317

Blagoveshchenskaya, A. D., Thomas, L., Feliciangeli, S. F., Hung, C. H. & Thomas, G. (2002). HIV-1 Nef downregulates MHC-I by a PACS-1- and PI3K-regulated ARF6 endocytic pathway. *Cell*, Vol.111, No.6, (December 2002), pp. 853-866, ISSN 0092-8674

Breuer, S., Gerlach, H., Kolaric, B., Urbanke, C., Opitz, N. & Geyer, M. (2006). Biochemical Indication for Myristoylation-Dependent Conformational Changes in HIV-1 Nef. *Biochemistry*, Vol.45, No.7, (Febraury 2006), pp. 2339-2349, ISSN 0006-2960

Brigino, E., Haraguchi, S., Koutsonikolis, A., Cianciolo, G. J., Owens, U., Good, R. A. & Day, N. K. (1997). Interleukin 10 is induced by recombinant HIV-1 Nef protein involving the calcium/calmodulin-dependent phosphodiesterase signal transduction pathway. *Proceedings of the National Academy of Sciences of the United States of America*, Vol.94, No.7, (April 1997), pp. 3178-3182, ISSN 0027-8424

Burtey, A., Rappoport, J. Z., Bouchet, J., Basmaciogullari, S., Guatelli, J., Simon, S. M., Benichou, S. & Benmerah, A. (2007). Dynamic interaction of HIV-1 Nef with the clathrin-mediated endocytic pathway at the plasma membrane. *Traffic*, Vol.8, No.1, (January 2007), pp. 61-76, ISSN 1398-9219

Campbell, T. D., Khan, M., Huang, M. B., Bond, V. C. & Powell, M. D. (2008). HIV-1 Nef protein is secreted into vesicles that can fuse with target cells and virions. *Ethnicity and disease*, Vol.18, (Spring), pp. S2-14-19, ISSN 1049-510X

Capobianchi, M. R., Ameglio, F., Cordiali Fei, P., Castilletti, C., Mercuri, F., Fais, S. & Dianzani, F. (1993). Coordinate induction of interferon alpha and gamma by recombinant HIV-1 glycoprotein 120. *AIDS Research and Human Retroviruses*, Vol.9, No.10, (October 1993), pp. 957-962, ISSN 0889-2229

Capobianchi, M. R., Ankel, H., Ameglio, F., Paganelli, R., Pizzoli, P. M. & Dianzani, F. (1992). Recombinant glycoprotein 120 of human immunodeficiency virus is a potent interferon inducer. *AIDS Research and Human Retroviruses*, Vol.8, No.5, (May 1992), pp. 575-579, ISSN 0889-2229

Chaudhry, A., Das, S. R., Hussain, A., Mayor, S., George, A., Bal, V., Jameel, S. & Rath, S. (2005). The Nef protein of HIV-1 induces loss of cell surface costimulatory molecules CD80 and CD86 in APCs. *Journal of Immunology*, Vol.175, No.7, (October 2005), pp. 4566-4574, ISSN 0022-1767

Creery, D., Angel, J. B., Aucoin, S., Weiss, W., Cameron, W. D., Diaz-Mitoma, F. & Kumar, A. (2002). Nef protein of human immunodeficiency virus and lipopolysaccharide induce expression of CD14 on human monocytes through differential utilization of interleukin-10. *Clinical and diagnostic laboratory immunology*, Vol.9, No.6, (November 2002), pp. 1212-1221, ISSN 1071-412X

Daniel, M. D., Kirchhoff, F., Czajak, S. C., Sehgal, P. K. & Desrosiers, R. C. (1992). Protective effects of a live attenuated SIV vaccine with a deletion in the nef gene. *Science*, Vol.258, No.5090, (December 1992), pp. 1938-1941, ISSN: 0036-8075

Das, S. R. & Jameel, S. (2005). Biology of the HIV Nef protein. *Indian Journal of Medical Research*, Vol.121, No.4, (April 2005), pp. 315-332, ISSN:0971-5916

Deacon, N. J., Tsykin, A., Solomon, A., Smith, K., Ludford-Menting, M., Hooker, D. J., McPhee, D. A., Greenway, A. L., Ellett, A., Chatfield, C. & al, e. (1995). Genomic structure of an attenuated quasi species of HIV-1 from a blood transfusion donor and recipients. *Science*, Vol.270, No.5238, (November 1995), pp. 988-991, ISSN: 0036-8075

Dennis, C. A., Baron, A., Grossmann, J. G., Mazaleyrat, S., Harris, M. & Jaeger, J. (2005). Co-translational myristoylation alters the quaternary structure of HIV-1 Nef in solution. *Proteins*, Vol.60, No.4, (September 2005), pp. 658-669, ISSN:0887-3585

Doehle, B. P., Hladik, F., McNevin, J. P., McElrath, M. J. & Gale, M. (2009). Human immunodeficiency virus type 1 mediates global disruption of innate antiviral signaling and immune defenses within infected cells. *Journal of Virology*, Vol.83, No.83, (October 2009), pp. 10395-10405, ISSN 0022-538X

Doms, R. W. & Trono, D. (2000). The plasma membrane as a combat zone in the HIV battlefield. *Genes and Development*, Vol.14, No.21, (November 2000), pp. 2677-2688, ISSN 0890-9369

Federico, M., Percario, Z., Olivetta, E., Fiorucci, G., Muratori, C., Micheli, A., Romeo, G. & Affabris, E. (2001). HIV-1 Nef activates STAT1 in human monocytes/macrophages through the release of soluble factors. *Blood*, Vol.98, No.9, (November 2001), pp. 2752-2761, ISSN 0006-4971

Foster, J.L, Denial, S.J., Temple, B.R.S. & Garcia, J.V. (2011) Mechanisms of HIV-1 Nef Function and Intracellular Signaling. J Neuroimmune Pharmacol (June 2011) Vol.6, No.2, pp. 230–246 ISSN 1557-1890

Fujii, Y., Otake, K., Tashiro, M. & Adachi, A. (1996a). Human immunodeficiency virus type 1 Nef protein on the cell surface is cytocidal for human CD4+ T cells. *FEBS Letters*, Vol.393, No.1, (September 1996), pp. 105-108, ISSN 0014-5793

Fujii, Y., Otake, K., Tashiro, M. & Adachi, A. (1996b). In vitro cytocidal effects of human immunodeficiency virus type 1 Nef on unprimed human CD4+ T cells without MHC restriction. *Journal of General Virology*, Vol.77, No.12, pp. 2943-2951, ISSN 0022-1317

Fujii, Y., Otake, K., Tashiro, M. & Adachi, A. (1996c). Soluble Nef antigen of HIV-1 is cytotoxic for human CD4+ T cells. *FEBS Letters*, Vol.393, No.1, (September 1996), pp. 93-96, ISSN 0014-5793

Fujinaga, K., Zhong, Q., Nakaya, T., Kameoka, M., Meguro, T., Yamada, K. & Ikuta, K. (1995). Extracellular Nef protein regulates productive HIV-1 infection from latency. *Journal of Immunology*, Vol.155, No.11, (December 1995), pp.5289-5298, ISSN 0022-1767

Geleziunas, R., Miller, M. D. & Greene, W. C. (1996). Unraveling the function of HIV type 1 Nef. *AIDS Research and Human Retroviruses*, Vol.12, No.17, (November 1996), pp. 1579-1582, ISSN 0889-2229

Geleziunas, R., Xu, W., Takeda, K., Ichijo, H. & Greene, W. C. (2001). HIV-1 Nef inhibits ASK1-dependent death signalling providing a potential mechanism for protecting the infected host cell. *Nature*, Vol.410, No.6830, (April 2001), pp. 834-838, ISSN 0028-0836

Gerlach, H., Laumann, V., Martens, S., Becker, C., Goody, R. & Geyer, M. (2010). HIV-1 Nef membrane association depends on charge, curvature, composition and sequence. *Nature chemical biology*, Vol.6, No.1, (January 2010), pp. 46-53 ISSN 1552-4469

Gessani, S., Puddu, P., Varano, B., Borghi, P., Conti, L., Fantuzzi, L. & Belardelli, F. (1994). Induction of beta interferon by human immunodeficiency virus type 1 and its gp120 protein in human monocytes-macrophages: role of beta interferon in restriction of virus replication. *Journal of Virology*, Vol.68, No.3, (March 1994), pp.1983-1986 ISSN 0022-538X

Geyer, M., Fackler, O. T. & Peterlin, B. M. (2001). Structure-function relationships in HIV-1 Nef. *EMBO Reports*, Vol.2, No.7, (July 2001), pp. 580-585, ISSN 1469-221X

Geyer, M., Munte, C. E., Schorr, J., Kellner, R. & Kalbitzer, H. R. (1999). Structure of the anchor-domain of myristoylated and non-myristoylated HIV-1 Nef protein. *Journal of Molecular Biology*, Vol.289, No.1, (May 1999), pp.123-138, ISSN 0022-2836

Greenberg, M. E., Bronson, S., Lock, M., Neumann, M., Pavlakis, G. N. & Skowronski, J. (1997). Co-localization of HIV-1 Nef with the AP-2 adaptor protein complex correlates with Nef-induced CD4 down-regulation. *EMBO Journal*, Vol.16, No.23, (December 1997), pp. 6964-6976, ISSN 0261-4189

Greenway, A. L., McPhee, D. A., Allen, K., Johnstone, R., Holloway, G., Mills, J., Azad, A., Sankovich, S. & Lambert, P. (2002). Human immunodeficiency virus type 1 Nef binds to tumor suppressor p53 and protects cells against p53-mediated apoptosis. *Journal of Virology*, Vol.76, No.6, (March 2002), pp. 2692-2702, ISSN 0022-538X

Grzesiek, S., Bax, A., Hu, J. S., Kaufman, J., Palmer, I., Stahl, S. J., Tjandra, N. & Wingfield, P. T. (1997). Refined solution structure and backbone dynamics of HIV-1 Nef. *Protein Science*, Vol.6, No.6, (June 1997), pp.1248-1263, ISSN 0961-8368

Gulizia, R. J., Collman, R. G., Levy, J. A., Trono, D. & Mosier, D. E. (1997). Deletion of nef slows but does not prevent CD4-positive T-cell depletion in human immunodeficiency virus type 1-infected human-PBL-SCID mice. *Journal of Virology*, Vol.71, No.5, (May 1997), pp. 4161-4164, ISSN 0022-538X

Hanna, Z., Kay, D. G., Rebai, N., Guimond, A., Jothy, S. & Jolicoeur, P. (1998). Nef harbors a major determinant of pathogenicity for an AIDS-like disease induced by HIV-1 in transgenic mice. *Cell*, Vol.95, No.2, (October 1998), pp. 163-175, ISSN 0092-8674

Huang, M. B., Jin, L. L., James, C. O., Khan, M., Powell, M. D. & Bond, V. C. (2004). Characterization of Nef-CXCR4 interactions important for apoptosis induction. *Journal of Virology*, Vol.78, No.20, (October 2004), pp. 11084-11096, ISSN 0022-538X

James, C. O., Huang, M. B., Khan, M., Garcia-Barrio, M., Powell, M. D. & Bond, V. C. (2004). Extracellular Nef protein targets CD4+ T cells for apoptosis by interacting with CXCR4 surface receptors. *Journal of Virology*, Vol.78, No.6, (March 2004), pp. 3099-3109, ISSN 0022-538X

Kaminchik, J., Margalit, R., Yaish, S., Drummer, H., Amit, B., Sarver, N., Gorecki, M. & Panet, A. (1994). Cellular distribution of HIV type 1 Nef protein: identification of domains in Nef required for association with membrane and detergent-insoluble cellular matrix. *AIDS Research and Human Retroviruses*, Vol.10, No.8, (August 1994), pp.1003-1010, ISSN 0889-2229

Kestler, H. W. r., Ringler, D. J., Mori, K., Panicali, D. L., Sehgal, P. K., Daniel, M. D. & Desrosiers, R. C. (1991). Importance of the nef gene for maintenance of high virus loads and for development of AIDS. *Cell*, Vol.65, No.4, (May 1991), pp. 651-662, ISSN 0092-8674

Kirchhoff, F., Greenough, T. C., Brettler, D. B., Sullivan, J. L. & Desrosiers, R. C. (1995). Brief report: absence of intact nef sequences in a long-term survivor with nonprogressive HIV-1 infection. *The New England Journal of Medicine*, Vol.332, No.4, (January 1995), pp. 228-232, ISSN 0028-4793

Lama, J. & Ware, C. F. (2000). Human immunodeficiency virus type 1 Nef mediates sustained membrane expression of tumor necrosis factor and the related cytokine LIGHT on activated T cells. *Journal of Virology*, Vol.74, No.20, (October 2000), pp. 9396-9402, ISSN 0022-538X

Lee, C. H., Saksela, K., Mirza, U. A., Chait, B. T. & Kuriyan, J. (1996). Crystal structure of the conserved core of HIV-1 Nef complexed with a Src family SH3 domain. *Cell*, Vol.85, No.6, (June 1996), pp. 931-942, ISSN 0092-8674

Lehmann, M. H., Walter, S., Ylisastigui, L., Striebel, F., Ovod, V., Geyer, M., Gluckman, J. C. & Erfle, V. (2006). Extracellular HIV-1 Nef increases migration of monocytes.

Experimental Cell Research, Vol.312, No.18, (November 2006), pp. 3659-3668, ISSN 0014-4827

Lenassi, M., Cagney, G., Liao, M., Vaupotic, T., Bartholomeeusen, K., Cheng, Y., Krogan, N. J., Plemenitas, A. & Peterlin, B. M. (2010). HIV Nef is secreted in exosomes and triggers apoptosis in bystander CD4+ T cells. *Traffic*, Vol.11, No.1, (January 2010), pp. 110-122, ISSN 1600-0854

Madrid, R., Janvier, K., Hitchin, D., Day, J., Coleman, S., Noviello, C., Bouchet, J., Benmerah, A., Guatelli, J. & Benichou, S. (2005). Nef-induced alteration of the early/recycling endosomal compartment correlates with enhancement of HIV-1 infectivity. *Journal of Biological Chemistry*, Vol.280, No.6, (Febraury 2005), pp. 5032-5044, ISSN 0021-9258

Malim, M. H. & Emerman, M. (2008). HIV-1 accessory proteins-ensuring viral survival in a hostile environment. *Cell Host and Microbe*, Vol.3, No.6, (June 2008), pp. 388-398, ISSN 1934-6069

Mangino, G., Percario, Z., Fiorucci, G., Vaccari, G., Manrique, S., Romeo, G., Federico, M., Geyer, M. & Affabris, E. (2007). In vitro treatment of human monocytes/macrophages with myristoylated recombinant Nef of human immunodeficiency virus type 1 leads to the activation of mitogen-activated protein kinases, IkappaB kinases, and interferon regulatory factor 3 and to the release of beta interferon. *Journal of Virology*, Vol.81, No.6, (March 2007), pp. 2777-2791, ISSN 0022-538X

Muratori, C., Cavallin, L. E., Krätzel, K., Tinari, A., De Milito, A., Fais, S., D'Aloja, P., Federico, M., Vullo, V., Fomina, A., Mesri, E. A., Superti, F. & Baur, A. S. (2009). Massive secretion by T cells is caused by HIV Nef in infected cells and by Nef transfer to bystander cells. *Cell Host and Microbe*, Vol.6, No.3, (September 2009), pp. 218-230, ISSN 1931-3128

Okada, H., Morikawa, S. & Tashiro, M. (1998). HIV-1 Nef binding protein expressed on the surface of murine blood cells. *Medical microbiology and immunology (Berlin)* 186, 201-207.

Okada, H., Takei, R. & Tashiro, M. (1997). HIV-1 Nef protein-induced apoptotic cytolysis of a broad spectrum of uninfected human blood cells independently of CD95(Fas). *FEBS Letters*, Vol.414, No.4, (March 1997), pp. 603-606, ISSN 0300-8584

Olivetta, E., Percario, Z., Fiorucci, G., Mattia, G., Schiavoni, I., Dennis, C., Jager, J., Harris, M., Romeo, G., Affabris, E. & Federico, M. (2003). HIV-1 Nef induces the release of inflammatory factors from human monocyte/macrophages: involvement of Nef endocytotic signals and NF-kappaB activation. *Journal of Immunology*, Vol.170, No.4, (February 2003), pp. 1716-1727, ISSN 0022-1767

Pantaleo, G., Graziosi, C., Butini, L., Pizzo, P. A., Schnittman, S. M., Kotler, D. P. & Fauci, A. S. (1991). Lymphoid organs function as major reservoirs for human immunodeficiency virus. *Proceedings of the National Academy of Sciences of the United States of America*, Vol.88, No.21, (November 1991), pp. 9838-9842, ISSN 0027-8424

Peng, G., Lei, K. J., Jin, W., Greenwell-Wild, T. & Wahl, S. M. (2006). Induction of APOBEC3 family proteins, a defensive maneuver underlying interferon-induced anti-HIV-1 activity. *Journal of Experimental Medicine*, Vol.203, No.1, (January 2006), pp. 41-46, ISSN 0022-1007

Percario, Z., Olivetta, E., Fiorucci, G., Mangino, G., Peretti, S., Romeo, G., Affabris, E. & Federico, M. (2003). Human immunodeficiency virus type 1 (HIV-1) Nef activates STAT3 in primary human monocyte/macrophages through the release of soluble factors: involvement of Nef domains interacting with the cell endocytotic machinery. *Journal of Leukocyte Biology*, Vol.74, No.5, (November 2003), pp. 821-832, ISSN 0741-5400

Peterlin, B. (2006). Nef: out and in? *Nature Immunology*, Vol.7, No.3, (March 2006), pp. 229-230, ISSN 1529-2908

Peterlin, B. M. & Trono, D. (2003). Hide, shield and strike back: how HIV-infected cells avoid immune eradication. *Nature reviews. Immunology*, Vol.3, No.2, (Febraury 2003), pp. 97-107, ISSN 1474-1733

Pitha-Rowe, I. F. & Pitha, P. M. (2007). Viral defense, carcinogenesis and ISG15: novel roles for an old ISG. *Cytokine Growth Factor Rev*, Vol.18, No.5-6, (October-December 2007), pp. 409-417, ISSN 1359-6101

Qiao, X., He, B., Chiu, A., Knowles, D. M., Chadburn, A. & Cerutti, A. (2006). Human immunodeficiency virus 1 Nef suppresses CD40-dependent immunoglobulin class switching in bystander B cells. *Nature Immunology*, Vol.7, No.3, (March 2006), pp. 302-310, ISSN 1529-2908

Quaranta, M. G., Camponeschi, B., Straface, E., Malorni, W. & Viora, M. (1999). Induction of Interleukin-15 production by HIV-1 Nef protein: a role in the proliferation of uninfected cells. *Experimental Cell Research*, Vol.250, No.1, (July 1999), pp. 112-121, ISSN 0014-4827

Quaranta, M. G., Mattioli, B., Giordani, L. & Viora, M. (2009). Immunoregulatory effects of HIV-1 Nef protein. *Biofactors*, Vol.35, No.2, (March-April 2009), pp. 169-174, ISSN 0951-6433

Quaranta, M. G., Mattioli, B., Spadaro, F., Straface, E., Giordani, L., Ramoni, C., Malorni, W. & Viora, M. (2003). HIV-1 Nef triggers Vav-mediated signaling pathway leading to functional and morphological differentiation of dendritic cells. The *FASEB Journal*, Vol.17, No.14, (November 2003), pp. 2025-2036, ISSN 0892-6638

Quaranta, M. G., Tritarelli, E., Giordani, L. & Viora, M. (2002). HIV-1 Nef induces dendritic cell differentiation: a possible mechanism of uninfected CD4(+) T cell activation. *Experimental Cell Research*, Vol.275, No.2, (May 2002), pp. 243-254, ISSN 0014-4827

Renkema, G. H. & Saksela, K. (2000). Interactions of HIV-1 NEF with cellular signal transducing proteins. *Frontiers in bioscience*, Vol.5, (Febraury 2000), pp. D268-283, ISSN 1093-9946

Roeth, J. F. & Collins, K. L. (2006). Human immunodeficiency virus type 1 Nef: adapting to intracellular trafficking pathways. *Microbiology and molecular biology reviews*, Vol.70, No.2, (June 2006), pp. 548-563, ISSN 1092-2172

Schindler, M., Münch, J., Kutsch, O., Li, H., Santiago, M. L., Bibollet-Ruche, F., Müller-Trutwin, M. C., Novembre, F. J., Peeters, M., Courgnaud, V., Bailes, E., Roques, P., Sodora, D. L., Silvestri, G., Sharp, P. M., Hahn, B. H. & Kirchhoff, F. (2006). Nef-mediated suppression of T cell activation was lost in a lentiviral lineage that gave rise to HIV-1. *Cell*, Vol.125, No.6, (June 2006), pp. 1055-1067, ISSN 0092-8674

Schindler, M., Würfl, S., Benaroch, P., Greenough, T. C., Daniels, R., Easterbrook, P., Brenner, M., Münch, J. & Kirchhoff, F. (2003). Down-modulation of mature major histocompatibility complex class II and up-regulation of invariant chain cell surface expression are well-conserved functions of human and simian immunodeficiency virus nef alleles. *Journal of Virology*, Vol.77, No.19, (October 2003), pp. 10548-10556, ISSN 0022-538X

Schwartz, O., Marechal, V., Le Gall, S., Lemonnier, F. & Heard, J. M. (1996). Endocytosis of major histocompatibility complex class I molecules is induced by the HIV-1 Nef protein. *Nature Medicine*, Vol.2, No.3, (March 1996), pp. 338-342, ISSN 1078-8956

Simmons, A., Aluvihare, V. & McMichael, A. (2001). Nef triggers a transcriptional program in T cells imitating single-signal T cell activation and inducing HIV virulence mediators. *Immunity*, Vol.14, No.6, (June 2001), pp. 763-777, ISSN 1074-7613

Sol-Foulon, N., Moris, A., Nobile, C., Boccaccio, C., Engering, A., Abastado, J. P., Heard, J. M., van Kooyk, Y. & Schwartz, O. (2002). HIV-1 Nef-induced upregulation of DC-SIGN in dendritic cells promotes lymphocyte clustering and viral spread. *Immunity*, Vol.16, No.1, (Janauary 2002), pp. 145-155, ISSN 1074-7613

Sowinski, S., Jolly, C., Berninghausen, O., Purbhoo, M. A., Chauveau, A., Köhler, K., Oddos, S., Eissmann, P., Brodsky, F. M., Hopkins, C., Onfelt, B., Sattentau, Q. & Davis, D. M. (2008). Membrane nanotubes physically connect T cells over long distances presenting a novel route for HIV-1 transmission. *Nature Cell Biology*, Vol.10, No.2, (Febraury 2008), pp. 211-219, ISSN 1476-4679

Speth, C., Schabetsberger, T., Mohsenipour, I., Stöckl, G., Würzner, R., Stoiber, H., Lass-Flörl, C. & Dierich, M. P. (2002). Mechanism of human immunodeficiency virus-induced complement expression in astrocytes and neurons. *Journal of Virology*, Vol.76, No.7, (April 2002), pp. 3179-3188, ISSN 0022-538X

Stacey, A. R., Norris, P. J., Qin, L., Haygreen, E. A., Taylor, E., Heitman, J., Lebedeva, M., DeCamp, A., Li, D., Grove, D., Self, S. G. & Borrow, P. (2009). Induction of a striking systemic cytokine cascade prior to peak viremia in acute human immunodeficiency virus type 1 infection, in contrast to more modest and delayed responses in acute hepatitis B and C virus infections. *Journal of Virology*, Vol.83, No.8, (April 2009), pp. 3719-3733, ISSN 0022-538X

Stove, V., Van de Walle, I., Naessens, E., Coene, E., Stove, C., Plum, J. & Verhasselt, B. (2005). Human immunodeficiency virus Nef induces rapid internalization of the T-cell coreceptor CD8alphabeta. *Journal of Virology*, Vol.79, No.17, (September 2005), pp. 11422-11433, ISSN 0022-538X

Stumptner-Cuvelette, P., Morchoisne, S., Dugast, M., Le Gall, S., Raposo, G., Schwartz, O. & Benaroch, P. (2001). HIV-1 Nef impairs MHC class II antigen presentation and surface expression. *Proceedings of the National Academy of Sciences of the United States of America*, Vol.98, No.21, (October 2001), pp. 12144-12149, ISSN 0027-8424

Swingler, S., Brichacek, B., Jacque, J. M., Ulich, C., Zhou, J. & Stevenson, M. (2003). HIV-1 Nef intersects the macrophage CD40L signalling pathway to promote resting-cell infection. *Nature*, Vol.424, No.6945, (July 2003), pp. 213-219, ISSN 0028-0836

Swingler, S., Mann, A., Jacque, J., Brichacek, B., Sasseville, V. G., Williams, K., Lackner, A. A., Janoff, E. N., Wang, R., Fisher, D. & Stevenson, M. (1999). HIV-1 Nef mediates lymphocyte chemotaxis and activation by infected macrophages. *Nature Medicine*, Vol.5, No.9, (September 1999), pp. 997-1003, ISSN 1078-8956

Szebeni, J., Dieffenbach, C., Wahl, S. M., Venkateshan, C. N., Yeh, A., Popovic, M., Gartner, S., Wahl, L. M., Peterfy, M., Friedman, R. M. & al, e. (1991). Induction of alpha interferon by human immunodeficiency virus type 1 in human monocyte-macrophage cultures. *Journal of Virology*, Vol.65, No.11, (November 1991), pp. 6362-6364, ISSN 0022-538X

Szilluweit, R., Boll, A., Lukowski, S., Gerlach, H., Fackler, O., Geyer, M. & Steinem, C. (2009). HIV-1 Nef perturbs artificial membranes: investigation of the contribution of the myristoyl anchor. *Biophysical journal*, Vol.96, No.8, (April 2009), pp. 3242-3250, ISSN 1542-0086

Tobiume, M., Fujinaga, K., Suzuki, S., Komoto, S., Mukai, S. & Ikuta, K. (2002). Extracellular Nef protein activates signal transduction pathway from Ras to mitogen-activated protein kinase cascades that leads to activation of human immunodeficiency virus from latency. *AIDS Research and Human Retroviruses*, Vol.18, No.6, (April 2002), pp. 461-467, ISSN 0889-2229

Varin, A., Manna, S. K., Quivy, V., Decrion, A. Z., Van Lint, C., Herbein, G. & Aggarwal, B. B. (2003). Exogenous Nef protein activates NF-kappa B, AP-1, and c-Jun N-terminal kinase and stimulates HIV transcription in promonocytic cells. Role in AIDS pathogenesis. *Journal of Biological Chemistry*, Vol.278, No.4, (Janauary 2003), pp. 2219-2227, ISSN 0021-9258

Witte, V., Laffert, B., Rosorius, O., Lischka, P., Blume, K., Galler, G., Stilper, A., Willbold, D., D'Aloja, P., Sixt, M., Kolanus, J., Ott, M., Kolanus, W., Schuler, G. & Baur, A. S. (2004). HIV-1 Nef mimics an integrin receptor signal that recruits the polycomb group protein Eed to the plasma membrane. *Molecular Cell*, Vol.13, No.2, (Janaury 2004), pp. 179-190, ISSN 1097-2765

Wolf, D., Witte, V., Laffert, B., Blume, K., Stromer, E., Trapp, S., d'Aloja, P., Schurmann, A. & Baur, A. S. (2001). HIV-1 Nef associated PAK and PI3-kinases stimulate Akt-independent Bad-phosphorylation to induce anti-apoptotic signals. *Nature Medicine*, Vol.7, No.11, (November 2001), pp. 1217-1224, ISSN 1078-8956

Wu, Y. & Marsh, J. W. (2001). Selective transcription and modulation of resting T cell activity by preintegrated HIV DNA. *Science*, Vol.293, No.5534, (August 2001), pp. 1503-1506, ISSN 0036-8075

Xu, W., Santini, P. A., Sullivan, J. S., He, B., Shan, M., Ball, S. C., Dyer, W. B., Ketas, T. J., Chadburn, A., Cohen-Gould, L., Knowles, D. M., Chiu, A., Sanders, R. W., Chen, K. & Cerutti, A. (2009). HIV-1 evades virus-specific IgG2 and IgA responses by targeting systemic and intestinal B cells via long-range intercellular conduits. *Nature Immunol*, Vol.10, No.9, (September 2009), pp. 1008-1017, ISSN 1529-2908

Xu, X. N., Laffert, B., Screaton, G. R., Kraft, M., Wolf, D., Kolanus, W., Mongkolsapay, J., McMichael, A. J. & Baur, A. S. (1999). Induction of Fas ligand expression by HIV involves the interaction of Nef with the T cell receptor zeta chain. *Journal of Experimental Medicine*, Vol.189, No.9, (May 1999), pp. 1489-1496, ISSN 0022-1007

Xu, X. N., Screaton, G. R., Gotch, F. M., Dong, T., Tan, R., Almond, N., Walker, B., Stebbings, R., Kent, K., Nagata, S., Stott, J. E. & McMichael, A. J. (1997). Evasion of cytotoxic T lymphocyte (CTL) responses by nef-dependent induction of Fas ligand (CD95L) expression on simian immunodeficiency virus-infected cells. *Journal of Experimental Medicine*, Vol.186, No.1, (July 1997), pp. 7-16, ISSN 0022-1007

Part 2

Innate Immunity

5

Human Defensins in HIV Infection: Friends or Foes?

Rachna Shah and Theresa L. Chang
Public Health Research Institute and Department of Microbiology and Molecular Genetics, University of Medicine and Dentistry of New Jersey-New Jersey Medical School
United States

1. Introduction

Defensins are antimicrobial peptides (AMPs) and play an important role in both innate and adaptive immune response (Ganz, 2002; Yang et al., 2004). Defensins display broad antimicrobial activities against bacteria, fungi and viruses (Ganz, 2003; Lehrer, 2004; Zanetti, 2004)·(Yang et al., 2004). Importantly, they also play a role in inflammation, tissue repair and angiogenesis (Kruse and Kristensen, 2008; Rehaume and Hancock, 2008). Increasing evidence indicates that the AMPs can act as a double-edged sword by providing protection against invading pathogens but at the same time causing potentially harmful inflammation or facilitating pathogen invasion. This review focuses on the role of human defensins in HIV infection. We will summarize the complex mechanisms by which defensins inhibit or enhance HIV infection in vitro, clinical evidence and studies in macaques with respect to the role of defensins in HIV transmission and pathogenesis.

2. Overview of human defensins

2.1 Defensins and their regulation

Defensins are positively charged peptides with β-sheet structures stabilized by three disulfide bonds between the cysteine residues (Ganz, 2003; Selsted and Ouellette, 2005). In humans, defensins are classified into two subfamilies: α-, and β- defensins, differing in their disulfide bond pairing. The linkages of Cys residues in α-defensins are Cys^1–Cys^6, Cys^2–Cys^4, Cys^3–Cys^5, whereas in β-defensins the linkages are Cys^1–Cys^5, Cys^2–Cys^4, Cys^3–Cys^6 (reviewed in Ganz, 2003; Yang et al., 2004; Yang et al., 2002). Despite variation in sequences and disulfide bond linkages, both families have similar structures (Hill et al., 1991; Hoover et al., 2001; Pardi et al., 1992; Szyk et al., 2006). Neutrophil α-defensins (HNPs 1-4) are mainly synthesized as a prepropeptide in promyelocytes, neutrophil precursor cells in the bone marrow, and the mature peptide is stored in primary granules of neutrophils (Ganz, 2003). Unlike HNPs, human α-defensin-5 (HD5) is released as a propeptide that is processed extracellularly (Ghosh et al., 2002; Porter et al., 2005). An additional class of mammalian defensins is the θ-defensin, originally found in rhesus monkeys (Tang et al., 1999). Primates including human, chimpanzees and gorillas contain pseudogenes of θ-defensin mRNAs with a conserved stop codon in the upstream of the signal sequence that prevents translation (Nguyen et al., 2003). It has a circular structure with the Cys residues linking

Cys^1-Cys^6, Cys^2-Cys^5, Cys^3-Cys^4 (Tang et al., 1999). The θ-defensins are formed by the fusion of two truncated α-defensin nonapeptides that are connected by fusion of the N- and C-termini (Leonova et al., 2001; Tang et al., 1999; Tran et al., 2002).

Human defensins are produced mainly by leukocytes and epithelial cells. HNPs 1-3 were first isolated from neutrophilic granulocytes (polymorphonucleated neutrophilic leukocytes; PMN), and account for 30-50% of total proteins in azurophil granules of neutrophils (Ganz et al., 1985). HNP4 comprising less than 2% of defensins in neutrophils has a relatively distinct sequence but similar structure with HNPs 1-3 (Ganz, 2003; Wilde et al., 1989). While neutrophils produce the highest amount of HNPs, these peptides can be found in other immune cells including natural killer cells, B cells, γδ T cells, and monocytes/macrophages, immature dendritic cells (Agerberth et al., 2000; Rodriguez-Garcia et al., 2007). In addition, cells can absorb and internalize HNPs intracellularly (Ganz, 1987; Mackewicz et al., 2003; Zaharatos et al., 2004), underlining the complexity in defining true HNP producing cells and the questions regarding the function of the up-taken defensins. HNPs have been detected in placenta, spleen, thymus, intestinal mucosa, saliva, and cervical mucus plugs (Agerberth et al., 2000; Cunliffe, 2003; Fellermann and Stange, 2001; Hein et al., 2002). HNPs can be released by chemokines, FCγ receptor cross-linking, phorbol myristate acetate (Chalifour et al., 2004; Ganz, 1987; Jan et al., 2006; Tanaka et al., 2003). Activation of toll-like receptors (TLRs) 2 and 5 by the outer membrane protein A of *Klebsiella pneumoniae* and flagellin of *Escherichia coli*, respectively, triggers the release of HNPs 1-3 by the $CD3^+CD56^+$ natural killer T cells (Chalifour et al., 2004). Additionally, direct interactions of *Mycobacterium bovis* BCG with eosinophils induces the production and release of HNPs 1-3 through TLR2 (Driss et al., 2008). Elevation of HNPs has been reported in the vaginal mucosa of women with *N. gonorrhoeae* (GC), *T. vaginalis, or C. trachomatis* (CT) (Simhan et al., 2007; Valore et al., 2006; Wiesenfeld et al., 2002), suggesting their role in mucosal immunity against infection *in vivo* (Heine et al., 1998; Wiesenfeld et al., 2002).

HD5, the most abundant AMPs in the small intestine, is constitutively expressed by paneth cells but can be found in other tissues such as the salivary glands, the female genital tract and the inflamed large bowel (Cunliffe et al., 2001; Fahlgren et al., 2003; Fellermann and Stange, 2001; George et al., 2008; Quayle et al., 1998; Salzman et al., 2007; Svinarich et al., 1997). Rhesus macaque, an animal model used for studying HIV pathogenesis, expresses six paneth cell defensins but their coding sequences are distinct from HD5 and HD6 (Tanabe et al., 2004). Analysis of intestinal specimens from patients with ileal Crohn's disease (CD), a chronic mucosal inflammation, suggests that NOD2 and Wnt signaling transcription factor Tcf-4 protein may modulate the level of HD5 gene expression (Wehkamp et al., 2004) (Wehkamp et al., 2007). HD5 is induced at the genital mucosa in patients with bacterial vaginosis, *GC* and *CT* infections (Fan et al., 2008; Porter et al., 2005), although the mechanism remains to be defined.

Six human β-defensins (HBD1, -2, -3, -4,-5,-6) have been identified and characterized (Pazgier et al., 2006; Yamaguchi et al., 2002; Yang et al., 2004). Although additional human β-defensins (Schutte et al., 2002) have been identified by gene-based searches. HBDs are expressed by epithelial cells and hematopeotic cells (Duits et al., 2002; Ganz, 2003; Yang et al., 2004). While HBD1 is often constitutively expressed, expression of HBD2 and HBD3 can be induced by viruses, bacteria, microbial products and pro-inflammatory cytokines, such as tumor-necrosis factor (TNF) and interleukin-1 (IL-1) (Duits et al., 2003; Ganz, 2003; Proud et al., 2004; Sorensen et al., 2005; Yang et al., 2001). HBD1, HBD2 and HBD3 have been detected in various epithelial tissues (Fellermann and Stange, 2001; Garcia et al., 2001; Harder et al., 2001). Both human α- and β-defensins have been found in breast milk (Armogida et al., 2004; Jia et al., 2001), suggesting a role for defensins in protecting infants from infection.

The mechanisms of induction of HBD1, HBD2 and HBD3 have been shown to be distinct from each other (Pazgier et al., 2006). HBD2 can be induced by TLR2, TLR3, TLR4, TLR7, NOD1 and NOD2 signaling in various epithelial cells and keratinocytes (Hertz et al., 2003; Nagy et al., 2005; Pivarcsi et al., 2005; Uehara et al., 2007; Vora et al., 2004). Stimulation of TLR3 has been shown to induce HBD1 and HBD2 expression in uterine epithelial cells (Schaefer et al., 2005). Induction of HBD2 and HBD3 but not HBD1 in bronchial epithelial cells in response to human rhinovirus infection is mediated by activation of nuclear factor-κB (NF-κB) but not of IL-1 (Proud et al., 2004). As TLR3 activation also induced HBD2 and HBD3, it is possible that intracellular double-stranded RNA generated during replication of rhinovirus may be involved in the regulation of HBDs (Duits et al., 2003; Proud et al., 2004). Similarly, HBD2 and HBD3 are induced in normal human oral epithelium cells, even in the absence of HIV-1 replication (Quinones-Mateu et al., 2003). Interestingly, a recent study reported that both X4- and R5-tropic viruses cannot induce HBD2 gene expression in the MatTeck oral tissue model nor primary gingival epithelial cells (Nittayananta et al., 2009). Additionally, high concentrations of X4 virus HIV-1_{Lai} block HBD2 gene expression by 50% (Nittayananta et al., 2009). In oral epithelium, TLR2 and NOD1/2 ligands synergistically activate NF-κB and induce HBD2 gene expression (Uehara and Takada, 2008). Cytokines such as IL-1 and IL-17 also play important roles in the regulation of HBD2 expression. Induction of HBD2 by IL-17A is mediated by PI3K pathway and MAPK pathway to activate NF-κB in airway epithelial cells, whereas regulation of HBD2 by the activation of NF-κB is not dependent on PI3K pathway in bronchial epithelial cell, (Huang et al., 2007; Jang et al., 2007; Kao et al., 2008), indicating that specific pathways involved in regulation of HBDs are cell type dependent.

2.2 Immunological and biological functions of defensins

Defensins have a wide range of functions in modulating innate and adaptive immunity(Yang et al., 2004) as well as biological aspects including metabolisms and angiogenesis (Coffelt and Scandurro, 2008; Joseph et al., 2008; Kruse and Kristensen, 2008; Liu et al., 2008; Rehaume and Hancock, 2008; Saraheimo et al., 2008). Both HNPs and HBDs exhibit chemotactic activity for T cells, monocytes and immature DCs and can induce production of cytokines and chemokines (Yang et al., 2004) (Chertov et al., 1996; Yang et al., 2000). HNP1 also regulates the release of IL-1β and enhances phagocytosis (Shi et al., 2007; Tecle et al., 2007). HBDs1-3 recruit memory T cells and immature DCs through binding to CCR6, the receptor for the CC-chemokine ligand 20 (CCL20; also known as MIP3α) (Yang et al., 1999; Zlotnik and Yoshie, 2000). HBD2 has multiple activities on mast cells, including induction of cell migration, degranulation and prostaglandin D_2 production (Niyonsaba et al., 2003). Murine β-defensin-2 can recruit bone-marrow-derived immature DCs through CCR6 and can induce DC maturation through TLR4 (Biragyn et al., 2002). HBD3 activate antigen-presenting cells such as monocytes and DCs through TLRs 1 and 2 (Funderburg et al., 2007). HBD3 activates antigen presenting cells (DCs and monocytes) via TLR1/2 (Funderburg et al., 2007). Defensins are frequently induced by pro-inflammatory cytokines or TLR activation (Ganz, 2003) (Klotman and Chang, 2006). Conversely, defensins can

induce cytokines and chemokines. HNPs upregulate the expression of CC-chemokines and IL-8 in macrophages and epithelial cells, respectively (Guo et al., 2004; Van Wetering et al., 1997). HBD2, known to be inducible in response to bacterial infection and pro-inflammatory cytokines (Ganz, 2003; Yang et al., 2004) can up-regulate IL-6, IL-8, IL-10, MCP-1, IL-1β, MIP-1β and RANTES in PBMCs (Boniotto et al., 2006). HD5 can induce IL-8 (Liu et al., 2007) that enhances HIV infection in cervical tissues (Narimatsu et al., 2005).
Defensins can bind to other host proteins to modulate immune or metabolic functions (Rehaume and Hancock, 2008). HNPs bind to low-density lipoprotein receptor-related proteins and interact with protein kinase Cα and β, leading to decreased smooth muscle contraction in response to phenylephrine (Nassar et al., 2002). HNPs also interact with adrenocorticotrophic hormone (ACTH) receptors and heparan sulfate-containing proteoglycan (HSPGs) to modulate other biological activities (Higazi et al., 1996; Higazi et al., 2000). HNP1 has been shown to inhibit the activity of conventional PKC isoforms in a cell-free system (Charp et al., 1988). This PKC inhibitory activity appears to be important for HNP1-mediated inhibition of HIV replication in primary $CD4^+$ T cells (Chang et al., 2005). As defensins display various biological functions, the roles of defensins in HIV-associated metabolic disorders or cancers in addition to HIV transmission and pathogenesis remain to be investigated.

3. Effect of defensins on HIV infection in vitro: Mechanism(s) of action

In contrary to the traditional role of defensins to defense host against pathogens, recent studies indicate that specific defensins can inhibit or enhance HIV infection. With respect to anti-HIV activities of defensins, these peptides have a dual role in antiviral activity. One aspect of antiviral activities involves direct interaction with viral envelopes possibly by disrupting virus envelopes similar to their antibacterial activity or by preventing viral entry. However, in contrast to anti-bacterial activities of defensins, there is no direct evidence supporting that defensins directly inactivate HIV virion by membrane disruption. The other involves indirect antiviral activity through interactions with potential target cells. These defensin–cell interactions are complex and at least in part mediated by interacting with cell surface glycoproteins and/or interfering with cell-signaling pathways that are required for viral replication. HD5 and HD6, induced in cervicovaginal epithelial cells in response to GC infection, enhance HIV infectivity (Klotman et al., 2008). The enhancing effect of HD5 and HD6 was more pronounced with R5 virus compared with X4 virus, indicating a potential clinical relevance as R5 virus is preferentially transmitted during primary infection. The specific mechanism is discussed as the following and activities of defensins and other antimicrobial peptides on HIV replication is summarized in Table 1.
The in vitro functions of defensins appear to be affected by factors such as the source of defensins, serum and salt. Different antiviral mechanisms of defensins may be operative in mucosal surfaces versus blood depending on the salt concentration or the presence of serum. This appears to be the case with the direct antiviral effect. Serum and salt conditions did alter the direct effect of defensins on the virion (Daher et al., 1986), (Chang et al., 2005; Quinones-Mateu et al., 2003). Some defensins (e.g. HNPs but not HD5 or HD6) at high concentrations are known to cause cytotoxicity in the absence of serum, which is associated with changes in cell membrane permeability, similar to their anti-bacterial activity. This cytotoxicity can be abolished by the presence of serum (Okrent et al., 1990 ;Van Wetering et

al., 1997) and defensin-mediated cytotoxicity may partially account for the antiviral effect (Mackewicz et al., 2003). While most defensins display potent direct antibacterial activities in conditions of low salt (Lehrer et al., 1993), neither a low concentration of salt nor the absence of serum are required for the chemotactic effects of defensins (Chertov et al., 1996; Yang et al., 1999). It is not clear whether other functions of defensins are altered depending on the environment.

Defensins	Effect	Mechanism	Reference
HNP1	Inhibit	Inactivates virion	Mackewicz et al,.2003; Chang et al.,2005
HNP1,HNP2	Inhibit	Up-regulate CC-chemokine production by macrophages	Guo et al.,2004
HNP1,HNP2	Inhibit	Bind to gp120 and CD4, block fusion	Furci et al.,2007;Wang et al.,2004
HNP1	Inhibit	Blocks viral nuclear import & transcription	Chang et al.,2005
HNP4	Inhibit	Bind to gp120 and CD4 (lectin independent)	Wang et al.,2004;Wu et al., 2005
HD5,HD6	Enhance	Enhance viral entry	Klotman et al.,2008
Cryptdin-3	Enhance	-	Tanabe et al.,2004
HBD2	Inhibit	Blocks early RT product formation	Sun et al.,2005
HBD2,HBD3	Inhibit	Down-regulate CXCR4 expression	Quinones-Mateu et al.,2003
Retrocyclin	Inhibit	Blocks viral entry	Cole et al.,2002; Munk et al.,2003
Retrocyclin	inhibit	Binds to gp120 and CD4	Cole et al.,2002; Wang et al.,2004 Munk et al.,2003;Wang et al,2003
Retrocyclin1	Inhibit	Blocks viral fusion	Gallo et al.,2006
RTD 1-3	Inhibit	Binds to gp120 and CD4	Wang et al.,2004

HNP = human neutrophil peptide; RTD = rhesus θ-defensin

Table 1. Effect of defensins on HIV infection

Inhibition of HIV replication by synthetic guinea-pig, rabbit and rat α-defensins was first reported in 1993 (Nakashima et al., 1993), when it was shown that these peptides could inhibit HIV-1 infection *in vitro* following viral entry into transformed $CD4^+$ T cells in the presence of serum (Nakashima et al., 1993). HNPs1-3 block HIV infection through multiple mechanisms (Furci et al., 2007; Zhang et al., 2002) (Chang et al., 2003; Mackewicz et al., 2003). HNPs1 -3 all have similar activities against HIV primary isolates (Wu et al., 2005), in contrast to their differential chemotactic activities on monocytes, where HNP3 has no effect (Territo et al., 1989). They can inhibit HIV-1 replication by a direct interaction with the virus as well by affecting multiple steps of HIV life cycle (Chang et al., 2003; Chang et al., 2005; Furci et al., 2007; Mackewicz et al., 2003; Wang et al., 2004). In the absence of serum, HNP1 has a direct effect on the virus prior to infection of a cell (Chang et al., 2005). In the presence of serum and at non-cytotoxic concentrations (low dose), HNP1 acts on primary CD4+ T cells and blocks HIV-1 infection at the steps of nuclear import and transcription by interfering with PKC signaling (Chang et al., 2005). The post-entry inhibitory effect of HIV infection occurs in primary CD4+ T cells and macrophages but not in several transformed T-cell lines (Chang et al., 2003; Chang et al., 2005). In the presence of serum, HNP1 did not affect expression of cell-surface CD4 and HIV-coreceptors on primary CD4+ T cells (Chang et al., 2005), whereas HNP2 down-regulates CD4 expression in the absence of serum (Furci et al., 2007). HNPs block HIV-mediated cell-cell fusion and the early steps of HIV infection by interacting with HIVgp120 and CD4 through their lectin-like properties (Furci et al., 2007). In macrophages, HNP1 and HNP2 upregulate the expression of CC-chemokines, which could contribute to inhibition of HIV through competition for receptors (Guo et al., 2004). CC-chemokines can also induce the release of HNPs from neutrophils by degranulation (Jan et al., 2006). Both effects could play a role *in vivo* in an innate immune response to HIV. At the mucosal surface, HNPs might work to directly inactivate the virions in the absence of serum; however, in the presence of serum, their inhibitory effect would largely be on the infected cell. HNPs1-3 have been reported to act as lectins and bind to HIV envelope glycoprotein gp120 and to CD4 with high affinity (Wang et al., 2004). The binding to gp120 is strongly attenuated by serum, thus accounting for the loss of the direct virion effect in the presence of serum. Interestingly, in contrast to HNPs1-3, HNP4 acts in a lectin-independent manner and does not bind to CD4 or HIV gp120 (Wang et al., 2004; Wu et al., 2005). However, HNP4 inhibits HIV replication more effectively than HNP1, -2 and -3 (Wu et al., 2005).

Other α-defensins, including HD5 and HD6, mouse paneth cell cryptdin-3 and cryptdin-4, and rhesus macaque myeloid α-defensin-3 (RMAD3) and RMAD4 have been tested for their ability to block HIV infection (Klotman et al., 2008; Tanabe et al., 2004). While HD5 did not exhibit any effect on X4 HIV-1_{LAI} infection of transformed CD4+ T cell lines (Tanabe et al., 2004), HD5 and HD6 significantly enhanced infectivity of HIV-1 R5 strains (Klotman et al., 2008). At high concentrations associated with cytotoxicity, RMAD4 blocks HIV replication, whereas, cryptdin-3 enhances viral replication. Studies on the molecular mechanism of the HIV enhancing effect of HD5 and HD6 indicate that defensins enhance HIV infection through promoting HIV attachment (Rapista et al., 2011). In addition, HD5 but not HD6 competes with heparan for binding to HIV. Importantly, these defensins have been shown to block in vitro anti-HIV activity of polyanionic microbicides, which have failed to protect women against HIV infection, and to interfere with anti-HIV activity of HIV entry and fusion inhibitors under specific conditions (Ding et al., 2011; Rapista et al., 2011).

The anti-HIV activities of HBD2 and HBD3 have been demonstrated under different conditions (Quinones-Mateu et al., 2003; Sun et al., 2005). Similar to HNP1 (Chang et al., 2005), HBD2 and HBD3 have dual anti-HIV activities through direct interactions with the virus and by altering the target cell. The binding of defensins to cellular membranes and HIV virions has been demonstrated by electron microscopy, although membrane disruption is not apparent (Quinones-Mateu et al., 2003). HBD2 does not affect viral fusion but inhibits the formation of early reverse transcribed HIV DNA products (Sun et al., 2005). There are conflicting reports on the downregulation of expression of HIV co-receptors by β-defensins. In studies reported by Sun *et al.* (Sun et al., 2005), HBD1 and HBD2 did not modulate cell-surface HIV co-receptor expression by primary CD4+ T cells, whereas Quinones-Mateu *et al.* (Quinones-Mateu et al., 2003) showed HBD2- and HBD3-mediated downregulation of surface CXCR4 but not CCR5 expression by peripheral blood mononuclear cells (PBMCs) at high salt conditions and in the absence of serum. Interestingly, HBD2 is constitutively expressed in healthy adult oral mucosa but the level seems to be diminished in HIV-infected individuals (Sun et al., 2005).

Retrocyclins, and RTD1, -2 and -3 act as lectins and can inhibit HIV entry (Cole et al., 2002; Munk et al., 2003; Wang et al., 2003; Wang et al., 2004). Retrocyclin and RTD1,-2 and -3 inhibit several HIV-1 X4 and R5 viruses including primary isolates (Munk et al., 2003; Wang et al., 2003; Wang et al., 2004). Unlike α- and β-defensins, retrocyclin does not appear to directly inactivate the HIV virion although it is not clear whether the experiments reported to date were performed under serum-free condition (Cole et al., 2002). Retrocyclin does however bind to HIV gp120 as well as CD4 with high affinity, which is consistent with inhibition of viral entry (Cole et al., 2002)·(Munk et al., 2003). This high-binding affinity to glycosylated gp120 and CD4 is mediated through interactions with their *O*-linked and *N*-linked sugars (Wang et al., 1998). Serum strongly reduces their binding to gp120 (Wang et al., 2004). RTD1 binds directly to the C-terminal heptad repeat of HIV envelope protein gp41, blocking formation of the six helix bundle required for fusion (Gallo et al., 2006). Recently, high concentrations of RTD1 and HNP1 have been shown to down-regulate CXCR4 in PBMCs in the absence of serum (Nittayananta et al., 2009). Studies on retrocyclin-1 analogues indicate that modification of this peptide can enhance its potency against HIV *in vitro* (Owen et al., 2004), suggesting their potential use as a microbicide.

4. Role of Defensins in HIV pathogenesis and transmission

Depending on the preparation of samples and analytical methods, the levels of defensins can be varied from one report to another. In addition, defensins have been found to interact with other cellular proteins in plasma (Higazi et al., 1996; Panyutich and Ganz, 1991; Panyutich et al., 1994), which may affect the measurement of defenisn levels by ELISA. In healthy donors, the plasma concentration of HNPs1-3 is ranging from ~150-500 ng/ml (Mukae et al., 2002). The levels of defensins in the plasma or at the mucosa are frequently elevated in patients with infections or diseases (Coffelt and Scandurro, 2008; Ihi et al., 1997). For examples, defensin levels in plasma from patients with sepsis reach 900-170,000 ng/ml (Panyutich et al., 1993). Using liquid chromatography-tandem mass spectrometry, the levels of HNPs in the saliva from healthy donors range from 1 to 10 ug/ml, whereas the level of HBDs 1-2 range from undetectable to 33 ng/ml (Gardner et al., 2009). The level of HNPs in cervicovaginal fluid from healthy women ranges from 250 ng/ml to 5 μg/ml depending on the laboratories (Levinson et al., 2009; Simhan et al., 2007).

HNPs1-3 The role of HNPs in HIV pathogenesis was first suggested that HNPs 1-3 were to account for the soluble anti-HIV activity of $CD8^+$ T cells (CAF) isolated from patients infected with HIV but remaining free of AIDS for a prolonged period (long-term nonprogressors, LTNPs) (Zhang et al., 2002). These peptides were detected in the media of stimulated $CD8^+$ T cells from normal healthy controls and LTNPs but not from HIV progressors. Subsequent studies on the cell source of defensins revealed that HNPs were probably produced by co-cultured monocytes and residual granulocytes of allogenic normal donor irradiated PBMCs that were used as feeder cells, but they were not produced by the $CD8^+$ T cells themselves (Mackewicz et al., 2003; Zaharatos et al., 2004). Using similar co-culture systems, levels of HNPs1-3 were measured in $CD8^+$ T-cell supernatants and cervical-vaginal mononuclear cells derived from HIV-exposed seronegative individuals, HIV-infected patients, and normal controls (Trabattoni et al., 2004). Higher levels of HNPs were found in CD8+ T cells from HIV-exposed seronegative individuals and HIV patients compared to normal controls.

D'Agostino et al. recently found that HIV-infected patients have a higher level of HNPs in plasma than healthy donors (D'Agostino et al., 2009). Using a co-culture system with radiated PBMCs, higher levels of HNPs in CD8+ T cells were found in patients with HIV infection compared to the healthy donors, and the intracellular HNP levels were further increased in stimulated CD8+ T cells. The intracellular level of HNPs in neutrophils is higher in HIV-infected patients than healthy donors. There is no significant difference in the plasma level of HNPs in HIV-infected patients with or without antiviral treatment (ART). However, reduction of HNPs in CD8+ T cell was found in HIV-infected patients on ART. Interestingly, this reduction in the HNP level was not found in HIV-infected patients on ART with virologic failure. In contrast to the report by D'Agostino et al., Rodriguez-Garcia et al. did not observe any association between plasma levels of HNPs and immunologic or virolgoic parameters (Rodriguez-Garcia et al., 2010). This report also described an increase in HNPs1-3 in dendritic cells, differentiated in vitro, in HIV controllers but not non-controllers compared to healthy controls. While it was suggested that increased HNPs1-3 production by dendritic cells in HIV-infected patients is associated with slower disease progression, analysis of specific immune cell subsets without further manipulation is needed to clarify the role of HNPs in HIV disease progression.

The association between production of HNPs1-3 in breast milk and transmission of HIV has also been investigated (Kuhn et al., 2005). In a case-controlled study of HIV-positive women, levels of HNPs in breast milk correlated with HIV RNA copy number in breast milk, which was a strong predictor of transmission. However, after adjusting for breast milk HIV copy number, higher levels of HNPs in breast milk were associated with a decreased incidence of intrapartum or postnatal HIV transmission. Bosire and colleagues performed similar studies to determine the correlation between the level of HNPs in breast milk and transmission risk in a cohort of 260 HIV-1-infected pregnant women in Nairobi followed for 12 months postpartum with their infants (Bosire et al., 2007). Analysis of breast milk from these women at month 1 postpartum demonstrated that women with detectable alpha-defensins and significantly higher mean breast milk HIV-1 RNA levels than women with undetectable alpha-defensins. Increased alpha-defensins concentrations in breast milk were also associated with subclinical mastitis and increased CC-chemokines in breast milk. Interestingly, in contrast to the report by Kuhn et al. (Kuhn et al., 2005), the level of defensins are not associated with vertical transmission, indicating a complex interplay between innate effectors, inflammation and HIV transmission.

There is a correlation between the abundance of several anti-HIV proteins, including HNPs1-3 and cell-associated HIV replication in lymphoid follicles compared with extrafollicular lymphoid tissue (Folkvord et al., 2005). Expression of these antiviral proteins is significantly lower in the follicular region, where HIV replication is concentrated, compared with the extrafollicular regions in lymph nodes from HIV-positive individuals.

Cationic peptides including defensins are required for anti-HIV activity of vaginal fluid from healthy women (Venkataraman et al., 2005). While it is well established that sexual transmitted infections (STIs) significantly increase the likelihood of HIV transmission (Chesson and Pinkerton, 2000; Cohen et al., 1997; Galvin and Cohen, 2004; Mabey, 2000; Plummer, 1998) and that levels of defensins including HNPs, HBDs and HD5 in genital fluid, are elevated in patients with STIs (Porter et al., 2005; Simhan et al., 2007; Valore et al.,

2006; Wiesenfeld et al., 2002), the role of defensins in HIV transmission seems to be complex. Studies using a cohort of HIV uninfected sex workers in Kenyan demonstrated the association between an increase in HNPs and LL-37 levels in the IgA-depleted cervicovaginal secretions from women with bacterial STIs and increase in HIV acquisition, despite that cervicovaginal secretions with high levels of HNPs and LL-37 exhibited anti-HIV activity in vitro (Levinson et al., 2009). This study underscores the complex role of defensins in HIV transmission at the vaginal mucosa and the urgent need to define the effect of elevated innate effectors on immune responses that contribute to enhanced HIV acquisition.

HBDs Significant correlations between the single-nucleotide polymorphism (SNPs) -44C/G and -20G/A in 5′ untranslated region of *DEFB1* (coding for HBD1) and a risk of perinatal transmission of HIV-1 in Italian and Brazilian populations, respectively (Braida et al., 2004; Milanese et al., 2006). The SNP -52G/G genotype is associated with reduced HIV-1 RNA in breast milk, but not in plasma in Mozabican HIV-infected women (Baroncelli et al., 2008). Interestingly, the functional analysis of promoter indicates that these SNPs suppress expression (Milanese et al., 2007). Studies on the role of HBD1 in mother-to-child transmission of HIV indicated that the -52G/G genotype and the -44/-52G haplotype exhibited a protective role against HIV infection in children, whereas the -52G/G genotype and the -44G/-52G haplotype were associated with low levels of HIV plasma viremia and a lower risk of maternal HIV transmission in mothers (Ricci et al., 2009). Although HBD1 does not exhibit any effect on HIV infection in vitro, the presence of SNP may affect HIV transmission by modulating immune response.

The role of defensins in protection against HIV infection has been studied in HIV-exposed seronegative (ESN) individuals. ESN expressed significantly greater mRNA copy numbers of HBD2 and 3 in oral mucosa than healthy controls, while no difference in mRNA copy numbers of HBD-1, 2 and 3 in vaginal and endocervical mucosa was observed between ESN and controls (Zapata et al., 2008). In addition, homozygosity for the A692G polymorphism is significantly more frequent in ESN than in seropositive individuals (Zapata et al., 2008). Sequence analysis of θ-defensin pseudogenes in ESN female sex-workers from Thailand revealed that all subjects had premature stop codons (Yang et al., 2005). Therefore, restoration of endogenous θ-defensin production does not account for the resistance to HIV-1 infection in these women.

5. Conclusion

Defensins play an important role in innate immune response. These peptides display versatile functions in modulating various immunological and biological aspects. Aberrant defensin expression has been associated with many human diseases (de Leeuw and Lu, 2007), although studies on the role of defensins in HIV pathogenesis and transmission in humans just began to reveal the complex functions of defensins in modulating HIV infection. While the innate immune system is evolutionarily conserved among multicellular organisms, it is challenging to find a suitable animal model to study the role of defensins in HIV pathogenesis and transmission due to complex diversity of defensins in mammals as well as apparent differences in mechanisms of action. Recently, increased expression of rhesus enteric a-defensins (REDs) in response to SIV infection was reported (Zaragoza et al., 2011). Additionally, decreased RED protein levels correlate with enteric opportunistic infection and advanced SIV disease. However, the primary sequences of RED and HD5 differ and it is not clear whether REDs could represent HD5. Future studies focusing on the development of a better animal model for studying innate immunity in HIV transmission and pathogenesis as well as careful assessments of immune responses in patients with reduced or elevated levels of defensins will shed light on the development of better strategies for HIV therapeutics.

6. References

Agerberth, B., J. Charo, J. Werr, B. Olsson, F. Idali, L. Lindbom, R. Kiessling, H. Jornvall, H. Wigzell, and G.H. Gudmundsson. 2000. The human antimicrobial and chemotactic peptides LL-37 and alpha-defensins are expressed by specific lymphocyte and monocyte populations. *Blood* 96:3086-3093.

Armogida, S.A., N.M. Yannaras, A.L. Melton, and M.D. Srivastava. 2004. Identification and quantification of innate immune system mediators in human breast milk. *Allergy Asthma Proc* 25:297-304.

Baroncelli, S., E. Ricci, M. Andreotti, G. Guidotti, P. Germano, M.C. Marazzi, S. Vella, L. Palombi, A. De Rossi, and M. Giuliano. 2008. Single-nucleotide polymorphisms in human beta-defensin-1 gene in Mozambican HIV-1-infected women and correlation with virologic parameters. *Aids* 22:1515-1517.

Biragyn, A., P.A. Ruffini, C.A. Leifer, E. Klyushnenkova, A. Shakhov, O. Chertov, A.K. Shirakawa, J.M. Farber, D.M. Segal, J.J. Oppenheim, and L.W. Kwak. 2002. Toll-like receptor 4-dependent activation of dendritic cells by beta-defensin 2. *Science* 298:1025-1029.

Boniotto, M., W.J. Jordan, J. Eskdale, A. Tossi, N. Antcheva, S. Crovella, N.D. Connell, and G. Gallagher. 2006. Human beta-defensin 2 induces a vigorous cytokine response in peripheral blood mononuclear cells. *Antimicrob Agents Chemother* 50:1433-1441.

Bosire, R., G.C. John-Stewart, J.M. Mabuka, G. Wariua, C. Gichuhi, D. Wamalwa, J. Ruzinski, R. Goodman, B. Lohman, D.A. Mbori-Ngacha, J. Overbaugh, and C. Farquhar. 2007. Breast milk alpha-defensins are associated with HIV type 1 RNA and CC chemokines in breast milk but not vertical HIV type 1 transmission. *AIDS Res Hum Retroviruses* 23:198-203.

Braida, L., M. Boniotto, A. Pontillo, P.A. Tovo, A. Amoroso, and S. Crovella. 2004. A single-nucleotide polymorphism in the human beta-defensin 1 gene is associated with HIV-1 infection in Italian children. *Aids* 18:1598-1600.

Chalifour, A., P. Jeannin, J.F. Gauchat, A. Blaecke, M. Malissard, T. N'Guyen, N. Thieblemont, and Y. Delneste. 2004. Direct bacterial protein PAMP recognition by human NK cells involves TLRs and triggers alpha-defensin production. *Blood* 104:1778-1783.

Chang, T.L., F. Francois, A. Mosoian, and M.E. Klotman. 2003. CAF-mediated human immunodeficiency virus (HIV) type 1 transcriptional inhibition is distinct from alpha-defensin-1 HIV inhibition. *J Virol* 77:6777-6784.

Chang, T.L., J. Vargas, Jr., A. DelPortillo, and M.E. Klotman. 2005. Dual role of alpha-defensin-1 in anti-HIV-1 innate immunity. *J Clin Invest* 115:765-773.

Charp, P.A., W.G. Rice, R.L. Raynor, E. Reimund, J.M. Kinkade, Jr., T. Ganz, M.E. Selsted, R.I. Lehrer, and J.F. Kuo. 1988. Inhibition of protein kinase C by defensins, antibiotic peptides from human neutrophils. *Biochem Pharmacol* 37:951-956.

Chertov, O., D.F. Michiel, L. Xu, J.M. Wang, K. Tani, W.J. Murphy, D.L. Longo, D.D. Taub, and J.J. Oppenheim. 1996. Identification of defensin-1, defensin-2, and CAP37/azurocidin as T-cell chemoattractant proteins released from interleukin-8-stimulated neutrophils. *J Biol Chem* 271:2935-2940.

Chesson, H.W., and S.D. Pinkerton. 2000. Sexually transmitted diseases and the increased risk for HIV transmission: implications for cost-effectiveness analyses of sexually transmitted disease prevention interventions. *J Acquir Immune Defic Syndr* 24:48-56.

Coffelt, S.B., and A.B. Scandurro. 2008. Tumors sound the alarmin(s). *Cancer Res* 68:6482-6485.

Cohen, M.S., I.F. Hoffman, R.A. Royce, P. Kazembe, J.R. Dyer, C.C. Daly, D. Zimba, P.L. Vernazza, M. Maida, S.A. Fiscus, and J.J. Eron, Jr. 1997. Reduction of concentration of HIV-1 in semen after treatment of urethritis: implications for prevention of sexual transmission of HIV-1. AIDSCAP Malawi Research Group. *Lancet* 349:1868-1873.

Cole, A.M., T. Hong, L.M. Boo, T. Nguyen, C. Zhao, G. Bristol, J.A. Zack, A.J. Waring, O.O. Yang, and R.I. Lehrer. 2002. Retrocyclin: a primate peptide that protects cells from infection by T- and M-tropic strains of HIV-1. *Proc Natl Acad Sci U S A* 99:1813-1818.

Cunliffe, R.N. 2003. Alpha-defensins in the gastrointestinal tract. *Mol Immunol* 40:463-467.

Cunliffe, R.N., F.R. Rose, J. Keyte, L. Abberley, W.C. Chan, and Y.R. Mahida. 2001. Human defensin 5 is stored in precursor form in normal Paneth cells and is expressed by some villous epithelial cells and by metaplastic Paneth cells in the colon in inflammatory bowel disease. *Gut* 48:176-185.

D'Agostino, C., M. Lichtner, C.M. Mastroianni, G. Ceccarelli, M. Iannetta, S. Antonucci, V. Vullo, and A.P. Massetti. 2009. In vivo release of alpha-defensins in plasma, neutrophils and CD8 T-lymphocytes of patients with HIV infection. *Curr HIV Res* 7:650-655.

Daher, K.A., M.E. Selsted, and R.I. Lehrer. 1986. Direct inactivation of viruses by human granulocyte defensins. *J Virol* 60:1068-1074.

de Leeuw, E., and W. Lu. 2007. Human defensins: turning defense into offense? *Infect Disord Drug Targets* 7:67-70.

Ding, J., A. Rapista, N. Teleshova, W. Lu, M.E. Klotman, and T.L. Chang. 2011. Mucosal human defensins 5 and 6 antagonize the anti-HIV activity of candidate polyanion microbicides. *J Innate Immun* 3:208-212.

Driss, V., F. Legrand, E. Hermann, S. Loiseau, Y. Guerardel, L. Kremer, E. Adam, G. Woerly, D. Dombrowicz, and M. Capron. 2008. TLR2-dependent eosinophil interactions with mycobacteria : role of {alpha}-defensins. *Blood*

Duits, L.A., P.H. Nibbering, E. van Strijen, J.B. Vos, S.P. Mannesse-Lazeroms, M.A. van Sterkenburg, and P.S. Hiemstra. 2003. Rhinovirus increases human beta-defensin-2 and -3 mRNA expression in cultured bronchial epithelial cells. *FEMS Immunol Med Microbiol* 38:59-64.

Duits, L.A., B. Ravensbergen, M. Rademaker, P.S. Hiemstra, and P.H. Nibbering. 2002. Expression of beta-defensin 1 and 2 mRNA by human monocytes, macrophages and dendritic cells. *Immunology* 106:517-525.

Fahlgren, A., S. Hammarstrom, A. Danielsson, and M.L. Hammarstrom. 2003. Increased expression of antimicrobial peptides and lysozyme in colonic epithelial cells of patients with ulcerative colitis. *Clin Exp Immunol* 131:90-101.

Fan, S.R., X.P. Liu, and Q.P. Liao. 2008. Human defensins and cytokines in vaginal lavage fluid of women with bacterial vaginosis. *Int J Gynaecol Obstet*

Fellermann, K., and E.F. Stange. 2001. Defensins -- innate immunity at the epithelial frontier. *Eur J Gastroenterol Hepatol* 13:771-776.

Folkvord, J.M., C. Armon, and E. Connick. 2005. Lymphoid follicles are sites of heightened human immunodeficiency virus type 1 (HIV-1) replication and reduced antiretroviral effector mechanisms. *AIDS Res Hum Retroviruses* 21:363-370.

Funderburg, N., M.M. Lederman, Z. Feng, M.G. Drage, J. Jadlowsky, C.V. Harding, A. Weinberg, and S.F. Sieg. 2007. Human -defensin-3 activates professional antigen-presenting cells via Toll-like receptors 1 and 2. *Proc Natl Acad Sci U S A* 104:18631-18635.

Furci, L., F. Sironi, M. Tolazzi, L. Vassena, and P. Lusso. 2007. Alpha-defensins block the early steps of HIV-1 infection: interference with the binding of gp120 to CD4. *Blood* 109:2928-2935.

Gallo, S.A., W. Wang, S.S. Rawat, G. Jung, A.J. Waring, A.M. Cole, H. Lu, X. Yan, N.L. Daly, D.J. Craik, S. Jiang, R.I. Lehrer, and R. Blumenthal. 2006. Theta-defensins prevent HIV-1 Env-mediated fusion by binding gp41 and blocking 6-helix bundle formation. *J Biol Chem* 281:18787-18792.

Galvin, S.R., and M.S. Cohen. 2004. The role of sexually transmitted diseases in HIV transmission. *Nat Rev Microbiol* 2:33-42.

Ganz, T. 1987. Extracellular release of antimicrobial defensins by human polymorphonuclear leukocytes. *Infect Immun* 55:568-571.

Ganz, T. 2002. Epithelia: not just physical barriers. *Proc Natl Acad Sci U S A* 99:3357-3358.

Ganz, T. 2003. Defensins: antimicrobial peptides of innate immunity. *Nat Rev Immunol* 3:710-720.

Ganz, T., M.E. Selsted, D. Szklarek, S.S. Harwig, K. Daher, D.F. Bainton, and R.I. Lehrer. 1985. Defensins. Natural peptide antibiotics of human neutrophils. *J Clin Invest* 76:1427-1435.

Garcia, J.R., F. Jaumann, S. Schulz, A. Krause, J. Rodriguez-Jimenez, U. Forssmann, K. Adermann, E. Kluver, C. Vogelmeier, D. Becker, R. Hedrich, W.G. Forssmann, and R. Bals. 2001. Identification of a novel, multifunctional beta-defensin (human beta-defensin 3) with specific antimicrobial activity. Its interaction with plasma membranes of Xenopus oocytes and the induction of macrophage chemoattraction. *Cell Tissue Res* 306:257-264.

Gardner, M.S., M.D. Rowland, A.Y. Siu, J.L. Bundy, D.K. Wagener, and J.L. Stephenson. 2009. Comprehensive defensin assay for saliva. *Anal Chem* 81:557-566.

George, M.D., J. Wehkamp, R.J. Kays, C.M. Leutenegger, S. Sabir, I. Grishina, S. Dandekar, and C.L. Bevins. 2008. In vivo gene expression profiling of human intestinal epithelial cells: analysis by laser microdissection of formalin fixed tissues. *BMC Genomics* 9:209.

Ghosh, D., E. Porter, B. Shen, S.K. Lee, D. Wilk, J. Drazba, S.P. Yadav, J.W. Crabb, T. Ganz, and C.L. Bevins. 2002. Paneth cell trypsin is the processing enzyme for human defensin-5. *Nat Immunol* 3:583-590.

Guo, C.J., N. Tan, L. Song, S.D. Douglas, and W.Z. Ho. 2004. Alpha-defensins inhibit HIV infection of macrophages through upregulation of CC-chemokines. *Aids* 18:1217-1218.

Harder, J., J. Bartels, E. Christophers, and J.M. Schroder. 2001. Isolation and characterization of human beta -defensin-3, a novel human inducible peptide antibiotic. *J Biol Chem* 276:5707-5713.

Hein, M., E.V. Valore, R.B. Helmig, N. Uldbjerg, and T. Ganz. 2002. Antimicrobial factors in the cervical mucus plug. *Am J Obstet Gynecol* 187:137-144.

Heine, R.P., H. Wiesenfeld, L. Mortimer, and P.C. Greig. 1998. Amniotic fluid defensins: potential markers of subclinical intrauterine infection. *Clin Infect Dis* 27:513-518.

Hertz, C.J., Q. Wu, E.M. Porter, Y.J. Zhang, K.H. Weismuller, P.J. Godowski, T. Ganz, S.H. Randell, and R.L. Modlin. 2003. Activation of Toll-like receptor 2 on human tracheobronchial epithelial cells induces the antimicrobial peptide human beta defensin-2. *J Immunol* 171:6820-6826.

Higazi, A.A., T. Ganz, K. Kariko, and D.B. Cines. 1996. Defensin modulates tissue-type plasminogen activator and plasminogen binding to fibrin and endothelial cells. *J Biol Chem* 271:17650-17655.

Higazi, A.A., T. Nassar, T. Ganz, D.J. Rader, R. Udassin, K. Bdeir, E. Hiss, B.S. Sachais, K.J. Williams, E. Leitersdorf, and D.B. Cines. 2000. The alpha-defensins stimulate proteoglycan-dependent catabolism of low-density lipoprotein by vascular cells: a new class of inflammatory apolipoprotein and a possible contributor to atherogenesis. *Blood* 96:1393-1398.

Hill, C.P., J. Yee, M.E. Selsted, and D. Eisenberg. 1991. Crystal structure of defensin HNP-3, an amphiphilic dimer: mechanisms of membrane permeabilization. *Science* 251:1481-1485.

Hoover, D.M., O. Chertov, and J. Lubkowski. 2001. The structure of human beta-defensin-1: new insights into structural properties of beta-defensins. *J Biol Chem* 276:39021-39026.

Huang, F., C.Y. Kao, S. Wachi, P. Thai, J. Ryu, and R. Wu. 2007. Requirement for both JAK-mediated PI3K signaling and ACT1/TRAF6/TAK1-dependent NF-kappaB activation by IL-17A in enhancing cytokine expression in human airway epithelial cells. *J Immunol* 179:6504-6513.

Ihi, T., M. Nakazato, H. Mukae, and S. Matsukura. 1997. Elevated concentrations of human neutrophil peptides in plasma, blood, and body fluids from patients with infections. *Clin Infect Dis* 25:1134-1140.

Jan, M.S., Y.H. Huang, B. Shieh, R.H. Teng, Y.P. Yan, Y.T. Lee, K.K. Liao, and C. Li. 2006. CC Chemokines Induce Neutrophils to Chemotaxis, Degranulation, and alpha-Defensin Release. *J Acquir Immune Defic Syndr* 41:6-16.

Jang, B.C., K.J. Lim, M.H. Suh, J.G. Park, and S.I. Suh. 2007. Dexamethasone suppresses interleukin-1beta-induced human beta-defensin 2 mRNA expression: involvement of p38 MAPK, JNK, MKP-1, and NF-kappaB transcriptional factor in A549 cells. *FEMS Immunol Med Microbiol* 51:171-184.

Jia, H.P., T. Starner, M. Ackermann, P. Kirby, B.F. Tack, and P.B. McCray, Jr. 2001. Abundant human beta-defensin-1 expression in milk and mammary gland epithelium. *J Pediatr* 138:109-112.

Joseph, G., L. Tarnow, A.S. Astrup, T.K. Hansen, H.H. Parving, A. Flyvbjerg, and J. Frystyk. 2008. Plasma alpha-defensin is associated with cardiovascular morbidity and mortality in type 1 diabetic patients. *J Clin Endocrinol Metab* 93:1470-1475.

Kao, C.Y., C. Kim, F. Huang, and R. Wu. 2008. Requirements for two proximal NF-kappaB binding sites and IkappaB-zeta in IL-17A-induced human beta-defensin 2 expression by conducting airway epithelium. *J Biol Chem* 283:15309-15318.

Klotman, M.E., and T.L. Chang. 2006. Defensins in innate antiviral immunity. *Nat Rev Immunol* 6:447-456.

Klotman, M.E., A. Rapista, N. Teleshova, A. Micsenyi, G.A. Jarvis, W. Lu, E. Porter, and T.L. Chang. 2008. Neisseria gonorrhoeae-Induced Human Defensins 5 and 6 Increase HIV Infectivity: Role in Enhanced Transmission. *J Immunol* 180:6176-6185.

Kruse, T., and H.H. Kristensen. 2008. Using antimicrobial host defense peptides as anti-infective and immunomodulatory agents. *Expert Rev Anti Infect Ther* 6:887-895.

Kuhn, L., D. Trabattoni, C. Kankasa, K. Semrau, P. Kasonde, F. Lissoni, M. Sinkala, M. Ghosh, C. Vwalika, G.M. Aldrovandi, D.M. Thea, and M. Clerici. 2005. Alpha-defensins in the prevention of HIV transmission among breastfed infants. *J Acquir Immune Defic Syndr* 39:138-142.

Lehrer, R.I. 2004. Primate defensins. *Nat Rev Microbiol* 2:727-738.

Lehrer, R.I., A.K. Lichtenstein, and T. Ganz. 1993. Defensins: antimicrobial and cytotoxic peptides of mammalian cells. *Annu Rev Immunol* 11:105-128.

Leonova, L., V.N. Kokryakov, G. Aleshina, T. Hong, T. Nguyen, C. Zhao, A.J. Waring, and R.I. Lehrer. 2001. Circular minidefensins and posttranslational generation of molecular diversity. *J Leukoc Biol* 70:461-464.

Levinson, P., R. Kaul, J. Kimani, E. Ngugi, S. Moses, K.S. MacDonald, K. Broliden, and T. Hirbod. 2009. Levels of innate immune factors in genital fluids: association of alpha defensins and LL-37 with genital infections and increased HIV acquisition. *Aids* 23:309-317.

Liu, C.Y., H.C. Lin, C.T. Yu, S.M. Lin, K.Y. Lee, H.C. Chen, C.L. Chou, C.D. Huang, P.C. Chou, W.T. Liu, C.H. Wang, and H.P. Kuo. 2007. The concentration-dependent chemokine release and pro-apoptotic effects of neutrophil-derived alpha-defensin-1 on human bronchial and alveolar epithelial cells. *Life Sci* 80:749-758.

Liu, H.Y., Q.F. Collins, F. Moukdar, D. Zhuo, J. Han, T. Hong, S. Collins, and W. Cao. 2008. Suppression of hepatic glucose production by human neutrophil alpha-defensins through a signaling pathway distinct from insulin. *J Biol Chem* 283:12056-12063.

Mabey, D. 2000. Interactions between HIV infection and other sexually transmitted diseases. *Trop Med Int Health* 5:A32-36.

Mackewicz, C.E., J. Yuan, P. Tran, L. Diaz, E. Mack, M.E. Selsted, and J.A. Levy. 2003. alpha-Defensins can have anti-HIV activity but are not CD8 cell anti-HIV factors. *Aids* 17:F23-32.

Milanese, M., L. Segat, and S. Crovella. 2007. Transcriptional effect of DEFB1 gene 5' untranslated region polymorphisms. *Cancer Res* 67:5997; author reply 5997.

Milanese, M., L. Segat, A. Pontillo, L.C. Arraes, J.L. de Lima Filho, and S. Crovella. 2006. DEFB1 gene polymorphisms and increased risk of HIV-1 infection in Brazilian children. *Aids* 20:1673-1675.

Mukae, H., H. Iiboshi, M. Nakazato, T. Hiratsuka, M. Tokojima, K. Abe, J. Ashitani, J. Kadota, S. Matsukura, and S. Kohno. 2002. Raised plasma concentrations of alpha-defensins in patients with idiopathic pulmonary fibrosis. *Thorax* 57:623-628.

Munk, C., G. Wei, O.O. Yang, A.J. Waring, W. Wang, T. Hong, R.I. Lehrer, N.R. Landau, and A.M. Cole. 2003. The theta-defensin, retrocyclin, inhibits HIV-1 entry. *AIDS Res Hum Retroviruses* 19:875-881.

Nagy, I., A. Pivarcsi, A. Koreck, M. Szell, E. Urban, and L. Kemeny. 2005. Distinct strains of Propionibacterium acnes induce selective human beta-defensin-2 and interleukin-8 expression in human keratinocytes through toll-like receptors. *J Invest Dermatol* 124:931-938.

Nakashima, H., N. Yamamoto, M. Masuda, and N. Fujii. 1993. Defensins inhibit HIV replication in vitro. *Aids* 7:1129.

Narimatsu, R., D. Wolday, and B.K. Patterson. 2005. IL-8 increases transmission of HIV type 1 in cervical explant tissue. *AIDS Res Hum Retroviruses* 21:228-233.

Nassar, T., S. Akkawi, R. Bar-Shavit, A. Haj-Yehia, K. Bdeir, A.B. Al-Mehdi, M. Tarshis, and A.A. Higazi. 2002. Human alpha-defensin regulates smooth muscle cell contraction: a role for low-density lipoprotein receptor-related protein/alpha 2-macroglobulin receptor. *Blood* 100:4026-4032.

Nguyen, T.X., A.M. Cole, and R.I. Lehrer. 2003. Evolution of primate theta-defensins: a serpentine path to a sweet tooth. *Peptides* 24:1647-1654.

Nittayananta, W., F. Hladik, M. Klausner, S. Harb, B.A. Dale, and R.W. Coombs. 2009. HIV type 1 fails to trigger innate immune factor synthesis in differentiated oral epithelium. *AIDS Res Hum Retroviruses* 25:1013-1021.

Niyonsaba, F., M. Hirata, H. Ogawa, and I. Nagaoka. 2003. Epithelial cell-derived antibacterial peptides human beta-defensins and cathelicidin: multifunctional activities on mast cells. *Curr Drug Targets Inflamm Allergy* 2:224-231.

Okrent, D.G., A.K. Lichtenstein, and T. Ganz. 1990. Direct cytotoxicity of polymorphonuclear leukocyte granule proteins to human lung-derived cells and endothelial cells. *Am Rev Respir Dis* 141:179-185.

Owen, S.M., D.L. Rudolph, W. Wang, A.M. Cole, A.J. Waring, R.B. Lal, and R.I. Lehrer. 2004. RC-101, a retrocyclin-1 analogue with enhanced activity against primary HIV type 1 isolates. *AIDS Res Hum Retroviruses* 20:1157-1165.

Panyutich, A., and T. Ganz. 1991. Activated alpha 2-macroglobulin is a principal defensin-binding protein. *Am J Respir Cell Mol Biol* 5:101-106.

Panyutich, A.V., E.A. Panyutich, V.A. Krapivin, E.A. Baturevich, and T. Ganz. 1993. Plasma defensin concentrations are elevated in patients with septicemia or bacterial meningitis. *J Lab Clin Med* 122:202-207.

Panyutich, A.V., O. Szold, P.H. Poon, Y. Tseng, and T. Ganz. 1994. Identification of defensin binding to C1 complement. *FEBS Lett* 356:169-173.

Pardi, A., X.L. Zhang, M.E. Selsted, J.J. Skalicky, and P.F. Yip. 1992. NMR studies of defensin antimicrobial peptides. 2. Three-dimensional structures of rabbit NP-2 and human HNP-1. *Biochemistry* 31:11357-11364.

Pazgier, M., D.M. Hoover, D. Yang, W. Lu, and J. Lubkowski. 2006. Human beta-defensins. *Cell Mol Life Sci* 63:1294-1313.

Pivarcsi, A., I. Nagy, A. Koreck, K. Kis, A. Kenderessy-Szabo, M. Szell, A. Dobozy, and L. Kemeny. 2005. Microbial compounds induce the expression of pro-inflammatory cytokines, chemokines and human beta-defensin-2 in vaginal epithelial cells. *Microbes Infect* 7:1117-1127.

Plummer, F.A. 1998. Heterosexual transmission of human immunodeficiency virus type 1 (HIV): interactions of conventional sexually transmitted diseases, hormonal contraception and HIV-1. *AIDS Res Hum Retroviruses* 14 Suppl 1:S5-10.

Porter, E., H. Yang, S. Yavagal, G.C. Preza, O. Murillo, H. Lima, S. Greene, L. Mahoozi, M. Klein-Patel, G. Diamond, S. Gulati, T. Ganz, P.A. Rice, and A.J. Quayle. 2005. Distinct defensin profiles in Neisseria gonorrhoeae and Chlamydia trachomatis urethritis reveal novel epithelial cell-neutrophil interactions. *Infect Immun* 73:4823-4833.

Proud, D., S.P. Sanders, and S. Wiehler. 2004. Human rhinovirus infection induces airway epithelial cell production of human beta-defensin 2 both in vitro and in vivo. *J Immunol* 172:4637-4645.

Quayle, A.J., E.M. Porter, A.A. Nussbaum, Y.M. Wang, C. Brabec, K.P. Yip, and S.C. Mok. 1998. Gene expression, immunolocalization, and secretion of human defensin-5 in human female reproductive tract. *Am J Pathol* 152:1247-1258.

Quinones-Mateu, M.E., M.M. Lederman, Z. Feng, B. Chakraborty, J. Weber, H.R. Rangel, M.L. Marotta, M. Mirza, B. Jiang, P. Kiser, K. Medvik, S.F. Sieg, and A. Weinberg. 2003. Human epithelial beta-defensins 2 and 3 inhibit HIV-1 replication. *Aids* 17:F39-48.

Rapista, A., J. Ding, B. Benito, Y.T. Lo, M.B. Neiditch, W. Lu, and T.L. Chang. 2011. Human defensins 5 and 6 enhance HIV-1 infectivity through promoting HIV attachment. *Retrovirology* 8:45.

Rehaume, L.M., and R.E. Hancock. 2008. Neutrophil-derived defensins as modulators of innate immune function. *Crit Rev Immunol* 28:185-200.

Ricci, E., S. Malacrida, M. Zanchetta, M. Montagna, C. Giaquinto, and A.D. Rossi. 2009. Role of beta-Defensin-1 Polymorphisms in Mother-to-Child Transmission of Human Immunodeficiency Virus Type 1. *J Acquir Immune Defic Syndr*

Rodriguez-Garcia, M., N. Climent, H. Oliva, V. Casanova, R. Franco, A. Leon, J.M. Gatell, F. Garcia, and T. Gallart. 2010. Increased alpha-defensins 1-3 production by dendritic cells in HIV-infected individuals is associated with slower disease progression. *PLoS One* 5:e9436.

Rodriguez-Garcia, M., H. Oliva, N. Climent, F. Garcia, J.M. Gatell, and T. Gallart. 2007. Human immature monocyte-derived dendritic cells produce and secrete alpha-defensins 1-3. *J Leukoc Biol* 82:1143-1146.

Salzman, N.H., M.A. Underwood, and C.L. Bevins. 2007. Paneth cells, defensins, and the commensal microbiota: a hypothesis on intimate interplay at the intestinal mucosa. *Semin Immunol* 19:70-83.

Saraheimo, M., C. Forsblom, K. Pettersson-Fernholm, A. Flyvbjerg, P.H. Groop, and J. Frystyk. 2008. Increased levels of alpha-defensin (-1, -2 and -3) in type 1 diabetic patients with nephropathy. *Nephrol Dial Transplant* 23:914-918.

Schaefer, T.M., J.V. Fahey, J.A. Wright, and C.R. Wira. 2005. Innate immunity in the human female reproductive tract: antiviral response of uterine epithelial cells to the TLR3 agonist poly(I:C). *J Immunol* 174:992-1002.

Schutte, B.C., J.P. Mitros, J.A. Bartlett, J.D. Walters, H.P. Jia, M.J. Welsh, T.L. Casavant, and P.B. McCray, Jr. 2002. Discovery of five conserved beta -defensin gene clusters using a computational search strategy. *Proc Natl Acad Sci U S A* 99:2129-2133.

Selsted, M.E., and A.J. Ouellette. 2005. Mammalian defensins in the antimicrobial immune response. *Nat Immunol* 6:551-557.

Shi, J., S. Aono, W. Lu, A.J. Ouellette, X. Hu, Y. Ji, L. Wang, S. Lenz, F.W. van Ginkel, M. Liles, C. Dykstra, E.E. Morrison, and C.O. Elson. 2007. A novel role for defensins in intestinal homeostasis: regulation of IL-1beta secretion. *J Immunol* 179:1245-1253.

Simhan, H.N., B.L. Anderson, M.A. Krohn, R.P. Heine, B. Martinez de Tejada, D.V. Landers, and S.L. Hillier. 2007. Host immune consequences of asymptomatic Trichomonas vaginalis infection in pregnancy. *Am J Obstet Gynecol* 196:59 e51-55.

Sorensen, O.E., D.R. Thapa, A. Rosenthal, L. Liu, A.A. Roberts, and T. Ganz. 2005. Differential regulation of beta-defensin expression in human skin by microbial stimuli. *J Immunol* 174:4870-4879.

Sun, L., C.M. Finnegan, T. Kish-Catalone, R. Blumenthal, P. Garzino-Demo, G.M. La Terra Maggiore, S. Berrone, C. Kleinman, Z. Wu, S. Abdelwahab, W. Lu, and A. Garzino-Demo. 2005. Human {beta}-Defensins Suppress Human Immunodeficiency Virus Infection: Potential Role in Mucosal Protection. *J Virol* 79:14318-14329.

Svinarich, D.M., N.A. Wolf, R. Gomez, B. Gonik, and R. Romero. 1997. Detection of human defensin 5 in reproductive tissues. *Am J Obstet Gynecol* 176:470-475.

Szyk, A., Z. Wu, K. Tucker, D. Yang, W. Lu, and J. Lubkowski. 2006. Crystal structures of human alpha-defensins HNP4, HD5, and HD6. *Protein Sci* 15:2749-2760.

Tanabe, H., A.J. Ouellette, M.J. Cocco, and W.E. Robinson, Jr. 2004. Differential effects on human immunodeficiency virus type 1 replication by alpha-defensins with comparable bactericidal activities. *J Virol* 78:11622-11631.

Tanaka, S., J.C. Edberg, W. Chatham, G. Fassina, and R.P. Kimberly. 2003. Fc gamma RIIIb allele-sensitive release of alpha-defensins: anti-neutrophil cytoplasmic antibody-induced release of chemotaxins. *J Immunol* 171:6090-6096.

Tang, Y.Q., J. Yuan, G. Osapay, K. Osapay, D. Tran, C.J. Miller, A.J. Ouellette, and M.E. Selsted. 1999. A cyclic antimicrobial peptide produced in primate leukocytes by the ligation of two truncated alpha-defensins. *Science* 286:498-502.

Tecle, T., M.R. White, D. Gantz, E.C. Crouch, and K.L. Hartshorn. 2007. Human neutrophil defensins increase neutrophil uptake of influenza A virus and bacteria and modify virus-induced respiratory burst responses. *J Immunol* 178:8046-8052.

Territo, M.C., T. Ganz, M.E. Selsted, and R. Lehrer. 1989. Monocyte-chemotactic activity of defensins from human neutrophils. *J Clin Invest* 84:2017-2020.

Trabattoni, D., S.L. Caputo, G. Maffeis, F. Vichi, M. Biasin, P. Pierotti, F. Fasano, M. Saresella, M. Franchini, P. Ferrante, F. Mazzotta, and M. Clerici. 2004. Human alpha Defensin in HIV-Exposed But Uninfected Individuals. *J Acquir Immune Defic Syndr* 35:455-463.

Tran, D., P.A. Tran, Y.Q. Tang, J. Yuan, T. Cole, and M.E. Selsted. 2002. Homodimeric theta-defensins from rhesus macaque leukocytes: isolation, synthesis, antimicrobial activities, and bacterial binding properties of the cyclic peptides. *J Biol Chem* 277:3079-3084.

Uehara, A., Y. Fujimoto, K. Fukase, and H. Takada. 2007. Various human epithelial cells express functional Toll-like receptors, NOD1 and NOD2 to produce anti-microbial peptides, but not proinflammatory cytokines. *Mol Immunol* 44:3100-3111.

Uehara, A., and H. Takada. 2008. Synergism between TLRs and NOD1/2 in oral epithelial cells. *J Dent Res* 87:682-686.

Valore, E.V., D.J. Wiley, and T. Ganz. 2006. Reversible deficiency of antimicrobial polypeptides in bacterial vaginosis. *Infect Immun* 74:5693-5702.

Van Wetering, S., S.P. Mannesse-Lazeroms, J.H. Dijkman, and P.S. Hiemstra. 1997a. Effect of neutrophil serine proteinases and defensins on lung epithelial cells: modulation of cytotoxicity and IL-8 production. *J Leukoc Biol* 62:217-226.

Van Wetering, S., S.P. Mannesse-Lazeroms, M.A. Van Sterkenburg, M.R. Daha, J.H. Dijkman, and P.S. Hiemstra. 1997b. Effect of defensins on interleukin-8 synthesis in airway epithelial cells. *Am J Physiol* 272:L888-896.

Venkataraman, N., A.L. Cole, P. Svoboda, J. Pohl, and A.M. Cole. 2005. Cationic polypeptides are required for anti-HIV-1 activity of human vaginal fluid. *J Immunol* 175:7560-7567.

Vora, P., A. Youdim, L.S. Thomas, M. Fukata, S.Y. Tesfay, K. Lukasek, K.S. Michelsen, A. Wada, T. Hirayama, M. Arditi, and M.T. Abreu. 2004. Beta-defensin-2 expression is regulated by TLR signaling in intestinal epithelial cells. *J Immunol* 173:5398-5405.

Wang, S.Z., P.K. Smith, M. Lovejoy, J.J. Bowden, J.H. Alpers, and K.D. Forsyth. 1998. The apoptosis of neutrophils is accelerated in respiratory syncytial virus (RSV)-induced bronchiolitis. *Clin Exp Immunol* 114:49-54.

Wang, W., A.M. Cole, T. Hong, A.J. Waring, and R.I. Lehrer. 2003. Retrocyclin, an antiretroviral theta-defensin, is a lectin. *J Immunol* 170:4708-4716.

Wang, W., S.M. Owen, D.L. Rudolph, A.M. Cole, T. Hong, A.J. Waring, R.B. Lal, and R.I. Lehrer. 2004. Activity of alpha- and theta-defensins against primary isolates of HIV-1. *J Immunol* 173:515-520.

Wehkamp, J., J. Harder, M. Weichenthal, M. Schwab, E. Schaffeler, M. Schlee, K.R. Herrlinger, A. Stallmach, F. Noack, P. Fritz, J.M. Schroder, C.L. Bevins, K. Fellermann, and E.F. Stange. 2004. NOD2 (CARD15) mutations in Crohn's disease are associated with diminished mucosal alpha-defensin expression. *Gut* 53:1658-1664.

Wehkamp, J., G. Wang, I. Kubler, S. Nuding, A. Gregorieff, A. Schnabel, R.J. Kays, K. Fellermann, O. Burk, M. Schwab, H. Clevers, C.L. Bevins, and E.F. Stange. 2007. The Paneth cell alpha-defensin deficiency of ileal Crohn's disease is linked to Wnt/Tcf-4. *J Immunol* 179:3109-3118.

Wiesenfeld, H.C., R.P. Heine, M.A. Krohn, S.L. Hillier, A.A. Amortegui, M. Nicolazzo, and R.L. Sweet. 2002. Association between elevated neutrophil defensin levels and endometritis. *J Infect Dis* 186:792-797.

Wilde, C.G., J.E. Griffith, M.N. Marra, J.L. Snable, and R.W. Scott. 1989. Purification and characterization of human neutrophil peptide 4, a novel member of the defensin family. *J Biol Chem* 264:11200-11203.

Wu, Z., F. Cocchi, D. Gentles, B. Ericksen, J. Lubkowski, A. Devico, R.I. Lehrer, and W. Lu. 2005. Human neutrophil alpha-defensin 4 inhibits HIV-1 infection in vitro. *FEBS Lett* 579:162-166.

Yamaguchi, Y., T. Nagase, R. Makita, S. Fukuhara, T. Tomita, T. Tominaga, H. Kurihara, and Y. Ouchi. 2002. Identification of multiple novel epididymis-specific beta-defensin isoforms in humans and mice. *J Immunol* 169:2516-2523.

Yang, C., L. Boone, T.X. Nguyen, D. Rudolph, K. Limpakarnjanarat, T.D. Mastro, J. Tappero, A.M. Cole, and R.B. Lal. 2005. theta-Defensin pseudogenes in HIV-1-exposed, persistently seronegative female sex-workers from Thailand. *Infect Genet Evol* 5:11-15.

Yang, D., A. Biragyn, D.M. Hoover, J. Lubkowski, and J.J. Oppenheim. 2004. Multiple roles of antimicrobial defensins, cathelicidins, and eosinophil-derived neurotoxin in host defense. *Annu Rev Immunol* 22:181-215.

Yang, D., A. Biragyn, L.W. Kwak, and J.J. Oppenheim. 2002. Mammalian defensins in immunity: more than just microbicidal. *Trends Immunol* 23:291-296.

Yang, D., Q. Chen, O. Chertov, and J.J. Oppenheim. 2000. Human neutrophil defensins selectively chemoattract naive T and immature dendritic cells. *J Leukoc Biol* 68:9-14.

Yang, D., O. Chertov, S.N. Bykovskaia, Q. Chen, M.J. Buffo, J. Shogan, M. Anderson, J.M. Schroder, J.M. Wang, O.M. Howard, and J.J. Oppenheim. 1999. Beta-defensins: linking innate and adaptive immunity through dendritic and T cell CCR6. *Science* 286:525-528.

Yang, D., O. Chertov, and J.J. Oppenheim. 2001. Participation of mammalian defensins and cathelicidins in anti-microbial immunity: receptors and activities of human defensins and cathelicidin (LL-37). *J Leukoc Biol* 69:691-697.

Zaharatos, G.J., T. He, P. Lopez, W. Yu, J. Yu, and L. Zhang. 2004. alpha-Defensins Released Into Stimulated CD8+ T-Cell Supernatants Are Likely Derived From Residual Granulocytes Within the Irradiated Allogeneic Peripheral Blood Mononuclear Cells Used as Feeders. *J Acquir Immune Defic Syndr* 36:993-1005.

Zanetti, M. 2004. Cathelicidins, multifunctional peptides of the innate immunity. *J Leukoc Biol* 75:39-48.

Zapata, W., B. Rodriguez, J. Weber, H. Estrada, M.E. Quinones-Mateu, P.A. Zimermman, M.M. Lederman, and M.T. Rugeles. 2008. Increased levels of human beta-defensins mRNA in sexually HIV-1 exposed but uninfected individuals. *Curr HIV Res* 6:531-538.

Zaragoza, M.M., S. Sankaran-Walters, D.R. Canfield, J.K. Hung, E. Martinez, A.J. Ouellette, and S. Dandekar. 2011. Persistence of gut mucosal innate immune defenses by enteric alpha-defensin expression in the simian immunodeficiency virus model of AIDS. *J Immunol* 186:1589-1597.

Zhang, L., W. Yu, T. He, J. Yu, R.E. Caffrey, E.A. Dalmasso, S. Fu, T. Pham, J. Mei, J.J. Ho, W. Zhang, P. Lopez, and D.D. Ho. 2002. Contribution of human alpha-defensin 1, 2, and 3 to the anti-HIV-1 activity of CD8 antiviral factor. *Science* 298:995-1000.

Zlotnik, A., and O. Yoshie. 2000. Chemokines: a new classification system and their role in immunity. *Immunity* 12:121-127.

6

Innate Immune Responses in HIV-Infection

Wilfried Posch, Cornelia Lass-Flörl and Doris Wilflingseder
Innsbruck Medical University, Division of Hygiene and Medical Microbiology
Austria

1. Introduction

The immune system comprises complex cellular and humoral systems, which are forming an interactive network to recognize and eradicate invading pathogens. Foreign molecules present on viruses, bacteria and parasites, but not on host cells, are discriminated from self through pathogen-associated molecular patterns. Upon entry of the pathogen into the body immediate non-specific immune responses are triggered and within a short time the innate immune system is completely activated. The innate immune system is composed of multiple humoral and cellular players, including cytokines, complement proteins, acute-phase proteins, dendritic cells, macrophages, NK cells, that co-operate in a complex to generate an efficient defense against infection (Figure 1). At best, these immediate innate immune responses are able to clear infection or bridge the period until the adaptive, specific immune response is taking effect.

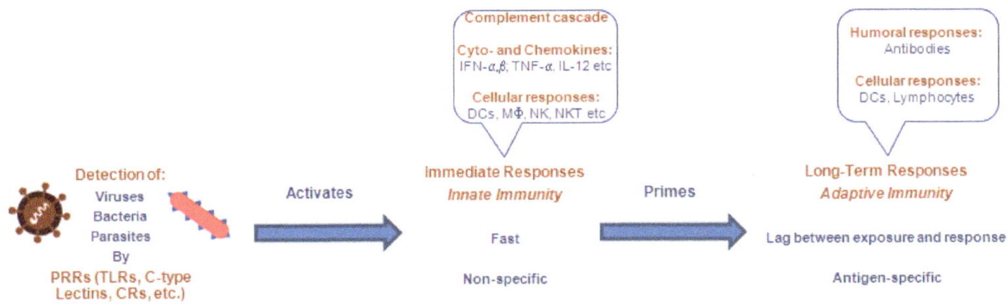

Fig. 1. Induction of Immune responses

Among the first components activated during the innate immune response is the complement system that together with interferons, cytokines and chemokines stimulate innate immune cells, such as dendritic cells (DCs), natural killer (NK) cells, natural killer T (NKT) cells, monocytes, or macrophages. These factors act in concert until the adaptive arm of immunity is established. Thus, to control the infection process in the acute phase a co-ordinated action of the innate immune elements is essential.

In the beginning of an infection viruses and microbes developed different strategies to avoid the attack of the innate immune system. Also the human immunodeficiency virus (HIV) is able to overcome innate and adaptive immune responses in infected individuals and thereby attenuates the immunity of the host. In the last years the interest in innate immune responses to control HIV infection significantly increased and this book chapter will describe various interactions and evasion strategies of HIV and innate immune elements with a special focus on complement and dendritic cells.

2. Interactions of HIV with humoral components of the innate immune system

Following entry of HIV into the host, humoral components of the innate immune system, such as complement system, interferons, cyto- and chemokines, are spontaneously activated and will be discussed here. Together with dendritic cells, which are among the first cells of the immune system to interact with HIV, the innate humoral components attract other cells of the immune system, e.g. NK cells or macrophages, to the sites of infection and a first line of defense is established. To ensure a logical configuration of the chapter, we will first summarize interactions of HIV with humoral components of the innate system and subsequently with cellular responses, although these actions cannot be separated and are proceeding in parallel at mucosal surfaces.

2.1 Interactions of HIV with the complement system

The complement system plays a crucial role during viral infection respecting both innate and adaptive immune responses. It constitutes the first barrier to control HIV propagation and can be activated via three different biochemical pathways: the classical, the MBL, and the lectin pathway (Fig. 2). The classical complement pathway was the first way to be identified, and activation of the classical pathway occurs when the first component of the pathway, C1, binds the Fc region of either natural or specific IgG antibody immune-complexed with viral antigen. The classical pathway is also triggered in an antibody-independent manner when C1 directly binds to virions or infected cells.

The alternative pathway is activated by direct recognition of certain microbial structures and the (mannan-binding) lectin (MBL) pathway is triggered by binding of terminal mannose residues on microbial glycoproteins and glycolipids (Fig. 2). All three pathways converge in the cleavage of C3, the main complement component, to the anaphylatoxin C3a and the opsonin C3b. This cleavage initiates a cascade of further activation events. C3b is covalently deposited on the microbial surface and joins with the C3 convertase to generate the C5 convertase. This convertase again cleaves C5 into C5a (anaphylatoxin) and C5b. C5b triggers the formation of the membrane attack complex (MAC), that consists of C5b, C6, C7, C8 and polymeric C9 molecules (Fig. 2). The formation of the MAC disrupts the microbial membrane, resulting in lysis of infected cells or pathogens (Stoiber et al., 2007; Speth et al., 2008). Figure 2 summarizes the activation events of the complement cascade using the example of a viral particle.

An appropriate control of the over 30 complement proteins, that are participating in the activation of the three different complement pathways, is crucial to prevent spontaneous activation and destruction of bystander cells. Thus, the complement system is tightly controlled by the 'regulators of complement activation' or RCAs. RCAs are present in fluid phase and also membrane-bound on the surface of host cells. Among the most important RCAs are secreted fH (factor H), C4bp (C4-binding protein), MCP (membrane-cofactor protein), CD55 (DAF), CD59, and CR1 (Spear et al., 1995; Spiller et al., 1997; Da Costa et al., 1999; Carroll, 2000).

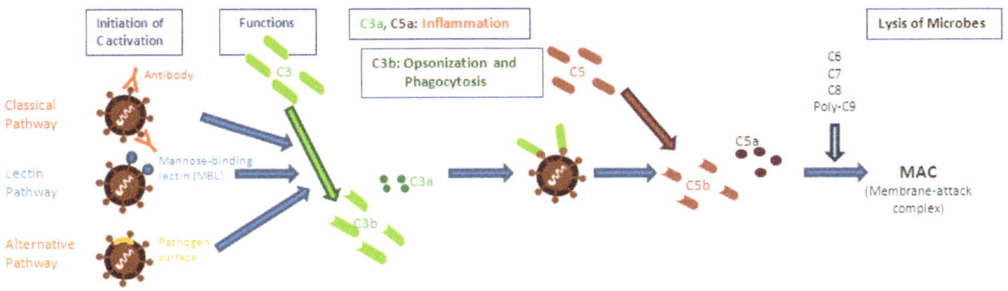

Fig. 2. Activation of Complement (C)

Upon entering the host HIV-1 spontaneaously activates the complement system via gp120 and gp41, even in the absence of HIV-specific antibodies, and is hence already coated with complement fragments at the initial stages of infection. After seroconversion, adaptive immunity is fully activated, as reflected by the generation of specific anti-HIV-1 antibodies and activated T cells. Activation of complement is strongly enhanced due to the Ab-C1 interactions, and deposition of complement fragments on virions dramatically increased by virus-bound Abs. Accordingly, opsonized infectious viral particles accumulate in HIV-1-positive individuals during the acute and chronic phase of infection and complement activation results in multifaceted outcomes. Despite the clearance and neutralization of HIV-1 virions by action of complement, it also accounts for the spread and maintenance of HIV during the infection. During the budding process, HIV acquires membrane-anchored RCAs such as CD59, CD55 and binds fH in fluid-phase (Frank et al., 1996). Therefore the virus is efficiently protected from complement-mediated lysis (CoML). Only at early stages of infection, CoML is suggested to contribute to the control of the virus before the adaptive immunity is fully activated. At later stages of infection, CoML seems to play a minor role in reducing the viral burden in infected individuals (Stoiber et al., 2007; Huber et al., 2008).

HIV that is not killed by complement-mediated lysis, persists covered with C3 fragments in the host. Thus, opsonized HIV accumulates in all so far tested compartments of the host, such as blood, lymphatic tissue (LT), brain, mothers milk, or seminal fluid and is able to interact with complement receptor (CR)-positive cells, e.g. DCs, macrophages, NK cells, B cells or follicular dendritic cells (FDCs). Opsonized virions were found to bind to complement receptor-expressing cells, which can promote enhanced viral infectivity and transmission *in vitro*.

Furthermore, it was shown that complement by itself or together with dendritic cells is involved in priming antiviral T cell immunity, therefore suggesting that complement not only triggers CoML but mediates adaptive immune responses (Kopf et al., 2002; Banki/Posch et al., 2010). C3-deficiency impeded priming of CD4$^+$ and CD8$^+$ T cells in an influenza virus model (Kopf et al., 2002), thus supporting this thesis. The exact mechanisms of complement-mediated T cell priming have not yet been resolved, but as recently shown, priming of naive CD8$^+$ T cells was significantly enhanced when DCs were exposed to complement-opsonized HIV compared to DCs stimulated with non-opsonized HIV (Banki/Posch et al., 2010). This was also confirmed *in vivo* using the Friend Murine Leukemia Virus model (Banki/Posch et al., 2010). Therefore, the failure to induce efficient T cell responses in the absence of complement can be explained by the fact that dendritic cells (DCs), which ingest C3-coated pathogens via CR3 or CR4, efficiently prime CD8$^+$ T cells, resulting in efficient activation of the adaptive immunity. Without C3 the antigen-presenting capacity of DCs, and consequently T cell priming, could be defective, which has to be further investigated. In addition, the appropriate cytokine environment for T cell priming could be altered in the absence of C3 and therefore weaken antigen-presentation.

Beside inducing T cell immunity, complement opsonization of HIV particles also accounts for the generation of a huge viral reservoir in infected individuals. This can be explained by the extracellular binding of C3d-opsonized HIV-particles to follicular dendritic cells (FDCs) in germinal centers (Kacani et al., 2000). Up to 90% of viral particles were shown to bind via C3d-CR2 interactions on FDCs, creating an additional reservoir for infectious HIV (Pantaleo, 1995; Haase, 1999).

In summary, HIV-complement interactions are very complex and contribute on the one hand to reduction of the viral load by lysis or neutralization due to opsonization, and on the other hand to spread of the virus by allowing attachment and maintenance to and on CR-expressing cells.

2.2 Induction of type I interferons and cytokines in acute HIV-infection

During the early stages of HIV infection, high-level viral replication, loss in $CD4^+$ T cell number and function, and an up-regulation of proinflammatory and immunoregulatory cytokines can be measured.As recently described, an ordered increase in plasma levels of multiple cytokines and chemokines was observed in acute HIV-infection (Stacey et al., 2009):

- Rapid and transient elevations in IFNα and IL-15 levels were succeeded by
- a large increase in inducible protein 10 (IP-10),
- rapid and sustained increases in tumor necrosis factor alpha (TNF-α) and monocyte chemotactic protein-1 (MCP-1),
- a more slowly induction of proinflammatory cytokines such as IL-6, IL-8, IL-12, and IFN-γ and
- late up-regulation of the immunoregulatory cytokine IL-10.

Plasmacytoid DCs (pDCs) act as the principal source of systemic IFNα production in many viral infections. pDCs were shown *in vitro* to produce cytokines following the endocytosis of HIV virions (Beignon et al., 2005) and they are responsible for early elevations in plasma IFNα, and together with myeloid dermal dendritic cells (DCs) in an early increase of IL-15, and TNFα levels. Myeloid DCs are made responsible for the slower and more-prolonged secretion of an array of cytokines including IL-6, IL-8, IL-12, IL-18, TNFα, and IL-10. This part of the chapter will review the most important facts about some of the cytokines and their functions in acute HIV infection.

Type I interferons and APOBEC3G in acute HIV infection

Interferons inhibit viral replication within host cells ("interfere"), but they do also have other functions, like activating immune cells, such as NK cells or macrophages, or up-regulating antigen-presentation to T cells. IFNα/β elicit potent antiviral activities in both virally infected and non-infected cells (Katze et al., 2002) and they additionally enhance the antiviral activity of NK cells and macrophages. Furthermore, IFNα/β induce maturation of immature pDCs, which is associated with increased expression of CD83, co-stimulatory molecules and enhanced secretion of cytokines, e.g. IFNα/β, TNFα and IL-6 (Cella et al., 1999) . IFN-secretion during infection causes symptoms like fever or aching muscles.

IFNα inhibits HIV replication, the mechanism by which it blocks replication of HIV *in vivo* are not known. The anti-HIV effects of IFNα were ascribed to a number of functions mediated by this cytokine, including inhibition of early steps in viral replication, inhibition of HIV gene expression, and effects on viral assembly and budding. HIV-1 activates plasmacytoid dendritic cells (pDCs) via toll like receptors (TLRs) and induces the secretion of IFNα. IFNα secretion is triggered from pDCs in acute HIV-infection via TLR7, TLR8 or TLR9 signaling (Beignon et al., 2005; Lee et al., 2006; Meier et al., 2007; Mandl et al., 2008; Zhang et al., 2009). TLRs are pattern recognition receptors (PRRs), which recognize conserved motifs specific for microorganisms. Certain viral proteins and viral single- or double-stranded RNAs are detected mainly by TLRs 7 [ssRNA]/8 [ssRNA]/9 [dsRNA] (Kadowaki et al., 2001; Diebold et al., 2004; Mandl et al., 2008). In acute HIV infection IFNα has a protective role, while chronic immune activation and inflammation associated with the production of type I interferon are major determinants of disease progression in primate lentivirus infections (Stoddard et al., 2010). IFNα drives the expression of several IFN regulatory factors (IRFs), and the induction of IFN-stimulated genes (ISGs) by an autocrine positive feedback loop. In turn, ISGs promote proliferation of immune cells and induce an antiviral state in cells.

IFNα was also demonstrated to potently induce APOBEC3G (Apolipoprotein B mRNA-editing enzyme-catalytic polypeptide-like 3G) to abrogate HIV Vif neutralization of APOBEC3 proteins (Peng et al., 2006). APOBEC3G, a cytidine deaminase, is an innate intracellular protein with lethal activity against HIV and exerts this intrinsic anti-HIV activity by introducing lethal G-to-A hypermutations in the viral genome (Casartelli et al., 2010). While HIV^+ patients with progressive disease show a significant decline in pDCs over time, long term non-progressors (LTNPs) maintain high levels of these cells and this may be of importance in the innate response in these patients.

TNF-α in acute HIV infection

TNF-α is a pro-inflammatory cytokine that mediates many inflammatory and immune functions (rev. in Armitage, 1994). It is produced by NK cells, macrophages, monocytes, T cells, B cells and neutrophils and exerts its actions via binding to TNF-R1 and TNF-R2. Attachment of HIV to TNF-R1 and subsequent activation of NFκB were demonstrated to significantly increase HIV-1 replication in cells of the macrophage lineage (Griffin et al., 1991; Naif et al., 1994; Herbein and Gordon, 1997). This enhancement was further amplified by IFN-γ (Han et al., 1996) and a positive autocrine TNF-α loop initiated by HIV-1 infection of monocyte-derived macrophages resulted in increased HIV-1 production (Esser et al., 1991, 1996, 1998). In contrast, ligation of TNF-α to TNF-R2 resulted in inhibition of HIV-1 replication (Herbein and Gordon, 1997).

Interleukins

IL-15 in acute HIV-infection

The activation of DCs by HIV determines a progressive accumulation of various cytokines, including IL-15, which subsequently acts as potent inducer of NK cell activation and cytotoxicity. DC-NK cell cross-talk represents a key mode of the cellular network regulating the links between innate and the adaptive immune response (Moretta, 2002; Moretta et al., 2006). IL-15 is produced during acute HIV-1 and SIV (simian immunodeficiency virus) infection and exerts an influence on viremia and viral set point. The viral set point was significantly increased during acute SIV-infection upon administration of IL-15. To identify cytokine biomarkers in plasma during acute HIV-1 infection that predict HIV disease progression, 30 cytokines were tested in 40 South African women in acute infection and 12 months post infection. Only a small panel of plasma cytokines during acute HIV-1 infection was predictive of long-term HIV disease prognosis in this group, namely IL-12p40, IL-12p70, IFN-γ, IL-7 and IL15. While IL-12p40, IL-12p70 and IFN-γ were significantly associated with lower viral load, IL-7 and IL-15 were associated with higher viral load (Roberts et al., 2010).

IL-6 in acute HIV-infection

IL-6 is a pro-inflammatory cytokine produced by macrophages, DCs, T and B cells in response to bacterial and viral infections. IL-6 mediates B cell stimulation, monocyte differentiation and induction of IL-4-producing cells (Rincon et al., 1997). It helps augmenting HIV-1 replication in macrophages and U1 cells (macrophage lineage) and enhances TNF-α-induced up-regulation of HIV-1 production (Poli et al., 1990; Poli and Fauci, 1992).

IL-10 in acute HIV-infection

IL-10 is an anti-inflammatory cytokine produced by monocytes/macrophages, DCs and activated T and B cells. This cytokine blocks macrophage activation and inhibits secretion of the pro-inflammatory cytokines IL-1, IL-6, IL-8, IL-12 or TNF-α (rev. in Moore et al, 2002). IL-10 was shown to interfere with HIV-infection at the early stages of HIV-1 infection although it does not alter CCR5 surface expression (Montaner et al., 1994; Wang et al., 1998). Pre-treatment of monocytes with IL-10 significantly decreased HIV-1 RNA expression and this inhibition of HIV replication was associated with down-modulation of IL-6- and TNF-a production by IL-10 (Weissman et al., 1994; Naif et al., 1994).

2.3 Induction of β-chemokines (MIP-1α, MIP-1β, RANTES) in acute HIV-infection

MIP-1α (CCL3) , MIP-1β (CCL4) and regulated upon activation normal T-cell expressed and secreted (RANTES, CCL5) were the first three factors of the β-chemokine family identified as suppressors of HIV infection (Cocchi et al., 1995). These chemokines have been identified to bind the G-protein coupled receptors CCR5, which acts as co-factor for macrophage-(R5) and dual-(R5X4)-tropic HIV-1 strains. Similarly, the ligand of CXCR4, SDF-1 (CXCL12) was shown to suppress infection with T cell-(X4-)tropic HIV strains (Bleul et al., 1996; Oberlin et al., 1996). Polymorphisms in the CCR5 locus, in particular a 32 bp gene deletion (CCR5Δ32) results in a decreased susceptibility to infection with macrophage-(R5)-tropic HIV-1 strains (Kramer et al., 2005). CCR5Δ32- heterocygotic individuals can be infected with R5-tropic HIV, but exhibit a significantly slower disease progression, whereas CCR5Δ32-homocygotic individuals are susceptible to infection with X4-tropic HIV-1 strains.

3. Interactions of HIV with cellular components of the innate immune system

Very little is known respecting the earliest events after HIV transmission in the genital tract or the rectal mucosa and most findings about these early events were acquired from *in vivo* models of SIV-infected macaques (Haase, 2005). The *in vivo* SIV models and *ex vivo* analyses in the human system pursue to identify cells and soluble factors involved in HIV-transmission (Haase, 2005; Hladik and McElrath, 2008). R5-tropic HIV-1 particles are selectively captured by epithelial cells and subsequently transfered to CCR5-expressing target cells underneath the epithelia. This could be responsible for the selective preferential transmission of R5-tropic HIV-1 strains (Meng et al., 2002). Langerhans cells (LCs) or other dendritic cells are present at the port of the mucosal entry site (in the underlying tissues of the vagina and cervix) and trap pathogens with their processes that extend to the luminal surface. Thus, viruses cross the mucosal barrier by attachment or infection of DCs, by transcytosis (M cells) or by infection of intraepithelial lymphocytes and macrophages (Fig. 3). Various cells of the innate immune system account for building the first line defense against HIV until the adaptive immune response is fully developed. Among those are LCs, myeloid DCs, pDCs, that recruite and activate NK cells (Fig. 3), macrophages, and NKT cells, which will be discussed in this part of the chapter.

3.1 Dendritic cells in acute HIV infection

Dendritic cells are the most potent antigen-presenting cells and can be divided into conventional myeloid DCs (LCs, dermal DCs, blood DCs) and plasmacytoid DCs (Table 1, adapted from *Altfeld et al., 2011*). They differ respecting their location, their C-type lectin and TLR expression, their role in HIV-infection, their cytokine production and their function (Table 1, Altfeld et al., 2011). As described very recently (Sabado et al., 2010), depletion of both, myeloid and plasmacytoid DCs from the circulation already occurs during the early

	Conventional DCs ($CD11c^+HLA\text{-}DR^+$)			Plasmacytoid DCs ($CD123^+HLA\text{-}DR^+$)
	Langerhans Cells	Dermal Dendritic Cells		
		$CD103^-$	$CD103^+$	
Location	Stratified squamous epithelium of the skin and oral and ano-genital mucosa	Dermis		Blood Secondary lymphoid organs Peripheral tissues (Skin, Lungs)
C-type lectin expression	Langerin	DC-SIGN DEC-205	Langerin DEC-205	BDCA-2
TLR expression	TLR2,3,5	TLR2,3,4,5		TLR7, 8, 9
Role in HIV-infection	Degradation of HIV in Birbeck granules	HIV shuttle and transfer	Unknown	•Production of type I interferons: antiviral and induction of bystander T cell death •Induction of Treg cells by HIV-induced IDO up-regulation •Recruitment of T cells to sites of HIV-infection, thus facilitating viral spread
Cytokine prodution	IL-1β, IL-6, IL-8, IL-12, IL-15, IL-23	IL-1β, IL-6, IL-8, IL-12, IL-15, IL-23		IFNα, IFNβ, IL-6, TNF
Function	•Prime Ag-specific T cells and B cells •NK cell activation by IL-12	•Prime Ag-specific T cells and B cells •NK cell activation by IL-12		•Treg induction • Plasma cell induction •NK cell activation by IFNs
Pathology during HIV-infection	•Reduced frequency in peripheral blood •Conflicting results respecting dysfunction and functionality	•Reduced frequency in peripheral blood •Conflicting results respecting dysfunction and functionality		•Reduced frequency in peripheral blood •Conflicting results respecting dysfunction and functionality

Table 1. DC-subsets and functions during HIV-infection (adapted from *Altfeld et al., 2011*, blood DCs not portrayed)

phases of HIV infection. The depletion from the circulation is suggested to be due to preferential re-distribution of both DC types from blood to lymphoid organs. This re-distribution is based on the ability of the DCs to up-regulate chemokine-receptor 7 (CCR7), that causes migration of DCs to the lymph nodes along a CCL19/CCL21 gradient. The reduction in circulating DC numbers was shown not to be transient, but also detectable in the chronic phase of infection and under highly-active antiretroviral therapy (Sabado et al., 2010). Restoration of circulating DCs might represent a key factor in providing an improved immune response against the virus.

3.1.1 Langerhans cells and HIV

Langerhans cells (LCs) build the first line defense against mucosal infections because they are situated ideally in mucosal tissues to catch pathogens (Fig. 3). LCs survey the basal and suprabasal layers of the stratified squamous epithelium of the skin and oral and ano-genital mucosa for invading pathogens (Katz et al., 1979; Romani et al., 1985; rev. in DeJong and Geijtenbeek, 2010). Upon capture of Ags, LCs start to mature, which is represented by up-regulation of CCR7, co-stimulatory molecules CD80/CD86/CD40, MHC class I and class II molecules and CD83 and by down-regulation of Langerin and E-cadherin (Merad et al., 2008). These mature LCs migrate to the lymph node to present the captured Ag to T cells, thus inducing an efficient immune response (Merad et al., 2008). Despite their important function in initiating adaptive immune responses, LCs additionally exert innate immune functions as recently shown (De Witte et al., 2007). LCs characteristically express a specific set of TLRs (TLR2, 3, 5), high levels of CD1a, the C-type lectin Langerin and intracellular Birbeck granules that might be crucial to their innate function (Valladeau et al., 2000; Liu, 2001; Flacher et al., 2006; Fahrbach et al., 2007, Romani et al., 2010). Langerin interacts with HIV-1 and other pathogens like fungi and bacteria. After heterosexual contact with an HIV-infected individuum, the chance to acquire HIV-1 is very low (0.01-0.1%) (Wu and KewalRemani, 2006) and LCs are the first cells to encounter HIV due to their location in the mucosal stratified epithelium. Attachment of HIV-gp120 to Langerin leads to internalization of the viral particle and subsequent degradation in the Birbeck granules, that are characteristic for LCs (De Witte et al., 2007). Thus, LCs are protected from infection with incoming, non-opsonized HIV particles and HIV-1 is not disseminated through the host (De Witte et al., 2007). Although LCs express the primary receptor for HIV-1, CD4, and the chemokine co-receptor CCR5, they are not productively infected by the virus. This is probably due to efficient capture of the virus by Langerin and targeting of HIV-1 to Birbeck granules, where it is degraded (De Witte et al., 2007). The rapid internalization of HIV-1 into LCs prevents also transmission to the main target cells of the virus, $CD4^+$ T cells. The degradation of HIV in Birbeck granules and the prevention of virus transfer to $CD4^+$ T cells renders Langerin as a protective anti-HIV barrier. When, in addition, sexually transmitted infections (STIs) are present, the anti-HIV-1-barrier of LCs is abrogated and HIV-1 transmission to $CD4^+$ T cells by LCs is promoted (DeJong et al., 2008, 2010; Ogawa et al., 2009). The by-passing of the anti-HIV-effect due to additional STIs results from direct interaction of the STIs with Langerin and therefore competition for HIV-1 binding, Langerin inhibition by high viral loads, lower Langerin surface expression by Poly(I:C) or HSV2 (DeJong et al., 2010), up-regulation of HIV entry receptors and down-regulation of restriction factors (Ogawa et al., 2009), or inflammation-induced TNF-α production by

Candida albicans or *Neisseria gonorrhoea* (DeJong et al., 2008). In summary, during acute co-infection the anti-viral function of LCs is significantly reduced due to competition for Langerin. This facilitates HIV-1 infection of LCs and thereby promotes HIV-1 transfer to and infection of CD4$^+$ T cells.

3.1.2 Dermal dendritic cells and HIV

In addition to LCs, interstitial dendritic cells are among the first cells to encounter HIV at mucosal surfaces (Fig. 3). They are underlying the epithelium and differ from LCs, since they do not contain Birbeck granules and express heterogenous amounts of CD1a (Bell et al., 1999). Interstitial DCs are localized in the dermis and oral, vaginal and colonic lamina propria (Pavli et al., 1990, 1993; Lenz et al., 1993; Nestle et al., 1993; McLellan et al., 1998). They are characterized by the expression of CD11c, high concentrations of various C-type lectin receptors, TLRs 2, 3, 4 and 5 and secretion of IL-1β, IL-6, IL-10, IL-12, IL-15, and IL-23 upon pathogenic stimulation (Liu, 2001). Also dermal dendritic cells can be functionally divided in immature and mature DCs (iDCs, mDCs) based on their T cell stimulatory capacity (Banchereau and Steinman, 1998). Following antigen exposure, iDCs undergo major changes and mature (described under 3.1.1). Upon entry of HIV into the host, the virus has to be transported from mucosal surfaces to lymphatic tissues, where it is transmitted to its primary targets, CD4$^+$ T lymphocytes. As mentioned above, this process is thought to be contrived by DCs. By clustering T cells, DCs may both activate antiviral immunity as well as facilitate spread of the virus. *In vitro* experiments showed that DCs efficiently capture and transfer HIV to T cells and initiated a vigorous infection (Pope et al., 1995; McDonald et al., 2003; Pruenster/Wilflingseder et al, 2005; Wilflingseder et al, 2007). These experiments imply that *in vivo* HIV exploits DCs at mucosal sites as shuttles to CD4$^+$ T cells in the lymph nodes. Preferential expression of CCR5 on immature LCs and DCs restricts the transmission of X4-tropic isolates at the site of infection. Additionally, *ex vivo* analyses revealed that X4-tropic HIV replicate worse in DCs and LCs compared to R5-tropic viruses (Granelli-Piperno et al, 1998; Kawamura et al, 2000; Ganesh et al, 2004). Productive infection of DCs and LCs with HIV is relatively inefficient compared to HIV-infection of CD4$^+$ T cells and HIV- or SIV-infected DCs are rarely detected *in vivo* (rev. in Piguet and Steinman, 2007). Virus is very efficiently transmitted to T cells either via de novo (*´cis´*-transfer) or without (*´trans´*-) infection despite the low-level productive infection of DCs (Turville et al, 2004). Especially C-type lectins such as Dendritic cell-specific ICAM-3-grabbing non-integrin (DC-SIGN) on dermal DCs was implicated in the transfer of HIV to T cells in the lymph nodes (Geijtenbeek et al., 2003; Turville et al., 2004). Similar to Langerin, DC-SIGN has high affinity for mannose and fucose structures. Dermal iDCs express the C-type lectin DC-SIGN and recently a second dermal DC subtype, expressing CD103 and Langerin, but no Birbeck granules, was described (Ginhoux et al., 2009). DC-SIGN captures low titres of HIV-1 through its interaction with the HIV-1 glycoprotein gp120 (Geijtenbeek et al., 2000) and this DC-SIGN/virus interaction protects HIV from degradation within the cells in contrast to the anti-viral action of Langerin on LCs (Geijtenbeek et al., 2000). DC-SIGN-complexed HIV-1 is stable and retains the infectivity for prolonged periods in contrast to DC-SIGN-bound antibody and probably other ligands that are internalized into lysosomal compartments for processing (Geijtenbeek et al., 2000; Engering et al., 2002). These studies suggest that DC-SIGN-bound HIV-1 particles hide near the cell membrane in DCs and are not degraded. After ligating DC-SIGN, HIV is indeed transported into non-lysosomal acidic organelles. Thereby, DC-SIGN effectively transmits HIV to CD4+ T cells and also leads to enhancement of infection in these co-cultures and facilitates '*trans*'-infection of the T cells (Geijtenbeek et al., 2000).

Besides C-type lectins, other molecules, such as adhesion molecules e.g. ICAM-1 (Pruenster/Wilflingseder et al, 2005) are described to further contribute to DC-HIV interaction. In all compartments tested so far (plasma, seminal fluid, lymphatic tissues), HIV is opsonized with C3 complement fragments and after seroconversion additionally with HIV-specific IgGs. Similar to the interaction of non opsonized HIV with C-type lectin receptors on DCs, receptors such as complement receptors (CRs) or Fc receptors (FcR) contribute to the attachment of the complement- or IgG-coated virus. If the virus is opsonized, the DC-SIGN- or ICAM-dependent interactions play a minor role for the attachment of HIV to DCs as well as the DC-mediated *cis* and *trans* HIV-infection (Pruenster/Wilflingseder et al, 2005). Complement-opsonization of HIV significantly enhanced the productive infection of DCs compared to non-opsonized HIV and also acted as an endogenous adjuvant for the DC-mediated induction of virus-specific CTLs (Wilflingseder et al., 2007; Banki/Posch et al., 2010). These results emphasize a role of DCs in combination with complement-coating of the virus in priming adaptive T cell responses. Vigorous *trans*-infection of CD4+ T cells by DCs was shown to be promoted by infectious synapse formation independent on the attachment mechanism (C-type lectin receptors, adhesion molecules, CRs [own unpublished observations]) (rev. by Piguet and Sattentau, 2004). The receptors involved in the HIV attachment have to be re-arranged and are recruited to the DC-T cell junctions (McDonald et al., 2003). Microscopic analyses of DC-CD4+ T cells revealed re-arrangement and recruitment of CD4 and chemokine-co-receptor to the infectious synapse on the T cell site and of HIV on the DC site (McDonald et al., 2003). Thereby, dermal DCs contribute not only to shuttle HIV from the mucosal site to the lymphatic tissue but also to efficiently transmit of HIV to its main targets, CD4+ T cells.

Beside the support of DCs in HIV dissemination, DCs produce high amounts of cytokines, such as IL-12 or interferons, which belong to the first line of the host defense against invading organisms. They are also able to activate NK cells via secretion of pro-inflammatory cytokines (IL-12, IL-15, IL-18) and other factors, thus enhancing their cytotoxicity to virally infected cells (Chehimi et al., 1989; Mellman and Steinman, 2001, Yu et al., 2001).

In terms of modulation of DC function by HIV infection *in vivo*, it is not clear if DC defects are resulting from the direct exposure to HIV or if they are due to production of host cell factors during infection. Circulating lipopolysaccharide (LPS) or other pathogen-derived factors were also implicated in chronic immune activation, which is monitored during HIV infection (Brenchley et al., 2006). Bacterial stimuli like LPS could result in maturation of iDCs thus rendering these cells tolerant to subsequent stimuli. *Ex vivo* tests of DCs from chronically infected individuals demonstrated that they were less potent in responding to other TLR stimuli as well as in stimulating T cell responses compared to DCs from non-infected individuals (Donaghy et al., 2003; Martinson et al., 2007).

DCs are furthermore involved in the generation of regulatory T cells and thus induce both, immunity and tolerance. DCs shown to induce tolerance are plasmacytoid DCs (pDCs). (Steinman, 2000).

3.1.3 pDCs and HIV

Plasmacytoid DCs or type 1 IFN-producing cells, are innate immune cells specialized in releasing massive amounts of IFNα and IFNβ upon viral challenge, including HIV (Fig. 3)

(Siegal et al., 1999). This blood DC population expresses high levels of HLA-DR and the characteristic markers BDCA-2 and CD123 (Table 1), but not CD11c, a marker of myeloid DCs (Table 1) (O´Doherty et al., 1994; Dzionek et al., 2001). pDCs are key initiators of the innate immune response *in vivo* and they can prime adaptive immunity due to the afore mentioned production of high type I interferon levels, especially upon exposure to viral products (Cella et al., 1999; Siegal et al, 1999). pDCs recognize pathogenic single-stranded RNA or unmethylated DNA mainly by TLR7 and TLR9. Due to the intracellular localization of these TLRs, the viruses have to be ingested by the cells and endosomal maturation must occur to activate NFkB- and MAPK-signals through MyD88. Once activated, pDCs mature and produce large amounts of pro-inflammatory and antiviral cytokines (Kadowaki et al., 2000; Ito et al., 2002; Colonna et al., 2004). pDCs do not only act as pro-inflammatory cells, but also provide negative regulatory signals and thereby induce tolerance (Ochando et al., 2006). pDCs express indoleamine 2,3-dioxygenase (IDO) and programmed death ligand 1 (PDL-1) that are associated with the negative modulation of T cell responses and regulatory T cell induction (Boasso et al., 2007, 2008; Chen et al., 2008). As shown, constant exposure of pDCs to HIV results in their chronic hyperactivation coming along with production of type I interferon and IDO, which exerts cytotoxic as well as suppressive effects on T cells (Herbeuval and Shearer, 2007). In acute HIV-infection pDCs recruit and activate NK cells to the sites of infection as well as to the lymph nodes (Gerosa et al., 2002; Megjugorac et al., 2004). The activation is due to IFNα released from pDCs, which was demonstrated to induce increased perforin expression in NK and $CD8^+$ T cells. The pDC-NK cell activation is bi-directional, since activated NK cells deplete immature pDCs to possibly select the more immunogenic mature pDCs at the sites on infection (Pertales et al., 2003a, 2003b; Ferlazzo and Munz, 2004). This process is called 'DC-editing' (Ferlazzo et al., 2002). Beside NK cell recruitment and activation, pDC-produced IFNα promotes maturation and migration of DCs.

pDCs are not as efficient in antigen-presentation as myeloid DCs and they are not located in high amounts at the site of pathogen entry. Due to their spontaneous antiviral and NK priming activity they are supposed to control the virus in the acute phase of infection and it is unlikely that they are involved in HIV capture, transport and transmission.

Deficiencies in pDC function were among the earliest observations of immune dysfunction in HIV-1 infection. Loss of pDCs in blood of chronically infected individuals has been ascribed to cell death and/or to a failure of bone marrow progenitors to differentiate into pDCs. Additionally, a low productive virus replication of IFNα-producing pDCs has been shown *in vivo* and *in vitro* by R5- and X4-tropic HIV variants (Donaghy et al., 2003; Schmidt et al, 2004). It is not known so far, if infection of pDCs plays a role for IFNα-secretion.

3.2 NK and NK T cells in acute HIV infection

Natural killer (NK) cells are lymphocytes deriving from bone marrow precursors. They circulate as mature populations in blood and spleen and are activated by type I interferons (Fig. 3). Classical NK cells do not express T cell antigen receptors (TCR) and are CD3-negative. They produce high levels of certain cyto- and chemokines, such as MIP-1α, MIP-1β, RANTES, TNFα, GM-CSF or IFN-γ and mediate significant levels of cytotoxic activity by exocytosis of granules containing perforin and granzymes. NK cells thus efficiently contribute to innate immune responses due to their spontaneous cytotoxic action against tumor and virus-infected targets. The direct cytotoxic activity of NK cells is regulated by the balance of activating and inhibitory NK cell receptors (Moretta et al, 2001; Moretta, 2002; Lanier, 2005) and they are able to kill HIV-infected target cells by direct lysis or by antibody-dependent cell-mediated cytotoxicity (ADCC) (Tasca et al, 2003; Bonaparte and Barker, 2004). ADCC is mediated in classical NK cells through their cell surface receptors for immunoglobulins (FcR). Additionally, NK cells initiate priming of the adaptive immunity due to their cross-talk with DCs. As mentioned above, NK cells activate DCs by cell-cell contact or secretion of cytokines and vice versa, DC-derived cytokines and membrane-bound molecules play a key role in NK cell activation (Zitvogel, 2002; Andrews et al, 2003; Ferlazzo et al, 2004; Cooper et al., 2004; Moretta et al, 2006; Newman et al, 2006). Their killer inhibitory receptors (KIRs), which transmit an inhibitory signal, if they encounter MHC class I molecules on a cell surface, are crucial in killing virus-infected cells. Two subsets of classical NK cells can be distinguished by their expression of CD16 and CD56. >95% of the NK cells belong to the $CD16^{high}CD56^{low}$ subset, which is responsible for the direct lysis of cells and the ADCC (Nagler et al, 1989; Caligiuri et al, 1990). The remaining 5% $CD16^{low/-}CD56^{high}$ subset produces high concentrations of IFN-γ and TNF-α, but this sub-population exerts a very low cytotoxic potential (Ahmad and Menezes, 1996). In HIV-infected individuals NK cell responses were shown to be impaired and the defects comprised cytotoxic activity of NK cells as well as secretion of CCR5-ligands MIP1α, MIP1β and RANTES (Scott-Algara et al, 1992; Mavilio et al, 2003; Kottilil, 2003). The HIV-mediated impairment of NK cells becomes manifest early after infection and continues during HIV progression and can be attributed to several factors:

HIV-infected individuals might have a down-regulation in intracellular perforin and granzyme A stores, which would account for the decreased cytotoxic capacity of NK cells in HIV-infection (Portales et al., 2003).

Another explanation might be the change in the expression patterns of various activating and inhibitory NK cell receptors during HIV-infection (DeMaria et al., 2003).

Chronic viral stimulation may also lead to inappropriate activation of peripheral NK cells, thus resulting in NK cell exhaustion or anergy (Alter et al., 2005; Mavilio et al., 2005).

Finally, $CD4^+$ NK cells may be a reservoir for HIV-1 *in vivo* and further investigation is necessary to explore this possibility.

A population of T cells sharing characteristics with classical NK cells has been identified based on expression of NK cell markers, and this population was named NK T cells (McDonald, 1995). NK T cells, a rare population of T lymphocytes, comprise only 0.01 ~ 1% of human peripheral blood mononuclear cells and play an important role in the innate immune defense (Motsinger et al, 2002). NK T cells are important immunoregulatory cells, producing both, high amounts of IFN-γ (⇨ double-negative NK T cells), a major T_H1 cytokine, and IL-4 and IL-13 (⇨ $CD4^+$ NK T cells), the major T_H2 type cytokines (Gumperz et al, 2002; Lee et al, 2002). Thus NK T cells may provide quicker help for a cell- (IFN-γ) or antibody-mediated (IL-4) response than conventional T cells through recruiting and stimulating other effector cells, such as NK cells, macrophages, DCs and conventional T cells. NK T cells can in addition act directly cytolytic through involving the perforin/granzymes and the Fas/FasL pathway (Metelitsa et al., 2001).

A semi-invariant TCR (NK T TCR) is expressed on NK T cells consisting of an invariant α-chain, and a restricted TCR-β-chain repertoire (rev. in Godfrey and Kronenberg, 2004). NK T cells recognize self or foreign glycolipids presented by the non-polymorphic MHC class I-like molecule CD1d (Bendelac et al, 1997; Joyce, 2001). NK T cells are stimulated by type I interferons or pro-inflammatory cytokines (IL-15, IL-12, IL-18). Therefore, also NK T cells need a cross-talk with DCs to be fully activated (pDCs ⇨ type I IFNs, DCs ⇨ IL-12).

Upon HIV-1 infection NK T cells are rapidly and selectively depleted from the circulation. The NK T cell numbers are dramatically reduced in HIV-infected individuals compared to healthy donors (Motsinger et al., 2002; Van der Vliet et al, 2004). *In vivo* studies showed that the decrease in NK T cell numbers significantly correlated with higher viral loads in infected individuals (Motsinger et al., 2002) and that these HIV-susceptible cells were rapidly destroyed *in vitro* by R5-tropic HIV-strains (Motsinger et al., 2002). The mature NK T phenotype is induced by persistent stimulation of the cells with unidentified self-Ags or Ag-independent mechanisms and the high expression of CCR5 on the surface renders NK T cells permissive for HIV. They are not only efficiently infected by HIV but also contribute to the viral spread due to activating resting by-stander CD4^{+} T cells (Unutmaz et al., 1999).

The rapid loss of NK T cells during early HIV-infection causes subsequent depletion of important immunoregulatory functions, which are involved in tumor immunity, defense against other invading pathogens and autoimmune diseases. This might facilitate establishment of other opportunistic infections or tumor development frequently detected at later stages of the disease. NKT cells are important cells of the innate immune system, which are selectively and rapidly depleted by HIV-1 infection. Stimulation of the surviving NK T cells is additionally impeded due to down-regulation of CD1d on antigen-presenting cells.

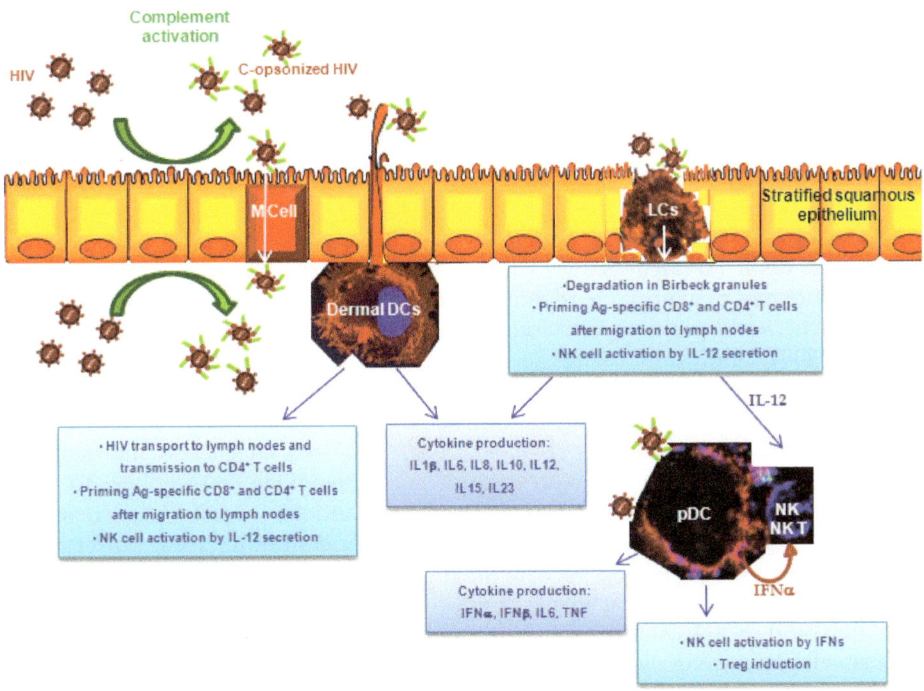

Fig. 3. Functions of DCs and NK/NK T cells during acute HIV infection

3.3 Macrophages in acute HIV infection

Macrophages resident at mucosal sites are proposed to play an important role during HIV-1 pathogenesis. Macrophages bridge innate and adaptive immunity similar to DCs, NK and NK T cells. They are recognizing, internalizing and degrading microorganisms and clear cell debris via TLRs, C-type lectins (Dectin-1), Fc receptors and complement receptor 3. Furthermore, macrophages present pathogen-derived peptides via MHC class II, thus initiating adaptive immune responses, and secret pro-inflammatory cytokines. Upon HIV-infection they are among the first cells encountered by the virus, but they are able to resist to HIV-mediated cytopathic effects. Therefore, macrophages are thought to serve as major cellular HIV reservoir together with latently infected resting $CD4^+$ T cells for long-term infection. Productively infected macrophages were detected in both untreated patients and those receiving antiretroviral therapy (ART), but the HIV infection within macrophages was not associated with virus-induced cytopathic effects (Koenig et al, 1986; Sharkey et al, 2000). The infectious virus is retained in macrophages for a prolonged period of time and the virus may be released from macrophages delayed and in a different compartment - thus macrophages contribute to persistence and spread of the virus (Crowe et al., 2003; Montaner et al., 2006; Carter and Ehrlich, 2008). As detected in NK or NK T cells, the functions of macrophages were found to be impaired by HIV-1 infection *in vitro* and *in vivo*. *In vivo* macrophages from HIV-infected individuals were found to be defective for phagocytosis of apopotic cells (Torre et al., 2002). *In vitro* HIV-1 impeded with phagocytosis via CR3 or FcR and also impaired internalization of *Candida albicans* and *Toxoplasma gondii* (Crowe et al., 1994; Kedzierska et al., 2002; Azzam et al., 2006; Leeansyah et al., 2007). As recently shown, Nef was a crucial factor in disrupting phagocytosis in HIV-1-infected cells (Mazzolini et al., 2010).

HIV and its accessory genes alter macrophage immune responses, macrophage cell cycle and enhance their own viral replication in macrophages (Margottin et al, 1998; Hassaïne et al, 2001; Federico et al, 2001; Coberley et al, 2004; Olivetta et al, 2005). HIV mediated a pro-inflammatory gene expression pattern in macrophages as demonstrated by microarray analyses, and this pro-inflammatory cytokine profile is suggested to enhance virus replication and persistence of chronically activated macrophages *in vivo*. In addition to up-regulation of pro-inflammatory cytokines, IFN- and NFκB-responsive cyto- and chemokines were increased upon HIV-1 infection. Up-regulation of these IFN- and NFκB-responsive cyto- and chemokines may promote recruitment of $CD4^+$ T cells and macrophages to sites of infection, which would promote the viral spread (Cicala et al, 2002; Izmailova et al, 2003; Woelk et al, 2004). Only low expression levels of CD4 are detected on the surface of macrophages; in contrast high levels of heparan sulfate proteoglycans (such as syndecan), macrophage mannose receptor (MR), and elastase are expressed (Nguyen and Hildreth, 2003; Bristow et al, 2003; De Parseval et al, 2005). HIV can attach and internalize into macrophages via these receptors. Expression of both chemokine co-receptors, CCR5 and CXCR4, was verified on primary human macrophages, and they can be infected with R5-, dual- and X4-tropic virus isolates *in vitro* and *in vivo* (Verani et al, 1998; Liu et al, 1996; Samson et al, 1998; Clapham and McKnight, 2002). Once ingested by macrophages, HIV accumulates in endocytic compartments similar to multivesicular bodies, which facilitate HIV assembly and escape immune surveillance (Kramer et al, 2005). This accumulation of HIV in the cytoplasmic vesicles of macrophages results in persistent storage of infectious virions and a delayed rapid infection of $CD4^+$ T cells (Sharova et al, 2005). When a virological synapse is formed between a macrophage and a T cell, the virus is efficiently transmitted. Therefore tissue macrophages were claimed to act as 'Trojan horse', that hide the virus from the immune system and disseminate the virus even after months.

3.4 Monocytes in acute HIV infection

Similar to DCs, LCs and macrophages, monocytes provide a first line of defense against invading pathogens and act as key mediators of innate immune mechanisms. On the other hand, they are also targets for monocyte-tropic pathogens, such as *Listeria*, cytomegalovirus and HIV (Drevets and Leenen, 2000). Monocytes express CD4, CCR5 and CXCR4 and are in particular susceptible to macrophage-tropic HIV strains. Similar to macrophages, monocytes are resistant to the cytopathic effects of HIV, they represent a key virus reservoir and may also disseminate HIV in different locations such as the brain (Kedzierska and Crowe, 2002; Crow et al., 2003). Early in acute infection, HIV and SIV enter the central nervous system (CNS) and macrophages and monocytes seem to play a crucial role in the neuropathogenesis of HIV-infection and to contribute to HIV-mediated dementia due to production of pro-inflammatory cytokines and neurotoxins (Chakrabarti et al., 1991; Kedzierska and Crowe, 2002). The induction of pro-inflammatory cytokines is thought to facilitate the entry of monocytes into the brain by disrupting the blood-brain and blood-cerebrospinal fluid barrier (Persidsky et al., 2000; Eugenin and Berman, 2003). In particular, CCL2 was associated with inflammation of the CNS (Mahad and Ransohoff, 2003). This cytokine is mainly secreted by monocytes and macrophages and initiates migration of T cells and other monocytes into the CNS and promotion of neuronal cell-death during HIV and SIV infection (Gartner and Liu, 2002; Fantuzzi et al., 2003). HIV-1 Tat activates microglial and perivascular cells to produce pro-inflammatory proteins, thereby leading to monocyte infiltration into the brain (Pu et al, 2003). Other features promoted by Tat following infection with HIV were chemotaxis of monocytes, their adhesion to the endothelium, and their recruitment into extra-vascular tissues. This modulation of the chemotactic activity seems to be mediated by the Tat cysteine-rich domain (Albini et al, 1998).

Thus, monocytes represent a prinicpal reservoir for HIV persistence due to the long storage period of infectious viral particles and infectious HIV was shown to be recovered from patients obtaining ART. HIV thus affects multiple immune functions of monocytes/macrophages (chemotaxis, phagocytosis, intracellular killing, APC function, cytokine production) and thereof allows establishment as well as re-activation of other opportunistic infections (Kedzierska and Crowe, 2002).

3.5 γδT cells in acute HIV infection

γδT cells are primarily situated in the gastrointestinal mucosa and play an important role in the first line of defense against viral, bacterial, and fungal pathogens. γδT cells make up 50% of all lymphocytes in the intraepithelial compartment and about 10% of lymphocytes in the lamina propria (James et al., 1986; Targan et al., 1995). γδT cells recognize soluble protein and non-protein Ags, but the mechanism of recognition remains elusive. γδT cells participate in the immune response to various viruses, including herpes simplex virus, Epstein-Barr virus, and HIV-1 (Maccario et al., 1995). Co-culture of γδT cells with HIV-1 infected lymphocytes resulted in increased cytotoxicity and production of HIV-1-suppresive mediators against the infected cells (Wallace et al., 1996; Poccia et al., 1999; Cipriani et al., 2000). HIV-1 infection is accompanied by significant changes in the blood and mucosal γδT cells during acute infection and, despite HAART, persist into the chronic phase, but the factors involved in these changes remain to be investigated.

4. Conclusions

In summary, innate immune responses contribute significantly to the first line of defense against invading HIV-1 particles on the one hand, but the virus has evolved different strategies to escape from the innate immune system on the other hand. While Langerhans Cells and plasmacytoid dendritic cells exert efficient antiviral actions by degrading the virus via Birbeck granules (LCs) or secreting high amounts of type I interferons (especially IFNα), interstitial dermal dendritic cells are suggested to contribute in viral transport and dissemination. The antiviral functions of LCs are also reversed upon co-infection with other STIs or microbes due to the competition of the pathogens for Langerin. The competition for Langerin allows attachment of HIV-1 to its main receptors, CD4 and the chemokine-co-receptor CCR5, on LCs and thus facilitates infection of LCs and subsequent transfer to $CD4^+$ T cells in the lymph nodes. This process of '*cis*'-infection of DCs, migration to the lymphatic tissues and transmission to $CD4^+$ T cells is also thought to be contrived by dermal DCs. The virus is furthermore efficiently protected against complement-mediated lysis due to acquisition of regulators of complement activation during the budding process from the host cell (CD55, CD59) and additionally in fluid-phase (fH). Thus, most of the virus is opsonized with C3-fragments *in vivo,* which allows interaction with complement-receptor expressing cells at mucosal surfaces. Therefore the host immune system itself has to reverse the protection of the virus against complement-mediated lysis. As recently demonstrated (Banki/Posch et al., 2010), complement-opsonization acts as endogenous adjuvant for the dendritic cell-mediated induction of retrovirus-specific CTLs *in vitro* and *in vivo,* which was the first evidence that specific CTLs are efficiently stimulated in a complement- and DC-dependent manner. This enhanced and efficient CTL-stimulatory capacity of DCs upon complement-opsonization of HIV may provide a host-cell protecting mechanism at the beginning of infection and understanding the exact interplay between differentially opsonized retroviral particles and APCs is of prime importance for DC-based vaccination strategies against retroviral infections. Not only benefits result from the complement opsonization of HIV- such complement-opsonized particles can also be ingested by CR3-expressing macrophages and monocytes, the major reservoirs of long-term HIV-persistence beside latently infected $CD4^+$ T cells. These cells facilitate HIV assembly and escape immune surveillance by hiding the particles from the immune system and by allowing efficient transfer of the particles to target cells in a delayed manner and another compartment. Instead of destroying the virus at the initial phases of infection, macrophages and monocytes seem to act as ´Trojan horse´ by actively contributing to the spread of HIV over long time periods. Beside LCs and pDCs, γδT cells, primarily located in the gastrointestinal mucosa, NK and NK T cells, that are activated by IFNα-secreted pDCs, build an important first line of defense against viral, bacterial, and fungal pathogens. HIV-1 counteracts this innate immune barrier by changing their functions and decreasing their numbers by yet mainly undefined mechanisms. The HIV-mediated loss in numbers of important innate immune cells, such as pDCs, NK and NK T cells or γδT cells, is associated with a modified cytokine microenvironment, which may additionally account for the chronic establishment of HIV-infection in the host. Because it is difficult identifying infected individuals very soon after exposure, little is known respecting the earliest events of HIV transmission in the genital tract or rectal mucosa. Most of the findings are deriving from *in vivo* models of SIV infection (rev. in Haase, 2005) and from *ex vivo* models aimed to identify cells and factors affecting the transmission of HIV (rev. in Hladik and McElrath, 2008). Even when using animal models the exact process how the virus infiltrates mucosal barriers to establish a productive infection in the host is extremely complex to evaluate. There are multiple innate soluble and cellular factors acting together upon entry of HIV into the host - yet, the innate mechanisms and even the specific adaptive immune responses fail to restrict the replication of HIV in most infected individuals indicating the selection of viral mutants that are able to efficiently escape these early and late cellular and humoral immune responses. In the last years, increasing evidence suggests that especially immunologic and virologic events occuring during primary infection irreversibly weaken the immune system, which is not able to restore and gradually fails to resist viral and opportunistic infections.

5. References

Ahmad, A, Menezes, J (1996) Antibody-dependent cellular cytotoxicity in HIV infections, *Faseb J.* 10:258-266

Albini, A et al., (1998) Identification of a novel domain of HIV tat involved in monocyte chemotaxis, *J Biol Chem* 273:15895-15900

Alter, G. et al. (2005) Sequential deregulation of NK cell subset distribution and function starting in acute HIV-1 infection, *Blood* 106, 3366–3369

Altfeld, M, Fadda, L, Frleta, D, Bhardwaj, N, (2011) DCs and NK cells: critical effectors in the immune response to HIV-1, *Nat Rev Immunol.* Mar;11(3):176-86

Andrews, DM, Scalzo, AA, Yokoyama, WM, Smyth, MJ, Degli-Esposti, MA (2003) Functional interactions between dendritic cells and NK cells during viral infection, *Nat Immunol* 4:175-181

Armitage, R, (1994) Tumor necrosis factor receptor superfamily members and their ligands. *Curr Opin Immunol*; 6: 407–413

Azzam, R, Kedzierska, K, Leeansyah, E, et al. (2006) Impaired complement-mediated phagocytosis by HIV type-1-infected human monocyte-derived macrophages involves a cAMP-dependent mechanism, *AIDS Res Hum Retroviruses* 22(7):619–629

Banchereau, J, Steinman, RM, (1998) Dendritic cells and the control of immunity, *Nature* 392:245-252

Bánki, Z*, Posch, W*, Ejaz, A, Oberhauser, V, Willey, S, Gassner, C, Stoiber, H, Dittmer, U, Dierich, MP, Hasenkrug, KJ, Wilflingseder, D, (2010) Complement as an endogenous adjuvant for dendritic cell-mediated induction of retrovirus-specific CTLs, *PLoS Pathog.* Apr 29;6(4):e1000891 *equal contribution

Beignon, AS, McKenna, K, Skoberne, M, Manches, O, DaSilva, I, Kavanagh, DG, Larsson, M, Gorelick, RJ, Lifson, JD, Bhardwaj, N, (2005) Endocytosis of HIV-1 activates plasmacytoid dendritic cells via Toll-like receptor-viral RNA interactions, *J Clin Invest.* Nov;115(11):3265-7

Bell, D, Young, JW, Banchereau, J, (1999) Dendritic cells, *Adv. Immunol* 72,255-324

Bendelac, A, et al.,(1997) Selection and adaptation of cells expressing major histocompatibility complex class I-specific receptors of the natural killer complex, *J Exp Med* Aug 4;186(3):349-51

Biggs, BA, Hewish, M, Kent, S, Hayes, K, Crowe, SM, (1995) HIV-1 infection of human macrophages impairs phagocytosis and killing of Toxoplasma gondii, *J Immunol.* 154(11):6132–6139

Bleul, CC, Farzan, M, Choe, H, Parolin, C, Clark-Lewis, I, Sodroski, J, Springer, TA, (1996) The lymphocyte chemoattractant SDF-1 is a ligand for LESTR/fusin and blocks HIV-1 entry, *Nature* 382:829-33

Boasso, A, Hardy, AW, Anderson, SA, Dolan, MJ, Shearer GM, (2008) HIV-induced type I interferon and tryptophan catabolism drive T cell dysfunction despite phenotypic activation *PLoS One* 3:e2961

Boasso, A, Herbeuval, JP, Hardy, AW, Anderson, SA, Dolan MJ, Fuchs D, Shearer GM, (2007) HIV inhibits CD4^{+} T-cell proliferation by inducing indoleamine 2,3-dioxygenase in plasmacytoid dendritic cells, *Blood* 109:3351-3359.

Bonaparte, MI, Barker, E, (2004) Killing of human immunodeficiency virus-infected primary T-cell blasts by autologous natural killer cells is dependent on the ability of the virus to alter the expression of major histocompatibility complex class I molecules, *Blood* 104:2087-2094

Brenchley, JM, *et al.*, (2006) Microbial translocation is a cause of systemic immune activation in chronic HIV infection, *Nature Med.* 12, 1365–1371

Bristow, CL, Mercatante, DR, Kole, R, (2003) HIV-1 preferentially binds receptors copatched with cell-surface elastase, *Blood.* Dec 15;102(13):4479-8

Caligiuri, MA, Zmuidzinas, A, Manley, TJ, Levine, H, Smith, KA, Ritz, J. (1990) Functional consequences of interleukin 2 receptor expression on resting human lymphocytes. Identification of a novel natural killer cell subset with high affinity receptors, *J Exp Med.* May 1;171(5):1509-26

Carroll, MC, (2000) A protective role for innate immunity in autoimmune disease, *Clin Immunol.* Apr;95(1 Pt 2):S30-8

Carter, CA, Ehrlich, LS, (2008) Cell biology of HIV-1 infection of macrophages. *Annu Rev Microbiol.* 62:425–443

Casartelli, N, Guivel-Benhassine, F, Bouziat, R, Brandler, S, Schwartz, O, Moris, A. (2010) The antiviral factor APOBEC3G improves CTL recognition of cultured HIV-infected T cells, *J Exp Med.* Jan 18;207(1):39-49

Cella, M, Jarrossay, D, Facchetti, F, Alebardi, O, Nakajima, H, Lanzavecchia, A, Colonna, M, (1999) Plasmacytoid monocytes migrate to inflamed lymph nodes and produce large amounts of type I interferon, *Nat. Med.* 5,919-923

Chakrabarti, L, Hurtrel, M, Maire, MA, Vazeux, R, Dormont, D, Montagnier, L, and Hurtrel B. (1991) Early viral replication in the brain of SIV-infected rhesus monkeys. *Am. J. Pathol.* 139:1273-1280.

Chehimi, J, Starr, SE, Kawashima, H, et al. (1989) Dendritic cells and IFN-alpha-producing cells are two functionally distinct non-B, non-monocytic HLA-DR+ cell subsets in human peripheral blood, *Immunology,* 1989;68:488

Chen, W, Liang, X, Peterson, AJ, Munn, DH, Blazar, BR, (2008) The indoleamine 2,3-dioxygenase pathway is essential for human plasmacytoid dendritic cell-induced adaptive T regulatory cell generation *J. Immunol.* 181:5396-5404

Cicala, C, Arthos, J, Selig, SM, Dennis, GJr, Hosack, DA, Van Ryk, D, Spangler, ML, Steenbeke, TD, Khazanie, P, Gupta, N, Yang, J, Daucher, M, Lempicki, RA, Fauci, AS, (2002) , *Proc Natl Acad Sci U S A.* Jul 9;99(14):9380-5

Cipriani, B, Borsellino, G, Poccia, F, Placido, R, Tramonti, D, Bach, S, Battistini, L, Brosnan, CF, (2000) Activation of C-C beta-chemokines in human peripheral blood $\gamma\delta$T cells by isopentenyl pyrophosphate and regulation by cytokines, *Blood* 95:39-4

Clapham, PR, McKnight, A, (2002) Cell surface receptors, virus entry and tropism of primate lentiviruses, *J Gen Virol.* Aug;83(Pt 8):1809-29

Coberley, CR, Kohler, JJ, Brown, JN, Oshier, JT, Baker, HV, Popp, MP, Sleasman, JW, Goodenow, MM, (2004) Impact on genetic networks in human macrophages by a CCR5 strain of human immunodeficiency virus type 1, *J Virol.* Nov;78(21):11477-86

Cocchi, F, DeVico ,AL, Garzino-Demo, A, Arya, SK, Gallo, RC, Lusso, P, (1995) Identification of RANTES, MIP-1 alpha, and MIP-1 beta as the major HIV-suppressive factors produced by CD8+ T cells, *Science* 270:1811-5

Colonna, M, Trinchieri, G, Liu, Y J, (2004) Plasmacytoid dendritic cells in immunity, *Nat. Immunol.* 5:1219-1226

Cooper, MA, Fehniger, TA, Fuchs, A, Colonna, M, Caligiuri, MA, (2004) NK cell and DC interactions, *Trends Immunol* 25:47-52

Crowe, S, Zhu, T, Muller, WA, (2003) The contribution of monocyte infection and trafficking to viral persistence, and maintenance of the viral reservoir in HIV infection, *J Leukoc Biol.* 2003;74(5):635–641

Crowe, SM, Vardaxis, NJ, Kent, SJ, et al., (1994) HIV infection of monocyte-derived macrophages in vitro reduces phagocytosis of Candida albicans, *J Leukoc Biol.* 56(3):318–327

Da Costa, XJ, Brockman, MA, Alicot, E, Ma, M, Fischer, MB, Zhou, X, Knipe, DM, Carroll, MC, (1999) Humoral response to herpes simplex virus is complement-dependent, *Proc Natl Acad Sci U S A* Oct 26;96(22):12708-12

De Jong, MA, *et al.*, (2008) TNF-alpha and TLR agonists increase susceptibility to HIV-1 transmission by human Langerhans cells ex vivo, *J. Clin. Invest.* 118 pp. 3440–3452

De Jong MA, et al., (2010) Herpes simplex virus type 2 enhances HIV-1 susceptibility by affecting Langerhans cell function, *J. Immunol.* 185 pp. 1633–1648

De Jong, MA, Geijtenbeek, TB (2010) Langerhans cells in innate defense against pathogens, *Trends Immunol.* Dec;31(12):452-9. Epub 2010 Oct 26

De Maria, A, et al., The impaired NK cell cytolytic function in viremic HIV-1 infection is associated with a reduced surface expression of natural cytotoxicity receptors (NKp46, NKp30 and NKp44), *Eur. J. Immunol.* 33, 2410–2418

De Parseval, A, Bobardt, MD, Chatterji, A, Chatterji, U, Elder, JH, David, G, Zolla-Pazner, S, Farzan, M, Lee, TH, Gallay, PA. (2005) , *J Biol Chem.* Nov 25;280(47):39493-504

De Witte, L, Nabatov, A, Pion, M, Fluitsma, D, de Jong, MA, de Gruijl, T, Piguet, V, van Kooyk, Y, Geijtenbeek, TB, (2007) Langerin is a natural barrier to HIV-1 transmission by Langerhans cells, *Nat Med.* Mar;13(3):367-71

Diebold, SS, Kaisho, T, Hemmi, H, Akira, S, Reis e Sousa, C, (2004) Innate antiviral responses by means of TLR7-mediated recognition of single-stranded RNA, *Science* Mar 5;303(5663):1529-31. Epub 2004 Feb 19

Donaghy, H, Gazzard, B, Gotch, F, Patterson, S, (2003) Dysfunction and infection of freshly isolated blood myeloid and plasmacytoid dendritic cells in patients infected with HIV-1, *Blood* 101, 4505–4511

Drevets, DA, and PJ Leenen (2000) Leukocyte-facilitated entry of intracellular pathogens into the central nervous system. *Microbes Infect.* 2:1609-1618.

Dzionek, A, Sohma, Y, Nagafune, J, Cella, M, Colonna, M, Facchetti, F, Gunther, G, Johnston, I, Lanzavecchia, A, Nagasaka, T, et al, (2001) BDCA-2, a novel plasmacytoid dendritic cell-specific type II C-type lectin, mediates antigen capture and is a potent inhibitor of interferon alpha/beta induction, *J. Exp. Med.* 194,1823-1834

Engering, A, et al.,(2002) The dendritic cell-specific adhesion receptor DC-SIGN internalizes antigen for presentation to T cells, *J. Immunol.* 168, 2118–2126

Esser, R, von Briesen, H, Brugger, M, et al., (1991) Secretory repertoire of HIV-infected human monocytes/macrophages, *Pathobiology* 59: 219–222

Esser, R, Glienke, W, von Briesen, H, Rubsamen-Waigmann, H, Andreesen, R, (1996) Differential regulation of proinflammatory and hematopoietic cytokines in human macrophages after infection with human immunodeficiency virus, *Blood* 88: 3474–3481

Esser, R, Glienke, W, Andreesen, R, et al., (1998) Individual cell analysis of the cytokine repertoire in human immunodeficiency virus-1-infected monocytes/macrophages by a combination of immunocytochemistry and in situ hybridization *Blood* 1998; 91:4752–4760

Eugenin, EA, and Berman JW. (2003) Chemokine-dependent mechanisms of leukocyte trafficking across a model of the blood-brain barrier. Methods 29:351-361.

Fantuzzi, L, Belardelli, F, and Gessani S. (2003) Monocyte/macrophage-derived CC chemokines and their modulation by HIV-1 and cytokines: a complex network of interactions influencing viral replication and AIDS pathogenesis. J. Leukoc. Biol. 74:719-725

Fahrbach, KM, et al. (2007) Activated CD34-derived Langerhans cells mediate transinfection with human immunodeficiency virus, *J. Virol.* 81, 6858–6868

Federico, M, Percario, Z, Olivetta, E, Fiorucci, G, Muratori, C, Micheli, A, Romeo, G, Affabris, E, (2001) HIV-1 Nef activates STAT1 in human monocytes/macrophages through the release of soluble factors, *Blood* Nov 1;98(9):2752-61

Ferlazzo, G. et al., (2002) Human dendritic cells activate resting natural killer (NK) cells and are recognized via the NKp30 receptor by activated NK cells, *J. Exp. Med.* 195, 343–351

Ferlazzo, G, Munz, C, (2004) NK cell compartments and their activation by dendritic cells, *J Immunol*, 172:1333

Ferlazzo, G, Thomas, D, Lin, SL, Goodman, K, Morandi, B, Muller, WA, Moretta, A, Münz, C, (2004) The abundant NK cells in human secondary lymphoid tissues require activation to express killer cell Ig-like receptors and become cytolytic, *J Immunol.* Feb 1;172(3):1455-62

Frank, I, Stoiber, H, Godar, S, Stockinger, H, Steindl, F, Katinger, HW, Dierich, MP, (1996) Acquisition of host cell-surface-derived molecules by HIV-1, *AIDS* Dec;10(14):1611-20

Ganesh, L, Leung, K, Loré, K, Levin, R, Panet, A, Schwartz, O, Koup, RA, Nabel, GJ, (2004) Infection of specific dendritic cells by CCR5-tropic human immunodeficiency virus type 1 promotes cell-mediated transmission of virus resistant to broadly neutralizing antibodies, *J. Virol.* Nov;78(21):11980-7

Gartner, S, and Liu Y.(2002) Insights into the role of immune activation in HIV neuropathogenesis. *J. Neurovirol.* 8:69-75.

Geijtenbeek, TB, et al. , (2000) DC-SIGN, a dendritic cell-specific HIV-1-binding protein that enhances trans-infection of T cells, *Cell* 100, 587–597

Geijtenbeek, TB, van Kooyk, Y, (2003) DC-SIGN: a novel HIV receptor on DCs that mediates HIV-1 transmission, *Curr Top Microbiol Immunol* 276:31-54

Geijtenbeek, TB, Gringhuis, SI, (2009) Signalling through C-type lectin receptors: shaping immune responses, *Nat. Rev. Immunol.* 9, pp. 465–479

Gerosa, F., Baldani-Guerra, B, Nisii, C, Marchesini, V, Carra, G, Trinchieri, G, (2002) Reciprocal activating interaction between natural killer cells and dendritic cells, *J. Exp. Med.* 195 (2002), pp. 327–333

Ginhoux, F, Liu, K, Helft, J, Bogunovic, M, Greter, M, Hashimoto, D, Price, J, Yin, N, Bromberg, J, Lira, SA, et al., (2009) The origin and development of nonlymphoid tissue CD103+ DCs, *J. Exp. Med.* 206:3115–3130

Godfrey, DI, Kronenberg, M, (2004) Going both ways: immune regulation via CD1d-dependent NKT cells *J Clin Invest.* Nov;114(10):1379-88

Granelli-Piperno, A, Delgado, E, Finkel, V, Paxton, W, Steinman, RM (1998) Immature dendritic cells selectively replicate macrophagetropic (M-tropic) human immunodeficiency virus type 1, while mature cells efficiently transmit both M- and T-tropic virus to T cells, *J Virol* 72:2733-2737

Granelli-Piperno, A, Shimeliovich, I, Pack, M, Trumpfheller, C, Steinman, RM, (2006) HIV-1 selectively infects a subset of nonmaturing BDCA1-positive dendritic cells in human blood, *J. Immunol.* 176, 991–998

Griffin, G, Leung, K, Folks, T, Kunkel, S, Nabel, G, (1991) Induction of NF-kappa B during monocyte differentiation is associated with activation of HIV-gene expression, *Res Virol* 142: 233–238

Haase, AT, (2005) Perils at mucosal front lines for HIV and SIV and their hosts, *Nat. Rev. Immunol.* 5:783–92

Han, X, Becker, K, Degen, H, Jablonowski, H, Strohmeyer, G, (1996) Synergistic stimulatory effects of tumour necrosis factor alpha and interferon gamma on replication of human immunodeficiency virus type 1 and on apoptosis of HIV-1-infected host cells, *EurJ Clin Invest* 26: 286–292

Hassaïne, G, Courcoul, M, Bessou, G, Barthalay, Y, Picard, C, Olive, D, Collette, Y, Vigne, R, Decroly, E, (2001) The tyrosine kinase Hck is an inhibitor of HIV-1 replication counteracted by the viral vif protein, *J Biol Chem.* May 18;276(20):16885-93

Herbein, G, Gordon, S. (1997) 55- and 75-kilodalton tumor necrosis factor receptors mediate distinct actions in regard to human immunodeficiency virus type 1 replication in primary human macrophages, *J Virol* 71: 4150–4156

Herbeuval, JP, Shearer, GM, (2007) HIV-1 immunopathogenesis: how good interferon turns bad, *Clin Immunol.* May;123(2):121-8

Hladik, F, McElrath, MJ, 2008) *Setting* the stage: host invasion by HIV, *Nat. Rev. Immunol.* 8:447–57

Huber, M, Olson, WC, Trkola, A, (2008) Antibodies for HIV treatment and prevention: window of opportunity?, *Curr Top Microbiol Immunol* 317:39-66

Ito, T, Amakawa, R, Kaisho, T, Hemmi, H, Tajima, K, Uehira, K, Ozaki, Y, Tomizawa, H, Akira, S, Fukuhara, S, (2002) Interferon-alpha and interleukin-12 are induced differentially by Toll-like receptor 7 ligands in human blood dendritic cell subsets, *J. Exp. Med.* 195:1507-1512

Izmailova, E, Bertley, FM, Huang, Q, Makori, N, Miller, CJ, Young, RA, Aldovini, A, (2003) HIV-1 Tat reprograms immature dendritic cells to express chemoattractants for activated T cells and macrophages, *Nat Med.* 2003 Feb;9(2):191-7

James, SP, Fiocchi, C, Graeff, AS, Strober, W, (1986) Phenotypic analysis of lamina propria lymphocytes. Predominance of helper-inducer and cytolytic T-cell phenotypes and deficiency of suppressor-inducer phenotypes in Crohn's disease and control patients, *Gastroenterology* 91:1483-1489

Joyce, S, (2001) Immune recognition, response, and regulation: how T lymphocytes do it, *Immunol Res.* 23(2-3):215-28

Kacani, L, Prodinger, WM, Sprinzl, GM, Schwendinger, MG, Spruth, M, Stoiber, H, Döpper, S, Steinhuber, S, Steindl, F, Dierich, MP, (2000) *Detachment of human immunodeficiency virus type 1 from germinal centers by blocking complement receptor type 2, J Virol* 74:7997-8002

Kadowaki, N, Antonenko, S, Lau, JY, Liu, YJ, (2000) Natural interferon alpha/beta-producing cells link innate and adaptive immunity, *J. Exp. Med.* 192:219-226

Kadowaki, N, Ho, S, Antonenko, S, Malefyt, RW, Kastelein, RA, Bazan, F, Liu, YJ, (2001) Subsets of human dendritic cell precursors express different toll-like receptors and respond to different microbial antigens, *J Exp Med.* Sep 17;194(6):863-9

Katz, SI, Tamaki, K, Sachs, DH, (1979) Epidermal Langerhans cells are derived from cells originating in bone marrow, *Nature* 282,324-326

Katze, MG, He, Y, Gale, M Jr, (2002) Viruses and interferon: a fight for supremacy *Nat Rev Immunol.* Sep;2(9):675-87

Kawamura, T, et al., (2008) Significant Virus Replication in Langerhans Cells following Application of HIV to Abraded Skin: Relevance to Occupational Transmission of HIV, *J Immunol* 180:3297-3304

Kedzierska, K, Crowe, SM, (2002) The role of monocytes and macrophages in the pathogenesis of HIV-1 infection, *Curr Med Chem* 9:1893-1903

Kedzierska, K, Ellery, P, Mak, J, Lewin, SR, Crowe, SM, Jaworowski, A, (2002) HIV-1 down-modulates gamma signaling chain of Fc gamma R in human macrophages: a possible mechanism for inhibition of phagocytosis, *J Immunol.* 168(6):2895–2903

Koenig, S, Gendelman, HE, Orenstein, JM, Dal Canto, MC, Pezeshkpour, GH, Yungbluth, M, Janotta, F, Aksamit, A, Martin, MA, Fauci, AS, (1986) Detection of AIDS virus in macrophages in brain tissue from AIDS patients with encephalopathy, *Science* Sep 5;233(4768):1089-93

Kopf, M, Abel, B, Gallimore, A, Carroll, M, Bachmann, MF, (2002) Complement component C3 promotes T-cell priming and lung migration to control acute influenza virus infection, *Nat Med.* Apr;8(4):373-8

Kottilil, S, (2003) Natural killer cells in HIV-1 infection: role of NK cell-mediated non-cytolytic mechanisms in pathogenesis of HIV-1 infection, *Indian J Exp Biol.* Nov;41(11):1219-25

Kramer, B, Pelchen-Matthews, A, Deneka, M, Garcia, E, Piguet, V, Marsh, M, (2005) HIV interaction with endosomes in macrophages and dendritic cells, *Blood Cells Mol Dis* 35:136-142

Kwon, DS, Kaufmann, DE, (2010) Protective and detrimental roles of IL-10 in HIV pathogenesis, *Eur Cytokine Netw.* Sep 1;21(3):208-14

Lanier, LL, (2005) NK cell recognition, *Annu Rev Immunol* 23:225-274

Lee, KW, Lee, Y, Kim, DS, Kwon, HJ, (2006) Direct role of NF-kappaB activation in Toll-like receptor-triggered HLA-DRA expression *Eur J Immunol.* May;36(5):1254-66

Leeansyah, E, Wines, BD, Crowe, SM, Jaworowski, A, (2007) The mechanism underlying defective Fcgamma receptor-mediated phagocytosis by HIV-1-infected human monocyte-derived macrophages, *J Immunol.* 178(2):1096–1104

Lenz, A, Heine, M, Schuler, G, Romani, N, (1993) Human and murine dermis contain dendritic cells. Isolation by means of a novel method and phenotypical and functional characterization, *J. Clin. Invest.* 92,2587-2596

Liu, R, Paxton, WA, Choe, S, Ceradini, D, Martin, SR, Horuk, R, MacDonald, ME, Stuhlmann, H, Koup, RA, Landau, NR, (1996) Homozygous defect in HIV-1 coreceptor accounts for resistance of some multiply-exposed individuals to HIV-1 infection, *Cell* Aug 9;86(3):367-77

Liu, YJ, (2001) Dendritic cell subsets and lineages, and their functions in innate and adaptive immunity, *Cell* 106, 259–262

Maccario, R, Comoli, P, Percivalle, E, Montagna, D, Locatelli, F, Gerna, G, (1995) Herpes simplex virus-specific human cytotoxic T-cell colonies expressing either gamma delta or alpha beta T-cell receptor: role of accessory molecules on HLA-unrestricted killing of virus-infected targets, *Immunology* 85:49-56

Mahad, DJ, and Ransohoff RM. (2003) The role of MCP-1 (CCL2) and CCR2 in multiple sclerosis and experimental autoimmune encephalomyelitis (EAE). *Semin. Immunol.* 15:23-32

Mandl, JN, Barry, AP, Vanderford, TH, Kozyr, N, Chavan, R, Klucking, S, Barrat, FJ, Coffman, RL, Staprans, SI, Feinberg, MB, (2008) Divergent TLR7 and TLR9 signaling and type I interferon production distinguish pathogenic and nonpathogenic AIDS virus infections, *Nat Med.* Oct;14(10):1077-87. Epub 2008 Sep 14

Margottin, F, Bour, SP, Durand, H, Selig, L, Benichou, S, Richard, V, Thomas, D, Strebel, K, Benarous, R, (1998) A novel human WD protein, h-beta TrCp, that interacts with HIV-1 Vpu connects CD4 to the ER degradation pathway through an F-box motif, *Mol Cell* Mar;1(4):565-74

Martinson, JA, et al., (2007) Dendritic cells from HIV-1 infected individuals are less responsive to Toll-like receptor (TLR) ligands, *Cell. Immunol.* 250, 75–84

Mavilio, D, et al., (2003) Natural killer cells in HIV-1 infection: dichotomous effects of viremia on inhibitory and activating receptors and their functional correlates, *Proc Natl Acad Sci U S A* 100:15011-15016

Mavilio, D. et al., (2005) Characterization of $CD56^-/CD16^+$ natural killer (NK) cells: a highly dysfunctional NK subset expanded in HIV-infected viremic individuals, *Proc. Natl Acad. Sci. USA* 102, 2886–2891

Mazzolini, J, Herit, F, Bouchet, J, Benmerah, A, Benichou, S, Niedergang, F, (2010) Inhibition of phagocytosis in HIV-1-infected macrophages relies on Nef-dependent alteration of focal delivery of recycling compartments *Blood* May 27;115(21):4226-36

McDonald, D, Wu, L, Bohks, SM, KewalRamani, VN, Unutmaz, D, Hope, TJ, (2003) Recruitment of HIV and its receptors to dendritic cell-T cell junctions, *Science* 300:1295-1297

McDonald, HR, (1995) NK1.1C T cell receptor-®/¯C cells: new clues to theirorigin, specificity, and function, *J. Exp.Med.* 182:633–38

McElrath, MJ, De Rosa, SC, Moodie, Z, Dubey, S, Kierstead, L, Janes, H, Defawe, OD, Carter, DK, Hural, J, Akondy, R, Buchbinder, SP, Robertson, MN, Mehrotra, DV, Self, SG, Corey, L, Shiver, JW, Casimiro, DR; Step Study Protocol Team, (2008) HIV-1 vaccine-induced immunity in the test-of-concept Step Study: a case-cohort analysis, *Lancet* Nov 29;372(9653):1894-905

McLellan, AD, Heiser, A, Sorg, RV, Fearnley, DB, Hart, DN, (1998) Dermal dendritic cells associated with T lymphocytes in normal human skin display an activated phenotype, *J. Invest. Dermatol.*111,841-849

Megjugorac, NJ, Young, HA, Amrute, SB, Olshalsky, SL, Fitzgerald-Bocarsly, P, (2004) Virally stimulated plasmacytoid dendritic cells produce chemokines and induce migration of T and NK cells, *J. Leukoc. Biol.* 75, pp. 504–514

Meier, A, Alter, G, Frahm, N, Sidhu, H, Li, B, Bagchi, A, Teigen, N, Streeck, H, Stellbrink, HJ, Hellman, J, van Lunzen, J, Altfeld, M, (2007) MyD88-dependent immune activation mediated by human immunodeficiency virus type 1-encoded Toll-like receptor ligands, *J Virol.* Aug;81(15):8180-91

Mellman, I, Steinman, RM, (2001) Dendritic cells: specialized and regulated antigen processing machines, *Cell* 106:255-258

Meng, G. et al., (2002) Primary intestinal epithelial cells selectively transfer R5 HIV-1 to CCR5+ cells, *Nat. Med.* 2, 150–156

Metelitsa, LS, Naidenko, OV, Kant, A, et al., (2001) Human NKT cells mediate antitumor cytotoxicity directly by recognizing target cell CD1d with bound ligand or indirectly by producing IL-2 to activate NK cells, *J Immunol* 167:3114–3122

Merad, M, et al., (2008) Origin, homeostasis and function of Langerhans cells and other langerin-expressing dendritic cells, *Nat. Rev. Immunol.* 8 pp. 935–947

Montaner, LJ, Crowe, SM, Aquaro, S, Perno, CF, Stevenson, M, Collman, RG, (2006) Advances in macrophage and dendritic cell biology in HIV-1 infection stress key understudied areas in infection, pathogenesis, and analysis of viral reservoirs, *J Leukoc Biol.* 2006;80(5):961–964

Moretta, A, (2002) Natural killer cells and dendritic cells: rendezvous in abused tissues, *Nat Rev Immunol.* Dec;2(12):957-64

Moretta, L, Bottino, C, Cantoni, C, Mingari, MC, Moretta, A, (2001) Human natural killer cell function and receptors, *Curr Opin Pharmacol.* Aug;1(4):387-91

Moretta, L, et al., (2006) Effector and regulatory events during natural killer-dendritic cell interactions, *Immunol Rev* 214:219-228

Motsinger, A, Haas, DW, Stanic, AK, Van Kaer, L, Joyce, S, Unutmaz, D, (2002) CD1d-restricted human natural killer T cells are highly susceptible to human immunodeficiency virus 1 infection, *J Exp Med.* Apr 1;195(7):869-79

Nagler, A, Lanier, LL, Cwirla, S, Phillips, JH, (1989) Comparative studies of human FcRIII-positive and negative natural killer cells, *J Immunol.* Nov 15;143(10):3183-91

Naif, H, Ho-Shon, M, Chang, J, Cunningham, AL, (1994) Molecular mechanisms of IL-4 effect on HIV expression in promonocytic cell lines and primary human monocytes, *J Leukoc Biol* 56: 335–339

Nestle, F, et al., (1993) Characterization of dermal dendritic cells obtained from normal human skin reveals phenotypic and functionally distinctive subsets, *J. Immunol.* 151,6535-6545

Newman, KC, Korbel, DS, Hafalla, JC, Riley, EM, (2006) Cross-talk with myeloid accessory cells regulates human natural killer cell interferon-gamma responses to malaria, *PLoS Pathog* 2:e118

Nguyen, DG, Hildreth, JE, (2003) Involvement of macrophage mannose receptor in the binding and transmission of HIV by macrophages, *Eur J Immunol* 33:483-493

Oberlin, E, Amara, A, Bachelerie, F, Bessia, C, Virelizier, JL, Arenzana-Seisdedos, F, Schwartz, O, Heard, JM, Clark-Lewis, I, Legler, DF, Loetscher, M, Baggiolini, M, Moser, B, (1996) The CXC chemokine SDF-1 is the ligand for LESTR/fusin and prevents infection by T-cell-line-adapted HIV-1, *Nature* 382:833-5

Ochando, JC, Homma, C, Yang, Y, Hidalgo, A, Garin, A, Tacke, F, Angeli, V, Li, Y, Boros, P, Ding, Y, Jessberger, R, Trinchieri, G, Lira, SA, Randolph, GJ, Bromberg, JS, (2006) Alloantigen-presenting plasmacytoid dendritic cells mediate tolerance to vascularized grafts, *Nat. Immunol.* 7:652-662

O'Doherty, U, Peng, M, Gezelter, S, Swiggard, WJ, Betjes, M, Bhardwaj, N, Steinman, RM (1994) Human blood contains two subsets of dendritic cells, one immunologically mature and the other immature, *Immunology* 82,487-493

Ogawa, Y, Kawamura, T, Kimura, T, Ito, M, Blauvelt, A, Shimada, S, (2009) Gram-positive bacteria enhance HIV-1 susceptibility in Langerhans cells, but not in dendritic cells, via Toll-like receptor activation, *Blood.* May 21;113(21):5157-66

Olivetta, E, Pietraforte, D, Schiavoni, I, Minetti, M, Federico, M, Sanchez, M, (2005) HIV-1 Nef regulates the release of superoxide anions from human macrophages, *Biochem J.* Sep 1;390(Pt 2):591-602

Pantaleo, G, et al., (1995) Studies in subjects with long-term nonprogressive human immunodeficiency virus infection, *N Engl J Med.* 332:209-216

Pavli, P, Woodhams, CE, Doe, WF, Hume, DA, (1990) Isolation and characterization of antigen-presenting dendritic cells from the mouse intestinal lamina propria, *Immunology* 70,40-47

Pavli, P, Hume, DA, Van De Pol, E, Doe, WF, (1993) Dendritic cells, the major antigen-presenting cells of the human colonic lamina propria, *Immunology* 78,132-141

Persidsky, Y, Zheng, J, Miller, D, and Gendelman, HE. (2000) Mononuclear phagocytes mediate blood-brain barrier compromise and neuronal injury during HIV-1-associated dementia. J. Leukoc. Biol. 68:413-422

Piguet, V, Sattentau, Q, (2004) Dangerous liaisons at the virological synapse, *J Clin Invest* 114:605-610

Piguet ,V, Steinman, RM, (2007) The interaction of HIV with dendritic cells: outcomes and pathways, *Trends Immunol.* 28:503-510

Poccia, F, Battistini, L, Cipriani, B, Mancino, G, Martini, F, Gougeon, ML, Colizzi, V, (1999) Phosphoantigen-reactive $V\gamma 9V\delta 2$ T lymphocytes suppress in vitro human immunodeficiency virus type 1 replication by cell-released antiviral factors including CC chemokines, *J. Infect. Dis.* 180:858-861

Poli, G, Bressler, P, Kinter, A, Duh, E, Timmer, WC, Rabson, A, Justement, JS, Stanley, S, Fauci, AS, (1990) Interleukin 6 induces human immunodeficiency virus expression in infected monocytic cells alone and in synergy with tumor necrosis factor alpha by transcriptional and post-transcriptional mechanisms, *J Exp Med.* Jul 1;172(1):151-8

Poli, G, Fauci, AS, (1992) The effect of cytokines and pharmacologic agents on chronic HIV infection, *AIDS Res Hum Retroviruses* Feb;8(2):191-7

Pope, M, Gezelter, S, Gallo, N, Hoffman, L, Steinman, RM. (2003) Low levels of HIV-1 infection in cutaneous dendritic cells promote extensive viral replication upon binding to memory CD4+ T cells, *J Exp Med.* Dec 1;182(6):2045-56

Portales, P, Reynes, J, Rouzier-Panis, R, et al., (2003) Perforin expression in T cells and virological response to PEG-interferon alpha2b in HIV-1 infection, *AIDS* 17:505

Portales, P. ,et al., (2003) Interferon-α restores HIV-induced alteration of natural killer cell perforin expression in vivo, *AIDS* 17, 495–504

Pruenster, M*, Wilflingseder, D*, et al., (2005) C-type lectin-independent interaction of complement opsonized HIV with monocyte-derived dendritic cells, *Eur J Immunol* 35:2691-2698

Pu, H, Tian, J, Flora, G, Lee, YW, Nath, A, Hennig, B, Toborek, M, (2003) HIV-1 Tat protein upregulates inflammatory mediators and induces monocyte invasion into the brain, *Mol Cell Neurosci.* Sep;24(1):224-37

Roberts, L, Passmore, JA, Williamson, C, Little, F, Bebell, LM, Mlisana, K, Burgers, WA, van Loggerenberg, F, Walzl, G, Djoba Siawaya, JF, Karim, QA, Karim, SS, (2010) Plasma cytokine levels during acute HIV-1 infection predict HIV disease progression, *AIDS*, Mar 27;24(6):819-31

Romani, N, Stingl, G, Tschachler, E, Witmer, MD, Steinman, RM, Shevach, EM, Schuler, G, (1985) The Thy-1-bearing cell of murine epidermis. A distinctive leukocyte perhaps related to natural killer cells, *J. Exp. Med.* 161,1368-1383

Romani, N. et al., (2010) Langerhans cells and more: langerin-expressing dendritic cell subsets in the skin, *Immunol.* Rev. 234, pp. 120–141

Sabado, RL, O'Brien, M, Subedi, A, et al., (2010) Evidence of dysregulation of dendritic cells in primary HIV infection, *Blood* 116(19):3839–3852

Samson, M, Libert, F, Doranz, BJ, Rucker, J, Liesnard, C, Farber, CM, Saragosti, S, Lapoumeroulie, C, Cognaux, J, Forceille, C, Muyldermans, G, Verhofstede, C, Burtonboy, G, Georges, M, Imai, T, Rana, S, Yi, Y, Smyth, RJ, Collman, RG, Doms, RW, Vassart, G, Parmentier, M, (1998) Resistance to HIV-1 infection in caucasian individuals bearing mutant alleles of the CCR-5 chemokine receptor gene, *Nature.* Aug 22;382(6593):722-5

Schmidt, B, Scott, I, Whitmore, RG, Foster, H, Fujimura, S, Schmitz, J, Levy, JA, (2004) Low-level HIV infection of plasmacytoid dendritic cells: onset of cytopathic effects and cell death after PDC maturation *Virology.* Nov 24;329(2):280-8

Scott-Algara, D, Vuillier, F, Cayota, A, Dighiero, G, (1992) Natural killer (NK) cell activity during HIV infection: a decrease in NK activity is observed at the clonal level and is not restored after in vitro long-term culture of NK cells, *Clin Exp Immunol.* 90(2):181-7

Sharkey, ME, Teo, I, Greenough, T, Sharova, N, Luzuriaga, K, Sullivan, JL, Bucy, RP, Kostrikis, LG, Haase, A, Veryard, C, Davaro, RE, Cheeseman, SH, Daly, JS, Bova, C, Ellison, RT 3rd, Mady, B, Lai, KK, Moyle, G, Nelson, M, Gazzard, B, Shaunak, S, Stevenson, M, (2000) Persistence of episomal HIV-1 infection intermediates in patients on highly active anti-retroviral therapy, *Nat Med.* Jan;6(1):76-81

Sharova, N, Swingler, C, Sharkey, M, Stevenson, M (2005) Macrophages archive HIV-1 virions for dissemination in trans, *Embo J.* 24:2481-2489

Siegal, FP, Kadowaki, N, Shodell, M, Fitzgerald-Bocarsly, PA, Shah, K, Ho, S, Antonenko, S, Liu, YJ, (1999) The nature of the principal type 1 interferon-producing cells in human blood, *Science* 284,1835-1837

Spear, GT, Lurain, NS, Parker, CJ, Ghassemi, M, Payne, GH, Saifuddin, M, (1995) Host cell-derived complement control proteins CD55 and CD59 are incorporated into the virions of two unrelated enveloped viruses. Human T cell leukemia/lymphoma virus type I (HTLV-I) and human cytomegalovirus (HCMV), *J Immunol.* Nov 1;155(9):4376-81

Speth, C, Prodinger, WM, Würzner, R, Stoiber, H, Dierich, MP, (2008) Complement In: Fundamental Immunology 6th edition, (ed Pauls). *Lippincott-Raven Philadelphia* New York, pp 1047-1078

Spiller, OB, Hanna, SM, Devine, DV, Tufaro, F, (1997) Neutralization of cytomegalovirus virions: the role of complement, *J Infect Dis.* Aug;176(2):339-47

Stacey, AR, Norris, PJ, Qin, L, Haygreen, EA, Taylor, E, Heitman, J, Lebedeva, M, DeCamp, A, Li, D, Grove, D, Self, SG, Borrow, P, (2009) Induction of a striking systemic cytokine cascade prior to peak viremia in acute human immunodeficiency virus type 1 infection, in contrast to more modest and delayed responses in acute hepatitis B and C virus infections, *J Virol.* 2009 Apr;83(8):3719-33

Steinman, RM, (2000) The dendritic cell advantage: New focus for immune-based therapies, *Drug News Perspect* 13:581-586

Stoiber, H, Banki, Z, Wilflingseder, D, Dierich, MP, (2007) Complement-HIV interactions during all steps of viral pathogenesis,*Vaccine* Jun 6;26(24):3046-54

Targan, SR, Deem, RL, Liu, M, Wang, S, Nel, A, (1995) Definition of a lamina propria T cell responsive state. Enhanced cytokine responsiveness of T cells stimulated through the CD2 pathway, *J. Immunol.* 154:664-675

Tasca, S, Tambussi, G, Nozza, S, Capiluppi, B, Zocchi, MR, Soldini, L, Veglia, F, Poli, G, Lazzarin, A, Fortis, C, (2003) Escape of monocyte-derived dendritic cells of HIV-1 infected individuals from natural killer cell-mediated lysis, *AIDS* Nov 7;17(16):2291-8

Torre, D, Gennero, L, Baccino, FM, Speranza, F, Biondi, G, Pugliese, A, (2002) Impaired macrophage phagocytosis of apoptotic neutrophils in patients with human immunodeficiency virus type 1 infection, *Clin Diagn Lab Immunol.* 9(5):983–986

Turville, SG, Santos, JJ, Frank, I, Cameron, PU, Wilkinson, J, Miranda-Saksena, M, Dable, J, Stössel, H, Romani, N, Piatak, M Jr, Lifson, JD, Pope, M, Cunningham, AL, (2004) Immunodeficiency virus uptake, turnover, and 2-phase transfer in human dendritic cells, *Blood* Mar 15;103(6):2170-9

Flacher, V, et al., (2006) Human Langerhans cells express a specific TLR profile and differentially respond to viruses and Gram-positive bacteria, *J. Immunol.* 177 pp. 7959–7967

Unutmaz, D, KewalRamani, VN, Marmon, S, Littman, DR, (1999) Cytokine signals are sufficient for HIV-1 infection of resting human T lymphocytes *J Exp Med.* Jun 7;189(11):1735-46

Valladeau, J, Ravel, O, Dezutter-Dambuyant, C, Moore, K, Kleijmeer, M, Liu, Y, Duvert-Frances, V, Vincent, C, Schmitt, D, Davoust, J, et al, (2000) Langerin, a novel C-type lectin specific to Langerhans cells, is an endocytic receptor that induces the formation of Birbeck granules, *Immunity* 12,71-81 van der Vliet, HJ, Molling, JW, von Blomberg, BM, Nishi, N, Kölgen, W, van den Eertwegh, AJ, Pinedo, HM, Giaccone ,G, Scheper, RJ, (2004) The immunoregulatory role of CD1d-restricted natural killer T cells in disease, *Clin Immunol.* Jul;112(1):8-23

Verani, A, Pesenti, E, Polo, S, Tresoldi, E, Scarlatti, G, Lusso, P, Siccardi, AG, Vercelli, D, (1998) CXCR4 is a functional coreceptor for infection of human macrophages by CXCR4-dependent primary HIV-1 isolates, *J Immunol.* Sep 1;161(5):2084-8

Wallace, M, Bartz, SR, Chang, WL, Mackenzie, DA, Pauza, CD, Malkovsky, M, (1996) Gamma delta T lymphocyte responses to HIV, *Clin. Exp. Immunol.* 103:177-184

Wang, J, Roderiquez, G, Oravecz, T, Norcross, MA, (1998) Cytokine regulation of human immunodeficiency virus type 1 entry and replication in human monocytes/macrophages through modulation of CCR5 expression,
J Virol. Sep;72(9):7642-7

Weissman, D, Poli, G, Fauci, AS, (1994) Interleukin 10 blocks HIV replication in macrophages by inhibiting the autocrine loop of tumor necrosis factor alpha and interleukin 6 induction of virus, *AIDS Res Hum Retroviruses,* Oct;10(10):1199-206

Wilflingseder, D, et al., (2007) IgG opsonization of HIV impedes provirus formation in and infection of dendritic cells and subsequent long-term transfer to T cells, *J Immunol* 178:7840-7848

Woelk, CH, et al., (2004) Interferon gene expression following HIV type 1 infection of monocyte-derived macrophages, *AIDS Res Hum Retroviruses* 20:1210-1222

Wu, L, KewalRamani, VN, (2006) Dendritic-cell interactions with HIV: infection and viral dissemination, *Nat. Rev. Immunol.* 6, pp. 859–868

Ogawa, Y, et al., Gram-positive bacteria enhance HIV-1 susceptibility in Langerhans cells, but not in dendritic cells, via Toll-like receptor activation, *Blood* 113 (2009), pp. 5157–5166

Yu, Y, Hagihara, M, Ando, K, et al., (2001) Enhancement of human cord blood CD34+ cell-derived NK cell cytotoxicity by dendritic cells, *J Immunol,* 2001;166:1590

Zitvogel, L, (2002) Dendritic and natural killer cells cooperate in the control/switch of innate immunity, J Exp Med 195:F9-14

Part 3

Host Factors in HIV Pathogenesis

7

Factors Contributing to HIV-1 Induced Pathogenesis in the Human Thymus

Bianca Blom[1], Marta Epeldegui[2] and Christel H. Uittenbogaart[2]
[1]*Academic Medical Center, University of Amsterdam*
Dept. Of Cell Biology & Histology, Amsterdam
[2]*UCLA AIDS Institute, David E. Geffen School of Medicine, University of California*
Department of Microbiology, Immunology & Molecular Genetics, Los Angeles, CA
[1]*The Netherlands*
[2]*USA*

1. Introduction

HIV infection is associated with a progressive loss of CD4+ T cells, leading to an acquired immunodeficiency syndrome (AIDS). The CD4+ T-cell depletion is due to the direct destruction of infected CD4+ T cells, as well as to an impaired production of T cells in the thymus. Our understanding of the exact role of the thymus in HIV-1 infection and HIV-1 pathogenesis remains incomplete, although substantial progress has been made over the last decade. *De Novo* generation of naïve human T cells occurs in the thymus, seeded with CD34+ progenitor cells, migrating from the bone marrow. These progenitor cells sequentially undergo a process of tightly controlled differentiation, including the rearrangement of T cell receptor genes, ultimately leading to the generation of functionally mature CD4+ and CD8+ single-positive (SP) T cells. Much has been learned of the types of cells in the thymus that are targets for CXCR4-tropic and CCR5-tropic HIV-1 isolates. Several groups provided evidence that HIV can infect thymocytes at various developmental stages. In addition, HIV activates the natural type-I-interferon (IFN)-producing plasmacytoid dendritic cells (pDC) that may induce bystander effects resulting in chronic immune activation. Evidence is also mounting that HIV induces abnormal development of regulatory T (Treg) cells in the thymus, either by direct infection or by enhancement of their survival and function, mediated by host-derived pro-inflammatory molecules. Collectively, these events compromise thymic function resulting in a decreased thymic output and a general decline in peripheral CD4+ T-cell numbers. Here we aim to discuss the cellular targets for CCR5-tropic and CXCR4-tropic HIV-1 isolates in the thymus, and how virus tropism relates to architectural differences observed in the HIV-infected thymus. In addition, we will discuss the role of pDC and Treg in HIV pathogenicity, and the impact of type I IFN on T cell regeneration. Finally, we will review the present status on the use of humanized mouse and non-human primate models to study HIV-1 infection of the thymus.

2. Thymic seeding progenitor cells

T cells uniquely complete their development in the specialized environment of the thymus, which in addition to TCRαβ T cells also supports development of functionally different types of T cells, including TCRγδ T cells, NKT cells, and regulatory T cells. The human thymus is seeded by hematopoietic progenitor cells that arrive via the blood and initially originate from the fetal liver (between week 6-20 of gestation) and later from the fetal bone marrow (from week 20 of gestation) and adult bone marrow. Our current understanding is that the thymus remains active through an advanced age, suggesting that thymic seeding progenitor cells (TSPs) should be present in adult blood. It is well established that all hematopoietic precursors in humans are present within a population of cells that express CD34 (Payne & Crooks, 2002), and this marker is useful in elucidating pathways in the development of particular hematopoietic lineages. In umbilical cord blood (UCB), CD34+CD45RA+CD7+ cells are found to have T, B, and NK and some granulocyte-macrophage (GM) precursor activities (Haddad et al., 2004; Hao et al., 2001). Phenotypically these cells resemble the $CD34^+CD38^{low}$ Early Thymic Progenitor cells (ETP), which are present within the thymus and have T cell, NK cell, and Dendritic Cell (DC) precursor activities (Res et al., 1996). The ETP have not yet undergone T cell receptor (TCR) gene rearrangements confirming that they form the most immature population in the thymus (Dik et al., 2005). This, together with the observation that ETP co-express CD10, makes it tempting to speculate that they are the direct progeny of the $CD34^+CD45RA^+CD7^+CD10^+CD38^{low}$ UCB cells (Hao et al., 2001). In addition, the notion that the human thymus harbors multipotential precursors indicates that T cell commitment takes place within this organ (Bhandoola et al., 2003). While these results are in line with data obtained in the mouse, more recent studies suggested that the murine thymus can be seeded not only by multipotent precursors, but also by precursor cells that are lineage restricted (Petrie & Kincade, 2005; Porritt et al., 2004). If that would be the case in humans, such lineage restricted cells should be present in UCB, but conflicting results were reported on this issue. One study failed to find evidence for the presence of TCR rearrangements in UCB $CD34^+$ cells (Blom et al., 1997), but another study reported the presence of complete TCRδ and partial TCRβ (Dβ-Jβ) rearrangements in $CD34^+CD7^+$ cord blood precursors (Ktorza et al., 1996). It is obvious that re-analysis preferentially by single-cell PCR analysis of the recently identified rare $CD34^+CD45RA^+CD7^+$ UCB population is required to solve this issue (Haddad et al., 2004; Hao et al., 2001). T cell–restricted precursors were convincingly identified in human bone marrow (Klein et al., 2003a), but whether these cells can migrate to the thymus is unclear. In the mouse it was demonstrated that for the proper seeding of progenitor cells into the thymus the collective action of the chemokine receptors CCR7 and CCR9 is required (Zlotoff et al., 2010). The role of these chemokine receptors to direct human progenitor cells into the thymus has not been established. In summary, at least a proportion of the precursors that seed the human thymus are multipotent. It remains elusive whether or not some of the precursors that migrate into the thymus are lineage restricted before entrance, and which signals control their thymic seeding.

3. Cellular stages in the development of early thymic progenitor cells into mature T Cells

In the thymus different regions can be distinguished, including the cortex and the medulla (Figure 1). The early steps in T cell development are induced in the cortex, which is characterized by a high cell density resulting from a high degree of proliferating immature thymocytes. In addition, an area of low cell density can be observed, which is known as the medulla. Based on phenotype and status of the TCR gene rearrangements we have gained significant insight in the various transitional stages of T cell development in the human thymus (Figure 2) (Spits et al., 1998; Spits, 2002). The ETP, lacking TCR rearrangements, are enclosed within a population of cells that express CD34, but lack CD1a expression. The downstream $CD34^+CD1a^+$ population is committed to the T cell lineage because they are unable to develop into non-T cells (Dalloul et al., 1999; Galy et al., 1993; Res & Spits, 1999; Spits et al., 1998). The cells that subsequently upregulate CD4 and downregulate CD34 are generally referred to as CD4 immature single-positive (CD4 ISP) (Hori et al., 1991). Downstream of the CD4 ISP subset are $CD4^+CD8\alpha^+\beta^-$ (early double-positive) and $CD4^+CD8\alpha^+\beta^+$ populations (Galy et al., 1993; Hori et al., 1991), which are the precursors of double-positive (DP) $TCR\alpha\beta^+$ cells. During the early stages in T cell development, the TCR loci undergo sequential rearrangements in the order of TCR$\delta > \gamma > \beta > \alpha$ (Blom et al., 1999; Dik et al., 2005; Verschuren et al., 1998). Depending on differences in the sensitivity of the assay used to measure TCRβ rearrangements productive TCRβ V-DJ rearrangements were either found in the $CD34^+CD1a^+$ cells (Dik et al., 2005) or in the CD4 ISP cells (Blom et al., 1999). It cannot be excluded, however, that a small contamination in the sorted $CD34^+CD1a^+$ cells in combination with a highly sensitive PCR detection assay was responsible for the positive signal (Dik et al., 2005). Only productive, in-frame TCRβ rearrangements result in the production of a TCRβ protein, which together with the CD3 subunits and the invariable pre-TCR-α (pTα) chain ensures cell surface expression of a pre-TCR. At this stage a process referred to as β-selection occurs in distinct populations of cells that differ in CD4 and CD8 expression. Both CD4 ISP and $CD4^+CD8\alpha^+\beta^-$ early double-positive subsets were found to contain intracytoplasmic (ic) $TCR\beta^-$ and $icTCR\beta^+$ cells (Blom et al., 1999; Carrasco et al., 1999). Ten to twenty percent of the CD4 ISP are $icTCR\beta^+$, and in contrast to the $TCR\beta^-$ CD4 ISP, these $icTCR\beta^+$ CD4 ISP are larger and express elevated levels of CD28 and CD71 (Taghon et al., 2009). A larger proportion is β-selected after upregulation of CD8β (Carrasco et al., 1999; Trigueros et al., 1998). Hence, these findings suggest that expression of a TCRβ protein and the ensuing β-selection occur within a certain developmental window and are not tightly coupled to regulation of CD4, CD8α, and CD8β expression.

Activation of the pre-TCR on the cell surface induces TCRβ-selection, which is a collective process leading to survival and proliferation of the cells, allelic exclusion, and induction of TCRα rearrangements (Spits, 2002). Subsequently, $CD4^+CD8^+$ DP T cells express a mature TCR$\alpha\beta$ complex on their cell surface, which is followed by positive and negative selection (Klein et al., 2009; Siggs et al., 2006). Positive selection mediated by the cortical thymic epithelial cells secures the survival of T cells that recognize self-major histocompatibility (MHC) antigens complexed with self-peptides with low/intermediate affinity. Conversely, high affinity self-peptide MHC complexes expressed by thymic dendritic cells (DC) in the medulla are pivotal for deletion of auto-reactive T cells, which is called negative selection. In the majority of cases when no interaction of TCR and MHC complexes can be established, the cells are unable to survive and die as a result of death by neglect. Positively selected thymocytes differentiate into T cells that express CD27 and CD45RA and high levels of CD3/TCR ($CD3^{hi}$) similar to naive T cells present in cord blood. Finally, lineage determination signals enforce the differentiation into either the helper $CD4^+$ T cell or cytotoxic $CD8^+$ T cells lineages.

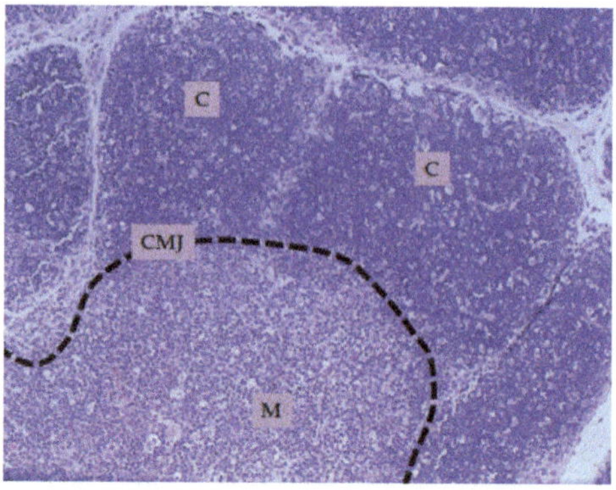

Fig. 1. Photomicrograph of the thymus. This section of human thymus (original magnification x10, courtesy of Dr. B. Jamieson, UCLA, Los Angeles, USA) was stained with hematoxylin/eosin and shows the cortex (C), which is a dense area of proliferating lymphocytes (thymocytes), and the medulla (M), where fewer cells localize and negative selection takes place. It is believed that progenitor cells enter the thymus at the cortico-medullary junction (CMJ) before migration into the cortex and commitment into the T cell lineage.

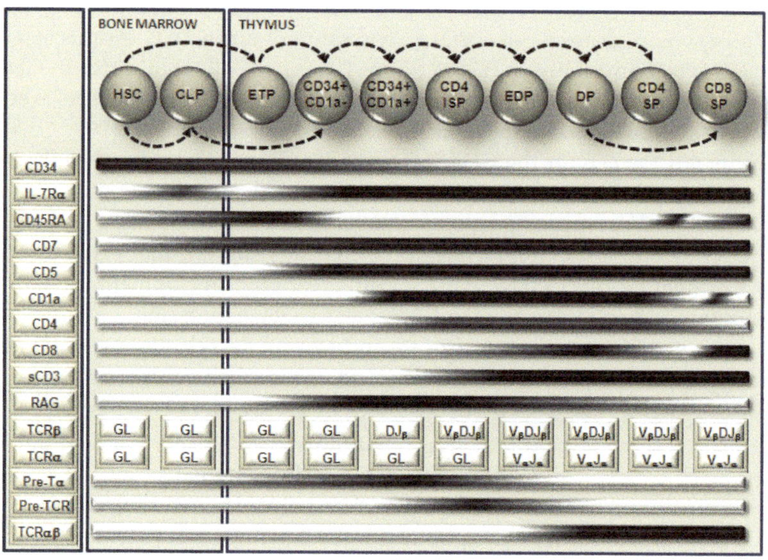

Fig. 2. Schematic model of human T cell development. Shown is the expression of cell surface markers on thymic progenitor cells and during the different stages of human T cell development in the thymus (black indicates expression, white indicates no expression). In addition, the status of T cell receptor (TCR) α and β gene rearrangements is shown. Hematopoietic stem cell (HSC), common lymphoid progenitor (CLP), early thymic progenitor (ETP), immature single positive (ISP), early double positive (EDP), single positive (SP), germline (GL), Diversity-Joining TCRβ (D-Jβ), Variable-DJ TCRβ (VβDJβ), Variable-Joining TCRα (VαJα).

4. Role of cytokines in T cell development

A role for interleukin (IL)-7 in the development of T cells in the thymus has been highlighted by many groups. The IL-7 receptor consists of two chains, IL-7Rα and gamma common (γc), which is also part of the receptors for IL-2, IL-4, IL-9, IL-15, and IL-21. Genetic defects in the genes encoding for γc (Noguchi et al., 1993; Russell et al., 1993), IL-7Rα (Giliani et al., 2005; Puel et al., 1998), or the Janus kinase Jak3, a component of the IL-7-induced signal transduction pathway (Macchi et al., 1995; Russell et al., 1995), account for the majority of severe combined immune deficiencies (SCID). This disease is characterized by strongly reduced numbers of T cells. The most frequent form of SCID is caused by mutations in the γc-encoding gene (reviewed in (Fischer et al., 2005)). In these patients, T and NK cells are absent, but in contrast to what is observed in γc-deficient mice, B cell development is normal (Noguchi et al., 1993; Russell et al., 1993). While IL-7Rα-deficient patients also display a profound T cell deficiency, they have near normal NK and B cell numbers (Giliani et al., 2005; Puel et al., 1998). This indicates that human T cell development, but not survival and proliferation of lymphoid precursors, specifically and critically depends on IL-7. The precise function of IL-7, which is produced by thymic epithelial cells, in human T cell development remains incompletely understood. Expansion and differentiation of developing T cells in a FTOC is inhibited by blocking the IL-7R signaling pathway using anti-IL-7 and anti-IL-7R antibodies (Pallard et al., 1999; Plum et al., 1996). This indicates that IL-7 has a crucial role in mediating survival and proliferation of human T cell precursors. It has been reported that this is likely mediated by IL-7-induced Phosphoinositide Kinase-3 (PI3K) activation through one tyrosine residue at position 449 in the cytoplasmic tail of the IL-7Rα chain (Pallard et al., 1999). Based on the notion that the distribution of subsets in the thymuses of IL-7Rα-deficient mice was near normal, it was argued that IL-7 does not appear to be critical for differentiation of mouse TCRαβ T cells in the thymus (Peschon et al., 1994). In humans, however, there is evidence that IL-7 is important for differentiation of human T cells. First, differentiation of $CD34^+$ precursors in a FTOC in the presence of anti-IL-7R antibody is almost completely blocked at the transition of $CD34^+CD1a^+$ cells into CD4 ISP (Plum et al., 1996). Second, according to one report, thymocytes from γc-deficient infants possess TCRβ D-J but lack V-DJβ rearrangements (Sleasman et al., 1994). Although a function of IL-7 in TCRβ rearrangements in human pre-T cells has yet to be confirmed, it may reflect the complete lack of T cells in many γc- and IL-7Rα-deficient patients (Giliani et al., 2005; Pesu et al., 2005). Conversely, IL-7 is required for peripheral T cell homeostasis in humans (Napolitano et al., 2001), which raises the alternative possibility that the combined defects in early T cell development and in T cell homeostasis are causal to the absolute T cell deficiency in γc-deficient patients. Collectively, these results indicate that IL-7 is indispensable for human T cell development, and moreover suggests that IL-7 is more critical for human than for mouse T cell development.

5. HIV tropism vs. thymic architecture

HIV can enter the cell through two major co-receptors, CXCR4 and CCR5, which are chemokine G-protein coupled receptors. Under physiological conditions CXCR4 ligates the chemokine CXCL12/SDF-1α, while CCR5 can be engaged by several chemokines, including RANTES (CCL5) or the macrophage inflammatory proteins MIP-1α (CCL3) and MIP-1β (CCL4) (Rossi & Zlotnik, 2000). Based on the expression pattern of these chemokine

receptors on leukocytes a clear distinction can be made between CXCR4 (X4)-tropic and CCR5 (R5)-tropic viruses (Deng et al., 1996; Dragic et al., 1996; Feng et al., 1996). In bone marrow, on average 40% of the $CD34^+$ progenitor cells express the chemokine receptor CXCR4 (Ishii et al., 1999). This subset was shown to have restricted lymphoid precursor activities, and resemble the $CD34^+CXCR4^+$ cells in neonatal UCB, which are likely the precursors of human CLPs (Haddad et al., 2004; Hao et al., 2001). CCR5 is expressed on the cell surface of only a minority of freshly isolated $CD34^+$ CB cells (1-21%), although at the intracellular level more than 80% of the $CD34^+$CB cells expressed abundant CCR5 receptors (Basu & Broxmeyer, 2009). While chemotaxis of $CD34^+$CB cells was not induced by the CCR5 ligands CCL3, CCL4 and CCL5, they transiently enhanced chemotaxis mediated by CXCL12, the ligand for CXCR4 (Basu & Broxmeyer, 2009). Whether $CD34^+$ cells can be infected by HIV has been the subject of great discussion through the years. Recently, Carter et al. (Carter et al., 2010) demonstrated that $CD34^+$ cells can be infected by both X4 and R5-tropic viruses *in vitro* as well as *in vivo*, thus potentially becoming a significant reservoir of HIV. In the thymus, both CXCR4 and CCR5 are expressed as well (Figure 3) (Berkowitz et al., 1998b; Gurney & Uittenbogaart, 2006; Kitchen & Zack, 1997; Kitchen & Zack, 1999; Pedroza-Martins et al., 1998; Zaitseva et al., 1998; Zamarchi et al., 2002; Zhang et al., 1998). Several studies have shown that expression of CXCR4 and CCR5 are modulated during thymocyte development (Berkowitz et al., 1998b; Gurney & Uittenbogaart, 2006; Zaitseva et al., 1998). CXCR4 is expressed on the majority of thymocytes at all stages of differentiation with the highest level of CXCR4 expression on the $CD34^+$ and CD4 ISP subsets (Berkowitz et al., 1998b; Hernandez-Lopez et al., 2002; Zaitseva et al., 1998). It was observed that CXCL12, in synergy with IL-7, mediates survival of these thymic progenitor subsets (Hernandez-Lopez et al., 2002). In accord with its co-receptor profile, CD4 ISP cells are infected with X4-tropic HIV-1, which has a cytopathic effect in the thymus resulting in a major depletion of cells (Gurney & Uittenbogaart, 2006; Kitchen & Zack, 1997). On more mature stages of T cell development CXCR4 is downregulated (Berkowitz et al., 1998b; Gurney & Uittenbogaart, 2006; Zaitseva et al., 1998). Notably, however, infected $CD8^+$ T cells are detected in the HIV-1 infected thymus, which can be explained by the observation that immature thymocytes, before they have differentiated into single positive thymocytes, can be infected by X4-tropic HIV-1 (Gurney & Uittenbogaart, 2006; Kitchen & Zack, 1997; Lee et al., 1997). Just prior to emigration from the thymus CXCR4 is again upregulated (Gurney & Uittenbogaart, 2006). Taken together, X4-tropic viruses can infect cells that are present in both the cortex and the medulla (Jamieson et al., 1995; Uittenbogaart et al., 1996). It is important to keep in mind that most of this work has been done with HIV laboratory strains that are highly cytopathic and may not be representative of what is happening *in vivo* in humans. This is enforced by the finding that HIV pediatric isolates from newborn children are not as cytopathic as the laboratory strains in infecting thymocytes at least *in vitro* (Pedroza-Martins et al., 1998).
Unlike CXCR4, the expression of CCR5 is much less widespread (Berkowitz et al., 1998a). CCR5 is detected on a relatively small proportion of thymocytes, including mature CD4 and CD8 single positive T cells which express CD27 but lack CD45RA (Berkowitz et al., 1998b; Gurney & Uittenbogaart, 2006), and is downregulated just prior to exiting the thymus (Berkowitz et al., 1998a; Gurney & Uittenbogaart, 2006). R5-tropic viruses are less cytopathic, which may at least in part be explained by the restricted co-receptor expression on a small subset, resulting in a much slower depletion of thymocytes (Jamieson et al., 1995). Moreover, the CCR5 expressing thymocytes are confined in the medullary area, which constrains prevalent replication of R5 viruses throughout the thymus (Berkowitz et al.,

1998a). Notably, like X4-tropic viruses, R5 strains are capable of depleting thymocytes leading to reduced cellularity in the thymus. One explanation can be that in addition to TCRαβ+ T cells, other CCR5+ cells are found in the thymus, including conventional DC (cDC), plasmacytoid DC (pDC), macrophages, CD161+ T cells and γδ T cells (Gurney et al., 2002; Gurney et al., 2004; Keir et al., 2002; Rozmyslowicz et al., 2010; Schmitt et al., 2006). Another explanation can be that pDC (see paragraph below) in response to the virus produce large amounts of type I IFNs (Gurney et al., 2004), which contributes to immune activation followed by cell death and T cell depletion. The pDC are likely more susceptible to R5-tropic HIV infection as they express CCR5 at higher levels compared to single positive thymocytes (Gurney et al., 2004). It was recently reported that IFN-α induced expression of CCR5 on CD4 ISP thymocytes, which consequently expands the tropism for R5-tropic viruses (Stoddart et al., 2010). This, together with the observation that thymi from HIV-infected individuals present with higher CCR5 expression on mature thymocytes as compared with thymocytes from uninfected individuals (Bandera et al., 2010), enforces the notion that immune activation has a detrimental role in thymic depletion.

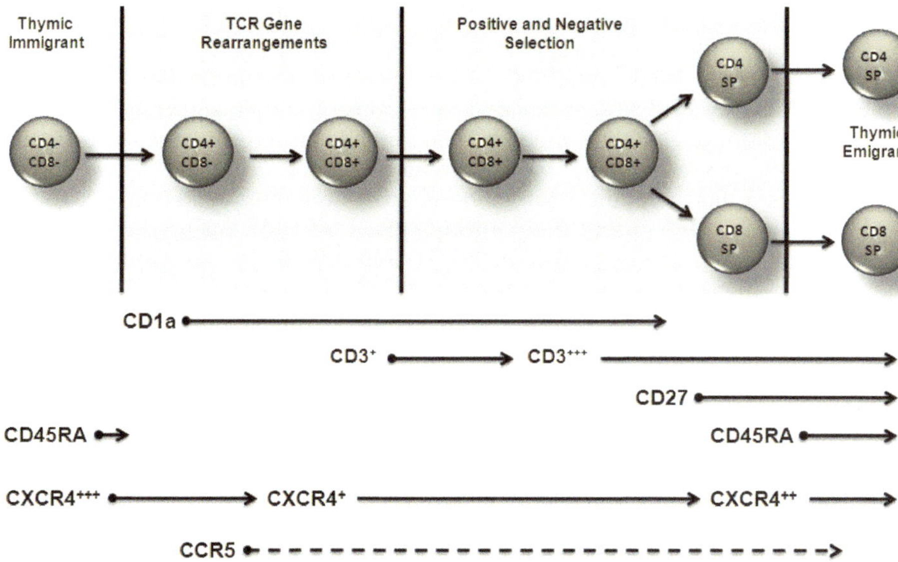

Fig. 3. Expression of chemokine receptors CXCR4 and CCR5 on cells at different stages during T cell development in the human thymus. The solid line arrows indicate high expression of the different cell surface markers, while the dotted line arrow indicates low expression. T cell receptor (TCR), single positive (SP).

6. Role of pDC in HIV pathogenesis in the thymus

Rare immune subsets like DC, play significant roles in the regulation of the immune system (Banchereau et al., 2000a; Banchereau et al., 2000b; Cella et al., 1999; Cella et al., 2000; Grouard et al., 1997; Kadowaki et al., 2000). Among the different types of DC subsets are pDC, which are present in cord and peripheral blood, T cell areas of the lymph nodes and in the medullary area of the thymus, and have the capacity to produce high levels of type I

IFN, i.e. IFNα and IFNβ, in response to viruses and other stimuli (Bendriss-Vermare et al., 2001; Cella et al., 1999; Foster et al., 2000; Kadowaki et al., 2000; Olweus et al., 1997; Res et al., 1999; Siegal et al., 1999; Vandenabeele et al., 2001). Type I IFNs are survival factors for pDC, while maturation of pDC depends on IL-3 (Grouard et al., 1997). Exposure of peripheral blood pDC to virus, or alternatively IFN-α or IL-3 either in combination with CD40L or TNF-α, leads to the appearance of pDC with a mature phenotype illustrated by the finding that they express increased levels of HLA Class II and costimulatory molecules (Kadowaki et al., 2000; Kohrgruber et al., 1999). PDC can differentiate *in vitro* into mature DC capable of stimulating $CD4^+$ naïve T cells to proliferate and differentiate, and depending on the environmental signals polarize T cells into T helper 2 (Th2) (Rissoan et al., 1999) or Th1 cells (Cella et al., 2000). Also, pDC have the ability to shape $CD8^+$ T cell responses either directly (Gilliet & Liu, 2002) or via crosspressentation (Hoeffel et al., 2007), and NKT cell responses (Kadowaki et al., 2001a). However, the central role of pDC *in vivo* is likely that of an IFN-α/β producing cell, and not an antigen presenting cell (Haeryfar, 2005).
In response to enveloped RNA and DNA viruses (Milone & Fitzgerald-Bocarsly, 1998), including live and inactivated HIV-1 (Beignon et al., 2005; Ferbas et al., 1994; Fong et al., 2002; Hardy et al., 2007; Yonezawa et al., 2003), human pDC are the main producers of IFN-α (Ferbas et al., 1994; Ishikawa et al., 2005; Milone & Fitzgerald-Bocarsly, 1998; Siegal et al., 1999). In contrast to conventional cDC, pDC do not produce interleukin-12 (IL-12) (Ito et al., 2006). The capacity of IFN-α production in response to virus is already present at the pro-pDC stage (Blom et al., 2000) and can be sustained during activation and maturation (Cella et al., 1999). IFN-α produced by pDC induces maturation of conventional cDC and thereby provides a link between innate and adaptive immunity (Ito et al., 2001). Several viral infections induce IFN-α, but the pathways that lead to IFN-α production are likely different. Recent reports suggest that in HIV-1 infection IFN-α production by pDC is stimulated through interaction of HIV-1 RNA with Toll like receptor (TLR)7 (Beignon et al., 2005; Hardy et al., 2007; O'Brien et al., 2011). Although it has been shown that pDC can be productively infected by R5-tropic and X4-tropic HIV-1 (Gurney et al., 2004; Keir et al., 2002), IFN-α production by pDC does not depend on productive HIV-1 infection (Beignon et al., 2005; Hardy et al., 2007). Furthermore, pDC express TLR9, which after engagement by oligodeoxynucleotides (ODNs) containing unmethylated CpG motifs mimicking bacterial DNA, activate the cells to secrete high levels of type I IFNs (Kadowaki et al., 2001b).
Development of pDC both in human and mouse depends on FLT3L (Blom et al., 2000; Gilliet et al., 2002). Furthermore, the Ets transcription factor Spi-B and the basic helix-loop-helix factor E2-2 are essential for the development of human pDC *in vitro* as well as *in vivo* (Cisse et al., 2008; Nagasawa et al., 2008; Schotte et al., 2003; Schotte et al., 2004). In the human thymus a cell type very similar to peripheral pDC was identified. These $CD3^-$ cells express CD4, CD45RA and high levels of CD123 and are localized at the cortico-medullary junction and in the medulla (Bendriss-Vermare et al., 2001; Olweus et al., 1997; Res et al., 1999; Schmitt et al., 2000; Vandenabeele et al., 2001). There are similarities but also differences between thymic and peripheral pDC. Both thymic and peripheral pDC respond, in addition to IL-3, also to GM-CSF (Ghirelli et al., 2010; Vandenabeele et al., 2001). Like the peripheral pDC, the thymic pDC have the capacity to develop into mature DC, but some differences were observed in the expression of certain cell surface antigens (Res et al., 1999). Thymic pDC consistently express CD2, CD5 and CD7, while peripheral pDC do not express CD7 and are heterogeneous with respect to the expression of CD2 and CD5 (Bendriss-Vermare et al., 2001; Res et al., 1999; Schmitt et al., 2006). Interestingly, thymic pDC constitutively

express low levels of IFN-α, which is upregulated by HIV-1 infection *in vivo* (Gurney et al., 2004). Moreover, thymic pDC produce less IFN-α upon infection with virus (Schmitt et al., 2006). These differences may imply either that thymic and peripheral pDC are different subsets, or that these alterations are enforced by the thymic microenvironment.

The role of pDC in controlling HIV-1 replication is still incompletely resolved. Several reports describe a decrease in frequency and function of peripheral blood pDC in HIV-1-infected patients (Chehimi et al., 2002; Donaghy et al., 2001; Feldman et al., 2001; Pacanowski et al., 2001; Soumelis et al., 2001). A decrease in pDC has been correlated with an increase in HIV-1 RNA virus load and opportunistic infections, suggesting that a loss of these cells may contribute to disease progression in HIV-1-infected patients (Donaghy et al., 2001; Siegal et al., 2001). This decrease in peripheral blood pDC may be due to HIV-1 induced cell death or migration of pDC from the peripheral blood to lymphoid tissues. In accord with the latter option, it was reported that HIV-1 infection induces pDC maturation resulting in expression of CCR7 and migration to lymph nodes (Schmidt et al., 2005), which is a major site of HIV-1 pathogenesis (Herbeuval et al., 2006). While pDC can suppress HIV-1 replication *in vitro* (Gurney et al., 2004; Yonezawa et al., 2003) and *ex vivo* (Meyers et al., 2007), pDC through their production of IFN-α have also been found to contribute to HIV pathogenesis by TRAIL-mediated apoptosis of uninfected $CD4^+$ T cells (Herbeuval et al., 2006). Recent data suggest that despite a decrease in pDC numbers in peripheral blood of HIV infected individuals, their production of TLR7/8 agonist induced cytokine/chemokine is even higher than that of pDC of non-infected individuals thereby contributing to chronic immune activation (Sabado et al., 2010). With respect to thymic pDC, these are also targets for CXCR4- and CCR5-tropic HIV as they express CD4 in addition to both CXCR4 and CCR5. Notably, the expression level of CCR5 on pDC is higher than on thymocytes, suggesting that pDC are more susceptible to CCR5-tropic HIV infection than thymocytes (Gurney et al., 2004; Ho Tsong Fang et al., 2008; Schmitt et al., 2000). Studies in the SCID-hu Thy/Liv mouse model (see paragraph on "Humanized mouse models to study HIV-1 immuno-pathogenesis") show that pDC are productively infected by HIV and that HIV infection induces IFN-α production resulting in upregulation of MHC-I and the interferon stimulated gene (ISG), MxA (Gurney et al., 2004; Keir et al., 2002; Schmitt et al., 2006). Recently, the suggestion was raised that as a consequence of upregulated MHC-I expression levels in the thymus, the generation of dysfunctional $CD8^+$ T cells with low expression of CD8 was induced resulting from altered negative selection (Favre et al., 2011). While no conclusive evidence was presented, when true this may have detrimental effects on thymopoiesis in the HIV-1-infected thymus, and contribute to the immunodeficiency of HIV disease.

7. Impact of IFN-alpha on T cell regeneration

Type I IFNs, including IFN-α and -β, are important cytokines that have been classically described to have an immunoregulatory function with central roles as antiviral mediators (Brassard et al., 2002; Grandvaux et al., 2002). However, type I IFNs have additional effects besides their well-known antiviral function. It has been shown that high concentrations of IFN-α interfered with T and B cell development in mice (Lin et al., 1998). In the thymus, an 80% decrease in the overall cellularity and a 50% reduction of the $CD4^+CD8^+$ DP population was observed (Lin et al., 1998). Considering the key role of IL-7 during T cell development (see paragraph above "Role of cytokines in T cell development") it was speculated that type

I IFNs might interfere with IL-7 signaling. Consistent with this it was shown that type I IFNs inhibited IL-7-driven expansion of $CD4^-CD8^-CD44^+CD25^+$ (also known as double negative (DN)2) cells in murine fetal thymus organ cultures (Su et al., 1997).
The main producers of type I IFNs are pDC, which express TLR7 and TLR9 enabling them to sense nucleic acids derived from viruses or bacteria (Kadowaki et al., 2001b; Cella et al., 1999; Kadowaki et al., 2000). In addition to secondary lymphoid organs and peripheral blood, pDC are present in the thymus, where they locate in the medulla and at the cortico-medullary junction (Bendriss-Vermare et al., 2001; Res et al., 1999; Vandenabeele et al., 2001). As this latter location is where TSP cells enter the thymus, it is conceivable that thymic pDC affect T cell development. In line with this it was demonstrated that IFN-α, when exogenously added as recombinant protein, impaired early human T cell development by interfering with the IL-7 signaling pathway (Schmidlin et al., 2006). Moreover, similar findings were observed when pDC were activated either by HIV-1 or the TLR9 agonist CpG-ODN in a co-culture setup in which thymic progenitor cells were induced to differentiate into both T cells and pDC (Schmidlin et al., 2006). Addition of neutralizing antibodies against type I IFNs in this system relieved the block in T cell development illustrating that type I IFNs produced by activated pDC have a detrimental effect on early T cell progenitor cells (Schmidlin et al., 2006). It remains largely elusive whether type I IFNs affect later stages of T cell development. This is not unlikely, however, given the architectural localization of pDC in the medulla, and the finding that the majority of thymocytes express the type I IFN receptor (CD118) on their surface (Keir et al., 2002). In fact, IFN-α was reported to interfere with IL-7-induced maturation at the transition of human $CD3^+CD1a^+$ to $CD3^{+/hi}CD1a^-$ thymocytes (Schmidlin et al., 2006). In addition, IFN-α induced the up-regulation of MHC class I expression in the thymus (Keir et al., 2002). This may cause adverse T cell selection in the thymus by changing the avidity of the TCR for MHC potentially depleting part of the mature $CD8^+$ T cell repertoire.

8. Role of regulatory T cells in HIV pathogenesis in the thymus

$CD4^+CD25^+$ regulatory T (Treg) cells are a distinct subset of $CD4^+$ T cells, which play a significant role in the generation and maintenance of peripheral tolerance (Maloy & Powrie, 2001; Sakaguchi, 2000; Sakaguchi, 2005). Although in humans Treg cells in the periphery constitute a small subset of the total T-cells (1%-2%) (Baecher-Allan et al., 2001), there is accumulating evidence that they play a significant role in the negative control of a broad spectrum of immune responses to antigens, such as in tumor immunity, organ transplantation, allergy, and microbial immunity (reviewed in (Sakaguchi, 2005)). Treg cells are identified by their constitutive expression of the alpha chain of the interleukin 2 (IL-2) receptor (CD25) and the presence of the forkhead/winged-helix transcription repressor FoxP3 (scurfin) (Baecher-Allan et al., 2001; Fontenot et al., 2003; Hori et al., 2003; Khattri et al., 2003; Yagi et al., 2004). There is mounting evidence that FoxP3 plays a crucial role in the development and function of human (Walker et al., 2003; Yagi et al., 2004) and murine (Fontenot et al., 2005) $CD4^+CD25^+$ Treg cells (reviewed in (Fontenot & Rudensky, 2005)). In addition to FoxP3, the cytokine IL-2 is essential for the development of Treg cells in the thymus and their maintenance in the periphery (reviewed in (Sakaguchi, 2005)). Although Treg cells show low levels of proliferation *in vitro* (Baecher-Allan et al., 2001), peripheral expansion of thymus-derived natural Treg (nTreg) cells ensures maintenance of the peripheral Treg pool in the adult mouse (Hori et al., 2002). In addition, antigen-dependent proliferation of Treg cells has been shown *in vivo* (Klein et al., 2003b; von Boehmer, 2005). The mechanism of T cell suppression by Treg cells is dependent on direct cell-cell contact (reviewed in (von Boehmer, 2005)). However, in addition to the direct effects of Treg cells, bystander effects include the production of cytokines (IL-10 and TGF-β) that have suppressive effects on immune responses (reviewed in (von Boehmer, 2005)).

In mice and rats as well as humans, nTreg cells develop intrathymically (Jordan et al., 2001; Kasow et al., 2004) and acquire their regulatory function while still in the thymus (Itoh et al., 1999; Saoudi et al., 1996; Stephens et al., 2001). Treg cells are continuously produced in the thymus as a distinct lineage contiguous with peripheral blood Treg cells (reviewed in (Fontenot et al., 2005; Sakaguchi, 2005)). There is recent evidence that thymic pDC play a role in the development of nTreg (Hanabuchi et al., 2010; Martin-Gayo et al., 2010). Both pDC and Treg cells are located closely together in the thymic medulla, which may suggest interactions between them (Martin-Gayo et al., 2010; Res et al., 1999; Watanabe et al., 2005). In addition to the induction of Treg cells by cDC activated with the IL-7 like cytokine thymic stromal lymphopoietin (TSLP) (Watanabe et al., 2005), FoxP3$^+$ Treg cells can also be induced in the thymus by pDC after these have been stimulated with TSLP (Hanabuchi et al., 2010). The role of TSLP activation of pDC in the development of thymic Treg is however still unclear as Martin-Gayo *et al.* found that thymic pDC were unresponsive to TSLP, but responsive to CD40L and IL-3 (Martin-Gayo et al., 2010). It is interesting to note that nTreg cells generated in the presence of cDC have opposite IL-10/TGF-β cytokine profiles from those generated wih pDC (Martin-Gayo et al., 2010). Thus, the interaction of pDC and cDC with Treg cells may play an important role in the development of tolerance in the thymus.

In contrast to adult peripheral blood, Treg cells in the human fetal and postnatal thymus (Annunziato et al., 2002; Cupedo et al., 2005; Kasow et al., 2004) and in cord blood (Takahata et al., 2004; Thornton et al., 2004) have a naïve phenotype, although they suppress the proliferation of CD25$^-$negative T cells, similar to Treg cells in the periphery. Treg cells identified by high expression of CD25 and FoxP3 are already present in the human fetal thymus and secondary lymphoid organs (Cupedo et al., 2005; Darrasse-Jeze et al., 2005). T cells expressing GITR, CTLA-4 and CD122 and high levels of CD25, corresponding to the phenotype of Treg cells, develop in the human thymus at the CD4$^+$CD8$^+$ stage during transition of CD27$^-$ to CD27$^+$ stage (Cupedo et al., 2005). When Treg cells leave the thymus and enter fetal secondary lymphoid tissues, lymph nodes and spleen, they acquire a memory/activated phenotype (Cupedo et al., 2005). In the normal functioning immune system there is a balance between the interactions of Treg cells and effector T cells, whereas deficiency of functional Treg cells leads to inappropriate immune responses to microbial infections and autoimmunity as exemplified in humans who suffer from the X-linked immunodeficiency syndrome (IPEX) with a mutation in FoxP3 (reviewed in (Fontenot et al., 2005; Sakaguchi, 2005)). In addition to CD4$^+$ Treg cells, CD8$^+$CD25$^+$ Treg cells have been identified in the thymus (Cosmi et al., 2003). The CD8$^+$CD25$^+$ Treg cells express FoxP3 mRNA, but lower levels of CD25 than the CD4$^+$ Treg cells (Cosmi et al., 2003).

There is ample evidence that Treg cells play a significant role in infectious diseases including viral infections (reviewed in (Belkaid & Rouse, 2005; Mills & McGuirk, 2004)). In humans, circulating peripheral Treg cells suppress CD4$^+$ and CD8$^+$ antiviral immune responses in chronic viral infections, such as HCV (Cabrera et al., 2004), CMV and HIV (Aandahl et al., 2004; Andersson et al., 2005; Eggena et al., 2005; Kinter et al., 2004; Oswald-Richter et al., 2004; Weiss et al., 2004). There is a clear measurable restoration of antiviral immune responses to CMV and HIV *in vitro* when CD4$^+$CD25$^+$ T cells are completely removed (Aandahl et al., 2004; Weiss et al., 2004). Although Treg cells produce immunosuppressive cytokines, IL-10 and TGF-β_1 in response to p24 antigen stimulation, the down modulation seen by $CD4^+CD25^+$ T cells is cell-cell contact dependent and independent of IL-10 and TGF-β_1 (Kinter et al., 2004; Weiss et al., 2004). The impact of Treg cells on HIV-1 infection is still unclear and may depend on the stage of infection. Early in viral infection, the proportion of Treg cells is unaltered as compared to normal controls (Aandahl et al., 2004). Elevated levels of circulating HIV specific $CD25^{hi}CD4^+$ T cells were observed in a majority of healthy, yet chronically, HIV infected individuals (Kinter et al., 2004). However, Treg cell numbers declined proportionately with the loss of $CD4^+$ T cells and disease progression (Kinter et al., 2004; Oswald-Richter et al., 2004). Treg cells were increased in tonsils, but decreased in the peripheral blood of untreated chronically HIV infected individuals, indicating that viral antigenic stimulation may have increased Treg cells in the lymphoid tissue and may have a detrimental effect on local immune responses (Andersson et al., 2005). A recent study in HIV infected individuals undergoing cardiac surgery showed that Treg cells were increased in the thymus of HIV-infected individuals as compared to uninfected individuals (Bandera et al., 2010). In a study of treatment naïve, chronically HIV infected individuals in Uganda, depletion of Treg cells was associated with immune activation (Eggena et al., 2005). The underlying mechanism suggests a complex balance between Treg cells and effector T cells. In summary, it will be of significant clinical value to determine at which stages of disease and in which tissues Treg cells have detrimental or protective effects on the immunopathology observed in HIV infection.

9. SIV pathogenic and non-pathogenic models

The use of animal models has been of great importance to study the thymus in HIV infection. In this regard the non-human primate models, and the SCID-hu and humanized mouse models, as discussed in the next section, are providing a great deal of knowledge on the role of the thymus in HIV infection. Studies in pathogenic and non-pathogenic models of simian immunodeficiency virus (SIV) infected non-human primates have further increased our understanding on the role of the thymus in HIV infection. In the non-pathogenic model SIV infection of its natural hosts (chimpanzees, sooty mangabeys, African green monkeys, and others) does not lead to depletion of $CD4^+$ T lymphocytes and AIDS, in contrast to the pathogenic model in which SIV infects its non-natural host (rhesus macaques) (reviewed in (Silvestri, 2008)). Effective innate immune responses including IFN-α and ISG are induced, but rapidly controlled in acute SIV infection of sooty mangabeys (SM) (Bosinger et al., 2009) and African Green monkeys (Diop et al., 2008; Jacquelin et al., 2009). However, acute SIV infection of rhesus macaques (RM) induces chronic immune activation and continuous expression of ISG (Bosinger et al., 2009). An increase in the ISG, MxA mRNA was found in lymphoid tissues, including the thymus, in SIV infected rhesus macaques. However, the elevated MxA levels did not correlate with control of viral infection in the animals (Abel et al., 2002) and are likely a sign of immune activation. Non-responsiveness to TGF-β1 was found to play a role in the lack of resolution of immune activation in rhesus macaques (Ploquin et al., 2006). Chronic immune activation was recognized many years ago as a major player in poor prognosis HIV infected individuals (Giorgi et al., 1999). Thus interference with immune activation was explored by administration of an antibody to the IFN-α receptor in SIV infected macaques, which reduced the loss of $CD4^+$ T cells in these animals (Tovey et al., 1994).

Studies of lymphoid tissues in SIV infected macaques have shed light on the differences between changes in T lymphocytes in peripheral blood and primary (thymus) and secondary lymphoid organs. In the thymus and secondary lymphoid organs proliferation of T lymphocytes and absolute CD4+ T lymphocytes were increased in acute SIV infection, but decreased in peripheral blood (Sopper et al., 2003). However in animals with first indication of AIDS, thymocytes were severely decreased (Sopper et al., 2003). Increased levels of thymocyte proliferation were also observed by Wykrzykowska *et al.* (Wykrzykowska et al., 1998) after an initial increase in apoptosis and depletion of thymic progenitors. Apoptosis in SIV infected macaques correlated with peak viremia and disruption of the apoptotic pathway (Rosenzweig et al., 2000). Pathogenicity of the virus on the level of apoptosis in the thymus was observed in macaques infected with a pathogenic and non-pathogenic HIV/SIV hybrid virus (SHIV) (Iida et al., 2000). Recent thymic emigrants can be determined by measuring T cell receptor excision circles (TRECs) in peripheral blood and provide a mirror of thymic function. Increased or stable levels of TRECs were found early after infection, but TREC levels decreased later when depletion of CD4+ thymocytes and apoptosis were observed in one of the animals (Sodora et al., 2002). Elevated TREC levels as compared to non-infected controls were observed in macaques infected with a less pathogenic SIVΔnef virus indicating that the thymus can maintain its function in the presence of low viral loads (Ho Tsong Fang et al., 2005). However the thymus as the major player in maintaining naïve peripheral CD4+ T cells has been disputed. Proliferation of peripheral T lymphocytes does also play a role in maintaining peripheral T cell homeostasis. Thymectomies of juvenile SIV infected macaques showed that TRECs in peripheral blood decreased after thymectomies. However, thymectomy in the SIV infected animals did not impact their clinical course or the ratio of CD45RA+ to CD45RA-CD4+ T cells (Arron et al., 2005).

10. Humanized mouse models to study HIV-1 immuno-pathogenesis

A small, easy-to-handle animal model that would facilitate the study of the pathophysiology of acute HIV-1 infection has been warranted after we were confronted with the HIV pandemic in the 1980s. Normal mice cannot be studied due to the limited species tropism of HIV, and therefore humanized mouse models have been instrumental to study HIV infections. Over the last decades significant progress has been made in the generation of humanized mouse models (Figure 4) with a functional human immune system, which has not only added to our insight into the development of human stem cells and the reconstitution of a human immune system in an *in vivo* setting, but also initiated studies on the preclinical testing of novel antiviral compounds, and the evaluation of vaccines.

Initially, humanized mice were generated using mice with the *scid* mutation in the C.B-17 mouse strain (Bosma et al., 1983). Such mice lack mature T and B cells due to a mutation in the *prkdc* gene, which is involved in rearrangement of TCR and Ig genes (Kirchgessner et al., 1995). Adoptive transfer of human peripheral blood lymphocytes (PBL) in C.B-17 SCID mice, which is commonly referred to as the human (hu) PBL-SCID model, resulted in the reconstitution of mature human T and B cells (Mosier et al., 1988). Although these transferred human lymphocytes only survived for a short period of time limiting long-term studies, hu-PBL-SCID mice have been used to study certain aspects of HIV-1 infection, including the importance of the state of activation of human CD4+ T cells at the time of primary infection in determining HIV-1 pathogenicity (Fais et al., 1999; Rizza et al., 1996). Resolutions to bypass the limited survival time of human lymphocytes were obtained by the transfer of human pluripotent progenitor cells ensuring development of multiple hematopoietic lineages. In such an optimized setting, human fetal thymic (FT) lobes and pieces of fetal liver (FL) were transplanted under the kidney capsule in C.B-17 SCID mice (McCune et al., 1988). In this hu-thymus (Thy)/liver (Liv) SCID mouse model almost exclusively T cells developed, which transiently migrated from the human thymus graft to the periphery. When compared to the first model, also this latter model suffers from the disadvantage that human T cell survival is reduced, although this is more apparent later after transplantation. This hu-Thy/Liv-SCID model has been extensively used for the analysis of human hematopoiesis, especially T cells, and as an animal model of HIV infection (McCune, 1997). HIV-1 injection in the thymic implant of hu-Thy/Liv-SCID mice resulted in significant HIV-1 infection not only in the Thy/Liv implant, but also in the spleen and peripheral blood, which indicated that HIV-1 infection could spread from the thymus to the peripheral lymphoid compartment (Kollmann et al., 1994). The effect of HIV-1 infection on thymocyte maturation and depletion depended upon the strain of HIV-1 infecting the thymus (Kollmann et al., 1995).

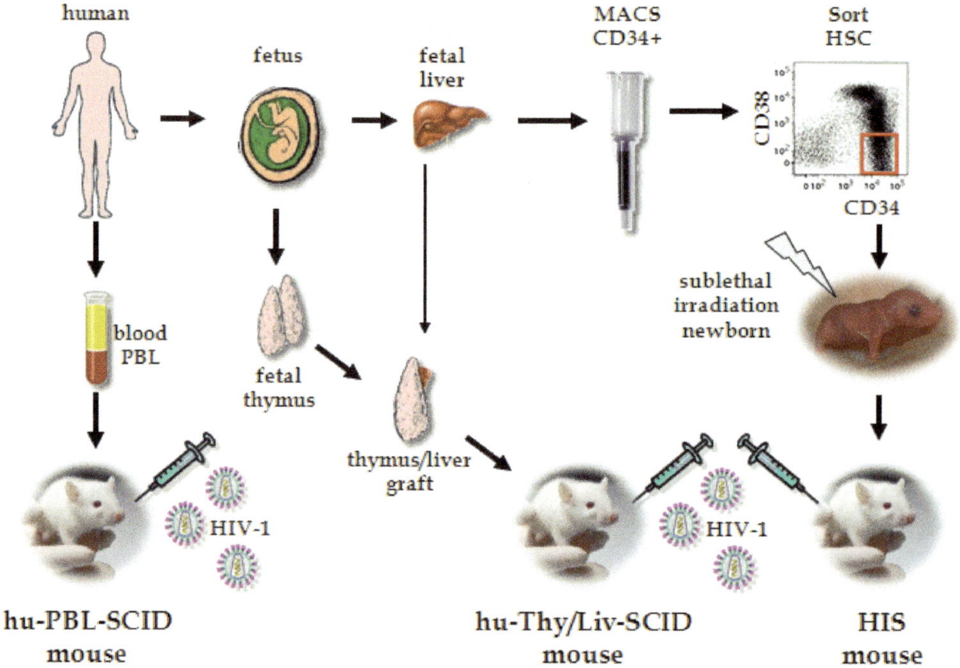

Fig. 4. Humanized mouse models to study HIV-1 infection *in vivo*. Several ways to generate humanized mouse models have been established (see text for further details). Human peripheral blood lymphocytes (hu-PBL) are injected in severe combined immunodeficient (SCID) mice to generate hu-PBL-SCID mice. Pieces of fetal liver (Liv) and thymus (Thy) can be grafted in SCID mice to generate the hu-Thy/Liv-SCID mouse. To create a human immune system (HIS) mouse, newborn immunodeficient mice are injected intrahepatically with CD34+CD38- human stem cells (HSC) after cell sorting from the fetal liver (or alternatively cord blood, bone marrow, mobilized peripheral blood, not shown).

To further optimize the humanized mouse model approaches were established to repopulate sublethally irradiated C.B-17 SCID mice with progenitor cells from human bone marrow or umbilical cord blood (Lapidot et al., 1992; Vormoor et al., 1994). In addition to development of T cells these mice also developed B cells and myeloid cells, which presented the potential to establish a humanized mouse model with a functional human immune system. Ablation of mouse NK cells further increased the frequency of thymopoiesis in animals reconstituted with human umbilical cord blood cells. This was not only demonstrated when using antibodies to deplete mouse NK cells (Kerre et al., 2002), but also when using recipient mice with a NK cell deficient genetic background (Greiner et al., 1998). Reconstitution of mice that are either defective in NK cell activity (non-obese diabetic (NOD)/SCID mice (Ogasawara et al., 2003) or NOD/SCID/$\beta 2m^{-/-}$ mice (Kollet et al., 2000) or have impaired NK cell development (NOD/SCID/$\gamma_c^{-/-}$ mice (Hiramatsu et al., 2003) were shown to have improved human T cell development. Despite their promise, however, repopulation of human T cells in the periphery of these mice are suboptimal (Hiramatsu et al., 2003; Kerre et al., 2002; Kollet et al., 2000). In addition to the genetic background, also the age of the mice upon reconstitution of HSC appears crucially important. Several groups observed that injection of human HSC to sublethally irradiated newborn BALB/c Rag2$^{-/-}$ $\gamma_c^{-/-}$ (BALB-Rag/γ) mice improved the reconstitution success rate (Gimeno et al., 2004; Traggiai et al., 2004). More than 80% of these humanized mice, either referred to as "human adaptive immune system Rag2$^{-/-}$ $\gamma_c^{-/-}$ mice" (huAIS-RG) (Traggiai et al., 2004) or "human immune system BALB-Rag2$^{-/-}$ $\gamma_c^{-/-}$" (HIS BALB-Rag/γ) (Gimeno et al., 2004), exhibited at least 10% or more human CD45$^+$ cells in peripheral blood and other lymphoid organs. Similar improvements were observed in newborn NOD/SCID/$\gamma_c^{-/-}$ (NOG) mice (Ishikawa et al., 2003; Ishikawa et al., 2005; Ito et al., 2002; Shultz et al., 2005) and to a lesser extent in newborn NOD/SCID/$\beta 2m^{-/-}$ mice when used as recipient of HSC (Kollet et al., 2000).
Part of the human CD4$^+$T cells in the spleen and peripheral blood of NOG mice express the co-receptors CXCR4 and CCR5 (Watanabe et al., 2007). In the thymus, CXCR4 is expressed on the majority of CD4$^+$CD8$^+$ thymocytes as well as on small numbers of CD4$^+$CD8$^-$ cells and CD4$^-$CD8$^+$ cells, while CCR5 was only expressed on a minor proportion of the thymocytes (Watanabe et al., 2007). Notably, early after HIV-1 infection of huNOG mice no viremia could be detected, and a detectable viral load was only observed late after infection using high doses of R5-tropic or X4-tropic HIV-1. No significant decline in the CD4/CD8 ratio was observed after R5-tropic virus infection of huNOG mice (Watanabe et al., 2007). Conversely, the HIS BALB-Rag/γ mice infected with a high dose R5-tropic HIV-1 did develop an inversion of the CD4/CD8 T-cell ratio in peripheral blood (Berges et al., 2006; Gorantla et al., 2007). After X4-tropic virus infection of huNOG mice a CD4$^+$ cell decline was detected at later time points (Watanabe et al., 2007). These findings suggest that humanized mice are less susceptible to low dose infection and undergo a slow course of CD4 T-cell depletion as compared to HIV-1 infected individuals. In addition, immune responses to HIV-1 infection in HIS mice generated from newborns are suboptimal resulting in only poor development of virus-specific antibodies and absence of HIV-specific T cell responses (An et al., 2007; Baenziger et al., 2006; Gorantla et al., 2007; Sato et al., 2010).
A more sophisticated HIS mouse model has been generated using NOD/SCID mice that were co-transplantated with human fetal Thy/Liv and CD34$^+$ HSC either from fetal liver (Lan et al., 2006; Tonomura et al., 2008) or bone marrow (BLT mice) (Melkus et al., 2006). BLT mice mounted stronger antigen-specific T-cell responses and T cell–dependent IgG production after in vivo antigen immunization (Melkus et al., 2006; Tonomura et al., 2008). Notably, a detectable viral load was observed in BLT mice after low dose infection with R5-

tropic virus, which was associated with the depletion of human CD4+ T cells in the blood (Brainard et al., 2009). Also, it was demonstrated that B cells in BLT mice were able to mount robust virus-specific antibody responses, although these responses were delayed as compared to adult human HIV infection (Brainard et al., 2009). Besides the intravenous route of HIV infection, HIS mice can be infected with HIV by relevant intravaginal and intrarectal routes (Berges et al., 2008; Denton et al., 2008; Sun et al., 2007). Taken together, this advanced humanized BLT mouse model shows great potential as a model to study HIV infection *in vivo* and holds promise for prospective studies to test the efficacy of candidate HIV vaccines and to validate the activity of antimicrobial agents acting at mucosal surfaces.

11. Summary and conclusion

Our knowledge of HIV infection of the thymus is primarily derived from animal models except for incidental reports of HIV infection *in vivo* in infants, children and adults (Bandera et al., 2010; Brunner et al., 2011; Calabro et al., 1995; Gaulton et al., 1997; Haynes et al., 1999; Rosenzweig et al., 1994). Indirect evidence of the impact of antiretroviral therapy on recovery of the thymus has been obtained through imaging studies and measurements of TRECs (Dion et al., 2007; Halnon et al., 2005; Lee et al., 2006; McCune et al., 1998 and reviewed in (Ho Tsong Fang et al., 2005)). It is clear that the thymus plays an important role in HIV infection and in the regeneration of naïve CD4+ T cells. Thymocytes, but also minor thymocyte subsets are targets for CCR5- and CXCR4-tropic HIV. These subsets include CD4+ TCRα/β, TCRγ/δ and CD161+ cells resembling NK-T cells (Gurney et al., 2002), Treg, cDC and pDC. Furthermore, pDC stimulated with HIV produce high levels of IFN-α, and thereby contribute to immune activation in particular when IFN-α levels are not controlled. Notably, insufficient T cell regeneration may not only be at the level of the thymus, but also at the level of hematopoietic stem cells. This is illustrated by the recent finding that the function and numbers of CD34+ hematopoietic stem cells in peripheral blood of HIV infected individuals are impaired despite control of viral replication (Sauce et al., 2011). Also, impaired progenitor cell function of umbilical cord blood CD34+ cells, including decreased cloning efficiency and generation of CD4+ T lymphocytes in fetal thymic organ culture, was observed in HIV-negative infants born to HIV-positive mothers (Nielsen et al., 2001). Consistent with these results, failure of hematopoiesis leading to impaired T cell regeneration was observed in SIV infected macaques and found to be unrelated to viral loads (Thiebot et al., 2005). Finally, a recent observation suggests that CD34+ cells can also be infected with HIV (Carter et al., 2010). Collectively, these results imply that HIV in addition to thymic destruction can also adversely affect thymic progenitor cells, likely caused by immune activation, and thereby contribute to T cell depletion in HIV infected individuals.

12. Acknowledgements

This work was supported by Grants from the National Institutes of Health (AI 080564, AI 52002, and AI 28697 (UCLA CFAR)), NIH Training grants T32-AR-053463 and T32-CA-009120 (to ME), and the Dutch Science Foundation (VIDI 917.66.310 to BB).

13. References

Aandahl, E. M., Michaelsson, J., Moretto, W. J., Hecht, F. M. & Nixon, D. F. (2004). Human CD4+ CD25+ regulatory T cells control T-cell responses to human immunodeficiency virus and cytomegalovirus antigens. *J.Virol.*, Vol. 78, No. 5, pp. (2454-2459)

Abel, K., Alegria-Hartman, M. J., Rothaeusler, K., Marthas, M. & Miller, C. J. (2002). The relationship between simian immunodeficiency virus RNA levels and the mRNA levels of alpha/beta interferons (IFN-alpha/beta) and IFN-alpha/beta-inducible Mx in lymphoid tissues of rhesus macaques during acute and chronic infection. *J.Virol.*, Vol. 76, No. 16, pp. (8433-8445)

An, D. S., Poon, B., Ho Tsong, F. R., Weijer, K., Blom, B., Spits, H., Chen, I. S. & Uittenbogaart, C. H. (2007). Use of a novel chimeric mouse model with a functionally active human immune system to study human immunodeficiency virus type 1 infection. *Clin.Vaccine Immunol.*, Vol. 14, No. 4, pp. (391-396)

Andersson, J., Boasso, A., Nilsson, J., Zhang, R., Shire, N. J., Lindback, S., Shearer, G. M. & Chougnet, C. A. (2005). The prevalence of regulatory T cells in lymphoid tissue is correlated with viral load in HIV-infected patients. *J.Immunol.*, Vol. 174, No. 6, pp. (3143-3147)

Annunziato, F., Cosmi, L., Liotta, F., Lazzeri, E., Manetti, R., Vanini, V., Romagnani, P., Maggi, E. & Romagnani, S. (2002). Phenotype, localization, and mechanism of suppression of CD4(+)CD25(+) human thymocytes. *J.Exp.Med.*, Vol. 196, No. 3, pp. (379-387)

Arron, S. T., Ribeiro, R. M., Gettie, A., Bohm, R., Blanchard, J., Yu, J., Perelson, A. S., Ho, D. D. & Zhang, L. (2005). Impact of thymectomy on the peripheral T cell pool in rhesus macaques before and after infection with simian immunodeficiency virus. *Eur.J.Immunol.*, Vol. 35, No. 1, pp. (46-55)

Baecher-Allan, C., Brown, J. A., Freeman, G. J. & Hafler, D. A. (2001). CD4+CD25high regulatory cells in human peripheral blood. *J.Immunol.*, Vol. 167, No. 3, pp. (1245-1253)

Baenziger, S., Tussiwand, R., Schlaepfer, E., Mazzucchelli, L., Heikenwalder, M., Kurrer, M. O., Behnke, S., Frey, J., Oxenius, A., Joller, H., Aguzzi, A., Manz, M. G. & Speck, R. F. (2006). Disseminated and sustained HIV infection in CD34+ cord blood cell-transplanted Rag2-/-gamma c-/- mice. *Proc.Natl.Acad.Sci.U.S.A*, Vol. 103, No. 43, pp. (15951-15956)

Banchereau, J., Briere, F., Caux, C., Davoust, J., Lebecque, S., Liu, Y. J., Pulendran, B. & Palucka, K. (2000a). Immunobiology of dendritic cells. *Annu.Rev.Immunol.*, Vol. 18, pp. (767-811)

Banchereau, J., Pulendran, B., Steinman, R. & Palucka, K. (2000b). Will the making of plasmacytoid dendritic cells in vitro help unravel their mysteries? *J.Exp.Med.*, Vol. 192, No. 12, pp. (F39-F44)

Bandera, A., Ferrario, G., Saresella, M., Marventano, I., Soria, A., Zanini, F., Sabbatini, F., Airoldi, M., Marchetti, G., Franzetti, F., Trabattoni, D., Clerici, M. & Gori, A. (2010). CD4+ T cell depletion, immune activation and increased production of regulatory T cells in the thymus of HIV-infected individuals. *PLoS.One.*, Vol. 5, No. 5, pp. (e10788)

Basu, S. & Broxmeyer, H. E. (2009). CCR5 ligands modulate CXCL12-induced chemotaxis, adhesion, and Akt phosphorylation of human cord blood CD34+ cells. *J.Immunol.*, Vol. 183, No. 11, pp. (7478-7488)

Beignon, A. S., McKenna, K., Skoberne, M., Manches, O., DaSilva, I., Kavanagh, D. G., Larsson, M., Gorelick, R. J., Lifson, J. D. & Bhardwaj, N. (2005). Endocytosis of HIV-1 activates plasmacytoid dendritic cells via Toll-like receptor-viral RNA interactions. *J.Clin.Invest,* Vol. 115, No. 11, pp. (3265-3275)

Belkaid, Y. & Rouse, B. T. (2005). Natural regulatory T cells in infectious disease. *Nat.Immunol.,* Vol. 6, No. 4, pp. (353-360)

Bendriss-Vermare, N., Barthelemy, C., Durand, I., Bruand, C., Dezutter-Dambuyant, C., Moulian, N., Berrih-Aknin, S., Caux, C., Trinchieri, G. & Briere, F. (2001). Human thymus contains IFN-alpha-producing CD11c(-), myeloid CD11c(+), and mature interdigitating dendritic cells. *J.Clin.Invest,* Vol. 107, No. 7, pp. (835-844)

Berges, B. K., Akkina, S. R., Folkvord, J. M., Connick, E. & Akkina, R. (2008). Mucosal transmission of R5 and X4 tropic HIV-1 via vaginal and rectal routes in humanized Rag2-/- gammac -/- (RAG-hu) mice. *Virology,* Vol. 373, No. 2, pp. (342-351)

Berges, B. K., Wheat, W. H., Palmer, B. E., Connick, E. & Akkina, R. (2006). HIV-1 infection and CD4 T cell depletion in the humanized Rag2-/-gamma c-/- (RAG-hu) mouse model. *Retrovirology.,* Vol. 3, pp. (76)

Berkowitz, R. D., Alexander, S., Bare, C., Linquist-Stepps, V., Bogan, M., Moreno, M. E., Gibson, L., Wieder, E. D., Kosek, J., Stoddart, C. A. & McCune, J. M. (1998a). CCR5- and CXCR4-utilizing strains of human immunodeficiency virus type 1 exhibit differential tropism and pathogenesis in vivo. *J.Virol.,* Vol. 72, No. 12, pp. (10108-10117)

Berkowitz, R. D., Beckerman, K. P., Schall, T. J. & McCune, J. M. (1998b). CXCR4 and CCR5 expression delineates targets for HIV-1 disruption of T cell differentiation. *J.Immunol.,* Vol. 161, No. 7, pp. (3702-3710)

Bhandoola, A., Sambandam, A., Allman, D., Meraz, A. & Schwarz, B. (2003). Early T lineage progenitors: new insights, but old questions remain. *J.Immunol.,* Vol. 171, No. 11, pp. (5653-5658)

Blom, B., Ho, S., Antonenko, S. & Liu, Y. J. (2000). Generation of interferon alpha-producing predendritic cell (Pre-DC)2 from human CD34(+) hematopoietic stem cells. *J.Exp.Med.,* Vol. 192, No. 12, pp. (1785-1796)

Blom, B., Res, P., Noteboom, E., Weijer, K. & Spits, H. (1997). Prethymic CD34+ progenitors capable of developing into T cells are not committed to the T cell lineage. *J.Immunol.,* Vol. 158, No. 8, pp. (3571-3577)

Blom, B., Verschuren, M. C., Heemskerk, M. H., Bakker, A. Q., Gastel-Mol, E. J., Wolvers-Tettero, I. L., van Dongen, J. J. & Spits, H. (1999). TCR gene rearrangements and expression of the pre-T cell receptor complex during human T-cell differentiation. *Blood,* Vol. 93, No. 9, pp. (3033-3043)

Bosinger, S. E., Li, Q., Gordon, S. N., Klatt, N. R., Duan, L., Xu, L., Francella, N., Sidahmed, A., Smith, A. J., Cramer, E. M., Zeng, M., Masopust, D., Carlis, J. V., Ran, L., Vanderford, T. H., Paiardini, M., Isett, R. B., Baldwin, D. A., Else, J. G., Staprans, S. I., Silvestri, G., Haase, A. T. & Kelvin, D. J. (2009). Global genomic analysis reveals rapid control of a robust innate response in SIV-infected sooty mangabeys. *J.Clin.Invest,* Vol. 119, No. 12, pp. (3556-3572)

Bosma, G. C., Custer, R. P. & Bosma, M. J. (1983). A severe combined immunodeficiency mutation in the mouse. *Nature,* Vol. 301, No. 5900, pp. (527-530)

Brainard, D. M., Seung, E., Frahm, N., Cariappa, A., Bailey, C. C., Hart, W. K., Shin, H. S., Brooks, S. F., Knight, H. L., Eichbaum, Q., Yang, Y. G., Sykes, M., Walker, B. D., Freeman, G. J., Pillai, S., Westmoreland, S. V., Brander, C., Luster, A. D. & Tager, A. M. (2009). Induction of robust cellular and humoral virus-specific adaptive immune responses in human immunodeficiency virus-infected humanized BLT mice. *J.Virol.,* Vol. 83, No. 14, pp. (7305-7321)

Brassard, D. L., Grace, M. J. & Bordens, R. W. (2002). Interferon-alpha as an immunotherapeutic protein. *J.Leukoc.Biol.,* Vol. 71, No. 4, pp. (565-581)

Brunner, J., Boehler, T., Ehemann, V., Kassam, S., Otto, H. & Sergi, C. (2011). Decreased Apoptosis Despite Severe CD4 Depletion in the Thymus of a Human Immunodeficiency Virus-1 Infected Child. *Klin.Padiatr.,* Vol.

Cabrera, R., Tu, Z., Xu, Y., Firpi, R. J., Rosen, H. R., Liu, C. & Nelson, D. R. (2004). An immunomodulatory role for CD4(+)CD25(+) regulatory T lymphocytes in hepatitis C virus infection. *Hepatology,* Vol. 40, No. 5, pp. (1062-1071)

Calabro, M. L., Zanotto, C., Calderazzo, F., Crivellaro, C., Del Mistro, A., De Rossi, A. & Chieco-Bianchi, L. (1995). HIV-1 infection of the thymus: evidence for a cytopathic and thymotropic viral variant in vivo. *AIDS Res.Hum.Retroviruses,* Vol. 11, No. 1, pp. (11-19)

Carrasco, Y. R., Trigueros, C., Ramiro, A. R., de Yebenes, V. G. & Toribio, M. L. (1999). Beta-selection is associated with the onset of CD8beta chain expression on CD4(+)CD8alphaalpha(+) pre-T cells during human intrathymic development. *Blood,* Vol. 94, No. 10, pp. (3491-3498)

Carter, C. C., Onafuwa-Nuga, A., McNamara, L. A., Riddell, J., Bixby, D., Savona, M. R. & Collins, K. L. (2010). HIV-1 infects multipotent progenitor cells causing cell death and establishing latent cellular reservoirs. *Nat.Med.,* Vol. 16, No. 4, pp. (446-451)

Cella, M., Facchetti, F., Lanzavecchia, A. & Colonna, M. (2000). Plasmacytoid dendritic cells activated by influenza virus and CD40L drive a potent TH1 polarization. *Nat.Immunol.,* Vol. 1, No. 4, pp. (305-310)

Cella, M., Jarrossay, D., Facchetti, F., Alebardi, O., Nakajima, H., Lanzavecchia, A. & Colonna, M. (1999). Plasmacytoid monocytes migrate to inflamed lymph nodes and produce large amounts of type I interferon. *Nat.Med.,* Vol. 5, No. 8, pp. (919-923)

Chehimi, J., Campbell, D. E., Azzoni, L., Bacheller, D., Papasavvas, E., Jerandi, G., Mounzer, K., Kostman, J., Trinchieri, G. & Montaner, L. J. (2002). Persistent decreases in blood plasmacytoid dendritic cell number and function despite effective highly active antiretroviral therapy and increased blood myeloid dendritic cells in HIV-infected individuals. *J.Immunol.,* Vol. 168, No. 9, pp. (4796-4801)

Cisse, B., Caton, M. L., Lehner, M., Maeda, T., Scheu, S., Locksley, R., Holmberg, D., Zweier, C., den Hollander, N. S., Kant, S. G., Holter, W., Rauch, A., Zhuang, Y. & Reizis, B. (2008). Transcription factor E2-2 is an essential and specific regulator of plasmacytoid dendritic cell development. *Cell,* Vol. 135, No. 1, pp. (37-48)

Cosmi, L., Liotta, F., Lazzeri, E., Francalanci, M., Angeli, R., Mazzinghi, B., Santarlasci, V., Manetti, R., Vanini, V., Romagnani, P., Maggi, E., Romagnani, S. & Annunziato, F. (2003). Human CD8+CD25+ thymocytes share phenotypic and functional features with CD4+CD25+ regulatory thymocytes. *Blood,* Vol. 102, No. 12, pp. (4107-4114)

Cupedo, T., Nagasawa, M., Weijer, K., Blom, B. & Spits, H. (2005). Development and activation of regulatory T cells in the human fetus. *Eur.J.Immunol.*, Vol. 35, No. 2, pp. (383-390)

Dalloul, A. H., Patry, C., Salamero, J., Canque, B., Grassi, F. & Schmitt, C. (1999). Functional and phenotypic analysis of thymic CD34+CD1a- progenitor-derived dendritic cells: predominance of CD1a+ differentiation pathway. *J.Immunol.*, Vol. 162, No. 10, pp. (5821-5828)

Darrasse-Jeze, G., Marodon, G., Salomon, B. L., Catala, M. & Klatzmann, D. (2005). Ontogeny of CD4+CD25+ regulatory/suppressor T cells in human fetuses. *Blood*, Vol. 105, No. 12, pp. (4715-4721)

Deng, H., Liu, R., Ellmeier, W., Choe, S., Unutmaz, D., Burkhart, M., Di Marzio, P., Marmon, S., Sutton, R. E., Hill, C. M., Davis, C. B., Peiper, S. C., Schall, T. J., Littman, D. R. & Landau, N. R. (1996). Identification of a major co-receptor for primary isolates of HIV-1. *Nature*, Vol. 381, No. 6584, pp. (661-666)

Denton, P. W., Estes, J. D., Sun, Z., Othieno, F. A., Wei, B. L., Wege, A. K., Powell, D. A., Payne, D., Haase, A. T. & Garcia, J. V. (2008). Antiretroviral pre-exposure prophylaxis prevents vaginal transmission of HIV-1 in humanized BLT mice. *PLoS.Med.*, Vol. 5, No. 1, pp. (e16)

Dik, W. A., Pike-Overzet, K., Weerkamp, F., de Ridder, D., de Haas, E. F., Baert, M. R., van der, S. P., Koster, E. E., Reinders, M. J., van Dongen, J. J., Langerak, A. W. & Staal, F. J. (2005). New insights on human T cell development by quantitative T cell receptor gene rearrangement studies and gene expression profiling. *J.Exp.Med.*, Vol. 201, No. 11, pp. (1715-1723)

Dion, M. L., Sekaly, R. P. & Cheynier, R. (2007). Estimating thymic function through quantification of T-cell receptor excision circles. *Methods Mol.Biol.*, Vol. 380, pp. (197-213)

Diop, O. M., Ploquin, M. J., Mortara, L., Faye, A., Jacquelin, B., Kunkel, D., Lebon, P., Butor, C., Hosmalin, A., Barre-Sinoussi, F. & Muller-Trutwin, M. C. (2008). Plasmacytoid dendritic cell dynamics and alpha interferon production during Simian immunodeficiency virus infection with a nonpathogenic outcome. *J.Virol.*, Vol. 82, No. 11, pp. (5145-5152)

Donaghy, H., Pozniak, A., Gazzard, B., Qazi, N., Gilmour, J., Gotch, F. & Patterson, S. (2001). Loss of blood CD11c(+) myeloid and CD11c(-) plasmacytoid dendritic cells in patients with HIV-1 infection correlates with HIV-1 RNA virus load. *Blood*, Vol. 98, No. 8, pp. (2574-2576)

Dragic, T., Litwin, V., Allaway, G. P., Martin, S. R., Huang, Y., Nagashima, K. A., Cayanan, C., Maddon, P. J., Koup, R. A., Moore, J. P. & Paxton, W. A. (1996). HIV-1 entry into CD4+ cells is mediated by the chemokine receptor CC-CKR-5. *Nature*, Vol. 381, No. 6584, pp. (667-673)

Eggena, M. P., Barugahare, B., Jones, N., Okello, M., Mutalya, S., Kityo, C., Mugyenyi, P. & Cao, H. (2005). Depletion of regulatory T cells in HIV infection is associated with immune activation. *J.Immunol.*, Vol. 174, No. 7, pp. (4407-4414)

Fais, S., Lapenta, C., Santini, S. M., Spada, M., Parlato, S., Logozzi, M., Rizza, P. & Belardelli, F. (1999). Human immunodeficiency virus type 1 strains R5 and X4 induce different pathogenic effects in hu-PBL-SCID mice, depending on the state of activation/differentiation of human target cells at the time of primary infection. *J.Virol.,* Vol. 73, No. 8, pp. (6453-6459)

Favre, D., Stoddart, C. A., Emu, B., Hoh, R., Martin, J. N., Hecht, F. M., Deeks, S. G. & McCune, J. M. (2011). HIV disease progression correlates with the generation of dysfunctional naive CD8(low) T cells. *Blood,* Vol. 117, No. 7, pp. (2189-2199)

Feldman, S., Stein, D., Amrute, S., Denny, T., Garcia, Z., Kloser, P., Sun, Y., Megjugorac, N. & Fitzgerald-Bocarsly, P. (2001). Decreased interferon-alpha production in HIV-infected patients correlates with numerical and functional deficiencies in circulating type 2 dendritic cell precursors. *Clin.Immunol.,* Vol. 101, No. 2, pp. (201-210)

Feng, Y., Broder, C. C., Kennedy, P. E. & Berger, E. A. (1996). HIV-1 entry cofactor: functional cDNA cloning of a seven-transmembrane, G protein-coupled receptor. *Science,* Vol. 272, No. 5263, pp. (872-877)

Ferbas, J. J., Toso, J. F., Logar, A. J., Navratil, J. S. & Rinaldo, C. R., Jr. (1994). CD4+ blood dendritic cells are potent producers of IFN-alpha in response to in vitro HIV-1 infection. *J.Immunol.,* Vol. 152, No. 9, pp. (4649-4662)

Fischer, A., Le Deist, F., Hacein-Bey-Abina, S., Andre-Schmutz, I., Basile, G. S., de Villartay, J. P. & Cavazzana-Calvo, M. (2005). Severe combined immunodeficiency. A model disease for molecular immunology and therapy. *Immunol.Rev.,* Vol. 203, pp. (98-109)

Fong, L., Mengozzi, M., Abbey, N. W., Herndier, B. G. & Engleman, E. G. (2002). Productive infection of plasmacytoid dendritic cells with human immunodeficiency virus type 1 is triggered by CD40 ligation. *J.Virol.,* Vol. 76, No. 21, pp. (11033-11041)

Fontenot, J. D., Gavin, M. A. & Rudensky, A. Y. (2003). Foxp3 programs the development and function of CD4+CD25+ regulatory T cells. *Nat.Immunol.,* Vol. 4, No. 4, pp. (330-336)

Fontenot, J. D., Rasmussen, J. P., Williams, L. M., Dooley, J. L., Farr, A. G. & Rudensky, A. Y. (2005). Regulatory T cell lineage specification by the forkhead transcription factor foxp3. *Immunity.,* Vol. 22, No. 3, pp. (329-341)

Fontenot, J. D. & Rudensky, A. Y. (2005). A well adapted regulatory contrivance: regulatory T cell development and the forkhead family transcription factor Foxp3. *Nat.Immunol.,* Vol. 6, No. 4, pp. (331-337)

Foster, G. R., Germain, C., Jones, M., Lechler, R. I. & Lombardi, G. (2000). Human T cells elicit IFN-alpha secretion from dendritic cells following cell to cell interactions. *Eur.J.Immunol.,* Vol. 30, No. 11, pp. (3228-3235)

Galy, A., Verma, S., Barcena, A. & Spits, H. (1993). Precursors of CD3+CD4+CD8+ cells in the human thymus are defined by expression of CD34. Delineation of early events in human thymic development. *J.Exp.Med.,* Vol. 178, No. 2, pp. (391-401)

Gaulton, G. N., Scobie, J. V. & Rosenzweig, M. (1997). HIV-1 and the thymus. *AIDS,* Vol. 11, No. 4, pp. (403-414)

Ghirelli, C., Zollinger, R. & Soumelis, V. (2010). Systematic cytokine receptor profiling reveals GM-CSF as a novel TLR-independent activator of human plasmacytoid predendritic cells. *Blood,* Vol. 115, No. 24, pp. (5037-5040)

Giliani, S., Mori, L., de Saint, B. G., Le Deist, F., Rodriguez-Perez, C., Forino, C., Mazzolari, E., Dupuis, S., Elhasid, R., Kessel, A., Galambrun, C., Gil, J., Fischer, A., Etzioni, A.

& Notarangelo, L. D. (2005). Interleukin-7 receptor alpha (IL-7Ralpha) deficiency: cellular and molecular bases. Analysis of clinical, immunological, and molecular features in 16 novel patients. *Immunol.Rev.,* Vol. 203, pp. (110-126)

Gilliet, M., Boonstra, A., Paturel, C., Antonenko, S., Xu, X. L., Trinchieri, G., O'Garra, A. & Liu, Y. J. (2002). The development of murine plasmacytoid dendritic cell precursors is differentially regulated by FLT3-ligand and granulocyte/macrophage colony-stimulating factor. *J.Exp.Med.,* Vol. 195, No. 7, pp. (953-958)

Gilliet, M. & Liu, Y. J. (2002). Generation of human CD8 T regulatory cells by CD40 ligand-activated plasmacytoid dendritic cells. *J.Exp.Med.,* Vol. 195, No. 6, pp. (695-704)

Gimeno, R., Weijer, K., Voordouw, A., Uittenbogaart, C. H., Legrand, N., Alves, N. L., Wijnands, E., Blom, B. & Spits, H. (2004). Monitoring the effect of gene silencing by RNA interference in human CD34+ cells injected into newborn RAG2-/- gammac-/- mice: functional inactivation of p53 in developing T cells. *Blood,* Vol. 104, No. 13, pp. (3886-3893)

Giorgi, J. V., Hultin, L. E., McKeating, J. A., Johnson, T. D., Owens, B., Jacobson, L. P., Shih, R., Lewis, J., Wiley, D. J., Phair, J. P., Wolinsky, S. M. & Detels, R. (1999). Shorter survival in advanced human immunodeficiency virus type 1 infection is more closely associated with T lymphocyte activation than with plasma virus burden or virus chemokine coreceptor usage. *J.Infect.Dis.,* Vol. 179, No. 4, pp. (859-870)

Gorantla, S., Sneller, H., Walters, L., Sharp, J. G., Pirruccello, S. J., West, J. T., Wood, C., Dewhurst, S., Gendelman, H. E. & Poluektova, L. (2007). Human immunodeficiency virus type 1 pathobiology studied in humanized BALB/c-Rag2-/-gammac-/- mice. *J.Virol.,* Vol. 81, No. 6, pp. (2700-2712)

Grandvaux, N., tenOever, B. R., Servant, M. J. & Hiscott, J. (2002). The interferon antiviral response: from viral invasion to evasion. *Curr.Opin.Infect.Dis.,* Vol. 15, No. 3, pp. (259-267)

Greiner, D. L., Hesselton, R. A. & Shultz, L. D. (1998). SCID mouse models of human stem cell engraftment. *Stem Cells,* Vol. 16, No. 3, pp. (166-177)

Grouard, G., Rissoan, M. C., Filgueira, L., Durand, I., Banchereau, J. & Liu, Y. J. (1997). The enigmatic plasmacytoid T cells develop into dendritic cells with interleukin (IL)-3 and CD40-ligand. *J.Exp.Med.,* Vol. 185, No. 6, pp. (1101-1111)

Gurney, K. B., Colantonio, A. D., Blom, B., Spits, H. & Uittenbogaart, C. H. (2004). Endogenous IFN-alpha production by plasmacytoid dendritic cells exerts an antiviral effect on thymic HIV-1 infection. *J.Immunol.,* Vol. 173, No. 12, pp. (7269-7276)

Gurney, K. B. & Uittenbogaart, C. H. (2006). Human immunodeficiency virus persistence and production in T-cell development. *Clin.Vaccine Immunol.,* Vol. 13, No. 11, pp. (1237-1245)

Gurney, K. B., Yang, O. O., Wilson, S. B. & Uittenbogaart, C. H. (2002). TCR gamma delta+ and CD161+ thymocytes express HIV-1 in the SCID-hu mouse, potentially contributing to immune dysfunction in HIV infection. *J.Immunol.,* Vol. 169, No. 9, pp. (5338-5346)

Haddad, R., Guardiola, P., Izac, B., Thibault, C., Radich, J., Delezoide, A. L., Baillou, C., Lemoine, F. M., Gluckman, J. C., Pflumio, F. & Canque, B. (2004). Molecular characterization of early human T/NK and B-lymphoid progenitor cells in umbilical cord blood. *Blood,* Vol. 104, No. 13, pp. (3918-3926)

Haeryfar, S. M. (2005). The importance of being a pDC in antiviral immunity: the IFN mission versus Ag presentation? *Trends Immunol.,* Vol. 26, No. 6, pp. (311-317)

Halnon, N. J., Jamieson, B., Plunkett, M., Kitchen, C. M., Pham, T. & Krogstad, P. (2005). Thymic function and impaired maintenance of peripheral T cell populations in children with congenital heart disease and surgical thymectomy. *Pediatr.Res.,* Vol. 57, No. 1, pp. (42-48)

Hanabuchi, S., Ito, T., Park, W. R., Watanabe, N., Shaw, J. L., Roman, E., Arima, K., Wang, Y. H., Voo, K. S., Cao, W. & Liu, Y. J. (2010). Thymic stromal lymphopoietin-activated plasmacytoid dendritic cells induce the generation of FOXP3+ regulatory T cells in human thymus. *J.Immunol.,* Vol. 184, No. 6, pp. (2999-3007)

Hao, Q. L., Zhu, J., Price, M. A., Payne, K. J., Barsky, L. W. & Crooks, G. M. (2001). Identification of a novel, human multilymphoid progenitor in cord blood. *Blood,* Vol. 97, No. 12, pp. (3683-3690)

Hardy, A. W., Graham, D. R., Shearer, G. M. & Herbeuval, J. P. (2007). HIV turns plasmacytoid dendritic cells (pDC) into TRAIL-expressing killer pDC and down-regulates HIV coreceptors by Toll-like receptor 7-induced IFN-alpha. *Proc.Natl.Acad.Sci.U.S.A,* Vol. 104, No. 44, pp. (17453-17458)

Haynes, B. F., Hale, L. P., Weinhold, K. J., Patel, D. D., Liao, H. X., Bressler, P. B., Jones, D. M., Demarest, J. F., Gebhard-Mitchell, K., Haase, A. T. & Bartlett, J. A. (1999). Analysis of the adult thymus in reconstitution of T lymphocytes in HIV-1 infection. *J.Clin.Invest,* Vol. 103, No. 4, pp. (453-460)

Herbeuval, J. P., Nilsson, J., Boasso, A., Hardy, A. W., Kruhlak, M. J., Anderson, S. A., Dolan, M. J., Dy, M., Andersson, J. & Shearer, G. M. (2006). Differential expression of IFN-alpha and TRAIL/DR5 in lymphoid tissue of progressor versus nonprogressor HIV-1-infected patients. *Proc.Natl.Acad.Sci.U.S.A,* Vol. 103, No. 18, pp. (7000-7005)

Hernandez-Lopez, C., Varas, A., Sacedon, R., Jimenez, E., Munoz, J. J., Zapata, A. G. & Vicente, A. (2002). Stromal cell-derived factor 1/CXCR4 signaling is critical for early human T-cell development. *Blood,* Vol. 99, No. 2, pp. (546-554)

Hiramatsu, H., Nishikomori, R., Heike, T., Ito, M., Kobayashi, K., Katamura, K. & Nakahata, T. (2003). Complete reconstitution of human lymphocytes from cord blood CD34+ cells using the NOD/SCID/gammacnull mice model. *Blood,* Vol. 102, No. 3, pp. (873-880)

Ho Tsong Fang, R., Colantonio, A. D. & Uittenbogaart, C. H. (2008). The role of the thymus in HIV infection: a 10 year perspective. *AIDS,* Vol. 22, No. 2, pp. (171-184)

Ho Tsong Fang, R., Khatissian, E., Monceaux, V., Cumont, M. C., Beq, S., Ameisen, J. C., Aubertin, A. M., Israel, N., Estaquier, J. & Hurtrel, B. (2005). Disease progression in macaques with low SIV replication levels: on the relevance of TREC counts. *AIDS,* Vol. 19, No. 7, pp. (663-673)

Hoeffel, G., Ripoche, A. C., Matheoud, D., Nascimbeni, M., Escriou, N., Lebon, P., Heshmati, F., Guillet, J. G., Gannage, M., Caillat-Zucman, S., Casartelli, N., Schwartz, O., De la, S. H., Hanau, D., Hosmalin, A. & Maranon, C. (2007). Antigen crosspresentation by human plasmacytoid dendritic cells. *Immunity.,* Vol. 27, No. 3, pp. (481-492)

Hori, S., Haury, M., Lafaille, J. J., Demengeot, J. & Coutinho, A. (2002). Peripheral expansion of thymus-derived regulatory cells in anti-myelin basic protein T cell receptor transgenic mice. *Eur.J.Immunol.,* Vol. 32, No. 12, pp. (3729-3735)

Hori, S., Nomura, T. & Sakaguchi, S. (2003). Control of regulatory T cell development by the transcription factor Foxp3. *Science,* Vol. 299, No. 5609, pp. (1057-1061)

Hori, T., Cupp, J., Wrighton, N., Lee, F. & Spits, H. (1991). Identification of a novel human thymocyte subset with a phenotype of CD3- CD4+ CD8 alpha + beta-1. Possible progeny of the CD3- CD4- CD8- subset. *J.Immunol.,* Vol. 146, No. 12, pp. (4078-4084)

Iida, T., Ichimura, H., Shimada, T., Ibuki, K., Ui, M., Tamaru, K., Kuwata, T., Yonehara, S., Imanishi, J. & Hayami, M. (2000). Role of apoptosis induction in both peripheral lymph nodes and thymus in progressive loss of CD4+ cells in SHIV-infected macaques. *AIDS Res.Hum.Retroviruses,* Vol. 16, No. 1, pp. (9-18)

Ishii, T., Nishihara, M., Ma, F., Ebihara, Y., Tsuji, K., Asano, S., Nakahata, T. & Maekawa, T. (1999). Expression of stromal cell-derived factor-1/pre-B cell growth-stimulating factor receptor, CXC chemokine receptor 4, on CD34+ human bone marrow cells is a phenotypic alteration for committed lymphoid progenitors. *J.Immunol.,* Vol. 163, No. 7, pp. (3612-3620)

Ishikawa, F., Livingston, A. G., Minamiguchi, H., Wingard, J. R. & Ogawa, M. (2003). Human cord blood long-term engrafting cells are CD34+ CD38-. *Leukemia,* Vol. 17, No. 5, pp. (960-964)

Ishikawa, F., Yasukawa, M., Lyons, B., Yoshida, S., Miyamoto, T., Yoshimoto, G., Watanabe, T., Akashi, K., Shultz, L. D. & Harada, M. (2005). Development of functional human blood and immune systems in NOD/SCID/IL2 receptor {gamma} chain(null) mice. *Blood,* Vol. 106, No. 5, pp. (1565-1573)

Ito, M., Hiramatsu, H., Kobayashi, K., Suzue, K., Kawahata, M., Hioki, K., Ueyama, Y., Koyanagi, Y., Sugamura, K., Tsuji, K., Heike, T. & Nakahata, T. (2002). NOD/SCID/gamma(c)(null) mouse: an excellent recipient mouse model for engraftment of human cells. *Blood,* Vol. 100, No. 9, pp. (3175-3182)

Ito, T., Amakawa, R., Inaba, M., Ikehara, S., Inaba, K. & Fukuhara, S. (2001). Differential regulation of human blood dendritic cell subsets by IFNs. *J.Immunol.,* Vol. 166, No. 5, pp. (2961-2969)

Ito, T., Kanzler, H., Duramad, O., Cao, W. & Liu, Y. J. (2006). Specialization, kinetics, and repertoire of type 1 interferon responses by human plasmacytoid predendritic cells. *Blood,* Vol. 107, No. 6, pp. (2423-2431)

Itoh, M., Takahashi, T., Sakaguchi, N., Kuniyasu, Y., Shimizu, J., Otsuka, F. & Sakaguchi, S. (1999). Thymus and autoimmunity: production of CD25+CD4+ naturally anergic and suppressive T cells as a key function of the thymus in maintaining immunologic self-tolerance. *J.Immunol.,* Vol. 162, No. 9, pp. (5317-5326)

Jacquelin, B., Mayau, V., Targat, B., Liovat, A. S., Kunkel, D., Petitjean, G., Dillies, M. A., Roques, P., Butor, C., Silvestri, G., Giavedoni, L. D., Lebon, P., Barre-Sinoussi, F., Benecke, A. & Muller-Trutwin, M. C. (2009). Nonpathogenic SIV infection of African green monkeys induces a strong but rapidly controlled type I IFN response. *J.Clin.Invest,* Vol. 119, No. 12, pp. (3544-3555)

Jamieson, B. D., Pang, S., Aldrovandi, G. M., Zha, J. & Zack, J. A. (1995). In vivo pathogenic properties of two clonal human immunodeficiency virus type 1 isolates. *J.Virol.*, Vol. 69, No. 10, pp. (6259-6264)

Jordan, M. S., Boesteanu, A., Reed, A. J., Petrone, A. L., Holenbeck, A. E., Lerman, M. A., Naji, A. & Caton, A. J. (2001). Thymic selection of CD4+CD25+ regulatory T cells induced by an agonist self-peptide. *Nat.Immunol.*, Vol. 2, No. 4, pp. (301-306)

Kadowaki, N., Antonenko, S., Ho, S., Rissoan, M. C., Soumelis, V., Porcelli, S. A., Lanier, L. L. & Liu, Y. J. (2001a). Distinct cytokine profiles of neonatal natural killer T cells after expansion with subsets of dendritic cells. *J.Exp.Med.*, Vol. 193, No. 10, pp. (1221-1226)

Kadowaki, N., Antonenko, S., Lau, J. Y. & Liu, Y. J. (2000). Natural interferon alpha/beta-producing cells link innate and adaptive immunity. *J.Exp.Med.*, Vol. 192, No. 2, pp. (219-226)

Kadowaki, N., Ho, S., Antonenko, S., Malefyt, R. W., Kastelein, R. A., Bazan, F. & Liu, Y. J. (2001b). Subsets of human dendritic cell precursors express different toll-like receptors and respond to different microbial antigens. *J.Exp.Med.*, Vol. 194, No. 6, pp. (863-869)

Kasow, K. A., Chen, X., Knowles, J., Wichlan, D., Handgretinger, R. & Riberdy, J. M. (2004). Human CD4+CD25+ regulatory T cells share equally complex and comparable repertoires with CD4+. *J.Immunol.*, Vol. 172, No. 10, pp. (6123-6128)

Keir, M. E., Stoddart, C. A., Linquist-Stepps, V., Moreno, M. E. & McCune, J. M. (2002). IFN-alpha secretion by type 2 predendritic cells up-regulates MHC class I in the HIV-1-infected thymus. *J.Immunol.*, Vol. 168, No. 1, pp. (325-331)

Kerre, T. C., De Smet, G., De Smedt, M., Zippelius, A., Pittet, M. J., Langerak, A. W., De Bosscher, J., Offner, F., Vandekerckhove, B. & Plum, J. (2002). Adapted NOD/SCID model supports development of phenotypically and functionally mature T cells from human umbilical cord blood CD34(+) cells. *Blood*, Vol. 99, No. 5, pp. (1620-1626)

Khattri, R., Cox, T., Yasayko, S. A. & Ramsdell, F. (2003). An essential role for Scurfin in CD4+CD25+ T regulatory cells. *Nat.Immunol.*, Vol. 4, No. 4, pp. (337-342)

Kinter, A. L., Hennessey, M., Bell, A., Kern, S., Lin, Y., Daucher, M., Planta, M., McGlaughlin, M., Jackson, R., Ziegler, S. F. & Fauci, A. S. (2004). CD25(+)CD4(+) regulatory T cells from the peripheral blood of asymptomatic HIV-infected individuals regulate CD4(+) and CD8(+) HIV-specific T cell immune responses in vitro and are associated with favorable clinical markers of disease status. *J.Exp.Med.*, Vol. 200, No. 3, pp. (331-343)

Kirchgessner, C. U., Patil, C. K., Evans, J. W., Cuomo, C. A., Fried, L. M., Carter, T., Oettinger, M. A. & Brown, J. M. (1995). DNA-dependent kinase (p350) as a candidate gene for the murine SCID defect. *Science*, Vol. 267, No. 5201, pp. (1178-1183)

Kitchen, S. G. & Zack, J. A. (1997). CXCR4 expression during lymphopoiesis: implications for human immunodeficiency virus type 1 infection of the thymus. *J.Virol.*, Vol. 71, No. 9, pp. (6928-6934)

Kitchen, S. G. & Zack, J. A. (1999). Distribution of the human immunodeficiency virus coreceptors CXCR4 and CCR5 in fetal lymphoid organs: implications for pathogenesis in utero. *AIDS Res.Hum.Retroviruses,* Vol. 15, No. 2, pp. (143-148)

Klein, F., Feldhahn, N., Lee, S., Wang, H., Ciuffi, F., von Elstermann, M., Toribio, M. L., Sauer, H., Wartenberg, M., Barath, V. S., Kronke, M., Wernet, P., Rowley, J. D. & Muschen, M. (2003a). T lymphoid differentiation in human bone marrow. *Proc.Natl.Acad.Sci.U.S.A,* Vol. 100, No. 11, pp. (6747-6752)

Klein, L., Hinterberger, M., Wirnsberger, G. & Kyewski, B. (2009). Antigen presentation in the thymus for positive selection and central tolerance induction. *Nat.Rev.Immunol.,* Vol. 9, No. 12, pp. (833-844)

Klein, L., Khazaie, K. & von Boehmer, H. (2003b). In vivo dynamics of antigen-specific regulatory T cells not predicted from behavior in vitro. *Proc.Natl.Acad.Sci.U.S.A,* Vol. 100, No. 15, pp. (8886-8891)

Kohrgruber, N., Halanek, N., Groger, M., Winter, D., Rappersberger, K., Schmitt-Egenolf, M., Stingl, G. & Maurer, D. (1999). Survival, maturation, and function of CD11c- and CD11c+ peripheral blood dendritic cells are differentially regulated by cytokines. *J.Immunol.,* Vol. 163, No. 6, pp. (3250-3259)

Kollet, O., Peled, A., Byk, T., Ben Hur, H., Greiner, D., Shultz, L. & Lapidot, T. (2000). beta2 microglobulin-deficient (B2m(null)) NOD/SCID mice are excellent recipients for studying human stem cell function. *Blood,* Vol. 95, No. 10, pp. (3102-3105)

Kollmann, T. R., Kim, A., Pettoello-Mantovani, M., Hachamovitch, M., Rubinstein, A., Goldstein, M. M. & Goldstein, H. (1995). Divergent effects of chronic HIV-1 infection on human thymocyte maturation in SCID-hu mice. *J.Immunol.,* Vol. 154, No. 2, pp. (907-921)

Kollmann, T. R., Pettoello-Mantovani, M., Zhuang, X., Kim, A., Hachamovitch, M., Smarnworawong, P., Rubinstein, A. & Goldstein, H. (1994). Disseminated human immunodeficiency virus 1 (HIV-1) infection in SCID-hu mice after peripheral inoculation with HIV-1. *J.Exp.Med.,* Vol. 179, No. 2, pp. (513-522)

Ktorza, S., Blanc, C., Laurent, C., Sarun, S., Verpilleux, M. P., Debre, P. & Schmitt, C. (1996). Complete TCR-delta rearrangements and partial (D-J) recombination of the TCR-beta locus in CD34+7+ precursors from human cord blood. *J.Immunol.,* Vol. 156, No. 11, pp. (4120-4127)

Lan, P., Tonomura, N., Shimizu, A., Wang, S. & Yang, Y. G. (2006). Reconstitution of a functional human immune system in immunodeficient mice through combined human fetal thymus/liver and CD34+ cell transplantation. *Blood,* Vol. 108, No. 2, pp. (487-492)

Lapidot, T., Pflumio, F., Doedens, M., Murdoch, B., Williams, D. E. & Dick, J. E. (1992). Cytokine stimulation of multilineage hematopoiesis from immature human cells engrafted in SCID mice. *Science,* Vol. 255, No. 5048, pp. (1137-1141)

Lee, J. C., Boechat, M. I., Belzer, M., Church, J. A., De Ville, J., Nielsen, K., Weston, S., Geng, Y., Dunaway, T., Kitchen, C. & Krogstad, P. A. (2006). Thymic volume, T-cell populations, and parameters of thymopoiesis in adolescent and adult survivors of HIV infection acquired in infancy. *AIDS,* Vol. 20, No. 5, pp. (667-674)

Lee, S., Goldstein, H., Baseler, M., Adelsberger, J. & Golding, H. (1997). Human immunodeficiency virus type 1 infection of mature CD3hiCD8+ thymocytes. *J.Virol.,* Vol. 71, No. 9, pp. (6671-6676)

Lin, Q., Dong, C. & Cooper, M. D. (1998). Impairment of T and B cell development by treatment with a type I interferon. *J.Exp.Med.,* Vol. 187, No. 1, pp. (79-87)

Macchi, P., Villa, A., Giliani, S., Sacco, M. G., Frattini, A., Porta, F., Ugazio, A. G., Johnston, J. A., Candotti, F., O'Shea, J. J. & . (1995). Mutations of Jak-3 gene in patients with autosomal severe combined immune deficiency (SCID). *Nature,* Vol. 377, No. 6544, pp. (65-68)

Maloy, K. J. & Powrie, F. (2001). Regulatory T cells in the control of immune pathology. *Nat.Immunol.,* Vol. 2, No. 9, pp. (816-822)

Martin-Gayo, E., Sierra-Filardi, E., Corbi, A. L. & Toribio, M. L. (2010). Plasmacytoid dendritic cells resident in human thymus drive natural Treg cell development. *Blood,* Vol. 115, No. 26, pp. (5366-5375)

McCune, J. M. (1997). Animal models of HIV-1 disease. *Science,* Vol. 278, No. 5346, pp. (2141-2142)

McCune, J. M., Loftus, R., Schmidt, D. K., Carroll, P., Webster, D., Swor-Yim, L. B., Francis, I. R., Gross, B. H. & Grant, R. M. (1998). High prevalence of thymic tissue in adults with human immunodeficiency virus-1 infection. *J.Clin.Invest,* Vol. 101, No. 11, pp. (2301-2308)

McCune, J. M., Namikawa, R., Kaneshima, H., Shultz, L. D., Lieberman, M. & Weissman, I. L. (1988). The SCID-hu mouse: murine model for the analysis of human hematolymphoid differentiation and function. *Science,* Vol. 241, No. 4873, pp. (1632-1639)

Melkus, M. W., Estes, J. D., Padgett-Thomas, A., Gatlin, J., Denton, P. W., Othieno, F. A., Wege, A. K., Haase, A. T. & Garcia, J. V. (2006). Humanized mice mount specific adaptive and innate immune responses to EBV and TSST-1. *Nat.Med.,* Vol. 12, No. 11, pp. (1316-1322)

Meyers, J. H., Justement, J. S., Hallahan, C. W., Blair, E. T., Sun, Y. A., O'Shea, M. A., Roby, G., Kottilil, S., Moir, S., Kovacs, C. M., Chun, T. W. & Fauci, A. S. (2007). Impact of HIV on cell survival and antiviral activity of plasmacytoid dendritic cells. *PLoS.One.,* Vol. 2, No. 5, pp. (e458)

Mills, K. H. & McGuirk, P. (2004). Antigen-specific regulatory T cells--their induction and role in infection. *Semin.Immunol.,* Vol. 16, No. 2, pp. (107-117)

Milone, M. C. & Fitzgerald-Bocarsly, P. (1998). The mannose receptor mediates induction of IFN-alpha in peripheral blood dendritic cells by enveloped RNA and DNA viruses. *J.Immunol.,* Vol. 161, No. 5, pp. (2391-2399)

Mosier, D. E., Gulizia, R. J., Baird, S. M. & Wilson, D. B. (1988). Transfer of a functional human immune system to mice with severe combined immunodeficiency. *Nature,* Vol. 335, No. 6187, pp. (256-259)

Nagasawa, M., Schmidlin, H., Hazekamp, M. G., Schotte, R. & Blom, B. (2008). Development of human plasmacytoid dendritic cells depends on the combined action of the basic helix-loop-helix factor E2-2 and the Ets factor Spi-B. *Eur.J.Immunol.,* Vol. 38, No. 9, pp. (2389-2400)

Napolitano, L. A., Grant, R. M., Deeks, S. G., Schmidt, D., De Rosa, S. C., Herzenberg, L. A., Herndier, B. G., Andersson, J. & McCune, J. M. (2001). Increased production of IL-7 accompanies HIV-1-mediated T-cell depletion: implications for T-cell homeostasis. *Nat.Med.*, Vol. 7, No. 1, pp. (73-79)

Nielsen, S. D., Jeppesen, D. L., Kolte, L., Clark, D. R., Sorensen, T. U., Dreves, A. M., Ersboll, A. K., Ryder, L. P., Valerius, N. H. & Nielsen, J. O. (2001). Impaired progenitor cell function in HIV-negative infants of HIV-positive mothers results in decreased thymic output and low CD4 counts. *Blood,* Vol. 98, No. 2, pp. (398-404)

Noguchi, M., Yi, H., Rosenblatt, H. M., Filipovich, A. H., Adelstein, S., Modi, W. S., McBride, O. W. & Leonard, W. J. (1993). Interleukin-2 receptor gamma chain mutation results in X-linked severe combined immunodeficiency in humans. *Cell,* Vol. 73, No. 1, pp. (147-157)

O'Brien, M., Manches, O., Sabado, R. L., Jimenez, B. S., Wang, Y., Marie, I., Rolnitzky, L., Markowitz, M., Margolis, D. M., Levy, D. & Bhardwaj, N. (2011). Spatiotemporal trafficking of HIV in human plasmacytoid dendritic cells defines a persistently IFN-alpha-producing and partially matured phenotype. *J.Clin.Invest,* Vol. 121, No. 3, pp. (1088-1101)

Ogasawara, K., Hamerman, J. A., Hsin, H., Chikuma, S., Bour-Jordan, H., Chen, T., Pertel, T., Carnaud, C., Bluestone, J. A. & Lanier, L. L. (2003). Impairment of NK cell function by NKG2D modulation in NOD mice. *Immunity.,* Vol. 18, No. 1, pp. (41-51)

Olweus, J., BitMansour, A., Warnke, R., Thompson, P. A., Carballido, J., Picker, L. J. & Lund-Johansen, F. (1997). Dendritic cell ontogeny: a human dendritic cell lineage of myeloid origin. *Proc.Natl.Acad.Sci.U.S.A,* Vol. 94, No. 23, pp. (12551-12556)

Oswald-Richter, K., Grill, S. M., Shariat, N., Leelawong, M., Sundrud, M. S., Haas, D. W. & Unutmaz, D. (2004). HIV infection of naturally occurring and genetically reprogrammed human regulatory T-cells. *PLoS.Biol.,* Vol. 2, No. 7, pp. (E198)

Pacanowski, J., Kahi, S., Baillet, M., Lebon, P., Deveau, C., Goujard, C., Meyer, L., Oksenhendler, E., Sinet, M. & Hosmalin, A. (2001). Reduced blood CD123+ (lymphoid) and CD11c+ (myeloid) dendritic cell numbers in primary HIV-1 infection. *Blood,* Vol. 98, No. 10, pp. (3016-3021)

Pallard, C., Stegmann, A. P., van Kleffens, T., Smart, F., Venkitaraman, A. & Spits, H. (1999). Distinct roles of the phosphatidylinositol 3-kinase and STAT5 pathways in IL-7-mediated development of human thymocyte precursors. *Immunity.,* Vol. 10, No. 5, pp. (525-535)

Payne, K. J. & Crooks, G. M. (2002). Human hematopoietic lineage commitment. *Immunol.Rev.,* Vol. 187, pp. (48-64)

Pedroza-Martins, L., Gurney, K. B., Torbett, B. E. & Uittenbogaart, C. H. (1998). Differential tropism and replication kinetics of human immunodeficiency virus type 1 isolates in thymocytes: coreceptor expression allows viral entry, but productive infection of distinct subsets is determined at the postentry level. *J.Virol.,* Vol. 72, No. 12, pp. (9441-9452)

Peschon, J. J., Morrissey, P. J., Grabstein, K. H., Ramsdell, F. J., Maraskovsky, E., Gliniak, B. C., Park, L. S., Ziegler, S. F., Williams, D. E., Ware, C. B., Meyer, J. D. & Davison, B. L. (1994). Early lymphocyte expansion is severely impaired in interleukin 7 receptor-deficient mice. *J.Exp.Med.,* Vol. 180, No. 5, pp. (1955-1960)

Pesu, M., Candotti, F., Husa, M., Hofmann, S. R., Notarangelo, L. D. & O'Shea, J. J. (2005). Jak3, severe combined immunodeficiency, and a new class of immunosuppressive drugs. *Immunol.Rev.,* Vol. 203, pp. (127-142)

Petrie, H. T. & Kincade, P. W. (2005). Many roads, one destination for T cell progenitors. *J.Exp.Med.,* Vol. 202, No. 1, pp. (11-13)

Ploquin, M. J., Desoutter, J. F., Santos, P. R., Pandrea, I., Diop, O. M., Hosmalin, A., Butor, C., Barre-Sinoussi, F. & Muller-Trutwin, M. C. (2006). Distinct expression profiles of TGF-beta1 signaling mediators in pathogenic SIVmac and non-pathogenic SIVagm infections. *Retrovirology.,* Vol. 3, pp. (37)

Plum, J., De Smedt, M., Leclercq, G., Verhasselt, B. & Vandekerckhove, B. (1996). Interleukin-7 is a critical growth factor in early human T-cell development. *Blood,* Vol. 88, No. 11, pp. (4239-4245)

Porritt, H. E., Rumfelt, L. L., Tabrizifard, S., Schmitt, T. M., Zuniga-Pflucker, J. C. & Petrie, H. T. (2004). Heterogeneity among DN1 prothymocytes reveals multiple progenitors with different capacities to generate T cell and non-T cell lineages. *Immunity.,* Vol. 20, No. 6, pp. (735-745)

Puel, A., Ziegler, S. F., Buckley, R. H. & Leonard, W. J. (1998). Defective IL7R expression in T(-)B(+)NK(+) severe combined immunodeficiency. *Nat.Genet.,* Vol. 20, No. 4, pp. (394-397)

Res, P., Martinez-Caceres, E., Cristina, J. A., Staal, F., Noteboom, E., Weijer, K. & Spits, H. (1996). CD34+CD38dim cells in the human thymus can differentiate into T, natural killer, and dendritic cells but are distinct from pluripotent stem cells. *Blood,* Vol. 87, No. 12, pp. (5196-5206)

Res, P. & Spits, H. (1999). Developmental stages in the human thymus. *Semin.Immunol.,* Vol. 11, No. 1, pp. (39-46)

Res, P. C., Couwenberg, F., Vyth-Dreese, F. A. & Spits, H. (1999). Expression of pTalpha mRNA in a committed dendritic cell precursor in the human thymus. *Blood,* Vol. 94, No. 8, pp. (2647-2657)

Rissoan, M. C., Soumelis, V., Kadowaki, N., Grouard, G., Briere, F., de Waal, M. R. & Liu, Y. J. (1999). Reciprocal control of T helper cell and dendritic cell differentiation. *Science,* Vol. 283, No. 5405, pp. (1183-1186)

Rizza, P., Santini, S. M., Logozzi, M. A., Lapenta, C., Sestili, P., Gherardi, G., Lande, R., Spada, M., Parlato, S., Belardelli, F. & Fais, S. (1996). T-cell dysfunctions in hu-PBL-SCID mice infected with human immunodeficiency virus (HIV) shortly after reconstitution: in vivo effects of HIV on highly activated human immune cells. *J.Virol.,* Vol. 70, No. 11, pp. (7958-7964)

Rosenzweig, M., Bunting, E. M. & Gaulton, G. N. (1994). Neonatal HIV-1 thymic infection. *Leukemia,* Vol. 8 Suppl 1, pp. (S163-S165)

Rosenzweig, M., Connole, M., Forand-Barabasz, A., Tremblay, M. P., Johnson, R. P. & Lackner, A. A. (2000). Mechanisms associated with thymocyte apoptosis induced by simian immunodeficiency virus. *J.Immunol.,* Vol. 165, No. 6, pp. (3461-3468)

Rossi, D. & Zlotnik, A. (2000). The biology of chemokines and their receptors. *Annu.Rev.Immunol.,* Vol. 18, pp. (217-242)

Rozmyslowicz, T., Murphy, S. L., Conover, D. O. & Gaulton, G. N. (2010). HIV-1 infection inhibits cytokine production in human thymic macrophages. *Exp.Hematol.,* Vol. 38, No. 12, pp. (1157-1166)

Russell, S. M., Keegan, A. D., Harada, N., Nakamura, Y., Noguchi, M., Leland, P., Friedmann, M. C., Miyajima, A., Puri, R. K., Paul, W. E. & . (1993). Interleukin-2 receptor gamma chain: a functional component of the interleukin-4 receptor. *Science,* Vol. 262, No. 5141, pp. (1880-1883)

Russell, S. M., Tayebi, N., Nakajima, H., Riedy, M. C., Roberts, J. L., Aman, M. J., Migone, T. S., Noguchi, M., Markert, M. L., Buckley, R. H., O'Shea, J. J. & Leonard, W. J. (1995). Mutation of Jak3 in a patient with SCID: essential role of Jak3 in lymphoid development. *Science,* Vol. 270, No. 5237, pp. (797-800)

Sabado, R. L., O'Brien, M., Subedi, A., Qin, L., Hu, N., Taylor, E., Dibben, O., Stacey, A., Fellay, J., Shianna, K. V., Siegal, F., Shodell, M., Shah, K., Larsson, M., Lifson, J., Nadas, A., Marmor, M., Hutt, R., Margolis, D., Garmon, D., Markowitz, M., Valentine, F., Borrow, P. & Bhardwaj, N. (2010). Evidence of dysregulation of dendritic cells in primary HIV infection. *Blood,* Vol. 116, No. 19, pp. (3839-3852)

Sakaguchi, S. (2000). Regulatory T cells: key controllers of immunologic self-tolerance. *Cell,* Vol. 101, No. 5, pp. (455-458)

Sakaguchi, S. (2005). Naturally arising Foxp3-expressing CD25+CD4+ regulatory T cells in immunological tolerance to self and non-self. *Nat.Immunol.,* Vol. 6, No. 4, pp. (345-352)

Saoudi, A., Seddon, B., Fowell, D. & Mason, D. (1996). The thymus contains a high frequency of cells that prevent autoimmune diabetes on transfer into prediabetic recipients. *J.Exp.Med.,* Vol. 184, No. 6, pp. (2393-2398)

Sato, K., Nie, C., Misawa, N., Tanaka, Y., Ito, M. & Koyanagi, Y. (2010). Dynamics of memory and naive CD8+ T lymphocytes in humanized NOD/SCID/IL-2Rgammanull mice infected with CCR5-tropic HIV-1. *Vaccine,* Vol. 28 Suppl 2, pp. (B32-B37)

Sauce, D., Larsen, M., Fastenackels, S., Pauchard, M., Ait-Mohand, H., Schneider, L., Guihot, A., Boufassa, F., Zaunders, J., Iguertsira, M., Bailey, M., Gorochov, G., Duvivier, C., Carcelain, G., Kelleher, A. D., Simon, A., Meyer, L., Costagliola, D., Deeks, S. G., Lambotte, O., Autran, B., Hunt, P. W., Katlama, C. & Appay, V. (2011). HIV disease progression despite suppression of viral replication is associated with exhaustion of lymphopoiesis. *Blood,* Vol.

Schmidlin, H., Dontje, W., Groot, F., Ligthart, S. J., Colantonio, A. D., Oud, M. E., Schilder-Tol, E. J., Spaargaren, M., Spits, H., Uittenbogaart, C. H. & Blom, B. (2006). Stimulated plasmacytoid dendritic cells impair human T-cell development. *Blood,* Vol. 108, No. 12, pp. (3792-3800)

Schmidt, B., Ashlock, B. M., Foster, H., Fujimura, S. H. & Levy, J. A. (2005). HIV-infected cells are major inducers of plasmacytoid dendritic cell interferon production, maturation, and migration. *Virology,* Vol. 343, No. 2, pp. (256-266)

Schmitt, C., Fohrer, H., Beaudet, S., Palmer, P., Alpha, M. J., Canque, B., Gluckman, J. C. & Dalloul, A. H. (2000). Identification of mature and immature human thymic dendritic cells that differentially express HLA-DR and interleukin-3 receptor in vivo. *J.Leukoc.Biol.,* Vol. 68, No. 6, pp. (836-844)

Schmitt, N., Nugeyre, M. T., Scott-Algara, D., Cumont, M. C., Barre-Sinoussi, F., Pancino, G. & Israel, N. (2006). Differential susceptibility of human thymic dendritic cell subsets to X4 and R5 HIV-1 infection. *AIDS,* Vol. 20, No. 4, pp. (533-542)

Schotte, R., Nagasawa, M., Weijer, K., Spits, H. & Blom, B. (2004). The ETS transcription factor Spi-B is required for human plasmacytoid dendritic cell development. *J.Exp.Med.,* Vol. 200, No. 11, pp. (1503-1509)

Schotte, R., Rissoan, M. C., Bendriss-Vermare, N., Bridon, J. M., Duhen, T., Weijer, K., Briere, F. & Spits, H. (2003). The transcription factor Spi-B is expressed in plasmacytoid DC precursors and inhibits T-, B-, and NK-cell development. *Blood,* Vol. 101, No. 3, pp. (1015-1023)

Shultz, L. D., Lyons, B. L., Burzenski, L. M., Gott, B., Chen, X., Chaleff, S., Kotb, M., Gillies, S. D., King, M., Mangada, J., Greiner, D. L. & Handgretinger, R. (2005). Human lymphoid and myeloid cell development in NOD/LtSz-scid IL2R gamma null mice engrafted with mobilized human hemopoietic stem cells. *J.Immunol.,* Vol. 174, No. 10, pp. (6477-6489)

Siegal, F. P., Fitzgerald-Bocarsly, P., Holland, B. K. & Shodell, M. (2001). Interferon-alpha generation and immune reconstitution during antiretroviral therapy for human immunodeficiency virus infection. *AIDS,* Vol. 15, No. 13, pp. (1603-1612)

Siegal, F. P., Kadowaki, N., Shodell, M., Fitzgerald-Bocarsly, P. A., Shah, K., Ho, S., Antonenko, S. & Liu, Y. J. (1999). The nature of the principal type 1 interferon-producing cells in human blood. *Science,* Vol. 284, No. 5421, pp. (1835-1837)

Siggs, O. M., Makaroff, L. E. & Liston, A. (2006). The why and how of thymocyte negative selection. *Curr.Opin.Immunol.,* Vol. 18, No. 2, pp. (175-183)

Silvestri, G. (2008). AIDS pathogenesis: a tale of two monkeys. *J.Med.Primatol.,* Vol. 37 Suppl 2, pp. (6-12)

Sleasman, J. W., Harville, T. O., White, G. B., George, J. F., Barrett, D. J. & Goodenow, M. M. (1994). Arrested rearrangement of TCR V beta genes in thymocytes from children with X-linked severe combined immunodeficiency disease. *J.Immunol.,* Vol. 153, No. 1, pp. (442-448)

Sodora, D. L., Milush, J. M., Ware, F., Wozniakowski, A., Montgomery, L., McClure, H. M., Lackner, A. A., Marthas, M., Hirsch, V., Johnson, R. P., Douek, D. C. & Koup, R. A. (2002). Decreased levels of recent thymic emigrants in peripheral blood of simian immunodeficiency virus-infected macaques correlate with alterations within the thymus. *J.Virol.,* Vol. 76, No. 19, pp. (9981-9990)

Sopper, S., Nierwetberg, D., Halbach, A., Sauer, U., Scheller, C., Stahl-Hennig, C., Matz-Rensing, K., Schafer, F., Schneider, T., ter, M., V & Muller, J. G. (2003). Impact of simian immunodeficiency virus (SIV) infection on lymphocyte numbers and T-cell turnover in different organs of rhesus monkeys. *Blood,* Vol. 101, No. 4, pp. (1213-1219)

Soumelis, V., Scott, I., Gheyas, F., Bouhour, D., Cozon, G., Cotte, L., Huang, L., Levy, J. A. & Liu, Y. J. (2001). Depletion of circulating natural type 1 interferon-producing cells in HIV-infected AIDS patients. *Blood,* Vol. 98, No. 4, pp. (906-912)

Spits, H. (2002). Development of alphabeta T cells in the human thymus. *Nat.Rev.Immunol.,* Vol. 2, No. 10, pp. (760-772)

Spits, H., Blom, B., Jaleco, A. C., Weijer, K., Verschuren, M. C., van Dongen, J. J., Heemskerk, M. H. & Res, P. C. (1998). Early stages in the development of human T, natural killer and thymic dendritic cells. *Immunol.Rev.,* Vol. 165, pp. (75-86)

Stephens, L. A., Mottet, C., Mason, D. & Powrie, F. (2001). Human CD4(+)CD25(+) thymocytes and peripheral T cells have immune suppressive activity in vitro. *Eur.J.Immunol.,* Vol. 31, No. 4, pp. (1247-1254)

Stoddart, C. A., Keir, M. E. & McCune, J. M. (2010). IFN-alpha-induced upregulation of CCR5 leads to expanded HIV tropism in vivo. *PLoS.Pathog.,* Vol. 6, No. 2, pp. (e1000766)

Su, D. M., Wang, J., Lin, Q., Cooper, M. D. & Watanabe, T. (1997). Interferons alpha/beta inhibit IL-7-induced proliferation of CD4- CD8- CD3- CD44+ CD25+ thymocytes, but do not inhibit that of CD4- CD8- CD3-. *Immunology,* Vol. 90, No. 4, pp. (543-549)

Sun, Z., Denton, P. W., Estes, J. D., Othieno, F. A., Wei, B. L., Wege, A. K., Melkus, M. W., Padgett-Thomas, A., Zupancic, M., Haase, A. T. & Garcia, J. V. (2007). Intrarectal transmission, systemic infection, and CD4+ T cell depletion in humanized mice infected with HIV-1. *J.Exp.Med.,* Vol. 204, No. 4, pp. (705-714)

Taghon, T., Van, d. W., I, De Smet, G., De Smedt, M., Leclercq, G., Vandekerckhove, B. & Plum, J. (2009). Notch signaling is required for proliferation but not for differentiation at a well-defined beta-selection checkpoint during human T-cell development. *Blood,* Vol. 113, No. 14, pp. (3254-3263)

Takahata, Y., Nomura, A., Takada, H., Ohga, S., Furuno, K., Hikino, S., Nakayama, H., Sakaguchi, S. & Hara, T. (2004). CD25+CD4+ T cells in human cord blood: an immunoregulatory subset with naive phenotype and specific expression of forkhead box p3 (Foxp3) gene. *Exp.Hematol.,* Vol. 32, No. 7, pp. (622-629)

Thiebot, H., Vaslin, B., Derdouch, S., Bertho, J. M., Mouthon, F., Prost, S., Gras, G., Ducouret, P., Dormont, D. & Le Grand, R. (2005). Impact of bone marrow hematopoiesis failure on T-cell generation during pathogenic simian immunodeficiency virus infection in macaques. *Blood,* Vol. 105, No. 6, pp. (2403-2409)

Thornton, C. A., Upham, J. W., Wikstrom, M. E., Holt, B. J., White, G. P., Sharp, M. J., Sly, P. D. & Holt, P. G. (2004). Functional maturation of CD4+CD25+CTLA4+CD45RA+ T regulatory cells in human neonatal T cell responses to environmental antigens/allergens. *J.Immunol.,* Vol. 173, No. 5, pp. (3084-3092)

Tonomura, N., Habiro, K., Shimizu, A., Sykes, M. & Yang, Y. G. (2008). Antigen-specific human T-cell responses and T cell-dependent production of human antibodies in a humanized mouse model. *Blood,* Vol. 111, No. 8, pp. (4293-4296)

Tovey, M. G., Lebon, P., Eid, P., Meyer, F., Hurtrel, B., Gresser, I., Venet, A., Girard, M. & Aubertin, A. M. (1994). Antibody to the human interferon-alpha receptor reduces the loss of CD4+ T cells in macaques infected with the simian immunodeficiency virus, SIVmac. *J.Interferon Res.,* Vol. 14, No. 5, pp. (287)

Traggiai, E., Chicha, L., Mazzucchelli, L., Bronz, L., Piffaretti, J. C., Lanzavecchia, A. & Manz, M. G. (2004). Development of a human adaptive immune system in cord blood cell-transplanted mice. *Science,* Vol. 304, No. 5667, pp. (104-107)

Trigueros, C., Ramiro, A. R., Carrasco, Y. R., de Yebenes, V. G., Albar, J. P. & Toribio, M. L. (1998). Identification of a late stage of small noncycling pTalpha- pre-T cells as immediate precursors of T cell receptor alpha/beta+ thymocytes. *J.Exp.Med.*, Vol. 188, No. 8, pp. (1401-1412)

Uittenbogaart, C. H., Anisman, D. J., Jamieson, B. D., Kitchen, S., Schmid, I., Zack, J. A. & Hays, E. F. (1996). Differential tropism of HIV-1 isolates for distinct thymocyte subsets in vitro. *AIDS*, Vol. 10, No. 7, pp. (F9-16)

Vandenabeele, S., Hochrein, H., Mavaddat, N., Winkel, K. & Shortman, K. (2001). Human thymus contains 2 distinct dendritic cell populations. *Blood*, Vol. 97, No. 6, pp. (1733-1741)

Verschuren, M. C., Blom, B., Bogers, A. J., Spits, H. & van Dongen, J. J. (1998). PJA-BP expression and TCR delta deletion during human T cell differentiation. *Int.Immunol.*, Vol. 10, No. 12, pp. (1873-1880)

von Boehmer, H. (2005). Mechanisms of suppression by suppressor T cells. *Nat.Immunol.*, Vol. 6, No. 4, pp. (338-344)

Vormoor, J., Lapidot, T., Pflumio, F., Risdon, G., Patterson, B., Broxmeyer, H. E. & Dick, J. E. (1994). Immature human cord blood progenitors engraft and proliferate to high levels in severe combined immunodeficient mice. *Blood*, Vol. 83, No. 9, pp. (2489-2497)

Walker, M. R., Kasprowicz, D. J., Gersuk, V. H., Benard, A., Van Landeghen, M., Buckner, J. H. & Ziegler, S. F. (2003). Induction of FoxP3 and acquisition of T regulatory activity by stimulated human CD4+. *J.Clin.Invest*, Vol. 112, No. 9, pp. (1437-1443)

Watanabe, N., Hanabuchi, S., Marloie-Provost, M. A., Antonenko, S., Liu, Y. J. & Soumelis, V. (2005). Human TSLP promotes CD40 ligand-induced IL-12 production by myeloid dendritic cells but maintains their Th2 priming potential. *Blood*, Vol. 105, No. 12, pp. (4749-4751)

Watanabe, S., Terashima, K., Ohta, S., Horibata, S., Yajima, M., Shiozawa, Y., Dewan, M. Z., Yu, Z., Ito, M., Morio, T., Shimizu, N., Honda, M. & Yamamoto, N. (2007). Hematopoietic stem cell-engrafted NOD/SCID/IL2Rgamma null mice develop human lymphoid systems and induce long-lasting HIV-1 infection with specific humoral immune responses. *Blood*, Vol. 109, No. 1, pp. (212-218)

Weiss, L., Donkova-Petrini, V., Caccavelli, L., Balbo, M., Carbonneil, C. & Levy, Y. (2004). Human immunodeficiency virus-driven expansion of CD4+CD25+ regulatory T cells, which suppress HIV-specific CD4 T-cell responses in HIV-infected patients. *Blood*, Vol. 104, No. 10, pp. (3249-3256)

Wykrzykowska, J. J., Rosenzweig, M., Veazey, R. S., Simon, M. A., Halvorsen, K., Desrosiers, R. C., Johnson, R. P. & Lackner, A. A. (1998). Early regeneration of thymic progenitors in rhesus macaques infected with simian immunodeficiency virus. *J.Exp.Med.*, Vol. 187, No. 11, pp. (1767-1778)

Yagi, H., Nomura, T., Nakamura, K., Yamazaki, S., Kitawaki, T., Hori, S., Maeda, M., Onodera, M., Uchiyama, T., Fujii, S. & Sakaguchi, S. (2004). Crucial role of FOXP3 in the development and function of human CD25+CD4+ regulatory T cells. *Int.Immunol.*, Vol. 16, No. 11, pp. (1643-1656)

Yonezawa, A., Morita, R., Takaori-Kondo, A., Kadowaki, N., Kitawaki, T., Hori, T. & Uchiyama, T. (2003). Natural alpha interferon-producing cells respond to human immunodeficiency virus type 1 with alpha interferon production and maturation into dendritic cells. *J.Virol.*, Vol. 77, No. 6, pp. (3777-3784)

Zaitseva, M. B., Lee, S., Rabin, R. L., Tiffany, H. L., Farber, J. M., Peden, K. W., Murphy, P. M. & Golding, H. (1998). CXCR4 and CCR5 on human thymocytes: biological function and role in HIV-1 infection. *J.Immunol.*, Vol. 161, No. 6, pp. (3103-3113)

Zamarchi, R., Allavena, P., Borsetti, A., Stievano, L., Tosello, V., Marcato, N., Esposito, G., Roni, V., Paganin, C., Bianchi, G., Titti, F., Verani, P., Gerosa, G. & Amadori, A. (2002). Expression and functional activity of CXCR-4 and CCR-5 chemokine receptors in human thymocytes. *Clin.Exp.Immunol.*, Vol. 127, No. 2, pp. (321-330)

Zhang, L., He, T., Talal, A., Wang, G., Frankel, S. S. & Ho, D. D. (1998). In vivo distribution of the human immunodeficiency virus/simian immunodeficiency virus coreceptors: CXCR4, CCR3, and CCR5. *J.Virol.*, Vol. 72, No. 6, pp. (5035-5045)

Zlotoff, D. A., Sambandam, A., Logan, T. D., Bell, J. J., Schwarz, B. A. & Bhandoola, A. (2010). CCR7 and CCR9 together recruit hematopoietic progenitors to the adult thymus. *Blood*, Vol. 115, No. 10, pp. (1897-1905)

8

Genetic Factors that Influence HIV Infection: The Role of the Major Histocompatibility Complex System

Daniel Pérez-Núñez[1] and Narcisa Martínez-Quiles[2]
[1]*Centro de Biología Molecular Severo Ochoa (CSIC-UAM), Madrid*
[2]*Department of Microbiology, Facultad de Farmacia*
Universidad Complutense de Madrid
Spain

1. Introduction

The HIV epidemic continues to be a major world-wide health and human problem as reflected in the AIDS epidemic updates from the World Health Organization (WHO). Highly active antiretroviral therapy (HAART) has improved health management, especially in developed countries, since it was first introduced in the mid-1990s. However, access to antiretroviral therapy in developing countries has been limited. Developing an effective vaccine is an on-going mission, the success of which depends on understanding key aspects of the immune response to HIV. Hence, studying the genetic components of the immune response to the HIV virus is essential.

The existence of genetic factors that modulate immune response to infectious diseases was described more than 10 years ago (Hill, 1998). We recommend various recent and extensive reviews that have focused on the immunobiology of HIV infection (Tripathi and Agrawal, 2007), the immune response to HIV (Chakrabarti and Simon, 2010; Miyazawa, et al. 2008) and specifically the innate response (Borrow and Bhardwaj 2008). Innate and adaptive immune responses play a decisive role during the initial stages of HIV infection and will also affect the progression of the disease. Definitive evidence that host genetics plays a role in the immune response to HIV is the fact that HIV-1 infection does not always progress to AIDS. A small percentage (less than 0.2%) of HIV-1 sero-positive patients is able to control the infection, meaning that they can maintain a viral load of fewer than 50 copies of HIV-1 RNA per ml over 10 years. These patients have been given different names: HIV controllers, HIV elite controllers, long-term non-progressors (LTNPs) or natural virus suppressors (Chakrabarti and Simon, 2010).

This chapter focuses on the influence exerted on HIV infection by the human major histocompatibility complex (MHC) system, also known as the human leukocyte antigen (HLA) system. The effect of the MHC system on HIV infection is crucial for development of an effective vaccine. We recommend several reviews on this subject that complement the present monograph (Carrington and O'Brien, 2003; Stephens, 2005; Miyazawa et al. 2008; Kaur and Mehra, 2009; Singh and Spector, 2009). In this chapter, we will first describe the most important and relevant characteristics of the MHC, then we will review the recent literature on the influence of the MHC on both horizontal and vertical (mother-to-infant) transmission. Finally, we highlight the molecular basis of the most important associations currently believed to exist between MHC and HIV transmission, with special emphasis on recent theories about how the MHC shapes the cytotoxic T cell (CTL) response and its relation to the appearance of HIV escape variants.

2. The human Major Histocompatibility Complex (MHC)

The MHC is located on the short arm of chromosome 6 and contains a large number of genes related to immune system function. Some MHC genes encode proteins that help to distinguish self and non-self components. They were first discovered in transplantation immunology and the gene products were called *antigens*. There are 3 major classes: Class I molecules are encoded by classical genes (A-C) and non-classical genes (E-G). Class II molecules are encoded by classical genes (DP, DQ, DR) and non-classical ones (DM, DOA, DOB). Class III molecules include components of the complement system and other immune system molecules.

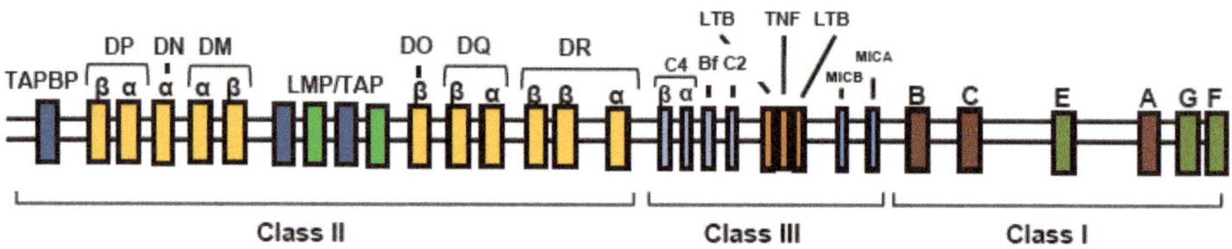

Fig. 1. Schematic of the Human Major Histocompatibility Complex (MHC).

2.1 The human MHC class I molecules

The class I protein comprises a α-polypeptide chain that associates with the invariant β chain β2 microglobulin (β2m). MHC class I molecules (A, B, C) present peptides mainly from inside the cell; for example, they present viral peptides when these are found in the cell cytoplasm. These peptides are produced by the proteasome, which breaks down proteins to fragments approximately 9 amino acids (AA) long. Viral, bacterial or self-peptides will be displayed in the binding cleft of the MHC molecule on the cell surface, in a process known as antigen presentation; the displayed fragments are recognized by $CD8^+$ or cytotoxic T cells (CTLs), which destroy infected cells. Each person expresses 3 MHC class I molecules (A, B, C) from each chromosome. Most nucleated cells express class I molecules. Many viruses reduce the expression of MHC class I molecules to hamper the immune response. This is the case of HIV, which down-regulates CD4 and HLA class I expression through its Nef protein (Greenberg et al., 1998). Compared to the HLA-A and -B loci, the HLA-C locus shows less polymorphism. In addition HLA-C proteins are expressed at lower levels on the cell surface, and seem to bind primarily to natural killer immunoglobulin-like receptors (KIRs).

Class Ia molecules show greater polymorphism and wider tissue distribution than class Ib molecules. Of the non-classical HLA class I molecules involved in HIV infection, HLA-G is the best studied. Alternative splicing of HLA-G gives rise to 7 isoforms, 4 membrane-bound (HLA-G 1-4) and 3 soluble (HLA-G 5-7). G5 and its membrane-bound counterpart G1 are proteolytically released from the membrane to give rise to the major soluble forms of HLA-

G. HLA-G is expressed in placental trophoblast cells as well as in the thymus, pancreas and other tissues. Its ectopic expression has been reported under various pathological conditions, including viral infections. It is currently accepted that HLA-G molecules exert immunosuppressive functions (Fainardi et al., 2011).

2.2 The human MHC class II molecules

These are encoded by three classical genes (HLA-DP, -DQ and -DR) and two non-classical ones (HLA-DM and -DO) (reviewed by (Handunnetthi et al., 2010)). This region includes other genes implicated in antigen processing, such as the genes encoding transporter associated with antigen processing protein 1 and 2 (TAP1 and TAP2). Class II molecules comprise α and β chains. Their expression is restricted mainly to thymic epithelial cells and bone marrow-derived antigen-presenting cells. The latter include B cells, macrophages (Mϕ) and dendritic cells (DCs). Differentiation of B cells into plasma cells, as well as differentiation of dendritic cells, is accompanied by down-regulation of MHC class II expression. On the contrary activation of T cells up-regulates their expression of class II molecules.

In the HLA-DR sub-region the gene DRA encodes 1 unpolymorphic α chain with only 1 common and 2 very rare alleles. The β chain is encoded by the very polymorphic DRB1 gene. There are 3 DRB1 paralogue genes: DRB3, DRB4 and DRB5, however DRB1 is expressed at a level five times higher than them. The MHC class II is highly polymorphic. For instance, there are over 500 different HLA DRB1 alleles in humans. The DRB loci are classified into 5 major haplogroups according to the number of functional genes (DRB1, 3, 4 and 5) and pseudogenes (DRB2, 6, 7, 8, 9) that are present (Table I).

Halogroup	Genes and Pseudogenes
DR1	DRB1, DRB6 and DRB9
DR8	DRB1 and DRB9
DR51	DRB1, DRB5, DRB6 and DRB9
DR52	DRB1, DRB2, DRB3 and DRB9
DR53	DRB1M DRB4M DRB7, DRB8 and DRB9
Families of DRB1 allelic lineage	**Genes**
DR1	HLA-DRB1*01 and *10
DR8	HLA-DRB1*08
DR51	HLA-DRB1*15 and *16
DR52	HLA-DRB1*03, *11, *13 and *14
DR53	HLA-DRB1*04, *07 and *09

Table 1. DRB loci classification in halogroups and DRB1 families.

Classical class II MHC genes are:

HLA-DP: α-chain encoded by the HLA-DPA1 locus (16 alleles) and β-chain encoded by the HLA-DPB1 locus (118 alleles).

HLA-DQ: α-chain encoded by the HLA-DQA1 locus (25 alleles) and β-chain encoded by the HLA-DQB1 locus (72 alleles).

HLA-DR: α-chain encoded by the HLA-DRA locus and 4 β-chains encoded by the HLA-DRB1, DRB3, DRB4, DRB5 loci.

The expression of MHC class II genes is tightly regulated, primarily at the transcriptional level. Their promoter contains regulatory elements collectively called the "SXY module", to which various proteins bind, including regulatory factor X (RFX) and the class II transactivator (CIITA) (Handunnetthi et al., 2010). Induction of CIITA and subsequent expression of the MHC class II isotype HLA-DR are hallmarks of $CD4^+$ T cell activation which, paradoxically, favors HIV replication. Interestingly, CIITA is able to inhibit HIV-1 in infected cells by blocking the function of the viral transactivators Tat and Tax (Tosi et al., 2009).

A key question about the influence of MHC on infectious disease is whether allele-specific sequence variation that affects the level of expression of HLA proteins can lead to class II-associated diseases. For instance, transcripts in resting peripheral B cells have been reported to be more abundant within the DR52 haplogroup than within the DR53 haplogroup. A vast number of self-antigens are expressed at high levels in the thymic epithelium. It is postulated that a general reduction of self-antigen expression in the thymus could result in loss of central tolerance, meaning that thymocytes with excessive reactivity to self-antigens escape elimination. Does this increase susceptibility to infectious diseases? In the case of HIV, it seems that MHC-II presentation, at least by monocytes/macrophages, is preserved during infection (Woc-Colburn et al., 2010).

Aside from the genes encoding the major antigens, a large number of other genes are located in the HLA complex (Fig. 1), many of which are involved in immune function. One significant characteristic of the HLA system is its tremendous polymorphism in the human population: there are many different alleles for each locus (ImmunoGeneTics HLA database: http://www.ebi.ac.uk./imgt/hal/atats.html). This implies that the chance of two unrelated individuals having identical HLA molecules on all loci is very low.

3. Historical perspective: HLA-disease association studies and HIV infection

The first reviews of HLA association with disease are from the late 1970s (Thomson and Bodmer, 1979) and early 1980s (Svejgaard et al., 1983), followed by other studies on HLA susceptibility to HIV infection (Scorza Smeraldi et al. ,1986; Just, 1995; Fauci, 1996; Buchacz et al. 1998) .

HLA genes exhibit "**linkage disequilibrium**", meaning that they are found together on the same chromosome at a higher frequency than expected according to their recombination distance. They are defined as a so-called "extended haplotype" or combination of alleles that are transmitted together as a unit. As with any gene frequently found in linkage disequilibrium with others, it is difficult to identify the specific HLA gene that is responsible for a given association observed in a population (Svejgaard et al., 1983).

Studies of HLA associations with infectious diseases must separate HLA effects from many **confounding factors,** which are other factors that independently affect the risk of developing the disease. If the prevalence of these other factors differs between the groups being compared, they will distort the observed association. In the case of HLA/HIV associations, confounding factors include the ethnicity of the population studied, the frequencies of the HLA alleles detected and the resolution of the typing methods used. HLA associations are considered to be "consistent" when a similar or equivalent association is observed across different ethnic groups (Tripathi and Agrawal, 2007).

3.1 HIV associations and ancestral haplotypes

Initial association analyses focused on **ancestral haplotypes.** An increased frequency of C4 null alleles was found in HIV-infected individuals, which could in fact reflect an indirect association with a discrete number of ancestral haplotypes (Cameron et al., 1990). At that time a series of studies focused on the A1-B8-DR3-DQ2 haplotype, also known as the 8.1 ancestral haplotype, which has been implicated in disease susceptibility (McNeil et al., 1996; Price et al., 1999). In addition, the HLA-B27 allele was found to be related to slow HIV disease progression (McNeil et al., 1996). Closer analysis of ancestral haplotypes points to a direct role of HLA-B35 in rapid HIV progression, and this allele is thought to be associated with disease susceptibility (Flores-Villanueva et al., 2003).

3.2 HIV infection and HLA frequencies of individual alleles

The proliferation of studies on associations between HLA frequencies and HIV infection made it clear to experts that it would be necessary to establish uniform research standards, such as more concrete definitions of HIV disease and its progression (Mann et al., 1992). Focusing on particular aspects of the disease, researchers were able to study a cohort of 106 homosexual men from Amsterdam and correlate certain alleles with different aspects of HIV pathogenesis, including skin rash (HLA-B62), rapid decline of CD4+ T lymphocytes to < 200/microL (HLA-B35), AIDS-related Kaposi's sarcoma (HLA-DR1) and opportunistic infections (HLA-DR3 and DQ2) (Klein et al., 1994). HLA disease associations studies were performed in different populations, such as in India (Shankarkumar, 2004), south India (Selvaraj et al., 2006) and southern Africa (Lombard et al., 2006).

An important milestone in demonstrating that HIV-1 disease progression is associated with MHC genes was the discovery of **HLA concordance** between hemophilic siblings: pairs that shared one or two haplotypes were significantly concordant in CD4+ T cell decline and AIDS status within 5 years of seroconversion, while no concordance was found in pairs sharing no haplotypes. This is strong evidence that HLA is a determining factor or at least a relevant marker of disease progression.

The expression level of HLA-G during HIV infection was found to be higher in monocytes from patients under HAART than from untreated individuals. Similarly, T cells from infected individuals express HLA-G. Different HLA-G alleles have been associated with protection (G-0105N9) and susceptibility (G-010108) (Fainardi et al. 2011).

Viral load is an important factor determining the progression of HIV-1 infection. The initial peak of infection is followed by a period when the level remains relatively stable; the level during this period is called the **"viral load set point" (VLS).** A recent study addressed the influence of genetic factors, including HLA genotype, on the VLS (Saathoff et al., 2010). The study population was from Tanzania and was composed of three groups: female bar workers and females and males from the general population. HLA alleles were classified as protective (A*0205, B*5801, B*8101, B*4201, B*5703), harmful (B*5802, B*4501, B*1801 and B*1503) or neutral (all others). The prevalence of elevated viral load was 40% lower among individuals with protective alleles than among those with neutral ones. The major conclusion from this study is that male gender and possessing harmful HLA alleles are associated with higher VLS.

HLA class II molecules are involved in presenting antigens to CD4+ T cells, which are central for establishing helper T responses. The HLA class II allele DRB1*1303 was associated with low plasma viral load in a cohort of 426 black South African females infected with HIV-1 clade C. This association was confirmed in a larger cohort of 1436 male European Americans infected with HIV-1 clade B, demonstrating that the association was independent of ethnicity and viral subtype. Whether the protective effect exerted by this allele is due to the development of CD4+ T cell responses has yet to be shown (Julg et al., 2010).

3.3 Advantage of heterozygous individuals

Heterozygosity of MHC genes has long been thought to confer an advantage in the battle against infectious agents, and possessing different alleles at class I and II loci should therefore represent a benefit for HIV-infected individuals. Carrington et al. (Carrington et al., 1999) corroborated this key immune system dogma by studying HIV infection. They found that maximum heterozygosity of HLA-A, -B, and -C genes delayed progression to AIDS, while individuals who were homozygous at one or more loci progressed rapidly to AIDS. Furthermore, they were able to conclude that B*35 and Cw*04 were consistently associated with rapid development of AIDS in Caucasians. This work led to the proposal of a "heterozygote advantage and B*35-Cw*04 disadvantage theory" (Carrington et al., 1999). In subsequent work, the researchers studied the role of TAP genes and HLA supertypes in resistance to HIV infection. They found that the B*35 Px alleles were a risk factor, while the presence of alanine at position 665 in TAP2 was associated with resistance. Whether this resistance was due to a higher efficiency in transporting peptides, or was a consequence of linkage disequilibrium, was not resolved (Liu et al., 2003). Further studies have sought to consolidate our understanding of HLA-B35 alleles as risk factors, and have extended the findings in Caucasians to other populations (Shankarkumar et al., 2003).

3.4 HLA supertypes

Several studies have focused on the analysis of HLA supertypes (Sidney et al., 2008), in which HLA alleles are functionally classified according to their peptide-binding specificities (MacDonald et al., 2001). An attempt was made to group different HLA-B antigens (identified in patients by serology) according to their peptide-anchoring pockets, in order to determine whether the abovementioned associations could be explained by differences in the peptide repertoire presented by those molecules (Itescu et al., 1995). Later on, it was proposed that HIV adapts to the most frequent alleles in the population, implying that the expression of rare supertypes confers an advantage (Trachtenberg et al., 2003).

3.5 Modern theories

A recent study that, in our opinion, is an important breakthrough in the field, proposed that it is not the contribution of only one "relevant" allele that governs disease susceptibility but rather the sum of small contributions from several alleles (Leslie et al., 2010). The authors of that study justified their reasoning based on the fact that after excluding subjects expressing any of the important HLA-B class I alleles that strongly affect HIV control (B*57, B*58, and B*18), HLA-B alleles continued to play the dominant role in the observed progression (Leslie et al., 2010). If true, this idea would help reconcile some of the disparities reported in the literature.

4. Vertical (mother-to-child) transmission of HIV-1

Perinatal HIV-1 infection constitutes a significant global health problem and prevention of transmission is a high public health priority (Matt and Roger, 2001; Ahmad, 2010; UNAIDS,

2010). Much progress has been made in the development and implementation of strategies designed to interrupt vertical transmission. Antiretroviral therapy in HIV-infected pregnant women has significantly reduced the rate of mother-to-child transmission in developed countries down to 1% (Coovadia, 2004). In developing countries, however, many women still have limited access to antiretrovirals, and HIV-1 infection in children remains a major concern, with approximately 500,000 new HIV-1 infected infants born every year worldwide (Ahmad, 2010; UNAIDS, 2010). Prevention of maternal-fetal transmission of HIV-1 is therefore a global priority, especially in developing countries.

Several lines of evidence suggest that host genetic factors are important determinants of both susceptibility to vertical transmission of HIV-1 and subsequent progression of AIDS in children (Matt and Roger, 2001). The identification of genetic markers linked with transmission and disease progression can help to define risk factors associated with vertical transmission and provide new insights into HIV-1 pathogenesis that can help in the development of an effective HIV-1 vaccine.

In addition, pediatric HIV infection offers a good opportunity to investigate the influence of host genetics on the evolution of HIV, since the virus has first been in contact with the mother's immune system and is then transmitted to a genetically related individual.

In children with perinatally acquired HIV-1 infection, the expression of clinical and immunologic signs of disease seems to follow a bimodal distribution. At the beginning of the original HIV epidemic in the 1980s and 1990s, approximately 15–20% of infected infants showed an early and severe course of disease and died within the first 2 years of life. The remaining children progressed more slowly and had a less severe course, surviving an average of 8 years or more (Blanche et al., 1994). Today, children perinatally infected with HIV-1 reach adolescence, largely because of advances in treatment over the past 10 years (Dollfus et al., 2010).

4.1 Routes of vertical HIV transmission

HIV-1 vertical transmission occurs mainly during the following stages (Ahmad, 2010):

1. *prepartum*, due to transplacental passage in utero,
2. *intrapartum*, due to exposure of infant skin and mucus membranes to maternal blood and vaginal secretions during delivery, and
3. *postpartum*, due to exposure to contaminated breastmilk during nursing

In the absence of prophylactic treatment, it is estimated that one-third of children are infected *in utero* (*prepartum*) and two-thirds are infected *intrapartum* or *postpartum* (Kuhn et al., 1997). Various factors appear to affect vertical transmission throughout the gestation period and it seems probable that an interplay of all factors occurs, with some factors more determinant than others during specific periods. For instance, factors protecting against *in utero* infection may be less efficient against delivery or breast-feeding transmission. A general and global strategy concerning all known factors must be used to prevent vertical transmission (Bongertz, 2001). A greater understanding of the role played by various risk factors for HIV-1 infection is crucial to designing new preventive and therapeutic strategies.

The risk of *prepartum* transmission depends on exposure of the fetus *in utero* to free virus or to HIV-infected maternal cells (Mittleman and Shearer, 1996), the risk of which is likely to be very high (Matt and Roger, 2001). Relatively few maternal cells are thought to enter the fetal circulation during gestation under normal circumstances. However, HIV-1 is known to infect cells within the placenta (Kesson et al., 1993). Intrauterine infection has therefore been suggested as a risk factor for mother-to-child transmission (Kuhn et al., 1999).

Certain conditions of delivery such as premature birth, low birth weight, early placental rupture or placental membrane inflammation seem to be related to increased risk of vertical transmission (Bongertz, 2001). Cesarean delivery is associated with a significant decrease in perinatal HIV transmission, from 55% to 80% (Welles et al., 2000). This result is likely to hold only for women with a sufficiently high viral load, since the transmission rate for women with undetectable viral loads is already low.

To avoid *postpartum* transmission, breastfeeding by HIV-infected women is not recommended because it is associated with an additional 15-20% risk of transmission of HIV-1 (Nduati et al., 2000).

In conclusion, it is now clear that the risk for vertical transmission and subsequent immune suppression depends on multiple factors in both the virus and the host (Singh and Spector, 2009). Several factors have been proposed to influence the risk of mother-to-child transmission and disease progression in children infected with HIV. These include high maternal viral load at birth (Shearer et al., 1997) and viral phenotype (De Rossi et al., 1997).

4.2 Maternal viral load and vertical HIV transmission

Higher maternal virus load is associated with an increase in the vertical HIV transmission rate (Cao et al., 1997; Rogers and Shaffer, 1999), although the correlation is modest. Treating HIV-infected pregnant women with the antiretroviral drug zidovudine was associated with a reduced rate of transmission (Connor et al., 1994), though the drug may not produce this effect by reducing viral load: a recent study found that zidovudine reduced vertical transmission despite a minimal effect on viral load (Melvin et al., 1997; Newberry and Kelsey, 2003). Whatever the mechanism of zidovudine, it remains generally true that risk of vertical transmission can be minimized if therapies known to reduce the patient's serum and vaginal viral loads are continued during pregnancy. Indeed, even if the risk of mother-to-child transmission is very low in women with low viral load, vertical transmission has been reported in women with all viral load levels (Newberry and Kelsey, 2003).

4.3 Viral phenotype and vertical HIV transmission

Viral phenotype is also a risk factor for vertical transmission. Genetic variability within HIV-1 is generated by reverse transcriptase during replication of the viral genome. The enzyme lacks 3′ proofreading ability. Consequently, rapid replication result in a high degree of virus polymorphism (Wei et al., 1995). This variability among virus phenotypes may allow the appearance of viral escape forms, so-called because they can escape the immune response (Pillay and Phillips, 2005), as well as allow the emergence of viral strains resistant to antiretroviral therapy (Biggar et al., 2002). Both of these viral forms may then be transmitted to the child. Viral phenotype is also a risk factor independent of reverse transcriptase: the frequency of appearance of resistance mutations depends on the HIV subtype (A, C and D) (Kantor et al., 2002).

4.4 Cytotoxic T lymphocytes (CTLs) and vertical HIV transmission

Various components of the immune system affect viral replication and therefore may participate in vertical transmission. Induction of suppressor and **cytotoxic T lymphocytes (CTLs)** and **neutralizing antibodies (NAbs)** are considered fundamental for a protective immune response against HIV (see Section 6) and have also been implicated in protection against vertical transmission (Bongertz, 2001).

Class I-restricted CTLs exert significant immune pressure on HIV-1 and may be an important factor in mother-to-child transmission (Pillay and Phillips, 2005). Recognition of peptide-MHC complexes by CTL receptor triggers a response that ends in the recognition and lysis of HIV-infected cells by CTLs, which blocks the propagation of HIV-1. There is an inverse correlation between plasma RNA viral load and levels of HIV-specific CTLs in patients infected by HIV-1 (Ogg et al., 1998). CTLs detect viral antigens that have been processed intracellularly. Peptides are cleaved and presented on the cell surface by MHC I molecules. Recognition of the peptide-MHC complex triggers a response that results in lysis of the infected cell. HIV-1-specific CTLs seem to contribute to the control of HIV-1, as do certain HLA class I alleles that encode the MHC molecules required for the presentation of these peptide fragments to CTLs. In particular, HLA-B27 and HLA-B57 are predicted to be involved in the control of both HIV infection and AIDS progression, while HLA-B35 is associated with rapid disease progression (Kaslow et al., 1996; Carrington et al., 1999).

The impact of CTL responses on vertical transmission in HIV-infected pregnant women has been investigated since the 1990s (Matt and Roger, 2001). CTL activity in the maternal peripheral circulation is similar to that in the non-pregnant state and CTLs can appear early in infants, where their presence correlates with slow progressive HIV disease (Pillay and Phillips, 2005). Consequently, an indirect role for CTLs in mother-to-child transmission has been proposed (Polycarpou et al., 2002). Moreover, levels of CTL precursor frequencies specific for *pol* and *nef* HIV variants were more frequently found during pregnancy in non-transmitting mothers than in transmitting ones (Jin et al., 1998). Because *nef* is transcribed early during the replication of HIV, a strong *nef*-specific CTL response may be important for the clearance of HIV soon after viral protein expression, thereby limiting further viral transmission. Interestingly, a *nef*-specific CTL response has also been observed in uninfected children born to HIV-positive women (De Maria et al., 1994). Importantly, $CD4^{+}$ T cells are critical in maintaining CTL activity against HIV-1 (Kalams and Walker, 1998), and their importance in vertical transmission has also been demonstrated (Plaeger et al., 1999).

Although it induces the CTL response, the virus cannot always be completely controlled. This is often due to mutations in viral peptides that allow virus to **escape CTL recognition via MHC class I molecules** (Pillay and Phillips, 2005). Vertical transmission of HIV-1 may imply that the transmitted virus is a CTL escape form; such forms have indeed been detected in infants (Pillay and Phillips, 2005). Mothers share at least 50% of their HLA alleles with their children but children may still respond differently than their mothers, depending on their HLA and their concordance with the mother's alleles. For example, if the mother and the child share the protective HLA-B27, transmission of virus to the child will be effective: since the virus is adapted to escape B27 recognition, the allele will not confer protection from HIV-1 on the child (Goulder et al., 2001). In contrast, if the child inherits the HLA B27 allele from the father, the child will be able to generate a strong response to viral epitopes. The viral escape mutation can be maintained in the HIV-1 population if it does not imply a fitness cost; if it does, the mutation will revert in the absence of immune pressure (see Section 6) (Allen et al., 2004).

4.5 Neutralizing antibodies (NAbs) and vertical HIV transmission

Although the CTL response is an important mediator of protective immunity and has been implicated in controlling virus load, the maternal CTL response is insufficient to determine the fate of HIV vertical transmission (Matt and Roger, 2001). Several other factors are important, including the ability of the mother to generate antibodies, particularly neutralizing antibodies (NAbs) that are able to block viral replication. In individuals infected with HIV-1, high levels of antibodies against the envelope viral proteins gp120 and gp41 are synthesized (Fig. 2). However, these antibodies do not seem to be very effective against HIV since they are not able to neutralize it *in vitro*. This is probably due to the high degree of glycosylation of these proteins (Reitter et al., 1998; Wyatt et al., 1998; Rudd et al., 2001). Nevertheless, there are other Nabs that can be generated rapidly in primary HIV infection (Richman et al., 2003). NAbs are thought to protect against vertical transmission, since they can pass through the placental barrier, they have been detected in mother's milk, and they are believed to be present during delivery (Bongertz, 2001). In general the presence of high amounts of NAbs is correlated with chronic, non-progressive disease (Pillay and Phillips, 2005).

High levels of NAbs are detected during pregnancy. Nevertheless, whether maternal NAbs and maternal humoral immunity in general play a role in vertical HIV transmission remains controversial. Several early reports indicated an association between maternal NAbs and protection against vertical transmission (Rossi et al., 1989; Devash et al., 1990; Louisirirotchanakul et al., 1999), but these observations were not confirmed (Bal et al., 1996; Hengel et al., 1998). Since selection for escape HIV-1 variants occurs during transmission, it is possible that non-neutralized variants are transmitted to the infant (Okamoto et al., 1997). Moreover it appears that the timing and mechanism of NAb activity during vertical transmission is important. A strong local NAb response is probably effective at controlling HIV multiplicity during pregnancy, but ineffective at blocking transmission of HIV-1-infected cells (Bongertz, 2001).

4.6 HIV coreceptors and vertical HIV transmission

In this section of the chapter, we will briefly describe non-MHC genetic factors that influence vertical transmission and then we will focus on the association between HLA polymorphism and vertical transmission.

In addition to CD4, HIV-1 uses other coreceptors to enter the T cell, and these have been identified as chemokine receptors (Cairns and D'Souza, 1998). The CCR5 chemokine receptor is mainly used by non-syncytium-inducing (NSI) HIV-1 strains, whereas syncytium-inducing strains use the SDF1 chemokine receptor CXCR4. Some strains also use additional chemokine receptors such as CCR2 and CX_3R1 (Cairns and D'Souza, 1998; Singh and Spector, 2009). A mutant CCR5 allele carrying a 32-bp deletion (CCR5-Δ32) was identified independently by several groups, and found to cause the loss of coreceptor activity (Dean et al., 1996; Liu et al., 1996; Samson et al., 1996). This allele has been identified as a natural polymorphism that reduces the risk of acquiring HIV-1 infection (McNicholl et al., 1997). Nevertheless, several studies about the role of this allele in mother-to-child transmission showed that CCR5-Δ32 heterozygosity alone does not protect against vertical transmission (Matt and Roger, 2001). Conversely, another genetic polymorphism, CCR5-59356-T, was strongly associated with a higher rate of vertical transmission of HIV-1 among black infants (Kostrikis et al., 1999).

The CCR2-64-I allele was shown to confer long-term protection in adults (Smith et al., 1997), but it was not associated with mother-to-child transmission (Mangano et al., 2000). A genetic polymorphism in the untranslated region of the SDF-1 gene in mothers was associated with increased risk of vertical transmission of HIV-1, mainly through breastfeeding (John et al., 2000).

4.7 MHC and vertical HIV transmission

Although vertical transmission of HIV-1 has been correlated with a wide range of viral and maternal features, the factors affecting this transmission have yet to be definitively identified (Matt and Roger, 2001). Efforts to explain why only a proportion of children born to HIV-infected mothers become infected have led to the discovery of important host genetic and delivery variables. One of the most relevant genetic factors is the MHC system, which, as mentioned above, plays a critical role in HIV transmission in both horizontal and vertical transmission. Since the 1990s, it has been known that certain HLA types are more susceptible or resistant to HIV-1 infection. In principle, HLA genotype may influence disease susceptibility *in utero* by affecting CTL response or other immune responses. HLA association with mother-to-child transmission has been found with class I, class II, and non-classical HLA alleles. A serologic HLA typing study of Scottish infants by Kilpatrick et al. (Kilpatrick et al., 1991) found that specific HLA haplotypes were associated either with protection or increased susceptibility to HIV-1 vertical transmission. In particular, the HLA-A3-B7-DR2 haplotype was associated with protection against HIV-1 infection, whereas the HLA-A1-B8-DR3 haplotype was associated with HIV-infected children. RFLP HLA-DRB1 analysis performed by Greggio et al. showed that certain DRB1-13 allele subtypes were associated with protection against vertical transmission of HIV-1 (Greggio et al., 1993). These findings were subsequently confirmed using molecular HLA typing methods. The HLA-DR2 allele (DRB1*1501) was not associated with mother-to-child transmission of HIV-1, while the HLA-DR3 (DRB1*03011) allele was positively associated with the occurrence of HIV-1 infection among American Caucasian infants (Winchester et al., 1995).

Among infected infants, MHC alleles can influence disease progression. For instance, the HLA DR3 haplotype (DRB1*0301-DQA*0501-DQB1*0201) was associated with the development of severe clinical manifestations and death in African-Americans, DPB1*0101 was associated with survival to at least two years of age, and DQB1*0604 was related with increased risk of infection (Just et al., 1995a). A study with Spanish children in Catalonia confirmed the association between the DQB1*0201 allele and severe clinical outcomes, but found that the DRB1*0301 allele showed a tendency to protect against disease progression (Just et al., 1996). The differences observed between these studies may be explained by ethnic differences among the children studied (Winchester et al., 1995; Just et al., 1996). Indeed, ethnicity appears to be an important variable for interpreting the effect of HLA alleles. For instance, the DRB1*13011 allele is significantly associated with a diminution in vertically transmitted HIV-1 infection in African-American children but not in American Caucasian children. Moreover, other HLA DR13 alleles (DRB1*1301, *1302, *1303) are associated with protection against HIV-1 transmission in African-American but not in Caucasian children (Winchester et al., 1995).

Altogether, these data suggest that the HLA DR3 haplotype is associated with both increased risk of vertical transmission of HIV-1 and pediatric disease progression (Just et al., 1995b; Winchester et al., 1995), while the HLA DR13 allele is associated with protection against HIV-1 infection (Winchester et al., 1995). However, the HLA DR3 (DRB1*03011) and HLA-A2 alleles show discordant effects between African-American and Caucasian ethnic groups.

These observations suggest that variations in the transport of virally encoded peptides to, or presentation by, MHC molecules may significantly influence the host response to HIV infection and mother-to-child transmission. However, the identity of the HLA alleles by itself does not determine risk of mother-to-child transmission. Rather, the concordance or discordance of HLA alleles between mother and child seems to be a key factor for vertical transmission.

HLA-G is a non-classical HLA molecule from MHC class Ib with a limited distribution in tissues, and it is selectively expressed in placental trophoblast cells in the maternal-fetal interphase (Kovats et al., 1990). HLA-G has been identified as a molecule involved in immune tolerance, and its main function appears to be to protect the fetus from maternal CTLs and natural killer (NK) cells (Hunt, Petroff et al. 2000). Because of its presence in the placenta, it is logical to suggest that HLA-G helps to determine vertical transmission of HIV-1, and that certain allelic mutations in the HLA-G gene increase or decrease protection of infants against *in utero* transmission. Indeed, a correlation between HLA-G variants and mother-to-child transmission was found in a study by Aikhionbare et al. (Aikhionbare et al., 2001). Discordance between mother and child for a mutation in exon 2 of HLA-G was significantly more common among non-transmitting than transmitting mother-child pairs. This suggests that mother-child pairs in which both carry the same mutation in HLA-G exon 2 may be at higher risk of vertical transmission of HIV-1. Nevertheless, another study with a bigger cohort of mother-child pairs in Zimbabwe did not find any relation between mother-child HLA-G concordance/discordance and either intrauterine or peripartum transmission (Matte et al., 2002). Moreover, the mutation in exon 2 of HLA-G (at codon 57) does not change the amino acid composition of the protein (silent mutation), so it is difficult to envisage how a silent mutation could have a direct influence on mother-child transmission of HIV-1. The significant association reported in the first study (Aikhionbare et al., 2001) may be attributed to their relatively small sample size. However, in more recent work, Aikhionbare et al. argued that the differences between the studies may be due to the homogeneous population in the Zimbabwe study, where 90% of the mother-child pairs belonged to the Shona ethnicity. They suggested that in such a homogeneous group, certain mutations may not play a role in disease protection, whereas they do in mixed populations. In addition, they identified several polymorphisms in HLA-G that may be associated with decreased risk of vertical transmission of HIV-1 (Aikhionbare et al., 2006).

An important milestone is the so-called "pattern of inheritance theory," based on the premise that HLA concordance between a mother and her infant can be a determinant of vertical transmission. A study showed that HLA class I antigen concordance between a mother and her child is associated with an increased risk of intrauterine HIV-1 transmission, whereas maternal-child HLA discordance results in protection against vertical transmission (MacDonald et al., 1998). This was confirmed in another study showing the association with HLA class I concordance, but not with HLA class II (Polycarpou et al., 2002). This was also shown in other studies where children who inherited one or more alleles associated with short-term disease progression progressed more rapidly to AIDS if they inherited the alleles from their fathers, but not if they inherited them from their mothers. The opposite situation also occurs: a protective allele may be effective in children only when it comes from the father and not from the mother (Kuhn et al., 2004). It has been proposed that fetal alloimmune responses directed against maternal HIV-infected cells or free virus bearing maternal MHC determinants may account for protection in some children (Mittleman and Shearer, 1996). Maternally derived cells carry HLA molecules on their surface, as well as infectious viral particles. Fetal cord blood leukocytes are able to recognize foreign maternal HLA and mount a strong immune response. Nevertheless, in cases in which maternal HLA antigens are similar or identical to fetal HLA, the fetal immune response is probably less potent or nonexistent (Mittleman and Shearer, 1996). This may explain why HLA concordance between a mother and her child is associated with an increased risk of intrauterine HIV transmission. A recent study of mother-child pairs in Spain suggests that HLA-B35 increases transmission risk, a finding that is also consistent with the pattern of inheritance theory (Arnaiz-Villena et al., 2009).

5. Other MHC-related factors that influence HIV transmission

5.1 Innate immune response

Although the innate immune response is an essential part of anti-viral responses, its role in HIV infection remains obscure (Biasin et al., 2010). Viruses are recognized by the immune system through receptors named "pattern recognition receptors" (PRRs) that bind to "pathogen-associated molecular patterns" (PAMPs), which are small pieces of the virus with a conserved "viral tag" that host cells identify as foreign. Viral proteins are recognized by Toll-like receptors (TLR) 2 and 4 in the plasma membrane, while viral nucleic acids are recognized by TLR 3, 7, 8 and 9, which are located in endosomal membranes. In this latter group, TLR7 and 8 recognize single-stranded viral RNA (v-ssRNA) from HIV. Studies on TLR signalling during HIV infection are scarce, even though it has been proposed that exposed but non-infected individuals mount stronger responses through TLR-initiated signalling (Biasin et al., 2010).

There are also cytoplasmic receptors such as RIG-I-like (RLR) and nucleotide-binding domain, leucine-rich receptors (NIRs) that have been implicated in the recognition of viruses. Signals from these receptors activate the cells that express them and initiate the production of interferons and inflammatory cytokines, including IL-1B and IL-18, which determine important aspects of the adaptive immune response, such as the CTL response. HIV is able to disrupt both TLR and RIG-1 signalling by depleting IRF3 interferon regulatory factor 3 (IRF-3) (Doehle et al., 2009). Type I interferons (IFN α/β) are especially crucial in early stages of viral infections. They promote an "antiviral state" by inducing the expression of hundreds of target genes, so-called interferon-stimulated genes (ISGs) (Baum and Garcia-Sastre, 2010). Plasmacitoid dendritic cells (pDCs) are the main natural INFα producers *in vivo*. This subpopulation appears to be depleted in chronic HIV infection (Soumelis et al., 2001).

5.2 NK responses

NKs are $CD3^+$ lymphocytes and they are divided into two major subgroups, NK regulatory or NK effector cells, depending on the levels of expression of CD56 and CD16. These cells play a prominent role during viral infections because they mediate early, non-adaptive responses against virus, and they modulate the activity of other effector cells of the innate and adaptive immune system. NKs exhibit cytolytic activity against cells infected with viruses and they secrete anti-viral products. Their cytolytic activity appears to involve receptors that bind MHC class I molecules. HIV-exposed but uninfected subjects have been reported to have enhanced NK functions and increased IFN-γ and TNF-α levels. During chronic HIV infection, NK cell cytotoxicity is reduced (Ahmad et al., 2001).

The ability of NKs to kill virally infected cells depends on a fine balance in the relative expression of inactivating and activating NK receptors (NKRs). Several studies have addressed the relationship between NK receptors that bind to MHC molecules, and viral load and NK activity during HIV infection (Ahmad et al., 2001; Gaudieri et al., 2005).

HLA-B molecules can be classified according to the presence of the mutually exclusive public epitopes Bw4 or Bw6 that are shared by various MHC molecules. However, only Bw4 is a ligand for KIRs, which are type I integral membrane glycoproteins. To date, 14 distinct KIR genes have been described (http://www.ebi.ac.uk.kir) (Paximadis et al., 2011). KIRs can have either activating or inhibitory functions. It has been shown that suppression of HIV-1 viremia is associated with homozygosity for HLA-Bw4. Furthermore, the Bw4-80I group, which has isoleucine at position 80, includes two alleles (B*57 and B*27) that are considered protective, as previously mentioned. KIR allele KIR3DS1, which is an activating receptor, binds HLA-B Bw4-80I molecules, and this binding was shown to delay progression to AIDS. Furthermore, coexpression of both alleles in the same individual reduces the risk of both infection and progression (Lopez-Vazquez et al., 2005; Boulet and Bernard 2008; Boulet et al., 2008).

The involvement of HLA-B Bw4/6 epitopes in transmission from infected men to their female sex partners was analyzed. Compared with men who were homozygous for Bw6, men who carried Bw4 were about half as likely to transmit HIV-1 to their female partner (Welzel et al., 2007). However, a more recent study that compared men homozygous for HLA-Cw1 or HLA-Cw2 attributed functional differences in human NK cell activity to distinct KIR/HLA genotypes, independently of KIR3DL1/HLA-Bw4 interactions (Ahlenstiel et al., 2008). It turns out that HLA-E and HLA-G are also important in the regulation of NK cell responses (Tripathi and Agrawal, 2007).

The simultaneous presence of the HLA-Bw4 epitope and both the HLA-B*57 and HLA-Cw*18 alleles correlated with low levels of viremia in 147 HIV-infected individuals in Brazil. The protective effect of HLA-Bw4 depended on the presence of HLA-B*57. In contrast to previous studies, the HLA-Bw4 epitope bearing isoleucine at position 80 did not confer a protective effect in the presence of the activating KIR3DS1 allele (Da Silva et al., 2011).

The associations most consistently observed between KIRs and HIV progression involves KIR3DS1 and KIR3DL. KIR and HLA class I alleles were studied in 224 South African mothers and their 222 infants, of whom 72 were infected and 150 uninfected (Paximadis et al., 2011). The frequencies of KIR2DL1 and KIR2DL3 were lower in intrapartum-transmitting (IP-T) mothers than in non-transmitting (NT) mothers. Homozygosity for KIR2DL3, alone or in combination with HLA-C heterozygosity (Cw1/Cw2), was more frequent in IP-T mothers than in NT ones. The combination of the KIR2DL3 allele and its ligand, HLA-Cw1 occurred less frequently in infected infants, as did homozygosity for KIR2DL3 in combination with HLA-Cw1/Cw2. It is noteworthy that these effects of genotype were more readily detectable after stratifying the sample based on low or high maternal viral load.

5.3 Chemokines

Since the discovery of CCR5 as an HIV entry cofactor (Dean et al., 1996), researchers have focused on chemokines as possible restriction/susceptibility factors (Alkhatib et al., 1996). Thus variants or haplotypes of CCL5, CCL2-CCL7-CCL1 and CCL3 have been consistently associated with differential susceptibility to infection or transmission (Telenti and McLaren, 2010). Polymorphism of chemokine receptors has, in turn, been linked to specific HLA alleles, such as CCR2 and HLA-B58; the latter is present in long-term survival women from Nairobi (Fang et al., 2004)

5.4 Other factors

CTL-associated antigen 4 (CTLA4) is a member of the immunoglobulin superfamily, and is expressed mainly on helper and regulatory T cells. After ligand binding it transmits an inhibitory signal to the cell. Single-nucleotide polymorphisms in the promoter region of the CTLA4 gene were analyzed in relationship to viral load and time to AIDS, but no clear association was established (Shao et al., 2006).

6. Contribution of HLA selection of CTL responses to HIV susceptibility or protection

Here we provide an overview of an important subject that is central to the struggle to develop a successful CTL-based HIV vaccine (Bangham et al., 2009). CTLs, also known as CD8+ T cells, eliminate HIV-infected cells through the recognition of antigenic peptides displayed by HLA class I molecules on the infected cell surface. HIV can evade T cell responses by mutating epitopes that are recognized by CTLs (Phillips et al., 1991) and then those HIV variants or "escape mutations" are selected if they maintain the fitness of the virus. This is called "fixation" of the mutation and it implies that the mutation confers some advantage for the virus against the CTL response. Significant efforts have been made to obtain a complete map of HIV epitopes recognized by CTLs and antibody-producing cells (http://www.hiv.lanl.gov), since this mapping is essential for vaccine development.

In general it is thought that most mutations occur in the initial phase of the infection when the virus is rapidly replicating and therefore is more likely to mutate. However, it appears that the mutations in some delayed escape variants occur later in the viral life cycle. One of the best documented examples of an HIV escape variant is a "gag epitope" recognized by the HLA-B27 molecule. Patients with HLA-B27 progress more slowly to AIDS than does the general HIV-infected population. Peptides that bind HLA-B27 very frequently have an arginine (R) at the second position. The HIV gag epitope$^{263\text{-}272}$ contains such arginine that when mutated, is no longer recognized by T cells. This escape mutation occurs in approximately 50% of HLA-B27-infected individuals after several years of infection. Why does it not appear at the beginning of the infection? Because the escape mutation R264K must be preceded by a first mutation, and then it subsequently appears together with a third. The mutation R264K has a fitness cost and thus the mutant virus tends to revert to the wild-type (WT) sequence in the absence of selection (i.e. HLA-B27). This was demonstrated by studying HLA-B27-negative babies born to HLA-B27-positive mothers infected with virus carrying the R264K mutation (Goulder et al., 2001); this study found that "HLA-mediated selective pressures on the virus in a transmitting mother-infant pair may undermine future HLA-mediated viral control in the child". Later the fitness cost was shown to be compensated by a third mutation in a position that binds an inhibitory receptor on dendritic cells (DCs). This example illustrates that escape mutations can be very complicated events, which may explain their late appearance in the course of the infection (McMichael et al., 2007).

There are well established examples of associations between expression of an HLA class I molecule and deviation from the consensus HIV sequence ("escape mutations"). The converse situation also exists, namely, association of certain HLAs with the WT or "preserved" sequence (Leslie et al., 2005). Therefore it was proposed that HIV-1 is adapting to HLA-restricted responses as a consequence of selection pressure (Moore et al., 2002; John et al., 2005). However, CTL escape mutants that revert following transmission to individuals

lacking the selecting MHC alleles have been identified. The obvious implication of these data is that some CTL responses can be evaded only by escape mutations that paradoxically reduce the replicative fitness of the virus (Leslie and Goulder, 2006). Study of the impact of HLA on HIV molecular evolution is further complicated by the "founder effect" of HIV strains (Bhattacharya et al., 2007; Klenerman and McMichael, 2007).
The question at the moment is to what extent is HIV adapting to HLA class I molecules? This issue was directly addressed in an international multi-cohort study, in which nine cohorts from 5 different continents were pooled, allowing the analysis of more than 2,800 subjects. They studied the HLA-B*51-restricted epitope TAFTIPSI, corresponding to residues 128-135 of reverse transcriptase, and they showed a strong correlation between the frequency of the escape mutation I135X and HLA-B*51 prevalence. Similarly, the frequencies of other well-defined CD8+ T-cell epitopes restricted by HLA-B*57 and HLA-B*27 correlated with the prevalence of the restricting HLA allele in the different cohorts, demonstrating strong evidence of HIV adaptation to HLA at the population level (Kawashima et al., 2009).

7. Summary: HLA molecules confer protection or susceptibility to HIV infection

The best way to identify protection or susceptibility factors is to study exposed but seronegative (ESN) individuals and HIV-infected LTNPs (Miyazawa et al., 2009). There are several possible factors that may determine how HLA molecules condition the anti-HIV immune response (Fig. 2). One obvious factor is the differences in peptide-binding repertoires among HLA molecules, which is the logic behind grouping the alleles in clusters or supertypes. Another factor is that HLA-DR polymorphism affects interaction with CD4 (Fleury et al., 1995), which implies that some HLA-DR molecules bind CD4+ lymphocytes more than others. Similarly, particular HLA molecules, such as HLA-B*27, HLA-B57, HLA-B*5701 (in Caucasians) and HLA-B*5703 (in Africans), are more likely to mediate successful control of HIV infection by activating CTL responses (den Uyl et al., 2004). HLA B*5701 was found to be a clear protective factor, but the protection could not be attributed to any quantitative differences in the total HIV-specific CD8+ T cell response (Migueles et al., 2000). In the case of HLA-B27, there are reports of CTL-protective response against p24 HIV protein, which has a relatively low rate of mutation (den Uyl et al., 2004). HIV-infected chimpanzees do not develop AIDS and therefore they have been used as a model to understand the influence of MHC on HIV disease. The peptide-binding groove of frequent chimpanzee MHC class I molecules, similarly to HLA-B*27/B*57, target similar conserved areas of HIV-1/SIV(cpz) (de Groot et al., 2010). Interestingly HLA-B*5701 is one of the major alleles responsible for hypersensitivity to the reverse transcriptase inhibitor abacavir (Mallal et al., 2002).
Various factors, including HLA that might confer protection or susceptibility, have been studied in a cohort of 30 LTNPs from Spain (Salgado et al., 2011b). For example, these investigators studied CCR5 and the *CCL3L1* gene, which encodes the MIP1a protein, an inhibitory CCR5 ligand. They found the B27 and B58 supertypes, as well as certain class I alleles, to be protective; the B7 supertype and other class I alleles were non-protective. No significant association with CCR5-Delta32 was found, probably because this mutation is rare among Spaniards. Similarly, CCL3K1 copy number did not influence the rate of progression.

Protective HLA-B and -C alleles were more frequent in LTNPs, though such an association was not observed with HLA-A alleles. In addition to HLA-B*5701 and -B*2705, the investigators found HLA-Cw0102, -Cw0602 and -Cw1203. The presence of allele combinations such as HLA B*5701-Cw0602, HLA B*2705-Cw0102, and HLA B*3801-Cw1203 showed the strongest association with non-progression.

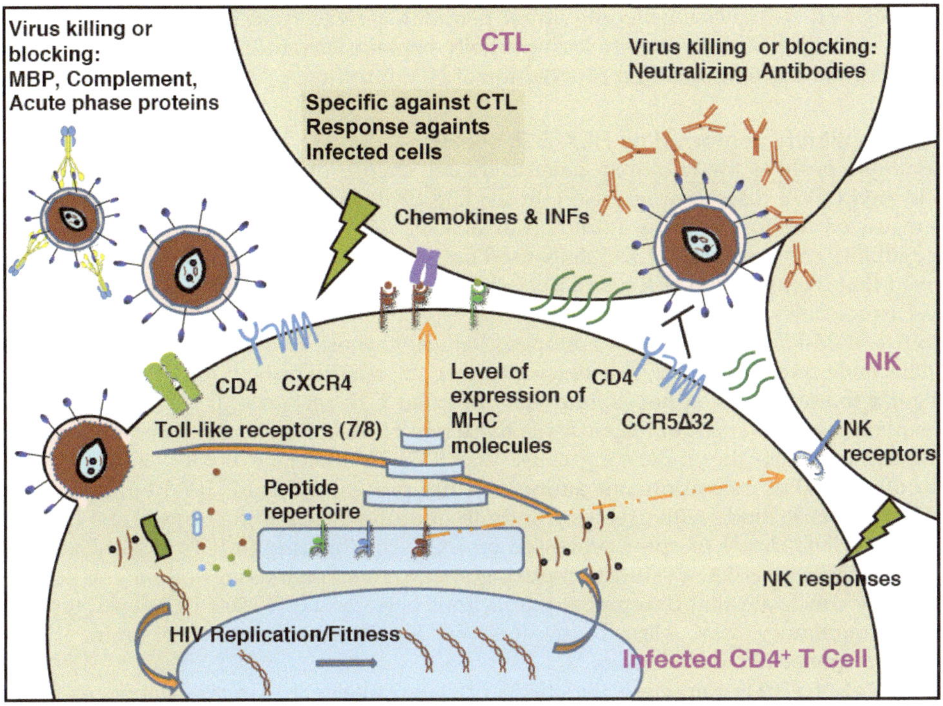

Fig. 2. Points where genetics influences HIV infection and its progression.

Although chimpanzees are susceptible to infection with HIV-1, they do not develop AIDS. A similar situation occurs when they are infected with the chimpanzee simian immunodeficiency virus (SIVcpz). Chimpanzee class I molecules are designated Patr-A, -B and -C, and like those of humans, they are polymorphic. However it has been proposed that their repertoire has been skewed by strong selective pressure exerted by HIV or an ancestral retrovirus of HIV. Therefore the chimpanzee has been used as a model system to understand resistance to progression to AIDS. Thus, the Patr peptide-binding repertoire has been analyzed and compared to the binding repertoire of human HLA-B*27 and B*57, two HLA molecules correlated with resistance in humans (Groot et al., 2010). This work showed that at least one Patr molecule in the study population recognizes conserved areas of the Gag protein that are also recognized by B*27 and B*57.

The mechanism of the protective effect exerted by HLA-B*58:01 was studied in South African individuals infected with HIV subtype-C (Chopera et al., 2011). One of the major conclusions of this work is that HLA-B*58:01 patients whose CTLs target the TW10 in the p24Gag viral epitope maintain higher CD4+ T cell numbers than those whose CTLs do not target that part of the epitope. However, escape mutations were detected early, as soon as two

weeks after infection. In addition, the escape mutations were accompanied in some cases by compensatory mutations that may limit the protective effect of the HLA-B*58:01 allele.
A correlation was found between the HLA peptide-binding affinities of 95 HLA class I alleles and sequence conservation of targeted viral regions in 52 human viruses, including HIV (Hertz et al., 2011). This analysis indicates that HLA-A alleles and those HLA-B alleles most closely related to chimpanzee alleles preferentially target peptides from DNA viruses, while other HLA-B alleles generally target peptides derived from RNA viruses. This is an important conclusion that may at least partially explain why it is primarily HLA-B alleles that determine susceptibility and progression of HIV infection.

7.1 Susceptibility conferred by HLA-B35 alleles

Individuals positive for HLA-B35 have a greater chance of becoming infected and show accelerated HIV-1 disease progression. In the late 1990s, numerous HIV mutations in HLA-B35-restricted epitopes were found (Kawana et al., 1999). Hence initial studies of susceptibility conferred by HLA-B35 focused on CTL responses (Jin et al., 2002). Later work showed that the increased risk was associated with the subset of HLA-B35 alleles known as B*35-Px molecules (Jin et al., 2002). Interestingly, some alleles in the alternative set of B*35 subtypes, B*35-PY, present HIV-1 epitopes identical to those of B*35-Px molecules, yet have no detectable impact on HIV-1 disease outcomes. In other words, both HLA-B35 subtypes recognize the same HIV epitopes, implying a similar CTL response. If that is true, how can we explain the differences in responses in these two HLA-B35 subsets? Differences in innate immunity could be the underlying cause: the B*35-PY molecule B*3501 and the B*35-Px molecule B*3503 differ by only one amino acid and present identical HIV-1 epitopes, yet the B*35-Px molecule binds with greater affinity to immunoglobulin-like transcript 4 (ILT4), an inhibitory MHC class I receptor expressed on DCs. This binding to ILT4 is associated with significantly stronger DC dysfunction during *in vitro* functional assays (Huang et al., 2009). That study concludes that differential interactions between HLA class I allele subtypes and immune regulatory MHC class I receptors on DCs is an important determinant of the immune response to the HIV virus.
Lazaryan et al. (2011) compared the effects of class I alleles in African-Americans infected with subtype B with those in Africans infected with subtype C. Among African-Americans, HLA alleles A*32, A*74, B*14 and B*45 were strongly associated with control of HIV infection. Furthermore, infrequent HLA-B alleles were associated with better disease outcome. This was consistent with a previous study by the same investigators, in which they found that relatively infrequent supertypes in African-Americans correlated with a better immunological profile. When the researchers took into account the known linkage disequilibrium among A, B and C alleles in their cohort, they detected that HLA-A*32 and A*74 were associated with favourable outcome. The protective effect of HLA-B*57 was also confirmed in this population, while B35 and B53 alleles were associated with poor outcome. These results are inconsistent with the previously described PX/PY theory (Huang et al., 2009) (section 7.1). Lazaryan et al. (2011) found that both B*5301 (PX) and B*3501 (PY), the most frequent alleles in their groups, were equally disadvantageous.

8. Hypersensitivity to anti-HIV drug treatment

The occurrence of hypersensitivity reactions to drugs used to treat HIV infection has complicated HIV treatment management. Antiretroviral drugs are currently grouped into 6 major classes:

- Nucleoside reverse transcriptase inhibitors (NRTIs)
- Non-nucleoside reverse transcriptase inhibitors (NNRTIs)
- Protease inhibitors (PIs)
- Entry inhibitors, further subdivided into fusion inhibitors and CCR5 inhibitors
- Integrase inhibitors

Most HIV patients receive therapy that combines various drugs, known as HAART. This complicates the diagnosis of drug hypersensitivity. In addition, allergic reactions to anti-HIV drugs usually occur with a delay of 1 to 6 weeks. Skin reactions are the most common manifestations, and they can vary from exanthema to systemic symptoms or syndromes that have received various names, such as drug-induced hypersensitivity syndrome (DIHS). Most of the drugs used to treat HIV infection produce hypersensitivity in a percentage of patients. We recommend to our readers an excellent recent review on the subject (Chaponda et al., 2011).

Genetic factors have been shown to play a role in some of the adverse effects of these drugs, especially in the case of **abacavir.** This NRTI induces hypersensitivity that is strongly associated with the MHC class I HLA*5701 allele (Mallal et al., 2002), implying a significant genetic component. Screening for HLAB*5701 has now become part of HIV treatment involving abacavir and has helped prevent adverse reactions.

9. New technologies

Historically, studies of HLA association with HIV infection have evolved in parallel with advances in technology. Initially HLA determinations were performed by serology, which has gradually been replaced by molecular techniques. We are now in the so-called "-omics" era: genomics and proteomic technologies, including microarrays, next-generation DNA sequencing and mass spectrometry, are important for identifying molecular markers in complex traits (Sharon et al., 2010), such as in HIV infection. The genetics of HIV susceptibility will most probably include frequent and rare variants, with each type of variant making different contributions to the specific aspect of the disease analyzed. This implies that the design of the study itself is a key factor that affects the consistency of the results. Therefore a large number of subjects is recommended in some instances (>1000 patients and >1000 controls) (Telenti and McLaren, 2010).

A whole-genome association study (WGAS) was performed to uncover the genetic factors that govern variations in viral load among individuals during the asymptomatic period of infection. Two polymorphisms were found, one located in an endogenous retroviral element occurring within the HLA-B57*01 allele, and another near the HLA-C gene (Fellay et al., 2007). More recently, a WGAS of a cohort of 2,554 HIV-infected Caucasian individuals excluded a role for any gene polymorphism outside the MHC complex, including the chemokine receptor gene cluster on chromosome 3 (Fellay et al., 2011). Viral control was associated with genetic variants that map near the HLA-B and -C loci, though variants also exist in the MHC region. The study detected in this cohort two previously described SNPs (Fellay et al., 2007) and found them to be associated with HLA-B*5701 and HLA-C (Fellay et al., 2011).

In a study of the association of HLA-C with HIV control, Kulkarni et al., (2011) reexamined the SNP -35, which lies 35 kb upstream of HLA-C (Fellay et al., 2007). This SNP was found to be in fact a marker of another polymorphism in the 3'-untranslated region (3'-UTR) of HLA-C. This polymorphism regulates the binding of a microRNA (miRNA), has-miR-148, to the 3'-UTR. This binding results in relatively low surface expression of HLA-C. MicroRNAs are RNAs that bind to the 3'-UTR to cause post-transcriptional repression, cleavage or destabilization. Even more, the 3'-UTR polymorphism of HLA-C that regulates binding by has-miR-148 is associated with HIV control.

Recently, the International HIV Controllers Study Group (Pereyra et al., 2010) analyzed a large cohort from multiple populations, comprising 974 controllers and 2,648 progressors. The study yielded 1,384,048 single-nucleotide polymorphisms (SNPs). In the largest group of 1,712 individuals of European ancestry, all SNPs that reached statistical significance were located in the MHC region, around class I genes. A similar clustering of SNPs occurred in other ethnic groups and across the entire sample population. When the HLA typing and the SNPs were considered together, through a process of "imputation" in which HLA type was inferred from a previous WGAS on diabetes, HLA B*57:01, B*27:05, B*14/Cw*08:02, B*52, and A*25 were identified as protective alleles, and B*35 and Cw*07 as risk alleles. These results are consistent with previous HLA association studies. The HIV Controllers study went a step further and analyzed whether the observed associations might be explained by the presence of specific AAs within the polymorphic positions on HLA molecules. Among a total of 372 polymorphic AA positions in class I and II, 286 were biallelic, accommodating two possible AAs, while the remaining 86 could accommodate more than two AAs. Interestingly position 97 was detected as the most polymorphic, with 6 alternatives. In fact, position 97 in HLA-B was more significant than any single SNP, and positions 67, 70 and 97, located in the binding groove, were better markers than any single classical HLA allele. Position 97 is located at the base of the binding groove and has an important contribution to peptide binding. Arginine is present at position 97 in HLA-B*35, a "risk molecule", while protective HLA molecules, such as B*5701, B*27:05 and B*14 possess valine, asparagine and tryptophan, respectively. A similar analysis performed on HLA-A showed a small but significant contribution of position 77, while for HLA-C the results were more difficult to interpret. This WGAS corroborated the importance of HLA-B peptide presentation for HIV susceptibility (Pereyra et al., 2010).

Novel genetic factors influencing plasma levels of HIV-RNA and cellular HIV-DNA in 605 HIV-1-infected individuals were investigated. Most of the SNPs were located in the 6p21 MHC region, near class I and II genes, except for two outside this region. One of them was located within the syndecan 2 gene (Dalmasso et al., 2008). Intriguingly, increased expression of syndecan isoform 1 -but not of isoform 2- has been implicated in microbial translocation in the gut that is associated with chronic stimulation of the immune system (Smith et al., 2010).

DNA microarrays were used to analyze gene expression patterns in CD3+ T cells from LTNPs and controls. They found that most up-regulated genes in rapid progressors localized to cellular organelles and were implicated in the regulation of DNA replication, cell cycle progression and DNA damage response. In contrast, most genes up-regulated in LTNPs were located at the plasma membrane and were involved in cytokine-cytokine receptor interaction, negative control of apoptosis and regulation of the actin cytoskeleton. This suggests that progressors mainly up-regulate markers of viral replication, while non-progressors do not (Salgado et al., 2010a).

Proteomics is now also being used to study host genetic factors in HIV response, though mostly in relation to specific aspects of the disease, such as neurological damage (reviewed by (Zhang et al., 2010)).

We would like to end this chapter by mentioning new trends in research on the genetics of HIV disease by mentioning the role of autophagy (Blanchet et al., 2010), and the cell skeleton or cytoskeleton (Harmon et al., 2010) during HIV infection and replication within the cells. A very recent and interesting report showed that a known tumour suppressor protein, the cyclin-dependent kinase inhibitor p21, has an important role in inhibiting various steps of HIV transcription in CD4+ T cells. Elite controllers showed increased expression of p21, which should effectively down-regulate HIV replication. Future studies should determine whether individuals expressing protective alleles such as HLA-B*57 express high levels of p21. These studies are necessary in light of the fact that the locus of the CDKN1A gene, which encodes p21, is located near the MHC class I genes (Chen et al., 2010). We are certain that genetic factors involved in these processes will be identified as susceptibility or protective factors in the near future.

Factor	Role in HIV infection	Reference (s)
HLA class I	Concordance between mother and child is associated with increased risk of HIV transmission. "Pattern of inheritance theory". Importance of AAs at position 97 in HLA-B and 77 in HLA-A molecules. HLA-B preferentially targets peptides derived from RNA viruses	MacDonald, et al., 1998; Polycarpou et al., 2002; Kuhn et al., 2004; Pereyra et al., 2010; Hertz et al., 2011
A25	Protection in disease progression	Pereyra et al., 2010
B27	Protection. Slow disease progression. Lower risk of infection and slow progression in vertical transmission. "Pattern of inheritance theory". CTL responses associated with HIV control	Kaslow et al., 1996, McNeil et al., 1996; Yap et al., 1996; Goulder et al., 2001; den Uyl et al., 2004; Groot et al., 2010 ; Pereyra et al., 2010 ; Salgado et al., 2011b
B35	Increase risk of infection and disease progression. Increased risk of vertical transmission. "Pattern of inheritance theory". Decreased number of CD4+ T lymphocytes. CTL responses associated with lack of HIV control. DC dysfunction	Klein et al., 1994; Carrington et al., 1999; Kawana et al, 1999; Jin et al., 2002; Flores-Villanueva et al., 2003; Liu et al., 2003; Arnaiz-Villena et al., 2009; Huang et al., 2009 ; Pereyra et al., 2010
B*51	CTL responses that control HIV replication. Viral mutations allow HIV escape	Kawashima et al., 2009
B*52	Protection in disease progression	Pereyra et al., 2010
B57	Protection. Slow disease progression. B*5701 in Caucasians and HLA-B*5703 in Africans, are more likely to mediate successful control of HIV infection by activating CTL responses	Kaslow et al., 1996; den Uyl et al., 2004; Fellay et al., 2007; Groot et al., 2010 ; Pereyra et al., 2010 ; Salgado et al., 2011b
B57*01	Hypersensitivity to *abacavir*.	Mallal et al., 2002

Factor	Role in HIV infection	Reference (s)
B58 and B58*01	Long survival in women in Nairobi. Protection against HIV infection. CTL responses	Fang et al., 2004 ; Chopera et al., 2011
Bw4	Protection in infection and disease progression. Suppression of viremia in homozygosis. Receptor for KIR (NK cells)	Lopez-Vazquez et al., 2005; Welzel et al., 2007; Boulet & Bernard, 2008; Boulet et al., 2008
HLA-C	Variation of viral load during asymptomatic period. Polymorphism at 3'UT region that binds microRNA decreasing its level of expression	Fellay et al., 2007; Kulkarni et al., 2011
Cw*04	Disease progression in Caucasian	Carrington et al., 1999
Cw*07	Risk of progression	Pereyra et al., 2010
DQB1*0201	Severe clinical outcome in children	Just et al., 1996
DR1	Kaposi's sarcoma	Klein et al., 1994
DR3, DRB1*0301	Opportunistic infections. Risk of infection in American Caucasian children.	Klein et al., 1994; Winchester et al., 1995
DR13, DRB1*130101, *1302, *1303	Protection in vertical transmission. DRB1*1303 associates with reduced viral loads	Greggio et al., 1993; Winchester et al., 1995; Julg et al., 2010
HLA-E	Implicated in NK cells responses	Tripathi & Agrawal, 2007
HLA-G	Discordance between mother and child for mutation in exon 2 has a higher frequency among non-transmitting mother-child pairs. Controversial role in vertical transmission. Implicated in NK cells responses	Aikhionbare et al., 2001; Matte et al., 2002; Aikhionbare et al., 2006; Tripathi et al., 2007; Fainardi et al., 2011
A3-B7-DR2	Protection in vertical transmission	Kilpatrick et al., 1991
A1-B8-DR3	Increased risk of vertical transmission	Kilpatrick et al., 1991
KIR2DL1, KIR2 DL3	Lower frequencies in intrapartum-transmitting (IP-T) mothers than in non-transmitting (NT) mothers	Paximadis et al., 2011
CCR5 (delta32), CCR2-64I	Correceptor for HIV, reduced risk of infection. CCR2-64-I allele was shown to confer long-term protection in adults	Dean et al., 1996; Liu et al., 1996; Samson et al., 1996 ; McNicholl et al., 1997; Smith et al., 1997

Table 2. Major factors associated with HIV infection and progression.

10. Acknowledgments

NMQ would like to acknowledge the support of the Spanish Ministry of Science and Innovation (MICINN-ISCIII; grant PS-09/00080).

11. References

Ahlenstiel, G., Martin, M. P., Gao, X., Carrington, M. & Rehermann, B. (2008). "Distinct KIR/HLA compound genotypes affect the kinetics of human antiviral natural killer cell responses." J Clin Invest 118(3): 1017-26.

Ahmad, N. (2010). "Molecular mechanisms of HIV-1 mother-to-child transmission and infection in neonatal target cells." Life Sci.

Ahmad, Sindhu, ST., Tran, P., Toma, E., Morisset, R., Menezes, J. & Ahmad, A.R. (2001). "Modulation of expression of the MHC class I-binding natural killer cell receptors, and NK activity in relation to viral load in HIV-infected/AIDS patients." J Med Virol 65(3): 431-40.

Aikhionbare, Hodge, T., Kuhn, L., Bulterys, M., Abrams, E.J. & Bond, V.C. (2001). "Mother-to-child discordance in HLA-G exon 2 is associated with a reduced risk of perinatal HIV-1 transmission." Aids 15(16): 2196-8.

Aikhionbare, Kumaresan, K., Shamsa, F., & Bond, V.C. (2006). "HLA-G DNA sequence variants and risk of perinatal HIV-1 transmission." AIDS Res Ther 3: 28.

Alkhatib, Combadiere, C., Broder, C.C., Feng, Y., Kennedy, P.E., Murphy, P.M & Berger E.A. (1996). "CC CKR5: a RANTES, MIP-1alpha, MIP-1beta receptor as a fusion cofactor for macrophage-tropic HIV-1." Science 272(5270): 1955-8.

Allen, Altfeld, M., Yu, X.G., O'Sullivan, K.M., Lichterfeld, M., Le Gall, S., John, M., Mothe, B.R., Lee, P.K., Kalife, E.T., Cohen, D.E., Freedberg, K.A., Strick, D.A., Johnston, M.N., Sette, A., Rosenberg, E.S., Mallal, S.A., Goulder, P.J., Brander, C. & Walker, B.D. (2004). "Selection, transmission, and reversion of an antigen-processing cytotoxic T-lymphocyte escape mutation in human immunodeficiency virus type 1 infection." J Virol 78(13): 7069-78.

Arnaiz-Villena, A., Martín-Villa, J.M., Amador, J.T., Cendoya-Matamoros, A., Tomé, M.I., Rivera, J.M. & Martinez-Quiles, N. (2009). "Risk of vertical HIV transmission combines the 'B35-Cw4 disadvantage' and the 'pattern of inheritance' theories of progression." Curr HIV Res 7(3): 314-9.

Bal, A.K., Miller, G., Viscarello, R. & Andiman, W.A. (1996). "Syncytium-inhibiting and neutralizing activity in maternal sera fail to prevent vertical transmission of human immunodeficiency virus type 1." Pediatr Infect Dis J 15(4): 315-20.

Bangham, C. R. (2009). "CTL quality and the control of human retroviral infections." Eur J Immunol 39(7): 1700-12.

Bashirova, A.A., Thomas, R. & Carrington, M. (2009). "HLA/KIR restraint of HIV: surviving the fittest." Annu Rev Immunol. 29:295-317.

Baum, A. & Garcia-Sastre, A. "Induction of type I interferon by RNA viruses: cellular receptors and their substrates." Amino Acids 38(5): 1283-99.

Bhattacharya, T., Daniels, M., Heckerman, D., Foley, B., Frahm, N., Kadie, C., Carlson, J., Yusim, K., McMahon, B., Gaschen, B., Mallal, S., Mullins, J.I., Nickle, D.C., Herbeck, J., Rousseau, C., Learn, G.H., Miura, T., Brander, C., Walker, B. & Korber, B. (2007). "Founder effects in the assessment of HIV polymorphisms and HLA allele associations." Science 315(5818): 1583-6.

Biasin, M., Clerici, M. & Piacentini, L. (2010). "Innate immunity in resistance to HIV infection." J Infect Dis 202 Suppl 3: S361-5.

Biasin, M., Piacentini, L., Lo Caputo, S., Naddeo, V., Pierotti, P., Borelli, M., Trabattoni, D., Mazzotta, F., Shearer, G.M. & Clerici, M. (2010). "TLR activation pathways in HIV-1-exposed seronegative individuals." J Immunol 184(5): 2710-7.

Biggar, R.J., Janes, M., Pilon, R., Roy, R., Broadhead, R., Kumwenda, N., Taha, T.E. & Cassol, S. (2002). "Human immunodeficiency virus type 1 infection in twin pairs infected at birth." J Infect Dis 186(2): 281-5.

Blanche, S., Mayaux, M.J., Rouzioux, C., Teglas, J.P., Firtion, G, Monpoux, F., Cicaru-Vigneron, N., Meier, F., Tricoire, J., Courpotin, C., Vilmer, E., Griscelli, C., Delfraissy, J.F. & the French Pediatric HIV Infection Study Group (1994). "Relation of the course of HIV infection in children to the severity of the disease in their mothers at delivery." N Engl J Med 330(5): 308-12.

Blanchet, Moris, A., Nikolic, D.S., Lehmann, M., Cardinaud, S., Stalder, R., Garcia, E., Dinkins, C., Leuba, F., Wu, L., Schwartz, O., Deretic, V. & Piguet, V. (2010). "Human immunodeficiency virus-1 inhibition of immunoamphisomes in dendritic cells impairs early innate and adaptive immune responses." Immunity 32(5): 654-69.

Bongertz, V. (2001). "Vertical human immunodeficiency virus type 1--HIV-1--transmission--a review." Mem Inst Oswaldo Cruz 96(1): 1-14.

Borrow, P. & Bhardwaj, N. (2008). "Innate immune responses in primary HIV-1 infection." Curr Opin HIV AIDS 3(1): 36-44.

Boulet, S. & Bernard, N.F. (2008). "Carrying certain KIR3DL1 alleles with HLA-B*57 is associated with protection from HIV infection." Med Sci (Paris) 24(12): 1030-2.

Boulet, S., Kleyman, M., Kim, J.Y., Kamya, P., Sharafi, S., Simic, N., Bruneau, J., Routy, J.P., Tsoukas, C.M., & Bernard, N.F. (2008). "A combined genotype of KIR3DL1 high expressing alleles and HLA-B*57 is associated with a reduced risk of HIV infection." Aids 22(12): 1487-91.

Buchacz, K.A., Wilkinson, D.A., Krowka, J.F., Koup, R.A. & Padian, N.S. (1998). "Genetic and immunological host factors associated with susceptibility to HIV-1 infection." Aids 12 Suppl A: S87-94.

Cairns, J. S. & D'Souza, M.P. (1998). "Chemokines and HIV-1 second receptors: the therapeutic connection." Nat Med 4(5): 563-8.

Cameron, P. U., Mallal, S.A., French, M.A. & Dawkins, R.L. (1990). "Major histocompatibility complex genes influence the outcome of HIV infection. Ancestral haplotypes with C4 null alleles explain diverse HLA associations." Hum Immunol 29(4): 282-95.

Cao, Y., Krogstad, P., Korber, B.T., Koup, R.A., Muldoon, M., Macken, C., Song, J.L., Jin, Z., Zhao, J.Q., Clapp, S., Chen, I.S., Ho, D.D. & Ammann, A.J. (1997). "Maternal HIV-1 viral load and vertical transmission of infection: the Ariel Project for the prevention of HIV transmission from mother to infant." Nat Med 3(5): 549-52.

Carrington, M., Nelson, G.W., Martin, M.P., Kissner, T., Vlahov, D., Goedert, J.J., Kaslow, R., Buchbinder, S., Hoots. K. & O'Brien, S.J. (1999). "HLA and HIV-1: heterozygote advantage and B*35-Cw*04 disadvantage." Science 283(5408): 1748-52.

Carrington, M. & O'Brien, S.J. (2003). "The influence of HLA genotype on AIDS." Annu Rev Med 54: 535-51.

Chaponda, M. & Pirmohamed, M. (2011). "Hypersensitivity reactions to HIV therapy." Br J Clin Pharmacol. 71(5):659-71.

Chakrabarti, L.A. & Simon, V. (2010). "Immune mechanisms of HIV control." Curr Opin Immunol 22(4): 488-96.

Chen, H., Li, C., Huang, J., Cung, T., Seiss, K., Beamon, J., Carrington, M.F., Porter, L.C., Burke, P.S., Yang, Y., Ryan, B.J., Liu, R., Weiss, R.H., Pereyra, F., Cress, W.D., Brass, A.L., Rosenberg, E.S., Walker, B.D., Yu, X.G. & Lichterfeld, M. (2011). "CD4+ T cells from elite controllers resist HIV-1 infection by selective upregulation of p21." J Clin Invest. 121(4): 1549-60.

Chopera, D.R., Mlotshwa, M., Woodman, Z., Mlisana, K., de Assis Rosa, D., Martin, D.P., Karim, S.A., Gray, C.M., Williamson, C. & the CAPRISA 002 Study Team. (2011) "Virological and immunological factors associated with HIV-1 differential disease progression in HLA-B*58:01 positive individuals." J Virol. 85(14):7070-7080

Connor, Sperling, R.S., Gelber, R., Kiselev, P., Scott, G., O'Sullivan, M.J., VanDyke, R., Bey, M., Shearer, W., Jacobson, R.L., Jimenez, E., O'Neill, E., Bazin, B., Delfraissy, J.F., Culnane, M., Coombs, R., Elkins, M., Moye, J., Stratton P. & Balsley, J., for the Pediatric AIDS Clinical Trials Group Protocol 076 Study Group (1994). "Reduction of maternal-infant transmission of human immunodeficiency virus type 1 with zidovudine treatment. Pediatric AIDS Clinical Trials Group Protocol 076 Study Group." N Engl J Med 331(18): 1173-80.

Coovadia, H. (2004). "Antiretroviral agents--how best to protect infants from HIV and save their mothers from AIDS." N Engl J Med 351(3): 289-92.

da Silva, E.M., Acosta, A.X., Santos, E.J., Netto, E.M., Lemaire, D.C., Oliveira, A.S., Barbosa, C.M., Bendicho, M.T., Galvão-Castro, B & Brites, C. (2010) "HLA-Bw4-B*57 and Cw*18 alleles are associated with plasma viral load modulation in HIV-1 infected individuals in Salvador, Brazil. "Braz J Infect Dis. 14(5):468-75.

Dalmasso, C., Carpentier, W., Meyer, L., Rouzioux, C., Goujard, C., Chaix, M.L., Lambotte, O., Avettand-Fenoel, V., Le Clerc, S., de Senneville, L.D., Deveau, C., Boufassa, F., Debré, P., Delfraissy, J.F., Broet, P., Theodorou, I. & ANRS Genome Wide Association 01. (2008). "Distinct genetic loci control plasma HIV-RNA and cellular HIV-DNA levels in HIV-1 infection: the ANRS Genome Wide Association 01 study." PLoS One 3(12): e3907.

de Groot, N. G., Heijmans, C.M., Zoet, Y.M., de Ru, A.H., Verreck, F.A., van Veelen, P.A., Drijfhout, J.W., Doxiadis, G.G., Remarque, E.J., Doxiadis, I.I., van Rood, J.J., Koning, F. & Bontrop, R.E.(2010). "AIDS-protective HLA-B*27/B*57 and chimpanzee MHC class I molecules target analogous conserved areas of HIV-1/SIVcpz." Proc Natl Acad Sci U S A 107(34): 15175-80.

De Maria, A., Cirillo, C. & Moretta, L. (1994). "Occurrence of human immunodeficiency virus type 1 (HIV-1)-specific cytolytic T cell activity in apparently uninfected children born to HIV-1-infected mothers." J Infect Dis 170(5): 1296-9.

De Rossi, A., Ometto, L., Masiero, S., Zanchetta, M. & Chieco-Bianchi, L. (1997). "Viral phenotype in mother-to-child HIV-1 transmission and disease progression of vertically acquired HIV-1 infection." Acta Paediatr Suppl 421: 22-8.

Dean, M., Carrington, M., Winkler, C., Huttley, G.A., Smith, M.W., Allikmets, R., Goedert, J.J., Buchbinder, S.P., Vittinghoff, E., Gomperts, E., Donfield, S., Vlahov, D., Kaslow, R., Saah, A., Rinaldo, C., Detels, R. & O'Brien, S.J. (1996). "Genetic restriction of HIV-1 infection and progression to AIDS by a deletion allele of the CKR5 structural gene. Hemophilia Growth and Development Study, Multicenter AIDS Cohort Study, Multicenter Hemophilia Cohort Study, San Francisco City Cohort, ALIVE Study." Science 273(5283): 1856-62.

den Uyl, D., van der Horst-Bruinsma, I.E. & van Agtmael, M. (2004). "Progression of HIV to AIDS: a protective role for HLA-B27?" AIDS Rev 6(2): 89-96.

Devash, Y., Calvelli, T.A., Wood, D.G., Reagan, K.J. & Rubinstein A. (1990). "Vertical transmission of human immunodeficiency virus is correlated with the absence of high-affinity/avidity maternal antibodies to the gp120 principal neutralizing domain." Proc Natl Acad Sci USA 87(9): 3445-9.

Doehle, B. P., F. Hladik, McNevin J.P., McElrath M.J. & Gale M. Jr. (2009). "Human immunodeficiency virus type 1 mediates global disruption of innate antiviral signaling and immune defenses within infected cells." J Virol 83(20): 10395-405.

Dollfus, C., Le Chenadec, J., Faye. A., Blanche. S., Briand, N., Rouzioux, C. & Warszawski, J. (2010). "Long-term outcomes in adolescents perinatally infected with HIV-1 and followed up since birth in the French perinatal cohort (EPF/ANRS CO10)." Clin Infect Dis 51(2): 214-24.

Fainardi, E., Castellazzi, M., Stignani, M., Morandi, F., Sana, G., Gonzalez, R., Pistoia, V., Baricordi, O.R., Sokal, E. & Peña, J. (2011). "Emerging topics and new perspectives on HLA-G". Cell Mol Life Sci. 68(3):433-51.

Fang, G., Kuiken C., Weiser B., Rowland-Jones S., Plummer F., Chen C.H., Kaul R.,Anzala A.O., Bwayo J., Kimani J, Philpott S.M., Kitchen C., Sinsheimer J.S., Gaschen B.,Lang D., Shi B., Kemal K.S., Rostron T., Brunner C., Beddows S., Sattenau Q., Paxinos E., Oyugi J. &Burger H. (2004). "Long-term survivors in Nairobi: complete HIV-1 RNA sequences and immunogenetic associations." J Infect Dis 190(4): 697-701.

Fauci, A. S. (1996). "Host factors and the pathogenesis of HIV-induced disease." Nature 384(6609): 529-34.

Fellay, J., K. V. Shianna, et al. (2007). "A whole-genome association study of major determinants for host control of HIV-1." Science 317(5840): 944-7.

Fellay, J., Frahm, N., Shianna, K.V., Cirulli, E.T., Casimiro, D.R., Robertson, M.N., Haynes, B.F., Geraghty, D.E., McElrath, M.J., Goldstein, D.B., National Institute of Allergy and Infectious Diseases Center for HIV/AIDS Vaccine Immunology & NIAID HIV Vaccine Trials Network (2011). "Host genetic determinants of T cell responses to the MRKAd5 HIV-1 gag/pol/nef vaccine in the step trial." J Infect Dis. 203(6):773-9

Fleury, S., Thibodeau, J., Croteau, G., Labrecque, N., Aronson, H.E., Cantin, C., Long, E.O. & Sékaly, R.P. (1995). "HLA-DR polymorphism affects the interaction with CD4." J Exp Med 182(3): 733-41.

Flores-Villanueva, P. O., Hendel, H., Caillat-Zucman, S., Rappaport, J., Burgos-Tiburcio, A., Bertin-Maghit, S., Ruiz-Morales, J.A., Teran, M.E., Rodriguez-Tafur & J., Zagury, J.F. (2003). "Associations of MHC ancestral haplotypes with resistance/susceptibility to AIDS disease development." J Immunol 170(4): 1925-9.

Gaudieri, S., Nolan, D., McKinnon, E., Witt, C.S., Mallal, S. & Christiansen, F.T. (2005). "Associations between KIR epitope combinations expressed by HLA-B/-C haplotypes found in an HIV-1 infected study population may influence NK mediated immune responses." Mol Immunol 42(4): 557-60.

Goulder, P. J., Brander, C., Tang, Y., Tremblay, C., Colbert, R.A., Addo, M.M., Rosenberg, E.S., Nguyen, T., Allen, R., Trocha, A., Altfeld, M., He, S., Bunce, M., Funkhouser, R., Pelton, S.I., Burchett, S.K., McIntosh, K., Korber, B.T. & Walker, B.D. (2001). "Evolution and transmission of stable CTL escape mutations in HIV infection." Nature 412(6844): 334-8.

Greenberg, M. E., Iafrate, A.J. & Skowronski, J. (1998). "The SH3 domain-binding surface and an acidic motif in HIV-1 Nef regulate trafficking of class I MHC complexes." Embo J 17(10): 2777-89.

Greggio, N. A., Cameran, M., Giaquinto, C., Zacchello, F., Koroliuk, D. & Colizzi, V. (1993). "DNA HLA-DRB1 analysis in children of positive mothers and estimated risk of vertical HIV transmission." Dis Markers 11(1): 29-35.

de Groot, N.G., Heijmans, C.M., Zoet, Y.M., de Ru, A.H., Verreck, F.A., van Veelen, P.A., Drijfhout, J.W., Doxiadis, G.G., Remarque, E.J., Doxiadis, I.I., van Rood, J.J., Koning, F. & Bontrop, R.E. (2010). "AIDS-protective HLA-B*27/B*57 and chimpanzee MHC class I molecules target analogous conserved areas of HIV-1/SIVcpz." Proc Natl Acad Sci U S A. 107(34):15175-80.

Handunnetthi, L., Ramagopalan, S.V., Ebers, G.C. & Knight, J.C. (2010). "Regulation of major histocompatibility complex class II gene expression, genetic variation and disease." Genes Immun 11(2): 99-112.

Harmon, B., Campbell, N. & Ratner, L. (2010). "Role of Abl kinase and the Wave2 signaling complex in HIV-1 entry at a post-hemifusion step." PLoS Pathog 6(6): e1000956.

Hengel, R. L., Kennedy, M.S., Steketee, R.W., Thea, D.M., Abrams, E.J., Lambert, G. & McDougal, J.S. (1998). "Neutralizing antibody and perinatal transmission of human immunodeficiency virus type 1. New York City Perinatal HIV Transmission Collaborative Study Group." AIDS Res Hum Retroviruses 14(6): 475-81.

Hertz, T., Nolan, D., James, I., John, M., Gaudieri, S., Phillips, E., Huang, J.C., Riadi, G., Mallal, S. & Jojic, N. (2011). "Mapping the landscape of host-pathogen coevolution: HLA class I binding and its relationship with evolutionary conservation in human and viral proteins." J Virol. 85(3):1310-21.

Hill, A. V. (1998). "The immunogenetics of human infectious diseases." Annu Rev Immunol 16: 593-617.

Huang, J., Goedert, J.J., Sundberg, E.J., Cung, T.D., Burke, P.S., Martin, M.P., Preiss, L., Lifson, J., Lichterfeld, M., Carrington, M. & Yu, X.G. (2009). "HLA-B*35-Px-mediated acceleration of HIV-1 infection by increased inhibitory immunoregulatory impulses." J Exp Med 206(13): 2959-66.

Hunt, J. S., Petroff, M.G., Morales, P., Sedlmayr, P., Geraghty, D.E. & Ober, C. (2000). "HLA-G in reproduction: studies on the maternal-fetal interface." Hum Immunol 61(11): 1113-7.

Itescu, S., Rose, S., Dwyer, E. & Winchester, R. (1995). "Grouping HLA-B locus serologic specificities according to shared structural motifs suggests that different peptide-anchoring pockets may have contrasting influences on the course of HIV-1 infection." Hum Immunol 42(1): 81-9.

Jin, X., Gao, X., Ramanathan, M.Jr, Deschenes, G.R., Nelson, G.W., O'Brien, S.J., Goedert, J.J., Ho, D.D., O'Brien, T.R. & Carrington, M. (2002). "Human immunodeficiency virus type 1 (HIV-1)-specific CD8+-T-cell responses for groups of HIV-1-infected individuals with different HLA-B*35 genotypes." J Virol 76(24): 12603-10.

Jin, X., Roberts, C.G., Nixon, D.F., Cao, Y., Ho, D.D., Walker, B.D., Muldoon, M., Korber, B.T. & Koup, R.A. (1998). "Longitudinal and cross-sectional analysis of cytotoxic T lymphocyte responses and their relationship to vertical human immunodeficiency virus transmission. ARIEL Project Investigators." J Infect Dis 178(5): 1317-26.

John, G. C., Rousseau, C., Dong, T., Rowland-Jones, S., Nduati, R., Mbori-Ngacha, D., Rostron, T., Kreiss, J.K., Richardson, B.A. & Overbaugh, J. (2000). "Maternal SDF1 3'A polymorphism is associated with increased perinatal human immunodeficiency virus type 1 transmission." J Virol 74(12): 5736-9.

John, M., Moore CB, James IR, Mallal SA.. (2005). "Interactive selective pressures of HLA-restricted immune responses and antiretroviral drugs on HIV-1." Antivir Ther 10(4): 551-5.

Julg, B., Moodley, E.S., Qi, Y., Ramduth, D., Reddy, S., Mncube, Z., Gao, X., Goulder, P.J., Detels, R., Ndung'u, T., Walker, B.D. & Carrington, M. (2011) "Possession of HLA class II DRB1*1303 associates with reduced viral loads in chronic HIV-1 clade C and B infection." J Infect Dis. 203(6):803-9.

Just, J. J. (1995a). "Genetic predisposition to HIV-1 infection and acquired immune deficiency virus syndrome: a review of the literature examining associations with HLA [corrected]." Hum Immunol 44(3): 156-69.

Just, J. J., Abrams, E., Louie, L.G., Urbano, R., Wara, D., Nicholas, S.W., Stein, Z., King, M.C. (1995b). "Influence of host genotype on progression to acquired immunodeficiency syndrome among children infected with human immunodeficiency virus type 1." J Pediatr 127(4): 544-9.

Just, J. J., Casabona, J., Bertrán, J., Montané, C., Fortuny, C., Rodrigo, C., Mur, A., Bosque, M., Jovane, L. & King, M.C. (1996). "MHC class II alleles associated with clinical and immunological manifestations of HIV-1 infection among children in Catalonia, Spain." Tissue Antigens 47(4): 313-8.

Kalams, S.A. & Walker, B.D. (1998). "The critical need for CD4 help in maintaining effective cytotoxic T lymphocyte responses." J Exp Med 188(12): 2199-204.

Kantor, R. & Lloyd, R. (2002). Comparaison of mother to child transmission (MTCT) and genotypic resistance in HIV-1 subtypes A, C and D and after single dose nevirapine (sd-NVP) in Africa. 9th Conference on Retroviruses and Opportunistic Infections. Seattle.

Kaslow, R. A., Carrington, M., Apple, R., Park, L., Muñoz, A., Saah, A.J., Goedert, J.J., Winkler, C., O'Brien, S.J., Rinaldo, C., Detels, R., Blattner, W., Phair, J., Erlich & H., Mann, D.L. (1996). "Influence of combinations of human major histocompatibility complex genes on the course of HIV-1 infection." Nat Med 2(4): 405-11.

Kaur, G. & Mehra, N. (2009). "Genetic determinants of HIV-1 infection and progression to AIDS: immune response genes." Tissue Antigens 74(5): 373-85.

Kawana, A., Tomiyama, H., Takiguchi, M., Shioda, T., Nakamura, T., Iwamoto, A. (1999). "Accumulation of specific amino acid substitutions in HLA-B35-restricted human immunodeficiency virus type 1 cytotoxic T lymphocyte epitopes." AIDS Res Hum Retroviruses 15(12): 1099-107.

Kawashima, Y., Pfafferott, K., Frater, J., Matthews, P., Payne, R., Addo, M., Gatanaga, H., Fujiwara, M., Hachiya, A., Koizumi, H., Kuse, N., Oka, S., Duda, A., Prendergast, A., Crawford, H., Leslie, A., Brumme, Z., Brumme, C., Allen, T., Brander, C., Kaslow, R., Tang, J., Hunter, E., Allen, S., Mulenga, J., Branch, S., Roach, T., John, M., Mallal, S., Ogwu, A., Shapiro, R., Prado, J.G., Fidler, S., Weber, J., Pybus, O.G., Klenerman, P., Ndung'u, T., Phillips, R., Heckerman, D., Harrigan, P.R., Walker, B.D., Takiguchi, M. & Goulder, P. (2009). "Adaptation of HIV-1 to human leukocyte antigen class I." Nature 458(7238): 641-5.

Kesson, A.M., Fear, W.R., Kazazi, F., Mathijs, J.M., Chang, J., King, N.J. & Cunningham, A.L. (1993). "Human immunodeficiency virus type 1 infection of human placental macrophages in vitro." J Infect Dis 168(3): 571-9.

Kilpatrick, D.C., Hague, R.A., Yap, P.L. & Mok, J.Y. (1991). "HLA antigen frequencies in children born to HIV-infected mothers." Dis Markers 9(1): 21-6.

Klein, M.R., Keet, I.P., D'Amaro, J., Bende, R.J., Hekman, A., Mesman, B., Koot, M., de Waal, L.P., Coutinho, R.A. & Miedema, F. (1994). "Associations between HLA frequencies and pathogenic features of human immunodeficiency virus type 1 infection in seroconverters from the Amsterdam cohort of homosexual men." J Infect Dis 169(6): 1244-9.

Klenerman, P. & McMichael, A. (2007). "AIDS/HIV. Finding footprints among the trees." Science 315(5818): 1505-7.

Kostrikis, L. G., Neumann, A.U., Thomson, B., Korber, B.T., McHardy, P., Karanicolas, R., Deutsch, L., Huang, Y., Lew, J.F., McIntosh, K., Pollack, H., Borkowsky, W., Spiegel, H.M., Palumbo, P., Oleske, J., Bardeguez, A., Luzuriaga, K., Sullivan, J., Wolinsky, S.M., Koup, R.A., Ho, D.D. & Moore, J.P. (1999). "A polymorphism in the regulatory region of the CC-chemokine receptor 5 gene influences perinatal transmission of human immunodeficiency virus type 1 to African-American infants." J Virol 73(12): 10264-71.

Kovats, S., Main, E.K., Librach, C., Stubblebine, M., Fisher, S.J. & DeMars, R. (1990). "A class I antigen, HLA-G, expressed in human trophoblasts." Science 248(4952): 220-3.

Kuhn, L., Abrams, E.J., Matheson, P.B., Thomas, P.A., Lambert, G., Bamji, M., Greenberg, B., Steketee, R.W. & Thea, DM. (1997). "Timing of maternal-infant HIV transmission: associations between intrapartum factors and early polymerase chain reaction results. New York City Perinatal HIV Transmission Collaborative Study Group." Aids 11(4): 429-35.

Kuhn, L., Abrams, E.J., Palumbo, P., Bulterys, M., Aga, R., Louie, L., Hodge, T.; Perinatal AIDS Collaborative Transmission Study. (2004). "Maternal versus paternal inheritance of HLA class I alleles among HIV-infected children: consequences for clinical disease progression." Aids 18(9): 1281-9.

Kuhn, L., Steketee, R.W., Weedon, J., Abrams, E.J., Lambert, G., Bamji, M., Schoenbaum, E., Farley, J., Nesheim, S.R., Palumbo, P., Simonds, R.J. & Thea, D.M. (1999). "Distinct risk factors for intrauterine and intrapartum human immunodeficiency virus transmission and consequences for disease progression in infected children. Perinatal AIDS Collaborative Transmission Study." J Infect Dis 179(1): 52-8.

Kulkarni, S., Savan, R., Qi, Y., Gao, X., Yuki, Y., Bass, S.E., Martin, M.P., Hunt, P., Deeks, S.G., Telenti, A., Pereyra, F., Goldstein, D., Wolinsky, S., Walker, B., Young, H.A. & Carrington, M. (2011). "Differential microRNA regulation of HLA-C expression and its association with HIV control." Nature. 472(7344):495-8.

Lazaryan, A., Song, W., Lobashevsky, E., Tang, J., Shrestha, S., Zhang, K., McNicholl, J.M., Gardner, L.I., Wilson, C.M., Klein, R.S., Rompalo, A., Mayer, K., Sobel, J., Kaslow, R.A.; HIV Epidemiology Research Study Group; Reaching for Excellence in Adolescent Care and Health Study Group. (2011). "The influence of human leukocyte antigen class I alleles and their population frequencies on human immunodeficiency virus type 1 control among African Americans". Hum Immunol. 72 (4):312-8.

Leslie, A., Kavanagh, D., Honeyborne, I., Pfafferott, K., Edwards, C., Pillay, T., Hilton, L., Thobakgale, C., Ramduth, D., Draenert, R., Le Gall, S., Luzzi, G., Edwards, A., Brander, C., Sewell, A.K., Moore, S., Mullins, J., Moore, C., Mallal, S., Bhardwaj, N., Yusim, K., Phillips, R., Klenerman, P., Korber, B., Kiepiela, P., Walker, B. & Goulder, P. (2005). "Transmission and accumulation of CTL escape variants drive negative associations between HIV polymorphisms and HLA." J Exp Med 201(6): 891-902.

Leslie, A., Matthews, P.C., Listgarten, J., Carlson, J.M., Kadie, C., Ndung'u, T., Brander, C., Coovadia, H., Walker, B.D., Heckerman, D. & Goulder, P.J. (2010) "Additive contribution of HLA class I alleles in the immune control of HIV-1 infection." J Virol 84(19): 9879-88.

Leslie, A.J. & Goulder, P.J. (2006). "HIV escape and attenuation by cytotoxic T lymphocytes." Curr Opin HIV AIDS 1(1): 34-39.

Liu, C., Carrington, M., Kaslow, R.A., Gao, X., Rinaldo, C.R., Jacobson, L.P., Margolick, J.B., Phair, J., O'Brien, S.J. & Detels, R. (2003). "Association of polymorphisms in human leukocyte antigen class I and transporter associated with antigen processing genes with resistance to human immunodeficiency virus type 1 infection." J Infect Dis 187(9): 1404-10.

Liu, R., Paxton, W.A., Choe, S., Ceradini, D., Martin, S.R., Horuk, R., MacDonald, M.E., Stuhlmann, H., Koup, R.A. & Landau, N.R. (1996). "Homozygous defect in HIV-1 coreceptor accounts for resistance of some multiply-exposed individuals to HIV-1 infection." Cell 86(3): 367-77.

Lombard, Z., Brune, A.E., Hoal, E.G., Babb, C., Van Helden, P.D., Epplen, J.T. & Bornman, L. (2006). "HLA class II disease associations in southern Africa." Tissue Antigens 67(2): 97-110.

Lopez-Vazquez, A., Miña-Blanco, A., Martínez-Borra, J., Njobvu, P.D., Suárez-Alvarez, B., Blanco-Gelaz, M.A., González, S., Rodrigo, L. & López-Larrea, C. (2005). "Interaction between KIR3DL1 and HLA-B*57 supertype alleles influences the progression of HIV-1 infection in a Zambian population." Hum Immunol 66(3): 285-9.

Louisirirotchanakul, S., Beddows, S., Cheingsong, R., Shaffer, N., Mastro, T.D., Likanonsakul, S., Wasi, C., Taylor, G.P. & Weber, J.N. (1999). "Role of maternal humoral immunity in vertical transmission of HIV-1 subtype E in Thailand." J Acquir Immune Defic Syndr 21(4): 259-65.

MacDonald, K. S., Embree, J., Njenga, S., Nagelkerke, N.J., Ngatia, I., Mohammed, Z., Barber, B.H., Ndinya-Achola, J., Bwayo, J. & Plummer, F.A. (1998). "Mother-child class I HLA concordance increases perinatal human immunodeficiency virus type 1 transmission." J Infect Dis 177(3): 551-6.

MacDonald, K. S., Matukas, L., Embree, J.E., Fowke, K., Kimani, J., Nagelkerke, N.J., Oyugi, J., Kiama, P., Kaul, R., Luscher, M.A., Rowland-Jones, S., Ndinya-Achola, J., Ngugi, E., Bwayo, J.J. & Plummer, F.A. (2001). "Human leucocyte antigen supertypes and immune susceptibility to HIV-1, implications for vaccine design." Immunol Lett 79(1-2): 151-7.

Mallal, S., Nolan, D., Witt, C., Masel, G., Martin, A.M., Moore, C., Sayer, D., Castley, A., Mamotte, C., Maxwell, D., James, I. & Christiansen, F.T. (2002). "Association between presence of HLA-B*5701, HLA-DR7, and HLA-DQ3 and hypersensitivity to HIV-1 reverse-transcriptase inhibitor abacavir." Lancet 359(9308): 727-32.

Mangano, A., Kopka, J., Batalla, M., Bologna, R. & Sen, L. (2000). "Protective effect of CCR2-64I and not of CCR5-delta32 and SDF1-3'A in pediatric HIV-1 infection." J Acquir Immune Defic Syndr 23(1): 52-7.

Mann, D. L., Carrington, M., O'Donnell, M., Miller, T. & Goedert, J. (1992). "HLA phenotype is a factor in determining rate of disease progression and outcome in HIV-1-infected individuals." AIDS Res Hum Retroviruses 8(8): 1345-6.

Matt, C. & Roger, M. (2001). "Genetic determinants of pediatric HIV-1 infection: vertical transmission and disease progression among children." Mol Med 7(9): 583-9.

Matte, C., Zijenah, L.S., Lacaille, J., Ward, B. & Roger, M. (2002). "Mother-to-child human leukocyte antigen G concordance: no impact on the risk of vertical transmission of HIV-1." Aids 16(18): 2491-4.

McMichael, A. J. (2007). "Triple bypass: complicated paths to HIV escape." J Exp Med 204(12): 2785-8.

McNeil, A. J., Yap, P.L., Gore, S.M., Brettle, R.P., McColl, M., Wyld, R., Davidson, S., Weightman, R., Richardson, A.M. & Robertson, J.R. (1996). "Association of HLA types A1-B8-DR3 and B27 with rapid and slow progression of HIV disease." Qjm 89(3): 177-85.

McNicholl, J. M., Smith, D.K., Qari, S.H. & Hodge, T. (1997). "Host genes and HIV: the role of the chemokine receptor gene CCR5 and its allele." Emerg Infect Dis 3(3): 261-71.

Melvin, A. J., Burchett, S.K., Watts, D.H., Hitti, J., Hughes, J.P., McLellan, C.L., King, P.D., Johnson, E.J., Williams, B.L., Frenkel, L.M. & Coombs, R.W. (1997). "Effect of pregnancy and zidovudine therapy on viral load in HIV-1-infected women." J Acquir Immune Defic Syndr Hum Retrovirol 14(3): 232-6.

Migueles, S. A., Sabbaghian, M.S., Shupert, W.L., Bettinotti, M.P., Marincola, F.M., Martino, L., Hallahan, C.W., Selig, S.M., Schwartz, D., Sullivan, J. & Connors, M. (2000). "HLA B*5701 is highly associated with restriction of virus replication in a subgroup of HIV-infected long term nonprogressors." Proc Natl Acad Sci U S A 97(6): 2709-14.

Mittleman, B.B. & Shearer, G.M. (1996). "Mother-to-infant transmission of HIV type 1: role of major histocompatibility antigen differences." AIDS Res Hum Retroviruses 12(15): 1397-400.

Miyazawa, M., Lopalco, L., Mazzotta, F., Lo Caputo, S., Veas, F. & Clerici, M; ESN Study Group. (2009). "The 'immunologic advantage' of HIV-exposed seronegative individuals." Aids 23(2): 161-75.

Miyazawa, M., Tsuji-Kawahara, S. & Kanari, Y. (2008). "Host genetic factors that control immune responses to retrovirus infections." Vaccine 26(24): 2981-96.

Moore, C. B., John, M., James, I.R., Christiansen, F.T., Witt, C.S. & Mallal, S.A. (2002). "Evidence of HIV-1 adaptation to HLA-restricted immune responses at a population level." Science 296(5572): 1439-43.

Nduati, R., John, G., Mbori-Ngacha, D., Richardson, B., Overbaugh, J., Mwatha, A., Ndinya-Achola, J., Bwayo, J., Onyango, F.E., Hughes, J., Kreiss, J. (2000). "Effect of breastfeeding and formula feeding on transmission of HIV-1: a randomized clinical trial." JAMA 283(9): 1167-74.

Newberry, Y. & Kelsey, J.J. (2003). "Mother to Child Transmission of HIV." Journal of Pharmacy Practice 16(3): 182-190.

Ogg, G. S., Jin, X., Bonhoeffer, S., Dunbar PR, Nowak MA, Monard S, Segal JP, Cao Y, Rowland-Jones SL, Cerundolo V, Hurley A, Markowitz M, Ho DD, Nixon DF, McMichael AJ. (1998). "Quantitation of HIV-1-specific cytotoxic T lymphocytes and plasma load of viral RNA." Science 279(5359): 2103-6.

Okamoto, Y., Shiosaki, K., Eda, Y., Tokiyoshi, S., Yamaguchi, Y., Gojobori, T., Hachimori, T., Yamazaki, S. & Hondo, M. (1997). "Father-to-mother-to-infant transmission of HIV-1: clonally transmitted isolate of infant mutates more rapidly than that of the mother and rapidly loses reactivity with neutralizing antibody." Microbiol Immunol 41(2): 131-8.

Paximadis, M., Minevich, G., Winchester, R., Schramm, D.B., Gray, G.E., Sherman, G.G., Coovadia, A.H., Kuhn, L. & Tiemessen, C.T. (2011). "KIR-HLA and maternal-infant HIV-1 transmission in sub-Saharan Africa." PLoS One. 6(2):e16541

Pereyra, F., Jia, X., McLaren, P.J., Telenti, A. & the International HIV Controllers Study Group (2010). "The major genetic determinants of HIV-1 control affect HLA class I peptide presentation." Science 330(6010): 1551-7.

Phillips, R. E., Phillips, R.E., Rowland-Jones, S., Nixon, D.F., Gotch, F.M., Edwards, J.P., Ogunlesi, A.O., Elvin, J.G., Rothbard, J.A., Bangham, C.R.M., Rizza, C.R. & McMichael, A.J. (1991). "Human immunodeficiency virus genetic variation that can escape cytotoxic T cell recognition." Nature 354(6353): 453-9.Pillay, T. & Phillips, R.E. (2005). "Adaptive evolution in perinatal HIV-1." Best Pract Res Clin Obstet Gynaecol 19(2): 211-29.

Plaeger, S., Bermudez, S., Mikyas, Y., Harawa, N., Dickover, R., Mark, D., Dillon, M., Bryson, Y.J., Boyer, P.J., Sinsheimer, J.S. "Decreased CD8 cell-mediated viral suppression and other immunologic characteristics of women who transmit human immunodeficiency virus to their infants." J Infect Dis 179(6): 1388-94.

Polycarpou, A., Ntais, C., Korber, B.T., Elrich, H.A., Winchester, R., Krogstad, P., Wolinsky, S., Rostron, T., Rowland-Jones, S.L., Ammann, A.J. & Ioannidis, J.P.; Ariel Project. (2002). "Association between maternal and infant class I and II HLA alleles and of their concordance with the risk of perinatal HIV type 1 transmission." AIDS Res Hum Retroviruses 18(11): 741-6.

Price, P., Witt, C., Allcock, R., Sayer, D., Garlepp, M., Kok, C.C., French, M., Mallal, S. & Christiansen, F. (1999). "The genetic basis for the association of the 8.1 ancestral haplotype (A1, B8, DR3) with multiple immunopathological diseases." Immunol Rev 167: 257-74.

Reitter, J. N., Means, R.E. & Desrosiers, R.C. (1998). "A role for carbohydrates in immune evasion in AIDS." Nat Med 4(6): 679-84.

Richman, D. D., Wrin, T., Little, S.J. & Petropoulos, C.J. (2003). "Rapid evolution of the neutralizing antibody response to HIV type 1 infection." Proc Natl Acad Sci U S A 100(7): 4144-9.

Rogers, M. F. & Shaffer, N. (1999). "Reducing the risk of maternal-infant transmission of HIV by attacking the virus." N Engl J Med 341(6): 441-3.

Rossi, P., Moschese, V., Broliden, P.A., Fundar, C., Quintin, I, Plebani, I., Giaquinto, C., Tovott, P.A., Ijunggren, K., Rosen, J., Wigzell, H., Jondal, M., & Wahrent, J. (1989). "Presence of maternal antibodies to human immunodeficiency virus 1 envelope glycoprotein gp120 epitopes correlates with the uninfected status of children born to seropositive mothers." Proc Natl Acad Sci U S A 86(20): 8055-8.

Rudd, P. M., Elliott, T., Cresswell, P., Wilson, I.A. & Dwek, R.A. (2001). "Glycosylation and the immune system." Science 291(5512): 2370-6.

Saathoff, E., Pritsch, M., Geldmacher, C., Hoffmann, O., Koehler, R.N., Maboko, L., Maganga, L., Geis, S., McCutchan, F.E., Kijak, G.H., Kim, J.H., Arroyo, M.A., Gerhardt, M., Tovanabutra, S., Robb, M.L., Williamson, C., Michael, N.L. & Hoelscher, M. (2010). "Viral and host factors associated with the HIV-1 viral load setpoint in adults from Mbeya Region, Tanzania." J Acquir Immune Defic Syndr. 54(3):324-30.

Salgado, M., López-Romero, P., Callejas, S., López, M., Labarga, P., Dopazo, A., Soriano, V. & Rodés, B. (2011a). "Characterization of host genetic expression patterns in HIV-infected individuals with divergent disease progression." Virology 411(1): 103-12.

Salgado, M., Simón, A., Sanz-Minguela, B., Rallón, N.I., López, M., Vicario, J.L., Benito,J.M. & Rodés, B. (2011b). "An additive effect of protective host genetic factors correlates with HIV nonprogression status." Acquir Immune Defic Syndr. 56(4):300-5.

Samson, M., Libert, F., Doranz, B.J., Rucker, J., Liesnard, C., Farber, C.M., Saragosti, S., Lapoumeroulie, C., Cognaux, J., Forceille, C., Muyldermans, G., Verhofstede, C., Burtonboy, G., Georges, M., Imai, T., Rana, S., Yi, Y., Smyth, R.J., Collman, R.G., Doms, R.W., Vassart, G. & Parmentier, M. (1996). "Resistance to HIV-1 infection in caucasian individuals bearing mutant alleles of the CCR-5 chemokine receptor gene." Nature 382(6593): 722-5.

Scorza Smeraldi, R., Fabio, G., Lazzarin, A., Eisera, N.B., Moroni, M. & Zanussi, C. (1986). "HLA-associated susceptibility to acquired immunodeficiency syndrome in Italian patients with human-immunodeficiency-virus infection." Lancet 2(8517): 1187-9.

Selvaraj, P., S. Swaminathan, S., Alagarasu, K., Raghavan, S., Narendran, G. & Narayanan P. (2006). "Association of human leukocyte antigen-A11 with resistance and B40 and DR2 with susceptibility to HIV-1 infection in south India." J Acquir Immune Defic Syndr 43(4): 497-9.

Shankarkumar, U. (2004). "HIV and human leukocyte antigen association--the Indian scenario." J HIV Ther 9(3): 60-4.

Shankarkumar, U., Thakar, M., Mehendale, S., Praranjape, R.S. & Mohanty, D. (2003). "Association of HLA B*3520, B*1801, and Cw*1507 with HIV-1 infection Maharashtra, India." J Acquir Immune Defic Syndr 34(1): 113-4.

Shao, W., Lazaryan A., Dorak M.T., Penman-Aguilar A., Wilson C.M., Margolick J.B., Goedert J.J., Prins M., Tang J. & Kaslow R.A. (2006). "Cohort- and time-specific associations of CTLA4 genotypes with HIV-1 disease progression." Aids 20(12): 1583-90.

Sharon, D., Chen, R. & Snyder, M. (2010). "Systems biology approaches to disease marker discovery." Dis Markers 28(4): 209-24.

Shearer, W. T., Quinn, T.C., LaRussa, P., Lew, J.F., Mofenson, L., Almy, S., Rich, K., Handelsman, E., Diaz, C., Pagano, M., Smeriglio, V., Kalish, L.A. (1997). "Viral load and disease progression in infants infected with human immunodeficiency virus type 1. Women and Infants Transmission Study Group." N Engl J Med 336(19): 1337-42.

Sidney, J., Peters, B., Frahm, N., Brander, C. & Sette, A. HLA class I supertypes: a revised and updated classification. BMC Immunol. 2008 22(9):1.

Singh, K.K. & Spector, S.A. (2009). "Host genetic determinants of human immunodeficiency virus infection and disease progression in children." Pediatr Res 65(5 Pt 2): 55R-63R.

Smith, A. J., Schacker, T.W., Reilly, C.S., Haase, A.T. (2010). "A role for syndecan-1 and claudin-2 in microbial translocation during HIV-1 infection." J Acquir Immune Defic Syndr 55(3): 306-15.

Smith, M. W., Dean, M., Carrington, M., Winkler, C., Huttley, G.A., Lomb, D.A., Goedert, J.J., O'Brien, T.R., Jacobson, L.P., Kaslow, R., Buchbinder, S., Vittinghoff, E., Vlahov, D., Hoots, K., Hilgartner, M.W., & O'Brien, S.J. (1997). "Contrasting genetic influence of CCR2 and CCR5 variants on HIV-1 infection and disease progression. Hemophilia Growth and Development Study (HGDS), Multicenter AIDS Cohort Study (MACS), Multicenter Hemophilia Cohort Study (MHCS), San Francisco City Cohort (SFCC), ALIVE Study." Science 277(5328): 959-65.

Soumelis, V., Scott, I., Gheyas, F., Bouhour, D., Cozon, G,, Cotte, L., Huang, L., Levy, J.A. & Liu, Y.J. (2001). "Depletion of circulating natural type 1 interferon-producing cells in HIV-infected AIDS patients." Blood 98(4): 906-12.

Stephens, H. A. (2005). "HIV-1 diversity versus HLA class I polymorphism." Trends Immunol 26(1): 41-7.

Svejgaard, A., Platz, P. & Ryder, L.P. (1983). "HLA and disease 1982--a survey." Immunol Rev 70: 193-218.

Telenti, A. & McLaren, P."Genomic approaches to the study of HIV-1 acquisition." J Infect Dis 202 Suppl 3: S382-6.

Thomson, G. & Bodmer, W. (1979). "HLA haplotype associations with disease." Tissue Antigens 13(2): 91-102.

Tosi, G., Bozzo, L. & Accolla, R.S. (2009). "The dual function of the MHC class II transactivator CIITA against HTLV retroviruses." Front Biosci 14: 4149-56.

Trachtenberg, E., Korber, B., Sollars, C., Kepler, T.B., Hraber, P.T., Hayes, E., Funkhouser, R., Fugate, M., Theiler, J., Hsu, Y.S., Kunstman, K., Wu, S., Phair, J., Erlich, H. & Wolinsky, S. (2003). "Advantage of rare HLA supertype in HIV disease progression." Nat Med 9(7): 928-35.

Tripathi, P. & Agrawal, S. (2007). "Immunobiology of human imunodeficiency virus infection." Indian J Med Microbiol 25(4): 311-22.

Tripathi, P. & Agrawal, S. (2007). "The role of human leukocyte antigen E and G in HIV infection." Aids 21(11): 1395-404.

UNAIDS (2010). UNAIDS report on the global AIDS epidemic.

Wei, X., Wei, X., Ghosh, S.K., Taylor, M.E., Johnson, V.A., Emini, E.A., Deutsch, P., Lifson, J.D., Bonhoeffer, S., Nowak, M.A., Hahn, B.H., Saag, M.S. & Shaw, G.M. (1995). "Viral dynamics in human immunodeficiency virus type 1 infection." Nature 373(6510): 117-22.

Welzel, T. M., Gao, X., Pfeiffer, R.M., Martin, M.P., O'Brien, S.J., Goedert, J.J., Carrington, M. & O'Brien, T.R. (2007). "HLA-B Bw4 alleles and HIV-1 transmission in heterosexual couples." Aids 21(2): 225-9.

Welles, S. L., Pitt, J., Colgrove, R., McIntosh, K., Chung, P.H., Colson, A., Lockman, S., Fowler, M.G., Hanson, C., Landesman, S., Moye, J., Rich, K.C., Zorrilla, C., Japour, A.J. (2000). "HIV-1 genotypic zidovudine drug resistance and the risk of maternal--infant transmission in the women and infants transmission study. The Women and Infants Transmission Study Group." Aids 14(3): 263-71.

Winchester, R., Chen, Y., Rose, S., Selby, J. & Borkowsky, W. (1995). "Major histocompatibility complex class II DR alleles DRB1*1501 and those encoding HLA-DR13 are preferentially associated with a diminution in maternally transmitted human immunodeficiency virus 1 infection in different ethnic groups: determination by an automated sequence-based typing method." Proc Natl Acad Sci U S A 92(26): 12374-8.

Woc-Colburn, L., Smultea, L., Ramachandra, L. & Canaday, D.H. (2010). "Preserved MHC class II antigen processing in monocytes from HIV-infected individuals." PLoS One 5(3): e9491.

Wyatt, R., Kwong, P.D., Desjardins, E., Sweet, R.W., Robinson, J., Hendrickson, W.A. & Sodroski, J.G. (1998). "The antigenic structure of the HIV gp120 envelope glycoprotein." Nature 393(6686): 705-11.

Zhang, L., Zhang, X., Ma, Q. & Zhou, H. (2010). "Host proteome research in HIV infection." Genomics Proteomics Bioinformatics 8(1): 1-9.

9

Impact of HIV Infection and HAART Therapy on CD4 T Helper Cell Subset Expression and Function

Christina Guzzo*, Nor Fazila Che Mat*, Xiubo Zhang* and Katrina Gee
Department of Biomedical and Molecular Sciences, Queen's University, Kingston, ON Canada

1. Introduction

1.1 Th cell development

Regulation of T helper (Th) cell differentiation and proliferation depends on which cytokines are present in the microenvironment of a naïve Th cell. Induction of specific transcription factors results in programming of the naïve Th0 cell into one of several subsets. Currently there are four well characterized Th cell subsets, namely Th1, Th2, Th17, and the T regulatory (Treg) cells (Figure 1). In this chapter we will be focusing on the Th1, Th17, and Treg cell populations. However, at this point it is also worth mentioning the relatively newly described Th9 and follicular (Tfh) cell subsets. Here we briefly discuss the differentiation pathways taken by a Th0 cell that ultimately results in the formation of these different subsets.

Since the early 1980's, the Th1/Th2 paradigm has been well-studied. Th1 cells are known for expression of the signature cytokine IFN-γ and resulting anti-viral activities. The necessary driving cytokine for these cells is IL-12 in conjunction with the Th1-specific transcription factor T-bet (Hsieh, Macatonia et al., 1993; Seder, Gazzinelli et al., 1993;Szabo, Sullivan et al., 2002). IL-27, related to IL-12, has been recently shown to play a role in the induction of Th1 cells, while also actively repressing development of other subsets. On the other hand, Th2 cells are largely recognized to support humoral immunity and are induced by the presence of IL-4 and resulting activation of the STAT6 transcription factor(Kaplan, Schindler et al., 1996;Kurata, Lee et al., 1999). Equally important is the activation of the GATA binding protein 3 (GATA-3), the main regular of Th2 development (Pai, Truitt et al., 2004;Zhu, Min et al., 2004). The newly defined Th17 cells have been implicated in a number of inflammatory disorders and are recognized as key Th cells that trigger massive proinflammatory responses. They are characterized by production of IL-17 and differentiation of these cells requires both tumor growth factor (TGF)-β and IL-6 which act together to promote development of the Th17 subset (Bettelli, Carrier et al., 2006; Mangan, Harrington et al., 2006). Additionally important to the generation of these cells is IL-23, which functions to aid in the development and proliferation of Th17 cells. The key transcription factors required belong to the retinoic acid-related orphan receptors (ROR)

---

* Authors contributed equally to this work.

family; both ROR-α and RORγt have been shown to be critical to Th17 development (Yang, Pappu et al., 2008). The Treg cell subset is crucial to the regulation of immune responses as these cells play a suppressive role, mainly via the expression of the anti-inflammatory cytokine IL-10. These cell subsets are unique from the other subsets as they can be formed either in the thymus (known as "naturally" occurring Tregs or nTreg) or as a result of TGF-β stimulation and T cell receptor (TCR) triggering (known as "inducible" Tregs or iTreg)(Murai, Krause et al., 2010). The main transcription factor for the development of these cells is Foxp3 which is only expressed in Treg cells (Zheng & Rudensky, 2007). Th9 cells have been recently identified as IL-21-dependent CD4 T cells producing IL-9, although a key function has yet to be identified for these cells, it appears that they may be involved in inflammation and allergy (Xing, Wu et al., 2011; Ma, Tangye et al., 2010; Wong, Ye et al., 2010). The Tfh cells are newly defined to be efficient producers of IL-10 and IL-21 (Suto, Kashiwakuma et al., 2008; Crotty, 2011). These cells generally express high levels of CXCR5 and are responsible for providing support for B cells (Crotty, 2011). Key to the differentiation of these cells, are IL-6 and IL-21 which mediate the induction of the transcription factor Bcl-6 (Nurieva, Chung et al., 2009).

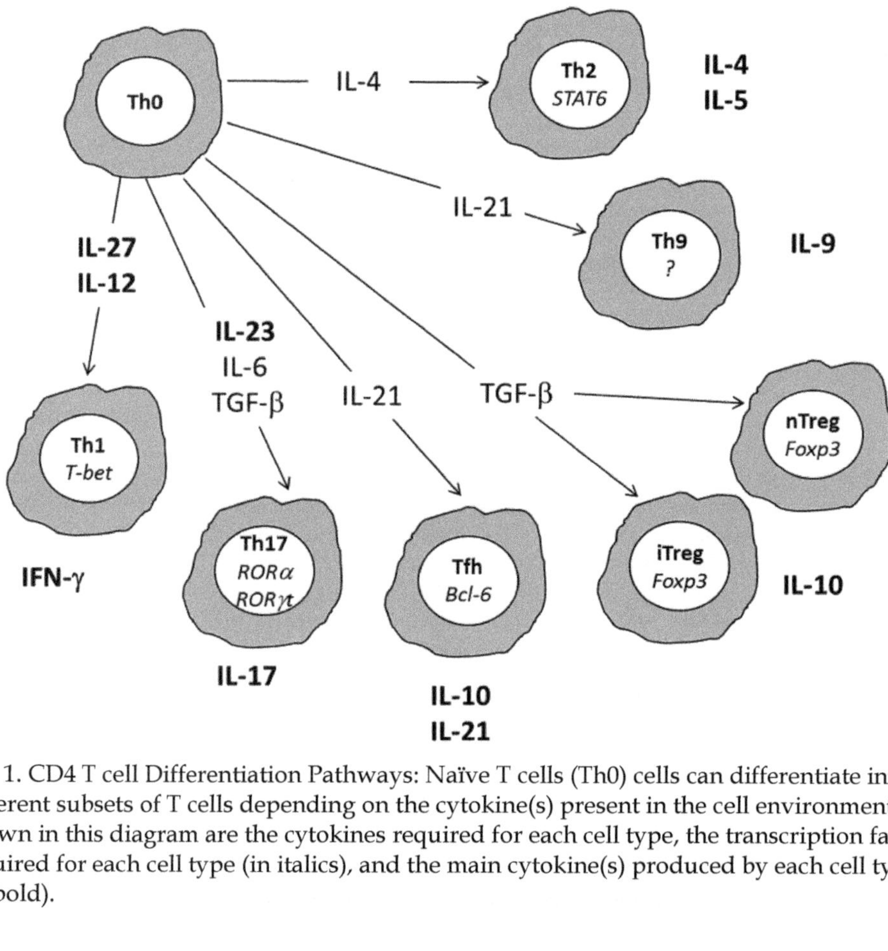

Fig. 1. CD4 T cell Differentiation Pathways: Naïve T cells (Th0) cells can differentiate into different subsets of T cells depending on the cytokine(s) present in the cell environment. Shown in this diagram are the cytokines required for each cell type, the transcription factors required for each cell type (in italics), and the main cytokine(s) produced by each cell type (in bold).

The IL-12 family of cytokines is composed of IL-12, IL-23, and IL-27, with each of these cytokines playing a different role in Th cell development. Proper regulation of the development and differentiation of CD4 T cells is critical to an effective immune response. As these cells are the main target of HIV infection, the resulting loss and imbalance of the Th cell subsets are a hallmark of HIV and AIDS. The remainder of this chapter will be devoted to a discussion of the impact of HIV infection on the function and expression of the IL-12 cytokine family members as it relates to Th cell differentiation and function with a focus on how Th1, Th17, and Treg CD4 T cell subsets are affected.

2. IL-12 and HIV infection

IL-12 is critically involved in generating cell-mediated immune responses to infectious agents, including HIV. Biologically active IL-12p70, a dimer of IL-12p35 and IL-12p40, is secreted by activated monocytes, macrophages, and dendritic cells. IL-12 expression drives the production and development of the Th1 subset of T cells, and is responsible for the induction of IFN-γ expression from these cells(Alber, Al-Robaiy et al., 2006).

IL-12 production is impaired in HIV-infected individuals and in cells infected *in vitro* with HIV (Chehimi, Starr et al., 1999; Daftarian, Diaz-Mitoma et al., 1995; Boucher, Parato et al., 2010;Buisson, Benlahrech et al., 2009). In terms of IL-12 receptor chain expression (IL-12Rβ1 and IL-12Rβ2), one study reported that resting peripheral blood mononuclear cells (PBMC) from HIV positive patients and HIV negative controls did not express IL-12Rβ1 or IL-12Rβ2 chains on their cell surface (Jones, Young et al., 2003). Upon examination of mRNA levels, the group found that levels of both receptor subunits were markedly reduced in HIV positive patients compared to HIV negative controls. Culture of activated cells with IL-12 resulted in upregulation of the IL-12Rβ2 chain suggesting that treatment with IL-12 may serve to recapitulate IL-12R levels and thus IL-12 responses (Jones, Young et al., 2003). In contrast, a recent study demonstrated that unstimulated CD4 T cells from HIV-1 positive patients expressed a two-fold increase of IL-12Rβ1 subunit compared with cells from HIV-1 negative controls (de Arquer, Pena et al., 2007). Similar to Jones et al (2003), this group found that stimulation of the CD4 T cells with IL-12 resulted in the enhancement of IL-12Rβ2. Together these two findings illustrate the potential importance of restoring IL-12 mediated responses, particularly in view of the role of IL-12 in Th1 cell differentiation and IFN-γ production.

The above observations suggest that although the virus inhibits IL-12 production, the immune cells attempt to bolster responses via upregulation of IL-12 receptor levels, which leads to speculation that treatment with IL-12 may be beneficial to patients. In *in vitro* models using T cells isolated from HIV patients, enhanced immune responses are observed upon treatment of these cells with recombinant IL-12 (Landay, Clerici et al., 1996). Vectors expressing IL-12 have also been used successfully in candidate vaccines in animal models (Chong, Egan et al., 2007; Boyer, Robinson,et al., 2005; Egan, Chong et al., 2005;Hirao, Wu et al., 2008). IL-12 is important for the priming of antigen-specific T cells, as demonstrated by a study using IL-12 deficient mice. Mice were immunized with HIV gp120 cDNA vectors and the cytotoxic T cell response in IL-12 deficient mice was significantly lower compared to wild type mice. Furthermore, reconstitution of IL-12 in the deficient mice was able to restore T cell responsiveness (Gupta et al., 2008). However, toxicity of IL-12 as a treatment option is a concern. Therefore, use of other cytokines which may have less toxicity, such as IL-23 or IL-27 is of interest. Additionally, treatment with anti-receptor or anti-cytokine antibodies to

IL-12 and IL-23 has proven useful in treatment of autoimmune diseases(Ding, Xu et al., 2008;Elson, Cong et al., 2007;Gottlieb, Cooper et al., 2007;Krueger, Langley et al., 2007). Treatment with recombinant IL-27 has also proven useful in an *in vitro* model of arthritis (Niedbala, Cai et al., 2008). Together, these points indicate alternative recombinant cytokine treatments could be applied in emerging HIV therapeutics.

3. IL-27 and HIV infection

IL-27 was first discovered in 2002 by Pflanz *et al.* as a novel member of the IL-12 family of cytokines (Pflanz, Timans et al., 2002). This family is comprised of molecules sharing subunits and receptor chain components; therefore, IL-27 and IL-12 have similar functions. IL-27 engages a heterodimeric receptor composed of gp130 and WSX-1 (Pflanz, Hibbert et al., 2004). Numerous immune cells respond to IL-27, as the IL-27 receptor can be found on endothelial cells, mast cells, activated B cells, monocytes, Langerhans cells, activated DCs, and polarized Th cells (Larousserie, Charlot et al., 2006; Lucas, Ghilardi et al., 2003; Pflanz, Hibbert et al., 2004;Ruckerl, Hessmann et al., 2006;Wirtz, Tubbe et al., 2006). Functionally, IL-27 exhibits pro- and anti-inflammatory properties and, thus, IL-27 can be regarded as an immunomodulatory cytokine. Recent evidence has indicated a role for IL-27 in the regulation of monocyte/macrophage function (Guzzo, Che Mat et al., 2010; Kalliolias & Ivashkiv, 2008), in addition to its well-characterized functions in T cells. IL-27, predominantly produced by activated monocytes and dendritic cells, can bridge innate and adaptive immunity by playing a key role in the activation of naïve T cells and differentiation to Th1 cells.

A role for IL-27 in the control of HIV replication was first described in 2007 (Fakruddin, Lempicki et al., 2007). This study evaluated the effects of HPV-VLPs (Human Papilloma Virus - Virus-Like Particles) on HIV-1 replication in PBMC, CD4 + T cells, and macrophages. Using the p24 antigen capture assay to assess viral replication, this study showed treatment with HPV-VLPs could suppress replication of both X4 and R5 strains of HIV-1. This suppression was independent of any effect on cell surface expression of CD4, CXCR4, or CCR5, as analyzed by surface staining and flow cytometry. Upon observing the anti-HIV effect of VLP treatment, the authors went on to perform DNA microarray analysis to look at gene expression profiles in PBMC and macrophages treated with VLPs. The authors noticed induction of interferon (IFN), IFN-stimulated genes (ISIGs), cytokines like IL-10, IP-10, IL-15, and most notably, IL-27. Thus, the anti-HIV effects seen with VLP treatment resulted from the release of suppressive factors following treatment of cells with HPV-VLPs. VLP-induced IL-27 expression and production in PBMC and macrophages was further confirmed and quantified using RT-PCR and ELISA, respectively. To tease out the specific role of IL-27 in suppression of HIV replication, the authors immunodepleted IL-27 from VLP-treated cell supernatants, and saw a significant reduction in the inhibition of HIV replication, indicating IL-27 secretion may be one factor contributing to the suppressive effects seen upon VLP treatment of HIV-infected cells. To confirm the direct effect of IL-27 on HIV replication, this study went on to treat cells with a recombinant IL-27 (rIL-27) dose response and showed increasing suppression of HIV replication in the presence of increasing rIL-27 doses. Furthermore, to determine the specificity of IL-27-mediated inhibition of HIV replication, the authors performed real-time RT-PCR to examine transcription of HIV RNA in the presence of IL-27. Results indicated a 60 – 80% decrease in HIV transcription in the presence of IL-27. Lastly, the authors performed DNA microarray analysis on PHA-stimulated CD4 + T cells in the presence or absence of IL-27 to compare gene induction profiles. Cells cultured in the presence of IL-27 showed significant upregulation of antiviral genes, including ISIGs, myxovirus resistance protein, and 2′-5′-oligoadenylate synthetase.

Shortly after the initial discovery of the IL-27 anti-HIV functions, the same research group examined the mechanisms of IL-27 antiviral activity compared to those of IFN-α, another key cytokine also known to inhibit HIV replication. In this study the activity and gene expression profiles of IL-27 and IFN-α were compared in human CD4 + T cells and macrophages (Imamichi, Yang et al., 2008). The authors performed a neutralization assay to define the role of IFN in IL-27-mediated inhibition of HIV replication. HIV-infected CD4 T cells and macrophages were treated with IL-27 in the presence/absence of an antibody cocktail containing neutralizing antibodies to each IFN. The antibody treatment did not affect HIV inhibition by IL-27, indicating that IFN is not an intermediate in the inhibition of HIV replication by IL-27. Of additional note, IL-27, like IFN-α, preferentially inhibited HIV replication in macrophages compared to CD4 T cells, as lower doses of these cytokines were required to get complete inhibition of HIV replication in macrophages compared to T cells. Using DNA microarray analysis, this study went on to compare the gene expression profiles of IL-27 and IFN-α in CD4 T cells and macrophages. From this experiment it was noted that both cytokines induced a similar profile of ISIGs and antiviral genes, with greater antiviral gene induction in the macrophages compared to CD4 T cells upon IL-27 stimulation. Of particular note, IL-27 significantly upregulated antiviral genes like myxovirus resistance 1 (MX1), oligoadenylate synthetase 2 (OAS2), and RNA-dependent protein kinase–eukaryotic initiation factor 2a kinase (PKR/EIF2AK) by greater than 2-fold in the macrophage cells. Furthermore, IL-27 also induced expression of apolipoprotein B messenger RNA-editing enzyme-catalytic polypeptide-like 3G (APOBEC3G) in macrophages, but not in CD4 T cells. The APOBEC proteins are key host cell-derived protective molecules, acting as anti-HIV proteins that function as cytidine deaminases to interfere with viral replication (Romani, Engelbrecht et al., 2009). Taken together, these results indicate that IL-27, like IFN-α, significantly induces multiple IFIGs and APOBEC3G in macrophages, resulting in the striking anti-HIV functions of these cytokines.

Subsequent to the initial studies on IL-27 functions in HIV infection, a separate research group set out to determine whether IL-27 directly or indirectly regulated expression of the APOBEC family of proteins (Greenwell-Wild, Vazquez et al., 2009). Since it had been previously shown that IFN-α could regulate expression of APOBEC, clinical trials commenced to explore the impact of IFN-α treatment on induction of APOBEC expression in the setting of HIV infection *et* (Neumann, Polis et al., 2007). However, the many negative side effects of IFN treatment led researchers to consider alternative mechanisms to induce APOBEC expression, in particular, mechanisms that minimize IFN toxicities associated with direct administration of this cytokine. Greenwell-Wild et al. (2009) showed that IL-27 could be a good alternative, as they showed IL-27 can induce APOBEC expression to curb HIV replication. This study attributed the anti-viral properties of IL-27 to the intermediary IL-27-induced IFN-α, which can then, in turn, coordinate anti-viral responses. Interestingly, this study investigated whether other IL-12 cytokine family members, namely IL-12 and IL-23, could suppress HIV replication. No significant reduction in HIV replication was observed with IL-12 or IL-23 treatments, indicating that the inhibition of HIV replication was selective to IL-27 in the IL-12 family of cytokines. This study went on to examine the kinetics of IL-27-induced APOBEC expression and found a 24 hour delay in the induction of expression by real-time PCR, suggestive of an intermediary in the induction of APOBEC expression. Since it was previously known that IFN-α could regulate APOBEC expression, IFN-α and IFN-β became likely agents for the intermediary molecules mediating IL-27-induced APOBEC expression. Greenwell-Wild et al. (2009) went on to show IL-27 can induce expression of both IFN-α and -β, and that these IFNs alone could inhibit HIV replication (p24 assay). Lastly, to confirm that IL-27 induces APOBEC expression through IFN, they blocked the IFN–α/β receptor (IFNAR) with neutralizing antibody, followed with IL-27 stimulation, and found no induction of APOBEC expression, indicating IFN is an intermediate requirement in IL-27-induced APOBEC expression. Furthermore, when IFN and IL-27 were added in unison to cell cultures, enhanced inhibition of HIV replication was observed, pointing to additional antiviral mechanisms under the regulation of these cytokines. Taken together, this study illustrates teamwork between two cytokines, IFN and IL-27, in the suppression of HIV.

So far we have reviewed how IL-27 can suppress HIV replication; however, limited studies have described how HIV can affect IL-27. The first study to investigate the impact of HIV infection on IL-27 investigated how clinical characteristics such as viral load, hepatitis C virus (HCV) co-infection, and CD4 T cell counts were associated with changes in circulating levels of IL-27 (Guzzo, Hopman et al., 2010). Guzzo *et al.* (2010) observed a modest negative correlation between IL-27 levels and HIV viral load, suggesting that circulating HIV virus may suppress IL-27 expression, a potential pathogenic mechanism for the virus to limit host anti-viral responses. Additionally, in this study, when patients were grouped according to those receiving HAART therapy and those naïve to HAART, no difference was found in IL-27 expression, illustrating no impact of HAART on IL-27 expression. Lastly, this study investigated if IL-27 expression was associated with changing CD4 T cell counts. A consistent trend was observed among patient groups, namely, IL-27 expression peaked with moderate declines in CD4 T cell counts (200-350), then decreased in the low CD4 T cell count (<200) patients. The study authors hypothesized that the initial boost in IL-27 signified the host response to viral insult (declining CD4 T cells), as the host upregulates the anti-HIV cytokine as a protective response. However, as HIV disease progresses, dysregulated immune responses and increasing viral loads renders the host unable to produce adequate IL-27, and the observation of decreased IL-27 with low CD4 T cells counts was observed. Overall, this study suggested that HIV viral load, HCV co-infection, and CD4 T cell counts are strongly associated with changes in circulating levels IL-27 in the HIV-infected host. This research was the first to report how HIV infection might affect expression of IL-27, and to date, only one other study has investigated the effect of HIV on IL-27 expression (Palermo, Patterson et al., 2011). Palermo et al. (2011) performed alternative AIDS vaccine strategies in rhesus macaques followed by viral challenge with adenovirus-expressing HIV-env, SIV-gag, or SIV-nef proteins. Following vaccination and viral challenge, global transcriptional profiling was performed to characterize any significant alterations in gene expression. At the time of peak viremia in the animals, gene expression profiles of the immunized groups were different from that of controls. Of particular note was an upregulation of IL-27 expression in the immunized group, indicating the protective host response to virus is a boost in the anti-viral cytokine, IL-27. This study reported significant differences in gene expression of a variety of immunological markers between treatment groups, suggesting new potential correlates of protection in HIV infection.

Taking into account the role of IL-27 in driving the differentiation of Th1 cells and keeping in mind the ability of IL-27 to inhibit HIV replication, it is clear that further understanding of the regulation of IL-27 expression and function during HIV infection is an important area of research. It is possible that the use of treatments that upregulate the expression of this cytokine may have a two-pronged beneficial effect: inhibition of virus replication and reinstating the Th1 CD4 T cell populations.

4. IL-23 and HIV infection

As discussed, the IL-12 family of cytokines regulates CD4 T cell development and immune responses. In particular, IL-23 is an IL-12 family member important in regulating the differentiation of the proinflammatory, IL-17-producing, Th17 cells. IL-23, a heterodimeric cytokine composed of covalently linked IL-12p40 and IL-23p19 subunits was originally discovered in 2000 and identified as a member of the IL-12-related cytokine family (Oppmann, Lesley et al., 2000). IL-23 is predominantly produced by activated myeloid cells such as activated monocytes, antigen-presenting cells, including dendritic cells and macrophages, T cells, B cells and endothelial cells (Oppmann, Lesley et al., 2000;Parham, Chirica et al., 2002;van Seventer, Nagai et al., 2002). IL-23 shares the IL-12p40 subunit with IL-12, and the IL-23-specific subunit, p19, forms a disulphide-linked heterodimer with the IL-12p40 subunit(Oppmann, Lesley et al., 2000). The high affinity IL-23 receptor complex is comprised of an IL-12Rβ1 (as found in IL-12 receptor) and a unique IL-23Rα subunit (Parham, Chirica et al., 2002). As mentioned in the previous section on IL-12, many studies have shown the effect of HIV infection on the production of IL-12 and IL-12 receptor expression; there is strong evidence suggesting that IL-12 production is impaired in cells infected *in vitro* with HIV and in HIV positive patients (Chehimi, Starr et al., 1994; Marshall, Chehimiet al., 1999;Daftarian, Diaz-Mitoma et al., 1995;Boucher, Parato et al., 2010; Buisson, Benlahrech et al., 2009). Since IL-12 and IL-23 share the p40 subunit as well as the IL-12Rβ1 receptor subunit, it is interesting to speculate on the impact of HIV on IL-23 function and the involvement of IL-23 in HIV pathogenesis.

The ability of immune cells to produce IL-23 during HIV infection has not been fully studied. Lee and colleagues were the first to demonstrate that spontaneously produced IL-23p19 and IFN-γ mRNA from PBMC are reduced in HIV positive patients who exhibited increased CD4 T cell counts while on long term HAART (Lee, French, & Price, 2004). The inability of the cells to produce "normal" levels of these key cytokines may compromise the immune response to opportunistic infections. A very recent study showed that LPS-induced IL-23 production by monocytes and dendritic cells from HIV positive patients was actually increased compared to HIV negative controls (Louis, Dutertre et al., 2010). This study included the first longitudinal analysis of IL-23 production during primary HIV infection. The authors found that the production of IL-23 was greatly increased and sustained during chronic infection. Interestingly, in response to simultaneous LPS and IFN-γ treatment, they also found that IL-23 production, but not IL-12p70 production correlated strongly with viral loads. This study indicates that HIV induces the production of IL-23, and that IL-23 may have an important role in controlling viral infection. However, taken together, these studies have conflicting results. In the study by Lee *et al.*, mRNA levels of p19 were examined whereas Louis et al. examined secreted IL-23, which may partially explain the observed discrepancy. In 2004, a study revealed that IL-23 has potent adjuvant effects on induction of epitope-specific cytotoxic T lymphocytes (CTLs) (Matsui, Moriya et al., 2004). The authors found that co-administration of an IL-23 expression plasmid in a prime-boost immunization enhanced the induction of Hepatitis C virus (HCV)-specific CTLs in mice. This finding suggests that

IL-23 might offer a new prophylactic and therapeutic strategy for vaccine development against infectious pathogens.
To date, the mechanism of how HIV affects the production of IL-23 is still not clear. However, a few studies have been reported on the molecular mechanism of the inhibitory action of HIV on IL-12, a related cytokine sharing the IL-12p40 subunit and IL-12Rβ1 receptor subunit with IL-23. An *in vitro* study showed that HIV infection of myeloid cells was able to disrupt MAP kinase activation and transcription factor binding to the IL-12p40 promoter(Chambers, Parks et al., 2004). This observation may be explained as a direct effect of HIV on the IL-12p40 promoter or may occur as a consequence of altered MAP kinase activation. Indeed, the authors demonstrated that the phosphorylation of JNK and p38 MAPK was impaired and the phosphorylation and degradation of IκBα was suppressed after HIV infection (Chambers, Parks, & Angel, 2004). Another *in vitro* study found that intracellular Nef inhibits LPS-induced IL-12p40 transcription by inhibiting the JNK-activated NF-κB without affecting AP-1 activity (Ma, Mishra et al., 2009). This result suggests that intracellular Nef selectively inhibits NF-κB activity (apart from other transcription factors, such as AP-1), resulting in the inhibition of IL-12p40 expression. Similar studies on the molecular mechanism of IL-23p19 regulation in the context of HIV infection have yet to be published.
It is well known that IL-23 is important for the development of a proinflammatory subset of T cells, Th17. Little is known about how HIV modulates the function of IL-23 and how HIV affects the main downstream functions of this cytokine in the promotion of Th17 cells. If HIV infection decreases IL-23 production, Th17 expansion and activation may be downregulated. To date, no study has examined the correlation between IL-23 and the IL-23/Th17 axis in HIV positive patients. Like IL-23, the roles of Th17 and IL-17 in HIV-replication and immunopathogenesis are not well understood. In the next section we will discuss the impact of HIV infection on Th17 cell regulation.

5. Th17 cells and HIV infection

The discovery of the Th17 subset has expanded our understanding of T cell mediated immunity, leading to a revision of the classical model of T cell populations. Th17 is a proinflammatory T cell population that is involved in host immune defense against pathogens not adequately handled by Th1 or Th2 cells. The Th17 subset is termed after its main effector proinflammatory cytokine, IL-17. The differentiation of Th17 subset is driven by the combination of TGF-β and IL-6 which upregulate the transcription factor RORγt (McGeachy, Chen et al., 2009). Th17 cells mediate inflammation through upregulation of chemokine and inflammatory cytokine expression, and recruitment of macrophages and neutrophils (Gaffen, Kramer et al., 2006;Korn, Bettelli et al., 2009). The inflammatory response is amplified by the presence of all these factors, resulting in a greater inflammation than the response from Th1/Th2 cells. Th17 cells have been demonstrated to be specifically involved in immunity against *Toxoplasma gondii, Candida albicans, Klebsiella pneumoniae* and *Mycobacterium tuberculosis* (Conti, Shen et al., 2009; Gaffen, Kramer, Yu, & Shen, 2006; Korn, Bettelli, Oukka, & Kuchroo, 2009). However a role for Th17 cells in the regulation of virus infection has been a recent focal area of research, particularly in the case of HIV.
Mucosal transmission of HIV is the main route of virus entry and site of initial virus infection. Th17 cells play important roles in the regulation of mucosal immunity, and they are found in

high concentration in the lamina propria of the GI tract (Hunt, 2010). Th17 cells prevent microbial translocation across mucosal surfaces by enhancing expression of antimicrobial peptides and mobilizing neutrophils to infected sites. At the same time, gut-associated lymphoid tissue (GALT) is a major reservoir for CD4 T cells, the source of Th17 cells, and a key site of HIV replication and CD4 T cell loss (Brenchley, Schacker et al., 2004;Mehandru, Poles et al., 2004). Pathogenic SIV as well as HIV infection results in rapid and significant Th17 loss from the GALT which would be expected to have deleterious effects on the regulation of microbial translocation (Brenchley, Schacker et al., 2004; Raffatellu, Santos et al., 2008). Indeed, HIV infection is correlated with increases in microbial translocation and mucosal inflammation (Gori, Tincati et al., 2008). This is supported by studies showing that plasma LPS levels, considered as an indication of microbial translocation, in HIV infected individuals are remarkably higher than uninfected individuals (Jiang, Lederman et al., 2009;d'Ettorre, Paiardini et al., 2011). Interestingly, SIV infected rhesus macaques exhibited Th17 depletion in ileal mucosa, resulting in a compromised mucosal barrier and susceptibility to *Salmonella* infection compared to that observed in uninfected macaques (Raffatellu, Santos, et al., 2008). Furthermore, in the same study, IL-17R deficient mice also had increased systemic dissemination of *Salmonella* from the gut. Together, this suggests that IL-17 deficiency may lead to impaired mucosal barrier function. An interesting report on Vδ1 T cells, T cells present in mucosal tissues expressing the γδ T cell receptor, demonstrated that HIV positive individuals exhibited an expanded population of these cells that produced both IFN-γ and IL-17 (Fenoglio, Poggi et al., 2009). This is of interest to mucosal immunity and HIV, as circulating Vδ1 T lymphocytes, resident cells in GALT, are increased in HIV-1 infection due to mucosal depletion and recirculation (Nilssen, Muller et al., 1996;Fenoglio, Poggi et al., 2009). Additionally, Fenoglio et al. (2009) showed that these cells were able to proliferate and produce IFN-γ and IL-17 in response to *C. albicans* and that these cells expressed markers for a memory T cell phenotype as well as the Th17 transcription factor RORC. The elevation of this subset of T cells in the context of HIV infection may represent a possible mechanism to compensate for impaired CD4 T cells, and in particular, that of Th17.

Studies elucidating the relationship between Th17 cells and HIV infection have yielded inconclusive results. The first report that associated HIV with IL-17 showed an increase of IL-17 production by CD4 T cells in peripheral blood of HIV patients both in cells left untreated or stimulated with PMA/ionomycin (Maek, Buranapraditkun et al., 2007). It was later shown that HIV-1 infected children with a plasma viral load of below 50 copies/ml (undetectable HIV) had enhanced IL-17 production in contrast to those with detectable HIV, which had no observable IL-17 production (Ndhlovu, Chapman et al., 2008). This suggested a possible impairment of Th17 cells in patients with detectable HIV levels and decreased IL-17 levels, and that restoration of Th17 cells could be possible through suppression of viremia. In 2008, Macal et al. showed that CD4 T cell restoration (>50%) could be achieved regardless of persistent proviral burden and previous HAART (Macal, Sankaran et al., 2008). This CD4 T cell restoration was associated with enhanced Th17 CD4 T cell accumulation. Additionally, HIV-1 and CMV specific IL-17 producing CD4 T cells are detectable in early HIV-1 infection, but are undetectable in chronic and non-progressive HIV-1 infection (Yue, Merchant et al., 2008). These experiments together suggest that IL-17 producing T cells are associated with viral load and disease progression. They also call into question of what impact the restoration of Th17 cells would have on the progression of HIV in the long run. If reconstitution is possible, increased Th17 levels may be beneficial in slowing the progression

of the disease towards AIDS, in particular with regard to the function of these cells to control possible fungal, parasitic, and bacterial opportunistic infections.
It is unclear if Th17 cells are preferentially targeted by HIV for infection. One study suggested preferential targeting of CCR6+CCR5+ Th17 cells by CCR5 tropic viruses *in vivo* (El Hed, Khaitan et al., 2010). CCR4+ CCR6+ and CXCR3+ CCR6+ T cells express cytokines and transcription factors specific for Th17 and Th1/Th17 lineages respectively. These markers contribute to gut and lymph node homing potential. These two types of cells are highly permissive to HIV replication in that while their frequency is diminished, they can recruit more CCR6+ T cells into sites of viral replication (Gosselin, Monteiro et al., 2010). Similarly, in SIV infection, $\alpha4\beta7^{hi}$CD4 memory T cells were found to harbour most Th17 cells and were significantly depleted (Kader, Wang et al., 2009). In SIV infected macaques, one group found that Th17 loss at mucosal surfaces predicted AIDS progression (Cecchinato, Trindade et al., 2008). Furthermore, there was a negative correlation between Th17 cell frequencies at mucosal sites and plasma virus level. Altogether these papers found that Th17 cells were preferentially depleted within a few weeks in HIV/SIV infection. Other reports show that Th17 cells may not be preferentially infected by HIV *in vivo*. Rather, CD4 T cell development was shown to be skewed away from the Th17 phenotype toward Th1 cell maturation in HIV patients (Brenchley, Paiardini et al., 2008) possibly leading to a significant loss of Th17 cells in the GI tract of HIV patients.
Although there is ample evidence to state that Th17 is important in HIV pathogenesis, it is still unclear how Th17 cells and IL-17 are regulated during HIV infection. Understanding how Th17 cells are dysregulated by HIV infection is crucial to restoring its population and function and it is possible that treatments designed to increase Th17 levels may be beneficial to HIV infection. This may be particularly important in the protection against opportunistic diseases, given that Th17 cells have been well characterized to protect against bacterial, parasitic, and fungal infections.

6. Treg in HIV infection

Treg cells function to prevent chronic immune activation and act in a suppressive manner to control immune activation. These cells are generally defined phenotypically as CD4, CD25+, and Foxp3+. It appears that within the setting of HIV infection, the Treg CD4 T cell population may be protective to the host by potentially suppressing HIV infection in conventional CD4 T cells as well as cytotoxic T cell activity (Moreno-Fernandez, Rueda et al., 2011;Kinter, McNally et al., 2007). The Treg population has been demonstrated to coordinate and maintain virus-specific immune responses (Rouse, Sarangi et al., 2006). Although Tregs have been shown to be infected by HIV, this may depend on the strain as well as host and viral properties. Moreno-Fernandez and colleagues (2009) demonstrated that X4 viruses exhibited a higher level of infection in Tregs at early time points compared to R5 viruses in Tregs and X4 viruses in effector T cells (Moreno-Fernandez, Zapata et al., 2009). A study which examined viral persistence in Treg cells found that these cells are preferentially targeted by HIV, as a greater number of Treg cells harboured more HIV DNA than non-Treg cells (Tran, de Goer de Herve MG et al., 2008). Of interest, the Foxp3 Treg transcription factor has been shown to enhance HIV gene expression via an NF-κB dependent mechanism(Holmes, Knudsen et al., 2007). Additionally, HIV-specific Treg cells have been detected (Kared, Lelievre et al., 2008;Torheim, Ndhlovu et al., 2009). Indeed, HIV has been shown to bind to Treg cells via gp120/CD4 interactions which has been correlated with increased suppressive activities, extended Treg survival, and upregulated homing receptors for peripheral lymph nodes and mucosal lymphoid tissues (Ji & Cloyd, 2009;Nilsson, Boasso et al., 2006). In the same study, it was shown that these Treg cells did not exhibit the same homing-induced apoptosis. Taken together, this suggests that the HIV-Treg interaction may contribute to upregulated levels of Tregs observed in lymphoid and mucosal compartments in HIV positive patients (Mozos, Garrido et al., 2007; Ji & Cloyd, 2009; Nilsson, Boasso et al., 2006).

Absolute numbers of Treg and Treg frequency during HIV infection is an area of contention in this field. However, it has been demonstrated that the relative frequency of Treg cells within the CD4 T cell population as a whole appears to increase during HIV infection while at the same time, the absolute numbers of Tregs decline(Schulze Zur, Thomssen et al., 2011). This is supported by several studies which indicated a gradual decline in Treg absolute numbers during HIV pathogenesis (Jiao, Fu et al., 2009; Prendergast, Prado et al., 2010; Thorborn, Pomeroy et al., 2010; Cao, Jamieson et al., 2009). In particular, in primary HIV infection in untreated individuals, HIV-specific Treg cells and suppressive activity decreased over a 24 month follow-up period (Kared, Lelievre et al., 2008). Interestingly, a recent study by Weis et al. (2010) demonstrated that Treg cells were able to control immune activation in patients on ART, however this control was lost during interruption of ART, an observation attributed to the decline in absolute Treg numbers(Weiss, Piketty et al., 2010).

Immune activation during HIV infection has been linked to HIV progression and negative outcomes during HIV infection (Douek, 2003; Kassiotis & O'Garra, 2008; Lawn, Butera et al., 2001; Terzieva, 2008). Tregs could be protective as they can control this immune hyperactivation especially during chronic infection (Fazekas de St & Landay, 2008; Belkaid & Rouse, 2005). On the other hand, excess Treg activity results in "over" suppression of immune responses resulting in too much immune suppression, leading to faster HIV progression and negative outcomes (Kinter, Horak et al., 2007). This point is also supported by a report showing that recombinant IL-2 treatment in a phase III trial actually enhanced Treg populations, possibly explaining why this treatment failed to elicit better clinical outcome (Weiss, Letimier et al., 2010). Treg depletion has been associated with an increase in immune activation (Eggena, Barugahare et al., 2005) and several important studies have demonstrated correlation of Treg proliferation and turnover with lower CD4 counts (Bi, Suzuki et al., 2009; Piconi, Trabattoni et al., 2010; Xing, Fu et al., 2010).

Interestingly, elite controllers, a rare population of individuals that can maintain undetectable HIV viral loads in the absence of HAART, demonstrated higher frequencies of Treg cells compared to individuals on HAART (Chase, Yang et al., 2008). On the other hand, Owen et al., showed that individuals on HAART had higher frequencies of Tregs compared to elite controllers (Owen, Heitman et al., 2010). In contrast yet again, more recent studies have demonstrated that elite controllers have a lower level of Treg cells compared to viremic individuals, but that this "low" level of Tregs is similar to that observed in HIV positive individuals with viral load controlled by HAART (Brandt, Benfield et al., 2011). In support of this, another group demonstrated that elite controllers had an even lower Treg frequency than HIV negative individuals (Hunt, Landay et al., 2011). In view of these studies it seems that the Treg frequency in elite controllers may vary according to the patient group examined and to which group the comparison is being made.

7. Th17 versus Treg in HIV infection

Since the main function of Th17 is to mediate inflammatory responses, and it is involved in autoimmune diseases, it is prudent that the response is kept under control to avoid damage to host tissue. Treg development is inexorably associated with Th17 development. IL-2, an important growth factor for T cells, is one of several cytokines that mediates the balance between Th17 and Tregs. *In vitro*, levels of Th17 were reduced in the presence of IL-2, while Treg numbers increased with IL-2 stimulation (Stockinger, 2007). The same is true with respect to HIV infection; a recent study demonstrated that administration of IL-2 to HIV patients on ART resulted in enhanced levels of CD4 T cells and Treg cells (Ndhlovu, Sinclair et al., 2010b). Overall enhancement of the CD4 T cell count was attributed to enhanced levels of naïve T cells. At the same time, this resulted in a decrease in Th17 cell frequency, although the absolute numbers of Th17 did not change. These results suggest then that IL-2 is important for driving the differentiation of CD4 T cells and is selective for Treg development while not affecting levels of Th17 cells already present.

As mentioned before, TGF-β function straddles the border between Treg and Th17 differentiation depending on the presence of IL-6. It is suggested that TGF-β is constitutively produced by the resting immune system to induce Tregs to limit the effect of activated memory T cells (Korn, Bettelli, Oukka, & Kuchroo, 2009). However, in the event that the immune system is triggered, IL-6 is induced to inhibit the production of Tregs and cause a switch towards Th17 development (Korn, Bettelli, Oukka, & Kuchroo, 2009). This supports the claim that both TGF-β and IL-6 must be present for Th17 differentiation. The parallel use of TGF-β in both Treg and Th17 subsets may be important in mediating the balance between the two. It has been suggested that Th17 and Treg share a reciprocal relationship (Bettelli, Carrier et al, 2006; Mucida, Park et al., 2007; Zhou, Lopes et al., 2008; Quintana, Basso et al., 2008). It has been shown that the observed rapid Th17 decline in acute HIV infection is predictive of the immune activation later seen in chronic infection. These studies also observed a loss of the Th17/Treg balance in pathogenic SIV infection (Lederer, Favre et al., 2009). More recently, Prendergast et al (2010) demonstrated a profound loss of Th17 cells before advanced disease, in contrast to a gradual decline of Treg cells (Prendergast, Prado et al,, 2010). In a recent review, B. Kanwar et al. suggest that it is the relative balance of these two subsets of T cells that is key to the regulation of progression of HIV/AIDS, as opposed to considering only the specific functions of either subset alone(Kanwar, Favre et al., 2010). Future work in this regard will be key to furthering our understanding of the impact of this virus on our immune system.

8. The "other" subsets: Th2, Th9, Tfh

As discussed above, clearly HIV infection impacts the function of Th1, Th17, and Treg cells. The antibody response supported by the Th2 T cell subset is critically important to anti-HIV immune responses, however the scope of this topic fell outside the realm of this chapter. Currently little is known about the impact of HIV infection on the development and function of Th9 and Tfh cells. It is interesting to speculate that the differentiation programming and functional effects of these cells are disrupted during infection and warrant further research in this regard.

9. Conclusion

In Figure 2, the overall effect of HIV infection on Th cell subset is illustrated. In actuality, it is likely that the mechanisms and impact of the virus on these cells is much more complex than portrayed here, however this diagram summarizes the general outcome of CD4 T cell differentiation in terms of Th1, Treg, and Th17 cells during HIV infection. Our immune systems consist of many complex processes that are interconnected and the effect of inhibiting or upregulating particular cell types will affect not only that particular cell type, but a multitude of other cells and cellular processes. As we further our understanding of HIV infection and HAART on the regulation of the differentiation of the CD4 T cell response, this will enhance our ability to design new treatment therapeutics and potential vaccine targets.

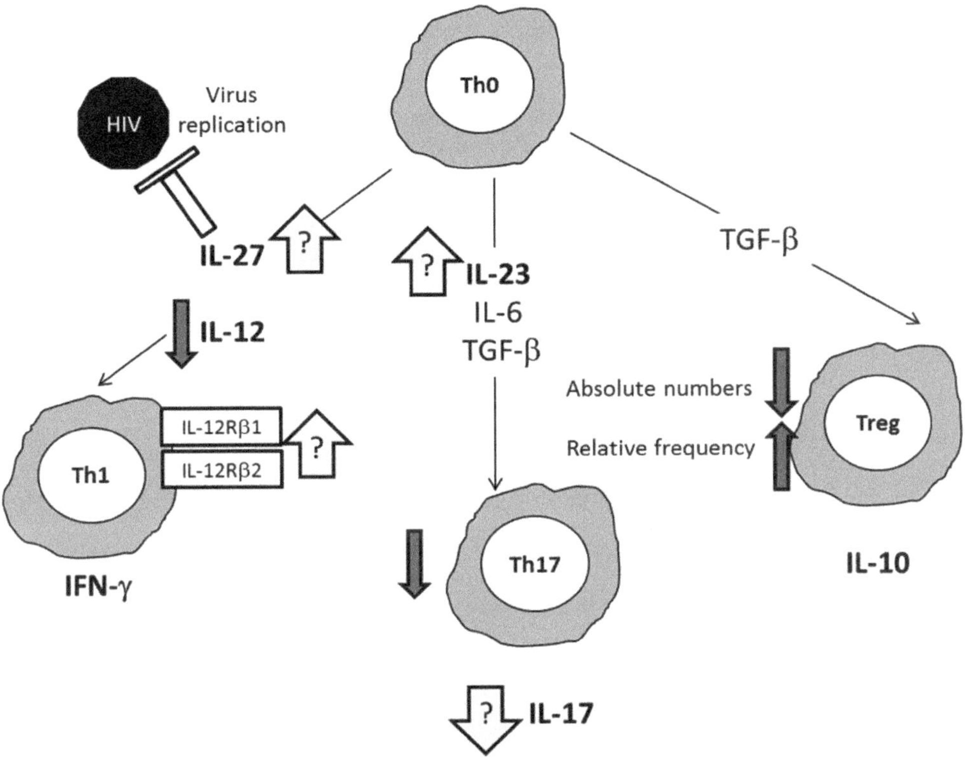

Fig. 2. Impact of HIV infection on the IL-12 family of cytokines and their respective effects on CD4 T cell development. Shown are the T helper (Th) subsets discussed in detail in this chapter. Cytokines that induce their differentiation are shown preceding the cell type, and effector cytokines are listed below each cell type. Dark arrows indicate well-defined increases (up arrow) or decreases (down arrows) in cytokines (IL-12) or Th cells (Th17 and Treg). Large arrows with question marks indicate increases (up arrows) or decreases (down arrow) in cytokine and receptor expression that are not well defined. Shown in the top left is the ability of IL-27 to inhibit HIV replication.

10. References

Alber, G., Al-Robaiy, S., Kleinschek, M., Knauer, J., Krumbholz, P., Richter, J., Schoeneberger, S., Schuetze, N., Schulz, S., Toepfer, K., Voigtlaender, R., Lehmann,

J., and Mueller, U. (2006). Induction of immunity and inflammation by interleukin-12 family members. *Ernst.Schering.Res.Found.Workshop.* 107-127.

Belkaid, Y. and Rouse, B. T. (2005). Natural regulatory T cells in infectious disease. *Nat Immunol.* 6, 353-360.

Bettelli, E., Carrier, Y., Gao, W., Korn, T., Strom, T. B., Oukka, M., Weiner, H. L., and Kuchroo, V. K. (2006). Reciprocal developmental pathways for the generation of pathogenic effector TH17 and regulatory T cells. *Nature* 441, 235-238.

Bi, X., Suzuki, Y., Gatanaga, H., and Oka, S. (2009). High frequency and proliferation of CD4+ FOXP3+ Treg in HIV-1-infected patients with low CD4 counts. *Eur.J.Immunol.* 39, 301-309.

Boucher, J. G., Parato, K. A., Frappier, F., Fairman, P., Busca, A., Saxena, M., Blahoianu, M. A., Ma, W., Gajanayaka, N., Parks, R. J., Kumar, A., and Angel, J. B. (2010). Disparate regulation of LPS-induced MAPK signaling and IL-12p40 expression between different myeloid cell types with and without HIV infection. *Viral Immunol.* 23, 17-28.

Boyer, J. D., Robinson, T. M., Kutzler, M. A., Parkinson, R., Calarota, S. A., Sidhu, M. K., Muthumani, K., Lewis, M., Pavlakis, G., Felber, B., and Weiner, D. (2005). SIV DNA vaccine co-administered with IL-12 expression plasmid enhances CD8 SIV cellular immune responses in cynomolgus macaques. *J.Med.Primatol.* 34, 262-270.

Brandt, L., Benfield, T., Mens, H., Clausen, L. N., Katzenstein, T. L., Fomsgaard, A., and Karlsson, I. (2011). Low level of regulatory T-cells and maintenance of balance between regulatory T-cells and TH17 cells in HIV-1-infected Elite Controllers. *J.Acquir.Immune.Defic.Syndr.*

Brenchley, J. M., Paiardini, M., Knox, K. S., Asher, A. I., Cervasi, B., Asher, T. E., Scheinberg, P., Price, D. A., Hage, C. A., Kholi, L. M., Khoruts, A., Frank, I., Else, J., Schacker, T., Silvestri, G., and Douek, D. C. (2008). Differential Th17 CD4 T-cell depletion in pathogenic and nonpathogenic lentiviral infections. *Blood.* 112, 2826-2835.

Brenchley, J. M., Schacker, T. W., Ruff, L. E., Price, D. A., Taylor, J. H., Beilman, G. J., Nguyen, P. L., Khoruts, A., Larson, M., Haase, A. T., and Douek, D. C. (2004). CD4+ T cell depletion during all stages of HIV disease occurs predominantly in the gastrointestinal tract. *J.Exp.Med.* %20;200, 749-759.

Buisson, S., Benlahrech, A., Gazzard, B., Gotch, F., Kelleher, P., and Patterson, S. (2009). Monocyte-derived dendritic cells from HIV type 1-infected individuals show reduced ability to stimulate T cells and have altered production of interleukin (IL)-12 and IL-10. *J.Infect.Dis.* 199, 1862-1871.

Cao, W., Jamieson, B. D., Hultin, L. E., Hultin, P. M., and Detels, R. (2009). Regulatory T cell expansion and immune activation during untreated HIV type 1 infection are associated with disease progression. *AIDS Res.Hum.Retroviruses.* 25, 183-191.

Cecchinato, V., Trindade, C. J., Laurence, A., Heraud, J. M., Brenchley, J. M., Ferrari, M. G., Zaffiri, L., Tryniszewska, E., Tsai, W. P., Vaccari, M., Parks, R. W., Venzon, D., Douek, D. C., O'Shea, J. J., and Franchini, G. (2008). Altered balance between Th17 and Th1 cells at mucosal sites predicts AIDS progression in simian immunodeficiency virus-infected macaques. *Mucosal.Immunol.* 1, 279-288.

Chambers, K. A., Parks, R. J., and Angel, J. B. (2004). Disruption of MAP kinase activation and nuclear factor binding to the IL-12 p40 promoter in HIV-infected myeloid cells. *Clin.Exp.Immunol.* 137, 329-340.

Chase, A. J., Yang, H. C., Zhang, H., Blankson, J. N., and Siliciano, R. F. (2008). Preservation of FoxP3+ regulatory T cells in the peripheral blood of human immunodeficiency virus type 1-infected elite suppressors correlates with low CD4+ T-cell activation. *J.Virol.* 82, 8307-8315.

Chehimi, J., Starr, S. E., Frank, I., D'Andrea, A., Ma, X., MacGregor, R. R., Sennelier, J., and Trinchieri, G. (1994). Impaired interleukin 12 production in human immunodeficiency virus-infected patients. *J.Exp.Med.* 179, 1361-1366.

Chong, S. Y., Egan, M. A., Kutzler, M. A., Megati, S., Masood, A., Roopchard, V., Garcia-Hand, D., Montefiori, D. C., Quiroz, J., Rosati, M., Schadeck, E. B., Boyer, J. D., Pavlakis, G. N., Weiner, D. B., Sidhu, M., Eldridge, J. H., and Israel, Z. R. (2007). Comparative ability of plasmid IL-12 and IL-15 to enhance cellular and humoral immune responses elicited by a SIVgag plasmid DNA vaccine and alter disease progression following SHIV(89.6P) challenge in rhesus macaques. *Vaccine* 25, 4967-4982.

Conti, H. R., Shen, F., Nayyar, N., Stocum, E., Sun, J. N., Lindemann, M. J., Ho, A. W., Hai, J. H., Yu, J. J., Jung, J. W., Filler, S. G., Masso-Welch, P., Edgerton, M., and Gaffen, S. L. (2009). Th17 cells and IL-17 receptor signaling are essential for mucosal host defense against oral candidiasis. *J.Exp.Med.* 206, 299-311.

Crotty, S. (2011). Follicular Helper CD4 T Cells (T(FH)). *Annu.Rev.Immunol.* 29:621-63., 621-663.

d'Ettorre, G., Paiardini, M., Zaffiri, L., Andreotti, M., Ceccarelli, G., Rizza, C., Indinnimeo, M., Vella, S., Mastroianni, C. M., Silvestri, G., and Vullo, V. (2011). HIV Persistence in the Gut Mucosa of HIV-Infected Subjects Undergoing Antiretroviral Therapy Correlates with Immune Activation and Increased Levels of LPS. *Curr.HIV.Res.*

Daftarian, M. P., Diaz-Mitoma, F., Creery, W. D., Cameron, W., and Kumar, A. (1995). Dysregulated production of interleukin-10 (IL-10) and IL-12 by peripheral blood lymphocytes from human immunodeficiency virus-infected individuals is associated with altered proliferative responses to recall antigens. *Clin.Diagn.Lab Immunol.* 2, 712-718.

de Arquer, G. R., Pena, R., Cabrera, C., Coma, G., Ruiz-Hernandez, R., Guerola, R., Clotet, B., Ruiz, L., Este, J. A., Calle, M. L., and Bofill, M. (2007). Skewed expression and up-regulation of the IL-12 and IL-18 receptors in resting and activated CD4 T cells from HIV-1-infected patients. *J.Leukoc.Biol.* 82, 72-78.

Ding, C., Xu, J., and Li, J. (2008). ABT-874, a fully human monoclonal anti-IL-12/IL-23 antibody for the potential treatment of autoimmune diseases. *Curr. Opin. Investig. Drugs* 9, 515-522.

Douek, D. C. (2003). Disrupting T-cell homeostasis: how HIV-1 infection causes disease. *AIDS Rev.* 5, 172-177.

Egan, M. A., Chong, S. Y., Megati, S., Montefiori, D. C., Rose, N. F., Boyer, J. D., Sidhu, M. K., Quiroz, J., Rosati, M., Schadeck, E. B., Pavlakis, G. N., Weiner, D. B., Rose, J. K., Israel, Z. R., Udem, S. A., and Eldridge, J. H. (2005). Priming with plasmid DNAs expressing interleukin-12 and simian immunodeficiency virus gag enhances the immunogenicity and efficacy of an experimental AIDS vaccine based on recombinant vesicular stomatitis virus. *AIDS Res.Hum.Retroviruses* 21, 629-643.

Eggena, M. P., Barugahare, B., Jones, N., Okello, M., Mutalya, S., Kityo, C., Mugyenyi, P., and Cao, H. (2005). Depletion of regulatory T cells in HIV infection is associated with immune activation. *J.Immunol.* 174, 4407-4414.

El Hed, A., Khaitan, A., Kozhaya, L., Manel, N., Daskalakis, D., Borkowsky, W., Valentine, F., Littman, D. R., and Unutmaz, D. (2010). Susceptibility of human Th17 cells to human immunodeficiency virus and their perturbation during infection. *J.Infect.Dis.* 201, 843-854.

Elson, C. O., Cong, Y., Weaver, C. T., Schoeb, T. R., McClanahan, T. K., Fick, R. B., and Kastelein, R. A. (2007). Monoclonal anti-interleukin 23 reverses active colitis in a T cell-mediated model in mice. *Gastroenterology* 132, 2359-2370.

Fakruddin, J. M., Lempicki, R. A., Gorelick, R. J., Yang, J., Adelsberger, J. W., Garcia-Pineres, A. J., Pinto, L. A., Lane, H. C., and Imamichi, T. (2007). Noninfectious papilloma virus-like particles inhibit HIV-1 replication: implications for immune control of HIV-1 infection by IL-27. *Blood* 109, 1841-1849.

Favre, D., Lederer, S., Kanwar, B., Ma, Z. M., Proll, S., Kasakow, Z., Mold, J., Swainson, L., Barbour, J. D., Baskin, C. R., Palermo, R., Pandrea, I., Miller, C. J., Katze, M. G., and McCune, J. M. (2009). Critical loss of the balance between Th17 and T regulatory cell populations in pathogenic SIV infection. *PLoS.Pathog.* 5, e1000295.

Fazekas de St, G. B. and Landay, A. L. (2008). Regulatory T cells in HIV infection: pathogenic or protective participants in the immune response? *AIDS.* 22, 671-683.

Fenoglio, D., Poggi, A., Catellani, S., Battaglia, F., Ferrera, A., Setti, M., Murdaca, G., and Zocchi, M. R. (2009). Vdelta1 T lymphocytes producing IFN-gamma and IL-17 are expanded in HIV-1-infected patients and respond to Candida albicans. *Blood.* 113, 6611-6618.

Gaffen, S. L., Kramer, J. M., Yu, J. J., and Shen, F. (2006). The IL-17 cytokine family. *Vitam.Horm.* 74:255-82., 255-282.

Gori, A., Tincati, C., Rizzardini, G., Torti, C., Quirino, T., Haarman, M., Ben Amor, K., van Schaik, J., Vriesema, A., Knol, J., Marchetti, G., Welling, G., and Clerici, M. (2008). Early impairment of gut function and gut flora supporting a role for alteration of gastrointestinal mucosa in human immunodeficiency virus pathogenesis. *J.Clin.Microbiol.* 46, 757-758.

Gosselin, A., Monteiro, P., Chomont, N., Diaz-Griffero, F., Said, E. A., Fonseca, S., Wacleche, V., El Far, M., Boulassel, M. R., Routy, J. P., Sekaly, R. P., and Ancuta, P. (2010). Peripheral blood CCR4+CCR6+ and CXCR3+CCR6+CD4+ T cells are highly permissive to HIV-1 infection. *J.Immunol.* 184, 1604-1616.

Gottlieb, A. B., Cooper, K. D., McCormick, T. S., Toichi, E., Everitt, D. E., Frederick, B., Zhu, Y., Pendley, C. E., Graham, M. A., and Mascelli, M. A. (2007). A phase 1, double-blind, placebo-controlled study evaluating single subcutaneous administrations of a human interleukin-12/23 monoclonal antibody in subjects with plaque psoriasis. *Curr.Med.Res.Opin.* 23, 1081-1092.

Greenwell-Wild, T., Vazquez, N., Jin, W., Rangel, Z., Munson, P. J., and Wahl, S. M. (2009). Interleukin-27 inhibition of HIV-1 involves an intermediate induction of type I interferon. *Blood.* 114, 1864-1874.

Guzzo, C., Che Mat, N. F., and Gee, K. (2010). Interleukin-27 induces a STAT1/3 and NF-kappaB dependent proinflammatory cytokine profile in human monocytes. *J.Biol.Chem.*

Guzzo, C., Hopman, W. M., Mat, N. F., Wobeser, W., and Gee, K. (2010). Impact of HIV infection, highly active antiretroviral therapy, and hepatitis C coinfection on serum interleukin-27. *AIDS.* 24, 1371-1374.

Hirao, L. A., Wu, L., Khan, A. S., Hokey, D. A., Yan, J., Dai, A., Betts, M. R., Draghia-Akli, R., and Weiner, D. B. (2008). Combined effects of IL-12 and electroporation enhances the potency of DNA vaccination in macaques. *Vaccine.* 26, 3112-3120.

Holmes, D., Knudsen, G., Mackey-Cushman, S., and Su, L. (2007). FoxP3 enhances HIV-1 gene expression by modulating NFkappaB occupancy at the long terminal repeat in human T cells. *J.Biol.Chem.* 282, 15973-15980.

Hsieh, C. S., Macatonia, S. E., Tripp, C. S., Wolf, S. F., O'Garra, A., and Murphy, K. M. (1993). Development of TH1 CD4+ T cells through IL-12 produced by Listeria-induced macrophages. *Science.* 260, 547-549.

Hunt, P. W. (2010). Th17, gut, and HIV: therapeutic implications. *Curr.Opin.HIV.AIDS.* 5, 189-193.

Hunt, P. W., Landay, A. L., Sinclair, E., Martinson, J. A., Hatano, H., Emu, B., Norris, P. J., Busch, M. P., Martin, J. N., Brooks, C., McCune, J. M., and Deeks, S. G. (2011). A low T regulatory cell response may contribute to both viral control and generalized immune activation in HIV controllers. *PLoS.One.* 6, e15924.

Hunter, C. A. (2005). New IL-12-family members: IL-23 and IL-27, cytokines with divergent functions. *Nat.Rev.Immunol.* 5, 521-531.

Imamichi, T., Yang, J., Huang, D. W., Brann, T. W., Fullmer, B. A., Adelsberger, J. W., Lempicki, R. A., Baseler, M. W., and Lane, H. C. (2008). IL-27, a novel anti-HIV cytokine, activates multiple interferon-inducible genes in macrophages. *AIDS* 22, 39-45.

Ji, J. and Cloyd, M. W. (2009). HIV-1 binding to CD4 on CD4+CD25+ regulatory T cells enhances their suppressive function and induces them to home to, and accumulate in, peripheral and mucosal lymphoid tissues: an additional mechanism of immunosuppression. *Int.Immunol.* 21, 283-294.

Jiang, W., Lederman, M. M., Hunt, P., Sieg, S. F., Haley, K., Rodriguez, B., Landay, A., Martin, J., Sinclair, E., Asher, A. I., Deeks, S. G., Douek, D. C., and Brenchley, J. M. (2009). Plasma levels of bacterial DNA correlate with immune activation and the magnitude of immune restoration in persons with antiretroviral-treated HIV infection. *J.Infect.Dis.* 199, 1177-1185.

Jiao, Y., Fu, J., Xing, S., Fu, B., Zhang, Z., Shi, M., Wang, X., Zhang, J., Jin, L., Kang, F., Wu, H., and Wang, F. S. (2009). The decrease of regulatory T cells correlates with excessive activation and apoptosis of CD8+ T cells in HIV-1-infected typical progressors, but not in long-term non-progressors. *Immunology.* 128, e366-e375.

Jones, M. L., Young, J. M., Huang, Q. R., Puls, R. L., Webber, C. A., and Benson, E. M. (2003). Interleukin 12-augmented T cell proliferation of peripheral blood mononuclear cells from HIV-seropositive individuals is associated with interleukin 12 receptor beta 2 upregulation. *AIDS Res.Hum.Retroviruses.* 19, 283-292.

Kader, M., Wang, X., Piatak, M., Lifson, J., Roederer, M., Veazey, R., and Mattapallil, J. J. (2009). Alpha4(+)beta7(hi)CD4(+) memory T cells harbor most Th-17 cells and are preferentially infected during acute SIV infection. *Mucosal.Immunol.* 2, 439-449.

Kalliolias, G. D. and Ivashkiv, L. B. (2008). IL-27 activates human monocytes via STAT1 and suppresses IL-10 production but the inflammatory functions of IL-27 are abrogated by TLRs and p38. *J.Immunol.* 180, 6325-6333.

Kanwar, B., Favre, D., and McCune, J. M. (2010). Th17 and regulatory T cells: implications for AIDS pathogenesis. *Curr.Opin.HIV.AIDS.* 5, 151-157.

Kaplan, M. H., Schindler, U., Smiley, S. T., and Grusby, M. J. (1996). Stat6 is required for mediating responses to IL-4 and for development of Th2 cells. *Immunity.* 4, 313-319.

Kared, H., Lelievre, J. D., Donkova-Petrini, V., Aouba, A., Melica, G., Balbo, M., Weiss, L., and Levy, Y. (2008). HIV-specific regulatory T cells are associated with higher CD4 cell counts in primary infection. *AIDS.* 22, 2451-2460.

Kassiotis, G. and O'Garra, A. (2008). Immunology. Immunity benefits from a little suppression. *Science.* 320, 1168-1169.

Kinter, A., McNally, J., Riggin, L., Jackson, R., Roby, G., and Fauci, A. S. (2007). Suppression of HIV-specific T cell activity by lymph node CD25+ regulatory T cells from HIV-infected individuals. *Proc.Natl.Acad.Sci.U.S.A.* 104, 3390-3395.

Kinter, A. L., Horak, R., Sion, M., Riggin, L., McNally, J., Lin, Y., Jackson, R., O'shea, A., Roby, G., Kovacs, C., Connors, M., Migueles, S. A., and Fauci, A. S. (2007). CD25+ regulatory T cells isolated from HIV-infected individuals suppress the cytolytic and nonlytic antiviral activity of HIV-specific CD8+ T cells in vitro. *AIDS Res.Hum.Retroviruses.* 23, 438-450.

Korn, T., Bettelli, E., Oukka, M., and Kuchroo, V. K. (2009). IL-17 and Th17 Cells. *Annu.Rev.Immunol.* 27:485-517., 485-517.

Krueger, G. G., Langley, R. G., Leonardi, C., Yeilding, N., Guzzo, C., Wang, Y., Dooley, L. T., and Lebwohl, M. (2007). A human interleukin-12/23 monoclonal antibody for the treatment of psoriasis. *N.Engl.J.Med.* 356, 580-592.

Kurata, H., Lee, H. J., O'Garra, A., and Arai, N. (1999). Ectopic expression of activated Stat6 induces the expression of Th2-specific cytokines and transcription factors in developing Th1 cells. *Immunity.* 11, 677-688.

Landay, A. L., Clerici, M., Hashemi, F., Kessler, H., Berzofsky, J. A., and Shearer, G. M. (1996). In vitro restoration of T cell immune function in human immunodeficiency virus-positive persons: effects of interleukin (IL)-12 and anti-IL-10. *J.Infect.Dis.* 173, 1085-1091.

Larousserie, F., Charlot, P., Bardel, E., Froger, J., Kastelein, R. A., and Devergne, O. (2006). Differential effects of IL-27 on human B cell subsets. *J.Immunol.* 176, 5890-5897.

Lawn, S. D., Butera, S. T., and Folks, T. M. (2001). Contribution of immune activation to the pathogenesis and transmission of human immunodeficiency virus type 1 infection. *Clin.Microbiol.Rev.* 14, 753-77, table.

Lederer, S., Favre, D., Walters, K. A., Proll, S., Kanwar, B., Kasakow, Z., Baskin, C. R., Palermo, R., McCune, J. M., and Katze, M. G. (2009). Transcriptional profiling in pathogenic and non-pathogenic SIV infections reveals significant distinctions in kinetics and tissue compartmentalization. *PLoS.Pathog.* 5, e1000296.

Lee, S., French, M. A., and Price, P. (2004). IL-23 and IFN-gamma deficiency in immunodeficient HIV patients who achieved a long-term increase in CD4 T-cell counts on highly active antiretroviral therapy. *AIDS.* 18, 1337-1340.

Louis, S., Dutertre, C. A., Vimeux, L., Fery, L., Henno, L., Diocou, S., Kahi, S., Deveau, C., Meyer, L., Goujard, C., and Hosmalin, A. (2010). IL-23 and IL-12p70 production by monocytes and dendritic cells in primary HIV-1 infection. *J.Leukoc.Biol.* 87, 645-653.

Lucas, S., Ghilardi, N., Li, J., and de Sauvage, F. J. (2003). IL-27 regulates IL-12 responsiveness of naive CD4+ T cells through Stat1-dependent and -independent mechanisms. *Proc.Natl.Acad.Sci.U.S.A* 100, 15047-15052.

Ma, C. S., Tangye, S. G., and Deenick, E. K. (2010). Human Th9 cells: inflammatory cytokines modulate IL-9 production through the induction of IL-21. *Immunol Cell Biol.* 88, 621-623.

Ma, W., Mishra, S., Gajanayaka, N., Angel, J. B., and Kumar, A. (2009). HIV-1 Nef inhibits lipopolysaccharide-induced IL-12p40 expression by inhibiting JNK-activated NFkappaB in human monocytic cells. *J.Biol.Chem.* %20;284, 7578-7587.

Macal, M., Sankaran, S., Chun, T. W., Reay, E., Flamm, J., Prindiville, T. J., and Dandekar, S. (2008). Effective CD4+ T-cell restoration in gut-associated lymphoid tissue of HIV-infected patients is associated with enhanced Th17 cells and polyfunctional HIV-specific T-cell responses. *Mucosal.Immunol.* 1, 475-488.

Maek, A. N., Buranapraditkun, S., Klaewsongkram, J., and Ruxrungtham, K. (2007). Increased interleukin-17 production both in helper T cell subset Th17 and CD4-negative T cells in human immunodeficiency virus infection. *Viral Immunol* 20, 66-75.

Mangan, P. R., Harrington, L. E., O'Quinn, D. B., Helms, W. S., Bullard, D. C., Elson, C. O., Hatton, R. D., Wahl, S. M., Schoeb, T. R., and Weaver, C. T. (2006). Transforming growth factor-beta induces development of the T(H)17 lineage. *Nature* 441, 231-234.

Marshall, J. D., Chehimi, J., Gri, G., Kostman, J. R., Montaner, L. J., and Trinchieri, G. (1999). The interleukin-12-mediated pathway of immune events is dysfunctional in human immunodeficiency virus-infected individuals. *Blood* 94, 1003-1011.

Matsui, M., Moriya, O., Belladonna, M. L., Kamiya, S., Lemonnier, F. A., Yoshimoto, T., and Akatsuka, T. (2004). Adjuvant activities of novel cytokines, interleukin-23 (IL-23) and IL-27, for induction of hepatitis C virus-specific cytotoxic T lymphocytes in HLA-A*0201 transgenic mice. *J.Virol.* 78, 9093-9104.

McGeachy, M. J., Chen, Y., Tato, C. M., Laurence, A., Joyce-Shaikh, B., Blumenschein, W. M., McClanahan, T. K., O'Shea, J. J., and Cua, D. J. (2009). The interleukin 23 receptor is essential for the terminal differentiation of interleukin 17-producing effector T helper cells in vivo. *Nat.Immunol.* 10, 314-324.

Mehandru, S., Poles, M. A., Tenner-Racz, K., Horowitz, A., Hurley, A., Hogan, C., Boden, D., Racz, P., and Markowitz, M. (2004). Primary HIV-1 infection is associated with preferential depletion of CD4+ T lymphocytes from effector sites in the gastrointestinal tract. *J.Exp.Med.* %20;200, 761-770.

Moreno-Fernandez, M. E., Rueda, C. M., Rusie, L. K., and Chougnet, C. A. (2011). Regulatory T cells control HIV replication in activated T cells through a cAMP-dependent mechanism. *Blood.*

Moreno-Fernandez, M. E., Zapata, W., Blackard, J. T., Franchini, G., and Chougnet, C. A. (2009). Human regulatory T cells are targets for human immunodeficiency Virus (HIV) infection, and their susceptibility differs depending on the HIV type 1 strain. *J.Virol.* 83, 12925-12933.

Mozos, A., Garrido, M., Carreras, J., Plana, M., Diaz, A., Alos, L., Campo, E., Garcia, F., and Martinez, A. (2007). Redistribution of FOXP3-positive regulatory T cells from lymphoid tissues to peripheral blood in HIV-infected patients. *J.Acquir.Immune.Defic.Syndr.* 46, 529-537.

Mucida, D., Park, Y., Kim, G., Turovskaya, O., Scott, I., Kronenberg, M., and Cheroutre, H. (2007). Reciprocal TH17 and regulatory T cell differentiation mediated by retinoic acid. *Science.* 317, 256-260.

Murai, M., Krause, P., Cheroutre, H., and Kronenberg, M. (2010). Regulatory T-cell stability and plasticity in mucosal and systemic immune systems. *Mucosal.Immunol.* 3, 443-449.

Ndhlovu, L. C., Chapman, J. M., Jha, A. R., Snyder-Cappione, J. E., Pagan, M., Leal, F. E., Boland, B. S., Norris, P. J., Rosenberg, M. G., and Nixon, D. F. (2008). Suppression of HIV-1 plasma viral load below detection preserves IL-17 producing T cells in HIV-1 infection. *AIDS* 22, 990-992.

Ndhlovu, L. C., Sinclair, E., Epling, L., Tan, Q. X., Ho, T., Jha, A. R., Eccles-James, I., Tincati, C., Levy, J. A., Nixon, D. F., Hecht, F. M., and Barbour, J. D. (2010b). IL-2 immunotherapy to recently HIV-1 infected adults maintains the numbers of IL-17 expressing CD4+ T (T(H)17) cells in the periphery. *J.Clin.Immunol.* 30, 681-692.

Ndhlovu, L. C., Sinclair, E., Epling, L., Tan, Q. X., Ho, T., Jha, A. R., Eccles-James, I., Tincati, C., Levy, J. A., Nixon, D. F., Hecht, F. M., and Barbour, J. D. (2010a). IL-2 immunotherapy to recently HIV-1 infected adults maintains the numbers of IL-17 expressing CD4+ T (T(H)17) cells in the periphery. *J.Clin.Immunol.* 30, 681-692.

Neumann, A., Polis, M., Rozenberg, L., Jackson, J., Reitano, K., McLaughlin, M., Koratich, C., Dewar, R., Masur, H., Haagmans, B., and Kottilil, S. (2007). Differential antiviral effect of PEG-interferon-alpha-2b on HIV and HCV in the treatment of HIV/HCV co-infected patients. *AIDS* 21, 1855-1865.

Niedbala, W., Cai, B., Wei, X., Patakas, A., Leung, B. P., McInnes, I. B., and Liew, F. Y. (2008). Interleukin-27 attenuates collagen-induced arthritis. *Ann.Rheum.Dis.*

Nilssen, D. E., Muller, F., Oktedalen, O., Froland, S. S., Fausa, O., Halstensen, T. S., and Brandtzaeg, P. (1996). Intraepithelial gamma/delta T cells in duodenal mucosa are related to the immune state and survival time in AIDS. *J.Virol.* 70, 3545-3550.

Nilsson, J., Boasso, A., Velilla, P. A., Zhang, R., Vaccari, M., Franchini, G., Shearer, G. M., Andersson, J., and Chougnet, C. (2006). HIV-1-driven regulatory T-cell accumulation in lymphoid tissues is associated with disease progression in HIV/AIDS. *Blood.* 108, 3808-3817.

Nurieva, R. I., Chung, Y., Martinez, G. J., Yang, X. O., Tanaka, S., Matskevitch, T. D., Wang, Y. H., and Dong, C. (2009). Bcl6 mediates the development of T follicular helper cells. *Science.* 325, 1001-1005.

Oppmann, B., Lesley, R., Blom, B., Timans, J. C., Xu, Y., Hunte, B., Vega, F., Yu, N., Wang, J., Singh, K., Zonin, F., Vaisberg, E., Churakova, T., Liu, M., Gorman, D., Wagner, J., Zurawski, S., Liu, Y., Abrams, J. S., Moore, K. W., Rennick, D., Waal-Malefyt, R., Hannum, C., Bazan, J. F., and Kastelein, R. A. (2000). Novel p19 protein engages IL-12p40 to form a cytokine, IL-23, with biological activities similar as well as distinct from IL-12. *Immunity.* 13, 715-725.

Owen, R. E., Heitman, J. W., Hirschkorn, D. F., Lanteri, M. C., Biswas, H. H., Martin, J. N., Krone, M. R., Deeks, S. G., and Norris, P. J. (2010). HIV+ elite controllers have low HIV-specific T-cell activation yet maintain strong, polyfunctional T-cell responses. *AIDS.* 24, 1095-1105.

Pai, S. Y., Truitt, M. L., and Ho, I. C. (2004). GATA-3 deficiency abrogates the development and maintenance of T helper type 2 cells. *Proc.Natl.Acad.Sci.U.S.A.* 101, 1993-1998.

Palermo, R. E., Patterson, L. J., Aicher, L. D., Korth, M. J., Robert-Guroff, M., and Katze, M. G. (2011). Genomic analysis reveals pre- and postchallenge differences in a rhesus macaque AIDS vaccine trial: insights into mechanisms of vaccine efficacy. *J.Virol.* 85, 1099-1116.

Parham, C., Chirica, M., Timans, J., Vaisberg, E., Travis, M., Cheung, J., Pflanz, S., Zhang, R., Singh, K. P., Vega, F., To, W., Wagner, J., O'Farrell, A. M., McClanahan, T., Zurawski, S., Hannum, C., Gorman, D., Rennick, D. M., Kastelein, R. A., de Waal, M. R., and Moore, K. W. (2002). A receptor for the heterodimeric cytokine IL-23 is composed of IL-12Rbeta1 and a novel cytokine receptor subunit, IL-23R. *J.Immunol.* 168, 5699-5708.

Peng, Q. L., Zhang, M. X., Li, G. Y., Liu, Y. X., Zhou, B. P., and Wang, H. (2010). [Loss of the balance between Th17 and Th1 populations in HIV/AIDS patients]. *Zhonghua Shi Yan.He.Lin.Chuang.Bing.Du Xue.Za Zhi.* 24, 17-20.

Pflanz, S., Hibbert, L., Mattson, J., Rosales, R., Vaisberg, E., Bazan, J. F., Phillips, J. H., McClanahan, T. K., de Waal, M. R., and Kastelein, R. A. (2004). WSX-1 and glycoprotein 130 constitute a signal-transducing receptor for IL-27. *J.Immunol.* 172, 2225-2231.

Pflanz, S., Timans, J. C., Cheung, J., Rosales, R., Kanzler, H., Gilbert, J., Hibbert, L., Churakova, T., Travis, M., Vaisberg, E., Blumenschein, W. M., Mattson, J. D., Wagner, J. L., To, W., Zurawski, S., McClanahan, T. K., Gorman, D. M., Bazan, J. F., de Waal, M. R., Rennick,

D., and Kastelein, R. A. (2002). IL-27, a heterodimeric cytokine composed of EBI3 and p28 protein, induces proliferation of naive CD4(+) T cells. *Immunity.* 16, 779-790.

Piconi, S., Trabattoni, D., Gori, A., Parisotto, S., Magni, C., Meraviglia, P., Bandera, A., Capetti, A., Rizzardini, G., and Clerici, M. (2010). Immune activation, apoptosis, and Treg activity are associated with persistently reduced CD4+ T-cell counts during antiretroviral therapy. *AIDS.* 24, 1991-2000.

Prendergast, A., Prado, J. G., Kang, Y. H., Chen, F., Riddell, L. A., Luzzi, G., Goulder, P., and Klenerman, P. (2010). HIV-1 infection is characterized by profound depletion of CD161+ Th17 cells and gradual decline in regulatory T cells. *AIDS.* %20;24, 491-502.

Quintana, F. J., Basso, A. S., Iglesias, A. H., Korn, T., Farez, M. F., Bettelli, E., Caccamo, M., Oukka, M., and Weiner, H. L. (2008). Control of T(reg) and T(H)17 cell differentiation by the aryl hydrocarbon receptor. *Nature.* 453, 65-71.

Raffatellu, M., Santos, R. L., Verhoeven, D. E., George, M. D., Wilson, R. P., Winter, S. E., Godinez, I., Sankaran, S., Paixao, T. A., Gordon, M. A., Kolls, J. K., Dandekar, S., and Baumler, A. J. (2008). Simian immunodeficiency virus-induced mucosal interleukin-17 deficiency promotes Salmonella dissemination from the gut. *Nat Med.* 14, 421-428.

Romani, B., Engelbrecht, S., and Glashoff, R. H. (2009). Antiviral roles of APOBEC proteins against HIV-1 and suppression by Vif. *Arch.Virol.* 154, 1579-1588.

Rouse, B. T., Sarangi, P. P., and Suvas, S. (2006). Regulatory T cells in virus infections. *Immunol.Rev.* 212, 272-286.

Ruckerl, D., Hessmann, M., Yoshimoto, T., Ehlers, S., and Holscher, C. (2006). Alternatively activated macrophages express the IL-27 receptor alpha chain WSX-1. *Immunobiology* 211, 427-436.

Schulze Zur, W. J., Thomssen, A., Hartjen, P., Toth, I., Lehmann, C., Meyer-Olson, D., Colberg, K., Frerk, S., Babikir, D., Schmiedel, S., Degen, O., Mauss, S., Rockstroh, J., Staszewski, S., Khaykin, P., Strasak, A., Lohse, A. W., Fatkenheuer, G., Hauber, J., and van Lunzen, J. (2011). Comprehensive analysis of frequency and phenotype of T regulatory cells in HIV infection: CD39 expression of FoxP3+ T regulatory cells correlates with progressive disease. *J.Virol.* 85, 1287-1297.

Seder, R. A., Gazzinelli, R., Sher, A., and Paul, W. E. (1993). Interleukin 12 acts directly on CD4+ T cells to enhance priming for interferon gamma production and diminishes interleukin 4 inhibition of such priming. *Proc.Natl.Acad.Sci.U.S.A.* 90, 10188-10192.

Stockinger, B. (2007). Good for Goose, but not for Gander: IL-2 interferes with Th17 differentiation. *Immunity.* 26, 278-279.

Suto, A., Kashiwakuma, D., Kagami, S., Hirose, K., Watanabe, N., Yokote, K., Saito, Y., Nakayama, T., Grusby, M. J., Iwamoto, I., and Nakajima, H. (2008). Development and characterization of IL-21-producing CD4+ T cells. *J.Exp.Med.* 205, 1369-1379.

Szabo, S. J., Sullivan, B. M., Stemmann, C., Satoskar, A. R., Sleckman, B. P., and Glimcher, L. H. (2002). Distinct effects of T-bet in TH1 lineage commitment and IFN-gamma production in CD4 and CD8 T cells. *Science* 295, 338-342.

Terzieva, V. (2008). Regulatory T cells and HIV-1 infection. *Viral Immunol.* 21, 285-291.

Thorborn, G., Pomeroy, L., Isohanni, H., Perry, M., Peters, B., and Vyakarnam, A. (2010). Increased sensitivity of CD4+ T-effector cells to CD4+CD25+ Treg suppression compensates for reduced Treg number in asymptomatic HIV-1 infection. *PLoS.One.* 5, e9254.

Torheim, E. A., Ndhlovu, L. C., Pettersen, F. O., Larsen, T. L., Jha, A. R., Torgersen, K. M., Kvale, D., Nixon, D. F., Tasken, K., and Aandahl, E. M. (2009). Interleukin-10-

secreting T cells define a suppressive subset within the HIV-1-specific T-cell population. *Eur.J.Immunol.* 39, 1280-1287.

Tran, T. A., de Goer de Herve MG, Hendel-Chavez, H., Dembele, B., Le Nevot, E., Abbed, K., Pallier, C., Goujard, C., Gasnault, J., Delfraissy, J. F., Balazuc, A. M., and Taoufik, Y. (2008). Resting regulatory CD4 T cells: a site of HIV persistence in patients on long-term effective antiretroviral therapy. *PLoS.One.* 3, e3305.

van Seventer, J. M., Nagai, T., and van Seventer, G. A. (2002). Interferon-beta differentially regulates expression of the IL-12 family members p35, p40, p19 and EBI3 in activated human dendritic cells. *J.Neuroimmunol.* 133, 60-71.

Villinger, F. and Ansari, A. A. (2010). Role of IL-12 in HIV infection and vaccine. *Eur.Cytokine Netw.* 21, 215-218.

Weiss, L., Letimier, F. A., Carriere, M., Maiella, S., Donkova-Petrini, V., Targat, B., Benecke, A., Rogge, L., and Levy, Y. (2010). In vivo expansion of naive and activated CD4+CD25+FOXP3+ regulatory T cell populations in interleukin-2-treated HIV patients. *Proc.Natl.Acad.Sci.U.S.A.* 107, 10632-10637.

Weiss, L., Piketty, C., Assoumou, L., Didier, C., Caccavelli, L., Donkova-Petrini, V., Levy, Y., Girard, P. M., Burgard, M., Viard, J. P., Rouzioux, C., and Costagliola, D. (2010). Relationship between regulatory T cells and immune activation in human immunodeficiency virus-infected patients interrupting antiretroviral therapy. *PLoS.One.* 5, e11659.

Wirtz, S., Tubbe, I., Galle, P. R., Schild, H. J., Birkenbach, M., Blumberg, R. S., and Neurath, M. F. (2006). Protection from lethal septic peritonitis by neutralizing the biological function of interleukin 27. *J.Exp.Med.* 203, 1875-1881.

Wong, M. T., Ye, J. J., Alonso, M. N., Landrigan, A., Cheung, R. K., Engleman, E., and Utz, P. J. (2010). Regulation of human Th9 differentiation by type I interferons and IL-21. *Immunol Cell Biol.* 88, 624-631.

Xing, J., Wu, Y., and Ni, B. (2011). Th9: a new player in asthma pathogenesis? *J.Asthma.* 48, 115-125.

Xing, S., Fu, J., Zhang, Z., Gao, Y., Jiao, Y., Kang, F., Zhang, J., Zhou, C., Wu, H., and Wang, F. S. (2010). Increased turnover of FoxP3high regulatory T cells is associated with hyperactivation and disease progression of chronic HIV-1 infection. *J.Acquir.Immune.Defic.Syndr.* 54, 455-462.

Yang, X. O., Pappu, B. P., Nurieva, R., Akimzhanov, A., Kang, H. S., Chung, Y., Ma, L., Shah, B., Panopoulos, A. D., Schluns, K. S., Watowich, S. S., Tian, Q., Jetten, A. M., and Dong, C. (2008). T helper 17 lineage differentiation is programmed by orphan nuclear receptors ROR alpha and ROR gamma. *Immunity.* 28, 29-39.

Yue, F. Y., Merchant, A., Kovacs, C. M., Loutfy, M., Persad, D., and Ostrowski, M. A. (2008). Virus-specific interleukin-17-producing CD4+ T cells are detectable in early human immunodeficiency virus type 1 infection. *J.Virol.* 82, 6767-6771.

Zheng, Y. and Rudensky, A. Y. (2007). Foxp3 in control of the regulatory T cell lineage. *Nat Immunol.* 8, 457-462.

Zhou, L., Lopes, J. E., Chong, M. M., Ivanov, I. I., Min, R., Victora, G. D., Shen, Y., Du, J., Rubtsov, Y. P., Rudensky, A. Y., Ziegler, S. F., and Littman, D. R. (2008). TGF-beta-induced Foxp3 inhibits T(H)17 cell differentiation by antagonizing RORgammat function. *Nature.* 453, 236-240.

Zhu, J., Min, B., Hu-Li, J., Watson, C. J., Grinberg, A., Wang, Q., Killeen, N., Urban, J. F., Jr., Guo, L., and Paul, W. E. (2004). Conditional deletion of Gata3 shows its essential function in T(H)1-T(H)2 responses. *Nat Immunol.* 5, 1157-1165.

10

Interactions of Infectious HIV-1 Virions with Erythrocytes: Implications for HIV-1 Pathogenesis and Infectivity

Zoltan Beck[1,2] and Carl R. Alving[1]
[1]*Division of Retrovirology, U.S. Military HIV Research Program, Walter Reed Army Institute of Research, Silver Spring, MD*
[2]*Henry M. Jackson Foundation for the Advancement of Military Medicine, Rockville, MD USA*

1. Introduction

According to widely held current paradigms of cellular infection and transmission of HIV-1 the virus first binds to a membrane receptor on a target cell, such as CD4 and a chemokine receptor (CCR5 or CXCR4) that serve as co-receptors. After penetration of the plasma membrane of the cell by the virus via receptor-mediated fusion, followed by insertion of the viral RNA and intracellular replication, the newly assembled virion buds from the host cell into the extracellular environment where it becomes a cell-free infectious virion. In accordance with this, it is widely believed that prior to infecting new target cells HIV-1 in blood exists mainly as cell-free infectious virions (Ho et al., 1989; Pan et al., 1993). Upon encountering a new target cell a new cycle leads to entry and infection of the new cell. In this chapter, we will review an alternative concept that HIV-1 can bind to human erythrocytes, and that erythrocyte-bound HIV-1 remains infectious and promotes *trans* infection of CD4(+) T cells. We further propose the general concept that is likely that virtually all infectious HIV-1 particles in blood are bound to circulating cells *in vivo*, rather than existing as cell-free circulating virus. We will review various mechanisms that might be involved in binding of infectious HIV-1 to erythrocytes, and the implications that *trans* infection by erythrocyte-bound HIV-1 might have for pathogenesis of HIV-1 and for vaccine development.

2. Binding of HIV-1 to erythrocytes: *In vitro* studies

Several studies have addressed the adherence of HIV-1 to erythrocytes *in vitro*. Olinger et al. (2000) suggested that HIV-1 binding to the surface of CD4(-) cells might be an important route for infection of T cells based on the ability of HIV-1 strain MN (T-cell line-adapted) and X4 and R5 primary isolates to bind to various cell types. Virus apparently bound *in vitro* both to isolated CD4(+) and CD4(-) cells, including peripheral blood mononuclear cells (PBMC), neutrophils, tonsillar mononuclear cells, platelets, and erythrocytes. Virus that had bound to CD4(-) cells was up to 17 times more infectious for T cells in co-cultures than was the same amount of cell-free virus. Enhanced infection of T cells by virus bound to CD4(-)

cells was not due to stimulatory signals provided by CD4(-) cells or infection of CD4(-) cells, and it was proposed that virus bound to the surface of CD4(-) cells was efficiently passed to CD4(+) T cells during cell-cell adhesion. Although the study by Olinger et al. (2000) did not investigate the mechanism of HIV-1 binding or the binding site on the CD4(-) cells, it was suggested that HIV-1 binds at relatively high levels to CD4(-) cells, including erythrocytes, and that cell-bound HIV-1 is highly infectious for T cells.

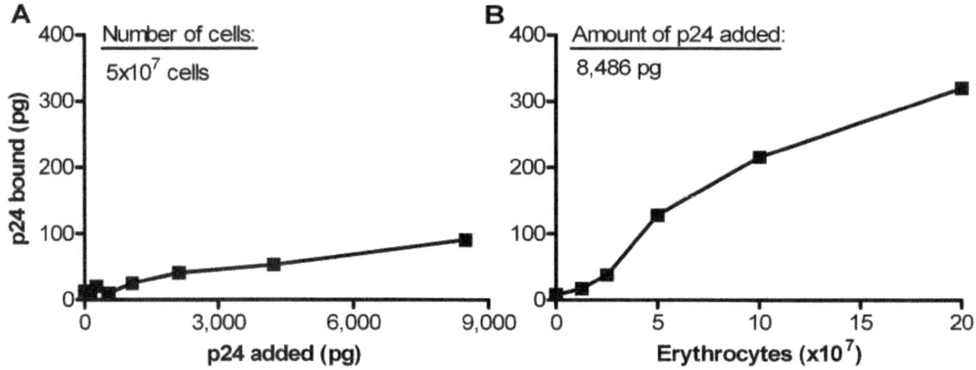

Fig. 1. Binding of a HIV-1 isolate to erythrocytes.

(A) Increasing amounts of HIV-1 isolate 90US_873 (as quantified by p24) were incubated with 5x107 erythrocytes and binding of p24 to the cells was determined. (B) Dose-dependent binding of the HIV-1 isolate (8,486 pg p24) with increasing numbers of erythrocytes. The experiment shown is representative of 3 separate experiments. In each experiment HIV-1 was bound to erythrocytes in triplicate, washed, and the triplicates were pooled for p24 determination. From Beck et al. (2009).

The binding of HIV-1 at 4°C *in vitro* to normal erythrocytes from 30 different individual donors was subsequently confirmed and found to be calcium dependent by Beck et al. (2009), and further confirmed by Garcia et al. (2011). As shown in Fig. 1A, the binding of p24 to 5 x 10^7 erythrocytes obtained from a selected individual donor exhibited a dose-response up to 8,486 pg of added p24 (the maximum amount of p24 in the HIV-1 stock that could be used in the assay); however when this latter amount of p24 was then incubated with increased numbers of erythrocytes, to a level of 20 x 10^7 (the maximum number of erythrocytes that could be used because of viscosity restraints in the assay), a further three-fold increase of p24 binding was observed (Fig. 1B) (Beck et al., 2009). At the highest ratio of erythrocytes/p24 there was no clear plateau in the amount of p24 binding, but it did appear likely that the binding pattern was in the form of a wide and relatively shallow sigmoid curve that might be approaching a plateau.

When the erythrocytes from 30 donors were examined, a mean of only 2.4% of the total added HIV-1 p24 was bound to the erythrocytes, but additional experiments further demonstrated that adsorption of the original HIV-1 preparation with erythrocytes removed essentially all (up to 97%) of the infectivity of HIV-1 for *trans* infection of CD4(+) PBMC (Beck et al., 2009). It was thus demonstrated that only a small fraction of the originally added p24 became bound to the erythrocytes, but this amount comprised virtually all of the infectious HIV-1 particles in the original preparation added to the cells.

From the data shown in Fig. 1 it seems clear that either the binding affinity of infectious HIV-1 particles for erythrocytes is extremely low, or the number of cells in the erythrocyte population that actually bind infectious HIV-1 particles is a very small number of the total cells present. However, because the binding to the cells survived several relatively vigorous washing techniques resulting in a p24-free supernatant, it would appear unlikely that the binding affinity to the cells was low. To estimate the approximate fraction of cells in the erythrocyte population that had the capacity to bind infectious HIV-1 particles, the following theoretical calculations can be considered. If one assumes that: (A) one infectious virion contains ~5,000 molecules of gag p24 (Briggs et al., 2004); and (B) the molecular weight of p24 is 24,000, then there are ~5,000 viruses per pg of p24. If one further assumes (C) that all of the infectious virions that were added to the erythrocytes were contained within 320 pg of p24 that were attached to 20 x 10^7 erythrocytes (Fig. 1B), then the calculation suggests that only approximately 1 infectious virion was bound per 125 erythrocytes. The data thus suggested that the binding of infectious HIV-1 particles to cells in the erythrocyte preparation was a relatively rare event, and perhaps fewer than 1% of the cells that were present in the erythrocyte pool had the capacity to bind HIV-1. However, it was also likely that binding to erythrocytes *per se* did occur because substantial binding was observed with erythrocyte ghosts prepared after the initial binding event was completed. Furthermore, binding was also observed directly with fresh erythrocyte ghosts (Beck et al., 2009).

2.1 Contaminating cell types as potential targets for binding of HIV-1 in erythrocyte preparations

Because <1% of the cells in the erythrocyte population appeared to bind the HIV-1, several possible circulating cell types could be suggested as candidates that might contain the observed HIV-1 binding site, including: myeloid-derived multipotent progenitor cells and long-lived hematopoietic stem cells (Carter et al., 2010; Carter et al., 2011); young erythrocytes or direct precursors of erythrocytes (such as reticulocytes); damaged but still circulating mature erythrocytes; aged erythrocytes near or at the end of their circulating life-span; and CD4(-) nucleated cells that were not removed during the preparation of the erythrocytes.

It is notable that platelets contain two C-type lectins, C-type lectin-like receptor 2 (CLEC-2) and dendritic cell-specific, ICAM-3 grabbing, nonintegrin (DC-SIGN), that are each surface-expressed proteins that exhibit calcium-dependent binding of infectious HIV-1 particles (Boukour et al., 2006; Chaipan et al., 2006; Flaujac et al., 2010). Although it has been suggested that platelets might represent a circulating reservoir for HIV-1, it has also been reported that internalization of HIV-1 by platelets might cause disrupt viral integrity (Boukour et al., 2006; Flaujac et al., 2010). Because platelets are notoriously sticky, it is possible that clumps of platelets might become bound as contaminants on a small number of erythrocytes either *in vitro* or *in vivo*, and because of the ability of platelets to bind HIV-1 these erythrocyte-platelet combinations might then serve as platforms for *trans* infection by attached HIV-1.

Hemolysis of the erythrocytes after the initial binding of HIV-1, followed by centrifugation to remove nucleated cells, revealed that a substantial amount of binding of p24 was found not only on the erythrocyte ghosts, but also on the small number of nucleated cells that contaminated the erythrocyte pool (Beck et al., 2009). Flow cytometry analysis of the erythrocyte population revealed only approximately 0.4% contamination by nucleated (nonhemolyzed) cells [0.07% CD4(+) and 0.33% CD4(-) cells]. However, based on the small numbers of nucleated cells in the erythrocyte population but the relatively high level of p24 binding to cells other than erythrocytes, it appeared that the binding of HIV-1 to leukocytes was stronger than binding of the HIV-1 to erythrocytes. Despite this, it was further demonstrated that when the initial incubation temperature of 4°C that was used for binding to erythrocytes was subsequently raised to 37°C, no detectable internalization of virus occurred over a period of 4 hours. Binding of p24 at 4°C, or even after 4 hours at 37°C, was substantially eliminated by treatment of the erythrocytes with EDTA. It was thus concluded that binding of the virus to sites on contaminating cells in the erythrocyte population that could be infected by HIV-1 did not account for any of the observed binding of HIV-1 (Beck et al., 2009).

3. Candidate binding sites on erythrocytes

The binding site (or sites) for infectious HIV-1 on erythrocytes, whether protein, carbohydrate, or lipid (including glycolipid or phospholipid), or combinations of these, have not yet been completely determined. In considering this problem, there is also the theoretical and practical difficulty of differentiating the binding of whole infectious virions from binding of defective virus particles or degradation products such as free p24.

The external cell membrane contains numerous proteins with many functions, and the literature on red cell proteins and their functions has been extensively reviewed (Anstee, 2011; Daniels, 2007; Denomme, 2004; Mohandas & Narla, 2005; Reid & Mohandas, 2004; Telen, 2005). At least 60 different erythrocytic surface proteins that could be candidates for binding of HIV-1 are classifiable into at least six categories based on their functions, namely: enzymes; membrane transporters; receptors; adhesion molecules; blood group antigens; and structural proteins. The functions of some of these proteins are known; in others their function can be assumed from the protein structure or from limited experimental evidence. Some of the proteins carry out only one specific function and some have more than one. Some might be evolutionary relics and may no longer have significant functions. Several membrane transporter glycoproteins are polymorphic, and are blood group antigens (such as Kidd, Gill, Rh, etc.). However other receptors and adhesion molecules have blood group function as well (Duffy, Lu, LW).

In pondering the possible binding sites, it is useful to remember that the complement-independent *in vitro* binding described above (section 2) required calcium, and many integrins or adhesion factors, including molecules in the C-type lectin-like domain superfamily such as DC-SIGN on dendritic cells and platelets, require calcium for binding to carbohydrates (Zelensky & Gready, 2005). The gp41 protein of HIV-1 contains a binding site for calcium that co-locates with a binding site for a glycosphingolipid (Ebenbichler et al., 1996; Yu et al., 2008). It is well-known that erythrocytes contain numerous glycosphingolipids, such as ganglioside GM3 (hematoside) and ceramide trihexoside (CTH or Gb3, also known as P^k blood group antigen) (Suzuki, 2009), and that binding of HIV-1 to these molecules, and to other glycolipids, can occur (Fantini et al., 2002; Alving, et al., 2006; Lund et al., 2009).

The above glycosphingolipids are possible candidate binding sites for HIV-1 on erythrocytes. However, binding to GM3 or Gb, or other glycosphingolipids, might initially seem unlikely because they are relatively small molecules and are hidden under overlying proteins in normal erythrocytes. Because of steric hindrance by overlying proteins they cannot even bind to specific antibodies (Alving, 2006). However, binding of antibodies to erythrocytic glycosphingolipids readily occurs when the erythrocytes have been damaged by proteolytic enzymes that remove some of the overlying proteins to unmask the underlying glycosphingolipid (Koscielak et al. 1968; Alving, 2006). In view of the observation that <1% of the cells in the *in vitro* erythrocyte population bound HIV-1 (see section 2), it is conceivable that the binding of HIV-1 to erythrocytes occurs to glycosphingolipids that are exposed on the small number of cells that are damaged, or that are at a critical point during the evolution from the reticulocyte stage to mature erythrocytes, or perhaps HIV-1 binds to erythrocytes that are senescent and are about to be removed from circulation.

3.1 Duffy blood group antigen on erythrocytes

The Duffy blood group antigen system was originally described in 1950 based on discovery of an alloantibody against an antigen denoted as Fy(a) in a patient with hemophilia who had received multiple transfusions (Cutbush et al., 1950). The Duffy antigen system consists of multimeric erythrocytic membrane surface proteins composed of different subunits in which glycoprotein D is the major subunit that carries the antigenic determinants as defined by anti-Fy(a), anti-Fy(b) antibodies (Tournamille et al., 1997). The Duffy antigen system achieved considerable prominence when it was discovered that it comprised the erythrocytic receptor site for binding and entry of merozoites of *Plasmodium vivax* and *Plasmodium knowlesi* into erythrocytes (Langhi & Bordin, 2006; Miller et al., 1976). Individuals lacking the Duffy phenotype were also found to be resistant to infection by strains of malaria that bind to Duffy antigen on erythrocytes, thus explaining the remarkable resistance to *P. vivax* malaria that occurs in large areas of West Africa. Because of the subsequent discovery that the Duffy antigen also binds to chemokines, resulting in the binding of cytokines to erythrocytes and endothelial cells and perhaps causing regulation of plasma cytokine levels, this blood group antigen family is now commonly known as the Duffy Antigen Receptor for Chemokines (DARC) (Smolarek et al., 2010). DARC belongs to a family of erythrocyte chemokine receptors that bind to interleukin 8 (IL-8), monocyte chemoattractant protein 1 (MCP-1), and RANTES, but that do not bind macrophage inflammatory protein 1α (MIP-1α) or MIP-1β.

In 1998, it was reported that HIV-1 could bind to DARC on erythrocytes *in vitro* and that erythrocyte-bound DARC could cause infection *in trans* of CD4(+) PBMC (Lachgar et al., 1998). In confirmation of this, based on an *in vitro* experimental study with erythrocytes containing or lacking the DARC phenotype, He et al. proposed that HIV-1 specifically binds to DARC on the surface of erythrocytes at 37°, and that this binding results in the *trans* infection of CD4(+) target cells by transfer of infectious HIV-1 to target cells from erythrocytes (He et al., 2008). Binding of HIV-1 particles to erythrocytes was inhibited by recombinant chemokines such as RANTES, but not by recombinant MIP-1α prior to incubation of the cells with HIV-1. It was suggested that RBCs may function as a reservoir for HIV-1 and it was postulated that DARC might be a receptor for HIV-1 on CD4(-) cell subsets such as neurons or endothelial cells. Although neither of these studies directly measured the binding of HIV-1 to DARC on erythrocytes, they provided evidence of increased infection of CD4(+) target cells when the CD4(+) target cells were co-incubated in the presence of DARC(+) erythrocytes, or co-incubated in the presence of DARC(+) erythrocytes that had been previously incubated with HIV-1 and then washed free of unbound HIV-1. Because this was not observed after co-incubation of HIV-1 with DARC(-) erythrocytes, the data were interpreted as evidence of infection *in trans*. It has recently been further reported that the HIV-1 strain MN gp120 envelope protein might exhibit sequence similarity to the binding domain of Duffy-binding protein of *P. vivax* (Bolton & Garry, 2011). The experimental conditions used for the reported binding of HIV-1 to DARC by He et al. (2008) differed from those used by Beck et al. (2009) in at least two ways: the HIV-1 preparation was incubated by He et al. with 10^7 erythrocytes (20-fold fewer than used by Beck et al. (2009)) and the initial incubation with HIV-1 was performed at 37° rather than 4°. He et al. (2008) reported that the DARC(+) erythrocytes caused infection *in trans* with 5- to 12-fold greater efficiency than DARC(−) erythrocytes. The larger number of erythrocytes employed by Beck et al. (2009) might therefore explain the binding of HIV-1 observed in the latter study with erythrocytes that were obtained from all donors, including both DARC(-) and DARC(+) erythrocytes. Although the preponderance of the above indirect evidence for HIV-1 binding to DARC supports the suggestion that DARC might enhance the binding of HIV-1 to erythrocytes, it does not negate other reports that adherence of infectious HIV-1 to erythrocytes can also occur through mechanisms that do not involve binding to DARC.

After the above laboratory demonstration of apparent DARC-dependent transfer of infectious HIV-1 from erythrocytes to CD4(+) target cells, He et al. (2008) further provided a detailed epidemiological survey, and a summary, of previously published genetic distributions of DARC(+) phenotype in different racial groups. Based on this survey, and based on a follow-on natural history study of HIV-1 infection (Kulkarni et al., 2009; Nibbs, 2009), they proposed that increased susceptibility to HIV-1 infection may be related to genetic occurrence of the DARC(+) phenotype, with a survival advantage to absence of the DARC phenotype, among Africans and African-Americans. They further concluded that after Duffy(+) individuals become infected with HIV-1 they had a decreased risk of disease progression (see editorial by Walton & Rowland-Jones, 2008).

The epidemiological conclusions that suggested racial predispositions to increased HIV-1 infection or decreased HIV-1 susceptibility among Africans and African-Americans were based on extrapolation from *in vitro* studies, and they caused considerable dissent from these concepts from numerous scientists engaged in large HIV research programs in which infectious patterns among Africans and African-Americans were being examined in detail (Horne et al., 2009; Julg et al., 2009; Walley et al., 2009; Winkler et al., 2009). This controversy relating to epidemiology of HIV-1 infection is interesting and still ongoing, but it is beyond the scope of the present discussion of the occurrence of binding of infectious HIV-1 particles to erythrocytes. At this time, the relative epidemiological importance from a practical standpoint of HIV-1 binding to erythrocytes having DARC(+)phenotypes is still not clear.

3.2 Complement receptors on erythrocytes

Circulating immune complexes (IC) are normally removed from blood through activation of the complement (C) cascade (Hebert, 1991; Schifferli et al., 1986). When the C cascade is activated by IC the production of C4 and C3b results in the binding of the IC to the C4/C3b receptor, also known as complement receptor type 1 (CR1 or CD35), that is present on the surface of the erythrocytes. The erythrocytes then transport the IC to fixed macrophages in the liver and spleen for removal from the circulation.

Complement-mediated binding of pathogen IC to erythrocytes is also well known, and the same mechanisms for removal of the pathogens take place. In the course of HIV-1 infection circulating IC inevitably appear that consist of induced antibodies that are bound to infectious HIV-1 particles (Morrow et al., 1986). Many authors have analyzed the role of C in HIV-1 infection (Aasa-Chapman et al., 2005; Beck et al., 2008; Gras et al., 1997; Huber &

Trkola, 2007; Legendre et al., 1996; Moir et al., 2000; Montefiori, 1997; Stoiber et al., 1997) and direct *in vitro* binding of HIV-1-erythrocyte IC to CR1 on erythrocytes, and even to recombinant CR1, has been demonstrated (Montefiori et al., 1994; Stoiber et al., 2008; Zhou & Montefiori, 1996)

To illustrate C-dependent binding of HIV-1-IC to erythrocytes, Horakova et al (2004). used radiolabeled HIV-1, and also prepared preformed HIV-1/anti-HIV-1 immune complexes (HIV-IC) that were opsonized in various human sera. The HIV-IC were purified using sucrose density gradient ultracentrifugation, and incubated with human erythrocytes. They observed immune adherence of the complexes to erythrocytes, and adherence was abolished when C was blocked. C-deficient sera indicated that both the classical and alternative pathways of C activation played a role. No adherence was seen in C1q-deficient serum, and the adherence of HIV-1 was reduced when the alternative pathway was blocked using anti-factor D Abs. The adherence could be inhibited by a mAb against CR1. At supraphysiological concentrations, purified C1q mediated the binding of a small fraction of HIV-1 and HIV-IC to erythrocytes.

4. Implications of binding of HIV-1 to erythrocytes for HIV-1 pathogenesis and vaccine development

The immune system serves as the primary defense against infection by pathogenic microorganisms. In the quest for development of an HIV-1 vaccine it is believed that neutralizing antibodies may be a useful, or even vital, requirement (Mascola & Montefiori, 2010). In addition, innate functions initiated by antibodies, including antibody-dependent complement activation, and Fc-receptor mediated antibody-dependent cell-mediated cytotoxicity (ADCC) or antibody-dependent cell-mediated viral inhibition (ADCVI) may also be mobilized, even by non-neutralizing antibodies (Asmal et al., 2011; Forthal & Moog, 2009). In the present context, the question arises whether erythrocytes may serve as an immunologically protected site for infectious HIV-1 virions that can cause HIV-1 infection of infection of HIV-1-susceptible cells *in trans*. To address the above question, Beck et al. (2011) studied the ability of two well-known broadly neutralizing human monoclonal IgG antibodies (mAbs), 4E10 and b12, to prevent *trans* infection of CD4(+) PBMC by erythrocyte-bound HIV-1 both in the presence and absence of complement (Fig. 2).

In the absence of C both of the mAbs neutralized *trans* infection of erythrocyte-bound virus less effectively than neutralization of cell-free virus, and at a low concentration 4E10 even caused enhanced *trans* infection, perhaps because of Fc-receptor mediated uptake of the virus by the PBMC. However, when cell-free HIV-1 was incubated with the 4E10 mAb in the presence of C, followed by incubation with erythrocytes, significant enhancement of *trans* infection occurred (Fig. 2). In contrast, if the HIV-1 was first pre-incubated with erythrocytes, and the 4E10 mAb and C were then added later, significant inhibition of *trans* infection was observed (Fig. 2).

The explanation for these different effects of C was explained by Beck et al. (2011) as being determined by different binding sites for HIV-1 on the erythrocyte. As illustrated in Fig. 3B, when cell-free HIV-1 was exposed to 4E10 and C, partial activation of the C cascade occurred and C3b was generated, as a result of which the viable infectious HIV-1 became bound to CR1 on the erythrocytes, leading to *trans* infection of PBMC. In contrast, as shown in Fig. 3A, when the HIV-1 was pre-attached to erythrocytes (presumably to a site other than CR1), then subsequent exposure to 4E10 and C caused complete activation of C, leading to generation of membrane attack complexes and killing of the HIV-1. Interestingly, the b12 mAb exhibited no C-dependent effects on erythrocyte-bound HIV-1, an observation that was compatible with previous absence of observed C effects in attempts to use b12 to inhibit mucosal infection in macaques.

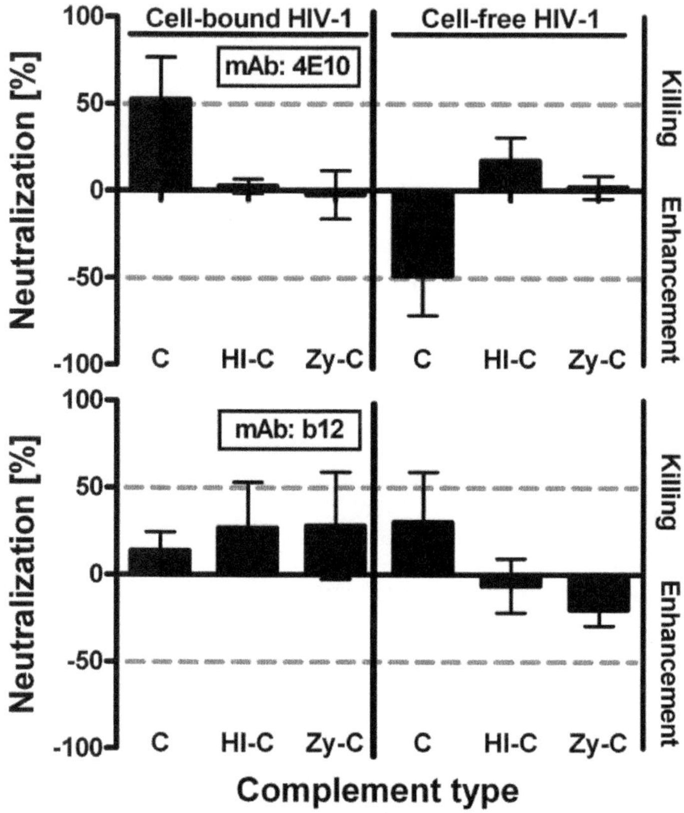

Fig. 2. Effects of antibody-dependent C activation on the trans infection of PBMC by erythrocyte-bound HIV-1-mAb complexes.

(A) Data with 4E10 are the mean±SEM of 8 experiments. (B) Data with b12 are the mean ± SEM of 6 experiments . The baselines represent the values obtained in the absence of C, heat-inactivated C (HI-C), or C inactivated by treatment with zymosan. (Zy-C). The dashed lines indicate the levels of 50% or−50%, defined as positive cutoffs for inhibition or enhancement of virus growth, respectively. In each case, 4E10 had been pre-incubated with the cell-bound or cell-free HIV-1, followed by addition of C, HI-C, or Zy-C, as indicated. From Beck et al. (2011).

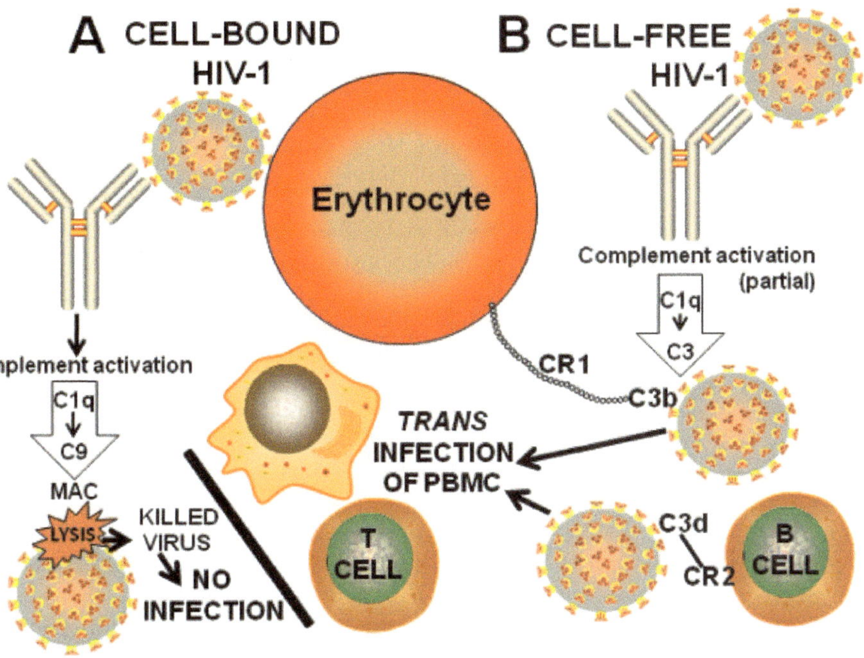

Fig. 3. Schematic representation of C-dependent neutralization of erythrocyte-bound virus, and C-dependent enhancement of infection of PBMC by cell-free virus.

(A) After antibody-independent and C-independent binding of HIV-1 to erythrocytes (Beck et al., 2009), binding of 4E10 (Fig. 4A), but not b12 (Fig. 4B), to the erythrocyte-bound HIV-1 results in C-dependent neutralization. (B) Binding of 4E10 (Fig. 4A), but not b12 (Fig. 4B), to cell-free HIV-1 results in C-dependent binding to CR1 on erythrocytes or B cells, or CR2 on B cells, with enhanced infection of PBMC through trans infection of PBMC by erythrocyte-bound or B cell-bound HIV-1. From Beck et al. (2011).

The conclusions by Beck et al. (2011) were that antibodies and C each represents a two-edged sword. Under certain circumstances, and depending on the individual antibody, inhibition or enhancement of *trans* infection of PBMC can be caused either by the antibody itself or by innate mediators such as Fc receptor binding or activation of C.

5. Does HIV-1 bind to erythrocytes *in vivo*?

In view of the considerable *in vitro* evidence that HIV-1 can bind to erythrocytes, the question naturally arises whether HIV-1 actually binds to erythrocytes *in vivo*. Three reports have examined whether HIV-1, or markers of the presence of HIV-1, can be detected on erythrocytes obtained from infected individuals. In the first study, Hess and colleagues reported that infectious HIV-1 was bound to erythrocytes via immune complexes (Hess et al., 2002; Levy, 2002). Hess et al. showed that HIV-1 RNA and infectious virus was bound to erythrocytes circulating in blood of HIV-1-infected patients. Even in infected individuals who lacked detectable plasma HIV-1 RNA, erythrocyte-associated HIV-1 was readily detected. They concluded that viral RNA was bound to immune complexes with a short half-life.

In a second study more highly purified erythrocytes were used from 13 HIV-1 infected but aviremic patients, 11 of whom were receiving ART and 2 of whom were "long-term nonprogressors" who were not receiving ART (Fierer et al., 2007). In this study, that used PCR detection techniques, the previous conclusions of Hess et al. (2002) were disputed in that virus was not detected on the purified erythrocytes (Fierer et al., 2007). Although the reason for the discrepancy with the previous study is unclear, Fierer et al. (2007) suggested that the previously studied cell population of Hess et al. (2002) might have contained a higher level of contaminating CD4(+) lymphocytes that were removed by Fierer et al by using more stringent purification techniques.

In a third recent study, the presence of p24-antigen bound to highly purified erythrocytes from HIV-1-positive individuals was reported (Garcia et al., 2011). In this study 51 out of the 71 patients with detectable plasma viral loads (pVL) showed erythrocyte-associated p24-antigen (Ag-E) whereas 13 showed p24-antigen in plasma (Ag-P). Twenty-two out of the 51 patients with Ag-E showed high pVL and undetectable Ag-P. The amount of erythrocyte-associated p24-antigen was not related to p24-antigen in plasma or pVL levels. Among the 41 patients with prior undetectable pVL, eight presented detectable pVL and erythrocyte-associated p24-antigen at the moment of the study. The other 33 showed undetectable pVL and 5 of these presented erythrocyte-associated p24-antigen. A positive relationship was found between the presence of erythrocyte-associated p24-antigen and the detectable pVL. This study thus confirmed the presence of erythrocyte-associated p24-antigen in HIV-1-infected individuals. Since erythrocyte-associated p24-antigen is not always related to pVL or p24-antigen in plasma, erythrocyte associated p24-antigen showed viral expression not represented in plasma.

Although the above three studies suggest that some degree of controversy exists, the preponderance of data now indicates that HIV-1 does bind to erythrocytes *in vivo*. In view of this it is reasonable to speculate whether such binding might result in hematologic abnormalities in HIV-1-infected patients. Changes in erythrocyte and lymphocyte membrane properties have been associated with infection, including changes in calcium signaling, decreased membrane fluidity, decreased acetylcholinesterase activity, and decreased intracellular calcium concentration (Martins-Silva et al., 2006). It was concluded that the observed changes were consistent with the hypothesis that erythrocytes were being maintained as a circulating *in vivo* reservoir of infectious virus and that this was causing adverse physical changes in the erythrocytes. Regardless of the exact mechanism(s) involved in causing these effects, it is apparent that anemia might be a potential sequel.

Anemia is reportedly the most common hematologic manifestation of HIV-1 infection (Claster, 2002). However, there can be multiple causes of anemia, including reduced erythrocyte production. As noted earlier (section 2.1), HIV-1 infects multipotent progenitor cells in the bone marrow that might affect reticulocyte production (Carter, et al., 2010). Anemia might also be secondary to a variety of causes such as drug-related anemia, parvovirus infection, and nutritional deficiencies, in addition to increased erythrocyte destruction. Clearly, appropriate therapies can address the various correctable causes of the clinical course of anemia. However, it should be noted that regardless of the underlying cause, anemia has been cited as an independent predictor of mortality and progress of disease among HIV-1-infected women in Tanzania (O'Brien et al., 2005).

6. Conclusion

From the above three studies it is evident that the question of HIV-1 binding to erythrocytes *in vivo* has generated some degree of controversy. Although the reasons for the failure of Fierer et al. (2007) to detect erythrocyte-bound HIV-1 are unknown, in view of the study by Hess et al., 2002 and the confirmatory results of Garcia et al. (2011), and when this it taken in the context of the several studies that have demonstrated binding of HIV-1 to erythrocytes *in vitro*, it seems likely that infectious HIV-1 virions are present on circulating erythrocytes in HIV-1 infected persons. In view of the recent *in vitro* evidence by Beck et al. (2011) that erythrocyte-bound HIV-1 may sometimes be more difficult to neutralize with antibodies than cell-free HIV-1, and that both inhibition and enhancement can occur with antibody-mediated innate immunity in the presence of C, it also seems likely that circulating erythrocytes may represent an attachment site for infectious HIV-1 that is relatively protected from attack by antibodies and C. It is possible that further research will identify means to induce antibodies that block *trans* infection by erythrocyte-bound HIV-1. A corollary of this is that development of a *trans* infection neutralization assay may also be useful as an *in vitro* correlate of protective immunity in addition to neutralization assays in which cell-free virus is the infecting agent.

7. Acknowledgement and disclaimer

This work was supported by a cooperative agreement (W81XWH-07-2-0067) between the Henry M. Jackson Foundation for the Advancement of Military Medicine, Inc., and the U.S. Department of Defense. The views and opinions expressed in this article are those of the authors and do not reflect the official policy of the Department of the Army, the Department of Defense, or the U.S. Government.

8. References

Aasa-Chapman, M. M., Holuigue, S., Aubin, K., Wong, M., Jones, N. A., Cornforth, D., Pellegrino, P., Newton, P., Williams, I., Borrow, P., & McKnight, A. (2005). Detection of antibody-dependent complement-mediated inactivation of both autologous and heterologous virus in primary human immunodeficiency virus type 1 infection. *Journal of Virology*, Vol.79, No.5, (March, 2005), pp. 2823-2830, ISSN 0022-538X

Alving, C. R. (2006). Antibodies to lipids and liposomes: immunology and safety. *Journal of Liposome Research*, Vol.16, No.3, (2006), pp. 157-166, ISSN 0898-2104

Alving, C. R., Beck, Z., Karasavva, N., Matyas, G. R., & Rao, M. (2006). HIV-1, lipid rafts, and antibodies to liposomes: implications for anti-viral-neutralizing antibodies. *Molecular Membrane Biology*, Vol.23, No.6, (November-December 2006), pp. 453-465, ISSN 0968-7688

Anstee, D. J. (2011). The functional importance of blood group-active molecules in human red blood cells. *Vox Sanguinis*, Vol.100, No.1, (January, 2011), pp. 140-149, ISSN 0042-9007

Asmal, M., Sun, Y., Lane, S., Yeh, W., Schmidt, S. D., Mascola, J. R., & Letvin, N. L. (2011). Antibody-dependent cell-mediated viral inhibition emerges after SIVmac251 infection of rhesus monkeys coincident with gp140 binding antibodies and is effective against neutralization-resistant viruses. *Journal of Virology*, Vol.85, No.11, (June, 2011), pp. 5465-5475, ISSN 0022-538X

Beck, Z., Brown, B. K., Matyas, G. R., Polonis, V. R., Rao, M., & Alving, C. R. (2011). Infection of human peripheral blood mononuclear cells by erythrocyte-bound HIV-1: Effects of antibodies and complement. *Virology*, Vol.412, No.2, (April 10, 2011), pp. 441-447, ISSN 0042-6822

Beck, Z., Brown, B. K., Wieczorek, L., Peachman, K. K., Matyas, G. R., Polonis, V. R., Rao, M., & Alving, C. R. (2009). Human erythrocytes selectively bind and enrich infectious HIV-1 virions. *PLoS One*, Vol.4, No.12, (2009), pp. e8297, ISSN 1932-6203

Beck, Z., Prohaszka, Z., & Fust, G. (2008). Traitors of the immune system-enhancing antibodies in HIV infection: their possible implication in HIV vaccine development. *Vaccine*, Vol.26, No.24, (June 6, 2008), pp. 3078-3085, ISSN 0264-0264-410

Bolton, M. J., & Garry, R. F. (2011). Sequence similarity between the erythrocyte binding domain 1 of the Plasmodium vivax Duffy binding protein and the V3 loop of HIV-1 strain MN reveals binding residues for the Duffy Antigen Receptor for Chemokines. *Virology Journal*, Vol.8, (January 31, 2011), pp. 45, doi:10.1186/1743-422X-8-45, ISSN 1743-422X

Boukour, S., Masse, J. M., Benit, L., Dubart-Kupperschmitt, A., & Cramer, E. M. (2006). Lentivirus degradation and DC-SIGN expression by human platelets and megakaryocytes. *Journal of Thrombosis and Haemostasis*, Vol.4, No.2, (February, 2006), pp. 426-435, ISSN 1538-7933

Briggs, J. A., Simon, M. N., Gross, I., Krausslich, H. G., Fuller, S. D., Vogt, V. M., & Johnson, M. C. (2004). The stoichiometry of Gag protein in HIV-1. *Nature Structural & Molecular Biology*, Vol.11, No.7, (July, 2004), pp. 672-675, ISSN 1545-9983

Carter, C. C., McNamara, L. A., Onafuwa-Nuga, A., Shackleton, M., Riddell, J. T., Bixby, D., Savona, M. R., Morrison, S. J., & Collins, K. L. (2011). HIV-1 Utilizes the CXCR4 chemokine receptor to infect multipotent hematopoietic stem and progenitor cells. *Cell Host & Microbe*, Vol.9, No.3, (March 17, 2011), pp. 223-234, ISSN 1931-3128

Carter, C. C., Onafuwa-Nuga, A., McNamara, L. A., Riddell, J. T., Bixby, D., Savona, M. R., & Collins, K. L. (2010). HIV-1 infects multipotent progenitor cells causing cell death and establishing latent cellular reservoirs. *Nature Medicine*, Vol.16, No.4, (April, 2010), pp. 446-451, ISSN 1078-8956

Chaipan, C., Soilleux, E. J., Simpson, P., Hofmann, H., Gramberg, T., Marzi, A., Geier, M., Stewart, E. A., Eisemann, J., Steinkasserer, A., Suzuki-Inoue, K., Fuller, G. L., Pearce, A. C., Watson, S. P., Hoxie, J. A., Baribaud, F., & Pohlmann, S. (2006). DC-SIGN and CLEC-2 mediate human immunodeficiency virus type 1 capture by platelets. *Journal of Virology*, Vol.80, No.18, (September, 2006), pp. 8951-8960, ISSN 0022-538X

Claster, S. (2002). Biology of anemia, differential diagnosis, and treatment options in human immunodeficiency virus infection. *The Journal of Infectious Diseases*, Vol.185, Supplement 2, (May 15 2002), pp. S105-S109, ISSN 022-1899

Cutbush, M., Mollison, P. L., & Parkin, D. M. (1950). A New Human Blood Group. *Nature*, Vol.165, No.4188, (1950), pp. 189-189, ISSN 0028-0836

Daniels, G. (2007). Functions of red cell surface proteins. *Vox Sanguinis*, Vol.93, No.4, (November, 2007), pp. 331-340, ISSN 0042-9007

Denomme, G. A. (2004). The structure and function of the molecules that carry human red blood cell and platelet antigens. *Transfusion Medicine Reviews*, Vol.18, No.3, (July, 2004), pp. 203-231, ISSN 0887-7963

Ebenbichler, C. F., Stoiber, H., Schneider, R., Patsch, J. R., & Dierich M. P. (1996). The human immunodeficiency virus type 1 transmembrane gp41 protein is a calcium-binding protein and interacts with the putative second-receptor molecules in a calcium-dependent manner. *Journal of Virology* Vol.70, No.3, (March 1996), pp. 1723-1728, ISSN 0022-538X

Fantini. J, Garmy. N, Mahfoud. R, & Yahi, N. (2002. Lipid rafts: structure, function and role in HIV, Alzheimer's and prion diseases. *Expert Reviews in Molecular Medicine*, Vol, 4, No. 27, (December 20 2002), pp. 1-22, ISSN 1462-3994

Fierer, D. S., Vargas, J., Jr., Patel, N., & Clover, G. (2007). Absence of erythrocyte-associated HIV-1 in vivo. *The Journal of Infectious Diseases*, Vol.196, No.4, (August 15, 2007), pp. 587-590, ISSN 022-1899

Flaujac, C., Boukour, S., & Cramer-Borde, E. (2010). Platelets and viruses: an ambivalent relationship. *Cellular and Molecular Life Sciences*, Vol.67, No.4, (February, 2010), pp. 545-556, ISSN 1420-682X

Forthal, D. N., & Moog, C. (2009). Fc receptor-mediated antiviral antibodies. *Current Opinion in HIV and AIDS*, Vol.4, No.5, (September, 2009), pp. 388-393, ISSN 1746-630X

Garcia, M. N., dos Ramos Farias, M. S., Avila, M. M., & Rabinovich, R. D. (2011). Presence of p24-antigen associated to erythrocyte in HIV-positive individuals even in patients with undetectable plasma viral load. *PLoS One*, Vol.6, No.1, (2011), pp. e14544, ISSN 1932-6203

Gras, G., Legendre, C., Richard, Y., & Dormont, D. (1997). Human immunodeficiency virus and the complement system. *Experimental and Clinical Immunogenetics*, Vol.14, No.1, (1997), pp. 11-15, ISSN 0254-9670

He, W., Neil, S., Kulkarni, H., Wright, E., Agan, B. K., Marconi, V. C., Dolan, M. J., Weiss, R. A., & Ahuja, S. K. (2008). Duffy antigen receptor for chemokines mediates trans-infection of HIV-1 from red blood cells to target cells and affects HIV-AIDS susceptibility. *Cell Host & Microbe*, Vol.4, No.1, (July 17, 2008), pp. 52-62, ISSN 1931-3128

Hebert, L. A. (1991). The clearance of immune complexes from the circulation of man and other primates. *American Journal of Kidney Diseases*, Vol.17, No.3, (March, 1991), pp. 352-361, ISSN 0272-6386

Hess, C., Klimkait, T., Schlapbach, L., Del Zenero, V., Sadallah, S., Horakova, E., Balestra, G., Werder, V., Schaefer, C., Battegay, M., & Schifferli, J. A. (2002). Association of a pool of HIV-1 with erythrocytes in vivo: a cohort study. *Lancet*, Vol.359, No.9325, (June 29, 2002), pp. 2230-2234, ISSN 0140-6736

Ho, D. D., Moudgil, T., & Alam, M. (1989). Quantitation of Human Immunodeficiency Virus Type-1 in the Blood of Infected Persons. *The New England Journal of Medicine*, Vol.321, No.24, (December 14, 1989), pp. 1621-1625, ISSN 0028-4793

Horakova, E., Gasser, O., Sadallah, S., Inal, J. M., Bourgeois, G., Ziekau, I., Klimkait, T., & Schifferli, J. A. (2004). Complement mediates the binding of HIV to erythrocytes. *Journal of Immunology*, Vol.173, No.6, (September 15, 2004), pp. 4236-4241, ISSN 0022-1767

Horne, K. C., Li, X., Jacobson, L. P., Palella, F., Jamieson, B. D., Margolick, J. B., Martinson, J., Turkozu, V., Visvanathan, K., & Woolley, I. J. (2009). Duffy antigen polymorphisms do not alter progression of HIV in African Americans in the MACS cohort. *Cell Host & Microbe*, Vol.5, No.5, (May 8, 2009), pp. 415-417; author reply 418-419, ISSN 1931-3128

Huber, M., & Trkola, A. (2007). Humoral immunity to HIV-1: neutralization and beyond. *Journal of Internal Medicine*, Vol.262, No.1, (July, 2007), pp. 5-25, ISSN 0954-6820

Julg, B., Reddy, S., van der Stok, M., Kulkarni, S., Qi, Y., Bass, S., Gold, B., Nalls, M. A., Nelson, G. W., Walker, B. D., Carrington, M., & Ndung'u, T. (2009). Lack of Duffy antigen receptor for chemokines: no influence on HIV disease progression in an African treatment-naive population. *Cell Host & Microbe*, Vol.5, No.5, (May 8, 2009), pp. 413-415; author reply 418-419, ISSN 1931-3128

Koscielak, J., Hakomori, S., & Jeanloz, R. W. (1968). Glycolipid antigen and its antibody. *Immunochemistry* Vol.5, No.5, (September 1968), pp. 441-455, ISSN 0019-2791

Kulkarni, H., Marconi, V. C., He, W., Landrum, M. L., Okulicz, J. F., Delmar, J., Kazandjian, D., Castiblanco, J., Ahuja, S. S., Wright, E. J., Weiss, R. A., Clark, R. A., Dolan, M. J., & Ahuja, S. K. (2009). The Duffy-null state is associated with a survival advantage in leukopenic HIV-infected persons of African ancestry. *Blood*, Vol.114, No.13, (September 24, 2009), pp. 2783-2792, ISSN 0006-4971

Lachgar, A., Jaureguiberry, G., Le Buenac, H., Bizzini, B., Zagury, J. F., Rappaport, J., & Zagury, D. (1998). Binding of HIV-1 to RBCs involves the Duffy antigen receptors for chemokines (DARC). *Biomedicine & Pharmacotherapy*, Vol.52, No.10, (1998), pp. 436-439, ISSN 0753-3322

Langhi, D. M., Jr., & Bordin, J. O. (2006). Duffy blood group and malaria. *Hematology*, Vol.11, No.5, (October, 2006), pp. 389-398, ISSN 1024-5332

Legendre, C., Gras, G., Krzysiek, R., Galanaud, P., Richard, Y., & Dormont, D. (1996). Mechanisms of opsonized HIV entry in normal B lymphocytes. *FEBS Letters*, Vol.381, No.3, (March 4, 1996), pp. 227-232, ISSN 0014-5793

Levy, J. A. (2002). HIV-1: hitching a ride on erythrocytes. *Lancet*, Vol.359, No.9325, (Jun 29, 2002), pp. 2212-2213, ISSN 0140-6736

Lund, N, Olsson, M. L., Ramkumar, S., Sakac, D., Yahalom, V., Levene, C., Hellberg, A., Ma, X. Z., Binnington, B., Jung, D., Lingwood, C. A., & Branch, D.R. (2009). The human P(k) histo-blood group antigen provides protection against HIV-1 infection. *Blood*, Vol.113, No.20, (May 14 2009), pp. 4980-4991, ISSN 0006-4971

Martins-Silva, J., Santos, N. C., Doroana, M., Duarte, N., Tavares, L., Antunes, F., & Saldanha, C. (2006). Changes in blood cell membrane properties in HIV type-1-infected patients. *AIDS Research and Human Retroviruses*, Vol.22, No.9, (September 2006), pp. 849-853, ISSN 0889-2229

Mascola, J. R., & Montefiori, D. C. (2010). The role of antibodies in HIV vaccines. *Annual Review of Immunology*, Vol.28, (March, 2010), pp. 413-444, ISSN 0732-0582

Miller, L. H., Mason, S. J., Clyde, D. F., & McGinniss, M. H. (1976). The resistance factor to Plasmodium vivax in blacks. The Duffy-blood-group genotype, FyFy. *The New England Journal of Medicine*, Vol.295, No.6, (August 5, 1976), pp. 302-304, ISSN 0028-4793

Mohandas, N., & Narla, A. (2005). Blood group antigens in health and disease. *Current Opinion in Hematology*, Vol.12, No.2, (March 2005), pp. 135-140, ISSN 1065-6251

Moir, S., Malaspina, A., Li, Y., Chun, T. W., Lowe, T., Adelsberger, J., Baseler, M., Ehler, L. A., Liu, S., Davey, R. T., Jr., Mican, J. A., & Fauci, A. S. (2000). B cells of HIV-1-infected patients bind virions through CD21-complement interactions and transmit infectious virus to activated T cells. *The Journal of Experimental Medicine*, Vol.192, No.5, (September 4, 2000), pp. 637-646, ISSN 0022-1007

Montefiori, D. C. (1997). Role of complement and Fc receptors in the pathogenesis of HIV-1 infection. *Springer Seminars in Immunopathology*, Vol.18, No.3, (1997), pp. 371-390, ISSN 0344-4325

Montefiori, D. C., Graham, B. S., Zhou, J. Y., Zhou, J. T., & Ahearn, J. M. (1994). Binding of human immunodeficiency virus type 1 to the C3b/C4b receptor CR1 (CD35) and red blood cells in the presence of envelope-specific antibodies and complement. National Institutes of Health AIDS Vaccine Clinical Trials Networks. *The Journal of Infectious Diseases*, Vol.170, No.2, (August, 1994), pp. 429-432, ISSN 022-1899

Morrow, W. J., Wharton, M., Stricker, R. B., & Levy, J. A. (1986). Circulating immune complexes in patients with acquired immune deficiency syndrome contain the AIDS-associated retrovirus. *Clinical Immunology and Immunopathology*, Vol.40, No.3, (September, 1986), pp. 515-524, ISSN 0090-1229

Nibbs, R. J. (2009). HIV: getting to the heart of DARCness. *Blood*, Vol.114, No.13, (September 24, 2009), pp. 2570-2571, ISSN 0006-4971

O'Brien, M. E., Kupka, R., Msamanga, G. I., Saathoff, E., Hunter, D. J., & Fawzi, W. W. (2005). Anemia is an independent predictor of mortality and immunologic progression of disease among women with HIV in Tanzania. *Journal of Acquired Immune Deficiency Syndromes*, Vol.40, No.2, (October 1 2005), pp. 219-225, ISSN 1077-9450

Olinger, G. G., Saifuddin, M., & Spear, G. T. (2000). CD4-Negative cells bind human immunodeficiency virus type 1 and efficiently transfer virus to T cells. *Journal of Virology*, Vol.74, No.18, (September, 2000), pp. 8550-8557, ISSN 0022-538X

Pan, L. Z., Werner, A., & Levy, J. A. (1993). Detection of plasma viremia in human immunodeficiency virus-infected individuals at all clinical stages. *Journal of Clinical Microbiology*, Vol.31, No.2, (February, 1993), pp. 283-288, ISSN 0095-1137

Reid, M. E., & Mohandas, N. (2004). Red blood cell blood group antigens: structure and function. *Seminars in Hematology*, Vol.41, No.2, (April, 2004), pp. 93-117, ISSN 0037-1963

Schifferli, J. A., Ng, Y. C., & Peters, D. K. (1986). The role of complement and its receptor in the elimination of immune complexes. *The New England Journal of Medicine*, Vol.315, No.8, (August 21, 1986), pp. 488-495, ISSN 0028-4793

Smolarek, D., Bertrand, O., Czerwinski, M., Colin, Y., Etchebest, C., & de Brevern, A. G. (2010). Multiple interests in structural models of DARC transmembrane protein. *Transfusion Clinique Et Biologique*, Vol.17, No.3, (September, 2010), pp. 184-196, ISSN 1246-7820

Stoiber, H., Banki, Z., Wilflingseder, D., & Dierich, M. P. (2008). Complement-HIV interactions during all steps of viral pathogenesis. *Vaccine*, Vol.26, No.24, (June 6, 2008), pp. 3046-3054, ISSN 0264-410X

Stoiber, H., Clivio, A., & Dierich, M. P. (1997). Role of complement in HIV infection. *Annual Review of Immunology*, Vol.15, (1997), pp. 649-674, ISSN 0732-0582

Suzuki, A. (2009). Tamio Yamakawa: Dawn of glycobiology. *Journal of Biochemistry*, Vol.146, No.2, (August, 2009), pp. 149-156, ISSN

Telen, M. J. (2005). Erythrocyte adhesion receptors: Blood group antigens and related molecules. *Transfusion Medicine Reviews*, vol.19, No.1, (January, 2005), pp. 32-44, ISSN 0887-7963

Tournamille, C., Le Van Kim, C., Gane, P., Blanchard, D., Proudfoot, A. E., Cartron, J. P., & Colin, Y. (1997). Close association of the first and fourth extracellular domains of the Duffy antigen/receptor for chemokines by a disulfide bond is required for ligand binding. *The Journal of Biological Chemistry*, Vol.272, No.26, (June 27, 1997), pp. 16274-16280, ISSN 0021-9258

Yu, H., Alfsen, A., Tudor, D., & Bomsel, M. (2008). The binding of HIV-1 gp41 membrane proximal domain to its mucosal receptor, galactosyl ceramide, is structure-dependent. *Cell Calcium*. Vol.43, No.1, (January, 2008), pp. 73-82, ISSN 0143-4160

Walley, N. M., Julg, B., Dickson, S. P., Fellay, J., Ge, D., Walker, B. D., Carrington, M., Cohen, M. S., de Bakker, P. I., Goldstein, D. B., Shianna, K. V., Haynes, B. F., Letvin, N. L., McMichael, A. J., Michael, N. L., & Weintrob, A. C. (2009). The Duffy antigen receptor for chemokines null promoter variant does not influence HIV-1 acquisition or disease progression. *Cell Host & Microbe*, Vol.5, No.5, (May 8, 2009), pp. 408-410; author reply 418-419, ISSN 1931-3128

Walton, R. T., & Rowland-Jones, S. L. (2008). HIV and chemokine binding to red blood cells--DARC matters. *Cell Host & Microbe*, Vol.4, No.1, (July 17, 2008), pp. 3-5, ISSN 1931-3128

Winkler, C. A., An, P., Johnson, R., Nelson, G. W., & Kirk, G. (2009). Expression of Duffy antigen receptor for chemokines (DARC) has no effect on HIV-1 acquisition or progression to AIDS in African Americans. *Cell Host & Microbe*, Vol.5, No.5, (May 8, 2009), pp. 411-413; author reply 418-419, ISSN 1931-3128

Zelensky, A. N., & Gready, J. E. The C-type lectin-like domain superfamily. (2005). *The FEBS Journal*, Vol.272, No.24, (December 2005), pp. 6179-6217, ISSN 1742-464X

Zhou, J., and Montefiori, D. C. (1996). Complement-activating antibodies in sera from infected individuals and vaccinated volunteers that target human immunodeficiency virus type 1 to complement receptor type 1 (CR1, CD35). *Virology*, Vol.226, No.1, (December 1, 1996), pp. 13-21, ISSN 0042-6822

Part 4

Co-Infection

11

Inducing Immune Protection Against *Trichomonas vaginalis*: A Novel Vaccine Approach to Prevent HIV Transmission

Sarah Cudmore, Jeffrey Smith and Gary Garber
University of Ottawa
Canada

1. Introduction

Human immunodeficiency virus (HIV) infection is a pandemic that affects all parts of the globe. Current treatments fail to cure disease and for this reason there is significant interest in producing a vaccine to prevent HIV transmission, but clinical trials have proved disappointing. For this reason it is important to consider alternative measures to control incidence and prevalence of the disease.

Trichomonas vaginalis is a highly prevalent and under-diagnosed sexually transmitted infection that facilitates transmission of and susceptibility to HIV infection (McClelland et al., 2007; Mavedzenge et al., 2010). Although current treatment is effective the disease is still poorly controlled and there are concerns about increasing levels of drug resistance (Upcroft & Upcroft, 2001). Efforts to research disease mechanisms and immune response with consideration to a rational vaccine design approach should be investigated as a potential method to reduce global incidence of *T. vaginalis* infection.

A reliable murine model of *T. vaginalis* infection has been established with symptoms in female mice mimicking those seen in women (from vaginitis/vulvitis and discharge to asymptomatic but culture-positive for infection). Using this model it has been shown that vaccinating mice (by injection of trichomonad cells with adjuvant) protects the animals from subsequent vaginal infection (Abraham et al., 1996). By studying immune responses in mice, factors that are critical for immunological protection can be elucidated to create a "blueprint" for an effective human vaccine.

Herein we provide an overview of the current understanding of *T. vaginalis* infection and epidemiology, methods of diagnosis and treatment, and implications of animal models for understanding disease mechanisms . We discuss how and why current *T. vaginalis* treatment protocols fail to control infection incidence with consideration as to how a *T. vaginalis* vaccine could overcome these obstacles and reduce disease burden. The association between *T. vaginalis* and HIV is examined and the potential for reducing HIV infection rates by lowering *T. vaginalis* incidence is elucidated.

A vaccine against *T. vaginalis* would provide long term protection that could be more successful than treatment in controlling the spread of this very common disease. As *T. vaginalis* infection is a clear risk factor for HIV acquisition, it is our belief that this approach would also be effective in ameliorating HIV incidence and prevalence, especially in areas such as South and Southeast Asia and sub-Saharan Africa where HIV and *T. vaginalis* are endemic (United Nations, 2009; World Health Organization, 2001).

2. *Trichomonas vaginalis*

2.1 Morphology

The basic structure of *T. vaginalis* as reviewed in Petrin et al. (1998) and Heine & McGregor (1993) is best described as a 10-20 µm ovoid organism with four free-moving flagella located at the anterior portion, and one recumbent flagellum attached to the body of the cell by a membrane that forms an axostyle running longitudinally from the anterior portion to the posterior forming a pointed tip. The flagella and undulating membrane contribute to the organism's characteristic jerky movements visualized under a common laboratory light microscope. Within the protozoan resides a nucleus with six chromosomes, a developed Golgi complex, but is devoid of mitochondria, peroxisomes or glycosomes, so instead contains hydrogenosomes typical of anaerobic protozoa and fungi. With respect to metabolic processes the parasitic nature of *T. vaginalis* owes to its inability to synthesize many nutrients and thus implicates a significant contribution of scavenged nutrients from hosts to survive (Heine & McGregor, 1993).

2.2 Genetics

Recently a draft genome sequence has been completed (Carlton et al., 2007) revealing a genome of approximately 160 Mb containing a core set of roughly 60,000 genes although it is suggested 39 Mb is repetitive genomic information as a result of enormous gene expansions. Important information will be derived from this data especially since gene regulation is not well understood and even now novel core promoter elements are being identified (Gomez et al., 2010; Smith et al., 2011) as well as hypothetical surface proteins from proteome analysis (de Miguel et al., 2010). Hypothetical surface proteins are of particular interest for extracellular parasites functioning to establish and maintain infection, and may shed light on current issues of classifying phenotypic differences for variable clinical presentation between hosts (Smith et al., 2011).

2.3 Epidemiology

T. vaginalis is an extracellular, anaerobic, parasitic protozoan that is the cause of trichomoniasis, the most common non-viral, curable STI with global incidence of at least 174 million cases per year (WHO, 2001), likely an immense underestimation of actual incidence. Nevertheless, to put this number into relative terms of other curable STI the global incidence of syphilis, chlamydia and gonorrhoea as reported by WHO (2001) were 12 million, 92 million and 62 million, respectively. The majority of cases are localized in regions of low income or lack of resources, especially health care. Other risk factors include *Neisseria gonorrhoeae* infection, *Chlamydia trachomatis* infection, risky sexual behaviours, older male partners (in terms of heterosexual couples), potential for non-sexual transmission by cultural habits such as shared bathing water, new or multiple sex partners, a history of STI, exchange of sex for payment, and drug use (Crucitti et al., 2011; Krashin et al., 2010; Sutton et al., 2007; Workowski & Berman, 2010).

2.4 Trichomoniasis

T. vaginalis resides in the squamous epithelium of the genital tract of both females and males with prevalence primarily within the reproductive years. General areas of infection in males include the urethra, external genitalia, prostate and epididymis. The vagina is the area most commonly infected for females though it should be noted that other areas of infection include the Bartholin's, Skene's and periurethral glands, bladder and cervix (Heine & McGregor, 1993; Petrin et al., 1998). The infection is followed by an incubation period prior to onset of symptoms, if any at all, with persistent infection commonly occurring in females whereas eventual resolution occurs in males whom mostly serve as carriers and spread the infection to other partners (Petrin et al., 1998; Van Der Pol et al, 2005).

A plethora of possible symptoms surrounds *T. vaginalis* infection. Rarely are all symptoms present nor are typical symptoms easily distinguishable from other urogenital infections. Additionally up to 50% of infected females and greater numbers in males are asymptomatic (Fouts & Kraus, 1980, as cited in Cudmore et al., 2004; Pastorek et al., 1996). While men and women usually present with malodorous discharge from the infected areas the most significant burden is found in women who may present with any of the following; high vaginal pH, bloody mucus, colpitis macularis, and vulvitis. Infection is associated with pelvic inflammatory disease, birth complications including premature rupture of the placental membrane, premature labour, low average birth-weight, and infertility, and increased transmission and contraction of HIV (Cotch et al, 1997; Mavedzenge et al., 2010; McClelland et al., 2008; Moodley et al., 2002; Pastorek et al., 1996; Wølner-Hanssen et al., 1989).

2.4.1 Treatment of trichmoniasis

Lossik (1990) describes the basics of metronidazole, a chemically modified form of the natural *Streptomyces* product azomycin from the family of nitroimidazoles, first synthesized in 1957 and finally marketed in 1960. Metronidazole is effectively administered as a single 2 g dose or 500 mg twice daily for seven days with average cure rates of 96% and 92%, respectively. Side effects are minimal and more adverse effects are the result of very high dosage and longer duration (Lossik, 1990). Upon diagnosis and treatment - typically females are diagnosed as male partners are less likely to observe or report symptoms - it is encouraged that sexual partners be tested and treated in concert as often these individuals are infected as well (up to 70% of male partners are also infected as reported by PCR testing in Seña et al., 2007). The treatment of trichomoniasis with this drug is highly effective although 5-10% of *T. vaginalis* isolates exhibit some degree of resistance as assayed in vitro (Upcroft & Upcroft, 2001).

Five years after the discovery of metronidazole the first metronidazole-refractory case of *T. vaginalis* isolated from a female patient was reported by Robinson (1962, as cited in Lossick, 1990). To avoid future difficulties with metronidazole resistance clinical and laboratory generated drug resistant isolates are under study to determine the mechanisms of resistance that can arise or have arisen (Upcroft & Upcroft, 2001). Alternatively, a *T. vaginalis* vaccine would sidestep the necessity to discover potential drug replacements in the event of epidemic resistance.

2.5 Phenotypic variance of clinical disease

In an attempt to define the phenotypic differences between clinical isolates causing symptomatic disease versus asymptomatic disease a number of areas are under investigation regarding host immune response and parasite-host interactions.

2.5.1 Host immune response

Scott et al. (2005) demonstrated that a symptomatic isolate of *T. vaginalis* induced only an IL-10 response in dendritic cells while a more diverse IL-12, IL-10 and IFN-α repertoire was produced in response to selected infectious mucosal bacteria. Within the findings a potential relationship is noted between an IL-10 only response and chronicity of infection. IL-10 alone contributes to inhibition of T helper type 1 (Th1) immunity and favours a Th2 response (Banchereau et al., 2000, as cited in Scott et al., 2005). Similar results of a lack of IL-12 induction in macrophages were previously reported by Chang et al. (2004). On the other hand, cytokines related to Th1 type response (IL-2 and IFN-gamma) have been noted to be more prevalent in the sera of mice infected with asymptomatic isolates than symptomatic isolates (Malla et al., 2007; Paintlia et al., 2002). Similar results have been found in other protozoal disease cytokine studies suggesting that in these cases Th1 mediated response may regulate disease and prevent overt clinical symptoms but not abolish infection (Agarwal et al., 1999, Bayraktar et al., 2005 and Campbell & Chadee, 1997, all as cited in Malla et al., 2007).

Yadav et al. (2005) investigated immunoglobulin kinetics of intravaginal trichomoniasis in a mouse model with asymptomatic and symptomatic clinical isolates. IgM, IgG (subclasses 1, 2a, 2b and 3) and IgA were measured in serum and from vaginal washes from mice infected with asymptomatic and symptomatic isolates. Titers of IgG, IgG1 and IgM of vaginal wash and serum samples were significantly greater in symptomatic infected mice than asymptomatic mice, while IgA responses were not statistically different for serum or vaginal washes of either asymptomatic or symptomatic isolates. These results are mostly in line with vaginal wash data from symptomatic infections in women showing IgG and IgA at detectable levels versus undetectable levels in asymptomatic women (Alderete, 1984, as cited in Yadav et al., 2005). Data from Paintlia et al. (2002) found greater IgA levels in both vaginal wash and serum samples of asymptomatic isolates infected in mice contradicting the aforementioned findings. These results may indicate complications with the model of study or are simply the intricacies of trichomonal infection. Thus, some antibodies may provide a method of predicting the severity of infection. Whether these findings are host dependent or mediated by phenotypic variance of *T. vaginalis* is yet to be elucidated.

2.5.2 Parasite-host interactions

Contact-independent mechanisms of damage correlated to symptomatic states of infection involve soluble factors shed from *T. vaginalis* including cell detaching factor (CDF), cysteine proteases and a haemolytic factor that is reliant on specific elevated vaginal pH in the range typically observed in clinical disease (Alderete & Garza, 1984; Fiori et al., 1996; Garber & Lemchuk-Favel, 1990).

Gene regulation is influenced by contact with epithelial cells (Kucknoor et al., 2005) and cytoadherence has been noted as a better predictor of in vivo pathogenicity than cytotoxicity by soluble factors (Escario et al., 1995). Unfortunately the pathogenic role of adhesion proteins such as AP65, AP51, AP33 and AP23 that have been associated with epithelial cell binding of *T. vaginalis* (Alderete & Garza, 1984; Arroyo et al., 1992) have not conclusively been elucidated. Midlej & Benchimol (2010) suggests that adherence may aid phagocytic capability and disruption of monolayers in which *T. vaginalis* literally mechanically disassembles and phagocytoses membranes of epithelial monolayers in vitro similar to previous findings in amoebae and macrophages during ingestion of tumour cells (Chambers & Weiser, 1969, as cited in Midlej & Benchimol, 2010; Martinez-Paolmo et al., 1985, as cited in Midlej & Benchimol, 2010). Particularly, whole, viable cells are not phagocytosed yet destruction of epithelial cell layers is observed suggesting necrotizing ability of *T. vaginalis*. Interestingly within Midlej & Benchimol's study (2010) an actin polymerization inhibitor significantly abrogated adherence while cytotoxicity remained relatively unaffected.

Another mechanism of interest is the availability of iron and its role in regulating immune evasion, and expression of adhesins and cysteine proteases (Lehker et al., 1991; Lehker & Alderete, 1992). Alternative pathway complement lysis allows destruction of trichomonads under low iron conditions assessed by Alderete et al. (1995). Upon supplementation of media with high levels of iron a cysteine proteinase capable of removing surface bound C3 is upregulated. Still not all cysteine proteases are upregulated as found in Kummer et al. (2008). Herein, the data provides an inverse correlation of iron abundance and presence of CP2, CP3, CP4 and CPT (collectively referred to as CP30) which are involved in apoptosis of human vaginal epithelial cells. Kummer et al. (2008) suggests this particular apoptotic mechanism may play a role in iron acquisition and is self-regulating upon iron uptake. Alvarez-Sánchez et al. (2007) also provide a negatively regulated soluble factor, CP65, under high iron conditions.

Understanding phenotypic variance will aid in understanding of the disease and elucidation of possibly novel mechanisms of regulation, as well as contribute to the strategies employed for development of a vaccine, a goal of ongoing research that will be discussed later.

2.6 Diagnosis

Before assessing the current diagnostic techniques available it is imperative to emphasize the difficulties of arriving at the diagnostic stage. Using a clinical syndromic approach a significant number of asymptomatic cases are missed. By not testing for nor treating asymptomatic infected individuals this enables the spread of disease and the lack of diagnosis results in underreported statistics of infection worldwide (Yin et al., 2008). Furthermore, in a prospective study Wiesenfeld & Macio (1999) found the available diagnostic tools such as simple wet mount microscopy, pH test or whiff test were often not used even under clinical suspicion of trichomoniasis. Ignoring the latter issue yet another problem arises. Diagnosis of cases investigated from clinical suspicion of trichomoniasis are at mercy of low sensitivity of current diagnostic standards as recent evaluations over the past decade have come to find (Lusk et al., 2010; Roth et al., 2011; Seña et al., 2007; Van Der Pol, 2007; Wendel et al., 2002). The most prevalent and most promising techniques will be reviewed below while a more detailed overview of guidelines for laboratory diagnosis and the methodology can be found in Domeika et al. (2010).

2.6.1 Culture and wet mount microscopy

Culture is considered the gold standard for diagnosis of *T. vaginalis*. Culture liquid is supplemented with antibiotics and samples are obtained from various locations such as vaginal/urethral discharge and swabs of known areas of infection. This technique requires as little as 10^2 trichomonads/mL (Garber, 2005). Unfortunately bacterial contamination remains an issue as well as lag growth phases of *T. vaginalis*. Additionally, this method is expensive and time consuming (Domeika et al., 2010) despite the availability of commercial culture systems (InPouch TV system: BioMed Diagnostics). Studies have found sensitivities ranging between 75-83% and specificity near 100% (Huppert et al., 2007; Nye et al., 2009; Wendel et al., 2002).

Wet mount is an attractive diagnostic tool due to its simplicity and cost effectiveness, and is consequently the most widely used (Huppert et al., 2007). This technique requires that samples are placed in physiological sterile saline and kept warm for immediate viewing under a common laboratory microscope. Positive detection is assessed by visualization of trichomonads exhibiting characteristic jerky movements (Domeika et al., 2010). Due to the requirement of at least 10^4 trichomonads/mL (Garber, 2005) this technique is not viable for urethral swab samples from males who typically yield low organism counts. Moreover, incorrect temperature or too much time elapsing between sampling and assessment results in loss of movement creating difficulty of differentiation from lymphocytes or nuclei of vaginal epithelial cells present in the sample (Garber, 2005). Sensitivities range from 52-61.5% and specificity near 100% (Huppert et al., 2007; Nye et al., 2009; Van Der Pol et al, 2006; Wendel et al., 2002).

2.6.2 Nucleic acid amplification test and transcription mediated amplification

Nucleic acid amplification testing (NAAT) and transcription mediated amplification (TMA) are recent, fairly labour intensive, highly sensitive but non-FDA approved diagnostic tools for detecting *T. vaginalis* which have been based on modifications of previous NAAT and TMA tests for infections such as chlamydia or gonorrhoea (Domeika et al., 2010; Van Der Pol et al, 2006). These tests may be conducted years after sample collection depending on proper storage conditions unlike wet mount which results in much less sensitivity unless maintained under strict time and temperature conditions (Van Der Pol et al, 2006). Despite high sensitivity for both male and female samples (Seña et al., 2007), greater than wet mount and culture (Crucitti et al., 2003; Lusk et al., 2010; Roth et al., 2011), in the range of 70-98% and specificity from 94-100% (Huppert et al., 2007; Nye et al., 2009; Seña et al., 2007; Wendel et al., 2002) this method is problematic as it is not point of care and remains unconfirmed for use in clinical settings.

2.6.3 Rapid antigen testing

Rapid antigen testing presents as probably the most promising technique despite requiring adequate technical skills and slightly less sensitivity than NAAT or TMA since it is inexpensive and can be employed at point of care (Domeika et al., 2010; Huppert et al., 2007). Also, this diagnostic tool is more sensitive than wet mount and culture microscopy. The rapid antigen test employed in Huppert (2007) obtained a sensitivity of 90% and specificity of 100%.

3. Murine model of infection and vaccination

An effective model for the study of *T. vaginalis* is pertinent not only to understand the disease in context of the findings discussed so far, which only skim the surface of the actual breadth of scientific knowledge for each topic, but also to encourage development of vaccine strategies especially given the underestimated prevalence of the disease, the largely asymptomatic population group that remains untreated and the lack of available drug treatment in low resource settings. Within this frame of mind a mouse model modified to its current state by our lab holds important implications for study of *T. vaginalis* pathogenicity and also serves as a vaccination model.

The murine model has been in development for some time coming to fruition as successfully demonstrating inducible protection upon vaccination against intravaginal challenge of *T. vaginalis* in BALB/c mice (Abraham et al., 1996).

First, estrogenization studies in rats appear to affect APC presentation in vaginal cells and uterine stromal cells negatively while increasing antigen presentation in the uterine epithelial cells through mechanisms not thoroughly understood (Wira et al., 2000).

Nevertheless estrogenization is pivotal for increasing experimental infection rates in mice. It is hypothesized estrogenization may induce a state of estrus that is more permissive to infection (Meysick & Garber, 1992). This hypothesis is in line with results also within Meysick & Garber (1992) that infection rates were increased, but duration was unaffected, thus a factor at timepoint zero of infection likely mediates the findings. Additionally, in the same study the vaginal flora of the mouse remained unaffected by treatment, an important factor as we will see in other studies. Interestingly as a side note estrogenization in mice affects CDF, a soluble cytotoxicity element secreted by *T. vaginalis* (Garber et al., 1991). This may complicate findings when used as a disease model.

Next, particular elements of the human vaginal environment have been thought to play a role in infection as noted by a decrease of *Lactobacillus* species levels and an associated increase of pH. Thus, through experimental inoculation of *Lactobacillus acidophilus* the mice would reflect more appropriately the human vaginal environment in terms of presence of lactobacilli and an associated pH decrease produced by products excreted by *L. acidophilus* (McGrory & Garber, 1992). With low percentages of natural incidence of lactobacilli in mice vaginas, an elevated pH and the disruption of these variables observed in human vaginas (Meysick & Garber, 1992) this factor of colonization was investigated. McGrory & Garber (1992) showed a significant increase in duration of trichomonal infection at day 24 post infection - 63-75% infected lactobacillus inoculated versus 0-25% infected controls. This suggests lactobacilli facilitate prolonged *T. vaginalis* infection.

Finally, the vaccination model (see Abraham et al., 1996) utilizes subcutaneous whole cell vaccination emulsified in adjuvant. While unfortunately the current adjuvants used (Freund's complete adjuvant and Freund's incomplete adjuvant) are not safe for human use, current preliminary work with human-safe FDA approved adjuvant aluminum hydroxide (Alhydrogel) has shown induction of serum immunoglobulin responses significantly greater than natural infection (unpublished observations). While this result is not entirely surprising it simply adds to validation for use of the current mouse model as a candidate for experimental vaccine development. Furthermore these mice when infected fall into categories of asymptomatic and symptomatic infection. Of the latter, typical symptoms include vulvitis, vaginitis and vaginal discharge.

Another similarity to human infection within the mouse model is that drug treatment resolution of infection and rechallenge does not confer any level of immune protection in mice as seen in humans (Abraham et al., 1996). On the other hand healthy skepticism is warranted in use of this current mouse model as suggested by Corbeil (1995). The actual pathogenic interactions of the murine vaginal epithelial cells with *T. vaginalis* are not characterized and similar protein binding adhesins mechanisms have not been demonstrated (Corbeil, 1995) which as previously noted was a significant correlate to symptomatic disease. Instead Corbeil suggests the use of a *Tritrichomonas foetus* bovine model.

4. Vaccinating against trichomonads

4.1 Bovine vaccine against *T. foetus*

The *T. foetus* bovine model cattle are a natural host to the parasite and infection occurs through natural means. In addition to its well characterized disease states a commercial vaccine is already available (Fort Dodge Laboratories, Fort Dodge, Iowa) based on previous work of immunization of bulls with whole cell or membrane fraction in oil adjuvant (Clark et al., 1983, as cited in Corbeil, 1995; Clark et al., 1984, as cited in Corbeil, 1995) and partial immunity in cows (Herr et al., as cited in Corbeil, 1995; Kvasnicka et al., 1989; Kvasnicka et al., 1992, as cited in Corbeil, 1995). The vaccines are not 100% protective, but significantly reduce transmission and infection rates among herds (Corbeil, 1995). Still this model may not be as attractive due to costs associated with purchase and husbandry of these animals whereas large sample numbers are obtainable, handling is easier and costs are within regular laboratory budgets to maintain mice. Also, while the host may be natural differences exist between *T. vaginalis* and *T. foetus* such as their ability to specifically induce lysis of human vascular endothelial cells and bovine vascular endothelial cells, respectively (Singh et al., 2004). As a last ironic note of difference it is the females that generally clear infection and the males that are asymptomatic carriers of *T. foetus* infection (Corbeil, 1995).

4.2 Developing a human vaccine against *T. vaginalis*

T. vaginalis presents an interesting challenge for providing immunity. It requires both mucosal immunity and consideration of mechanisms surrounding chronicity. Notably a vaccine obstacle is the surface heterogeneity of *T. vaginalis* inadvertently downregulating potent immunogenic proteins or glycoproteins (Alderete et al., 1986). Between phenotypic expression differences and strain differences between asymptomatic and symptomatic isolates an immunogen will be required to elicit robust immune response against a variable spectrum of antigens upon infectious challenge. The immunological activation necessarily must be sufficient enough to provide resolution without drug treatment especially in females.

Theoretically speaking the approach may seem easy such as vaccinating against a protein involved in sequestering resources given the parasitic nature of the infection. Even if a recombinant immunogenic protein can be purified and produced consistently the delivery method is problematic as many routes of vaccination exist. While some routes are more desirable than others, depending on the adjuvant of choice the options to produce an appropriate response via a given route become far and few between. While applying our expanding knowledge of adjuvant mechanisms and adjuvant-mediated immune response skew (O'Hagan & De Gregorio, 2009) may seem an obvious path, it neglects to consider the importance of understanding of the infection processes that mediate immune evasion or are the reason natural immunity fails in the first place. This gap emphasizes our need for a consistent laboratory model for study of pathogenesis and the mechanisms of function to facilitate adjuvant selection and even antigen selection as a subunit vaccine alone may not work. Lastly, in design of a vaccine we must consider the target demographic. In this case there is a strong need to service low resource communities especially those sub-Saharan Africa areas with high incidence and prevalence of both *T. vaginalis* and HIV infection (World Health Organization, 2001).

Progress in development of a bovine vaccine rather than a human vaccine has been strongly driven by economical factors of commercial farming involving loss of calves in utero (Kvasnicka et al., 1989). If it is commercial revenue or cost associated with the disease that drives funding for research then one must consider the 1.52-2.05 fold increased risk of HIV-1 acquisition (Mavedzenge et al., 2010; McClelland et al., 2008) and the costs associated with drug therapy of both trichomoniasis and HIV.

5. Rationale for a human *T. vaginalis* vaccine

5.1 Failure to control *T. vaginalis* with current treatment

The current treatment for trichomoniasis is oral metronidazole or tinidazole, either as a single 2g dose, or 500mg twice a day for 5 to 7 days (WHO, 2003). Treatment of a patient's current sexual partners has often been recommended but there is some question as to the efficacy of partner therapy. The Centers for Disease Control and Prevention (CDC) do not recommend patient delivered partner treatment (PDPT) for trichomoniasis as they have not found sufficient evidence that PDPT significantly impacts rates of *T. vaginalis* infection (Centers for Disease Control and Prevention, 2006). Additionally, there are barriers associated with PDPT. Having multiple partners or a new partner are predictors for trichomoniasis (Peterman et al., 2006), so PDPT may be ineffective as it may be difficult or undesirable to provide multiple partners with treatment, and a partner obtained after treatment has been completed obviously could not have been the source of initial infection and therefore will not receive treatment. Additionally, a study of HIV positive women who were provided with PDPT showed that 25% did not deliver treatment to their partners. Reasons for not delivering medication included being unable to contact a partner, not wanting to see a partner again, and being afraid of a partner's reaction. Fear of a partner's reaction was not limited to revealing *T. vaginalis* infection, but was also associated with having a partner who was unaware of the woman's HIV infection status (Gatski et al., 2010). This is particularly disturbing in light of the fact that the presence *of T. vaginalis* can lead to an increased risk of the partner contracting HIV, while at the same time ignorance about HIVpositive status may mean that the partner is more willing to engage in unprotected sex.

Because trichomoniasis is endemic in resource-limited settings, diagnosis is generally made purely on the basis of symptoms without any clinical testing. Syndromic treatment then is prescribed based on the most likely cause of illness. Because the symptoms of *T. vaginalis* infection are similar to other non-ulcerative STIs (urethritis in men, vaginitis and discharge in women) (Petrin et al., 1998) the disease is frequently misdiagnosed and the inappropriate drug is prescribed. Despite of the fact that WHO guidelines indicate metronidazole or tinidazole therapy is recommended in all cases of vaginal discharge (WHO, 2003), trichomoniasis is still under-diagnosed and under-treated.

A study in India showed that using the relatively inexpensive InPouch culture kit to test for *T. vaginalis* at the point of care increased would have increased the correct treatment of trichomoniasis from 51% (syndromic treatment, no testing performed) to 82% (based on InPouch results) (Madhivanan et al., 2009). Unfortunately, culture testing requires 3 to 7 days of incubation to confirm the presence or absence of trichomonads, and this time frame may not be acceptable to patients who need to travel to reach medical facilities.

Another problem with syndromic management of trichomoniasis is that treatment guidelines are clear for women only. In India, a country where metronidazole treatment for vaginal discharge is part of syndromic management, high rates of *T. vaginalis* infection were still found in women, and also in many men. Current guidelines recommend treating for trichomoniasis in men only if symptoms of urethritis persist after treatment for gonorrhoea and chlamydia (WHO, 2003). Introducing metronidazole as a part of syndromic treatment for men presenting with non-ulcerative genital infection has been recommended (Becker et al., 2010), however this will still not address the problem of asymptomatic carriers.

Poor control of trichomoniasis is not solely a problem in developing countries. A study in the United States showed that the prevalence of *T. vaginalis* infection is approximately 3% in women between the ages of 14 and 49. This infection rate doubles in the poorly educated and economically disadvantaged, and nearly quadruples in black women (Allsworth et al., 2009). Additionally persistent, subclinical *T. vaginalis* infections have been reported even after seemingly successful treatment. A study on HIV positive women diagnosed with trichomoniasis showed that despite reported compliance with metronidazole treatment regimen and putative successful cure (negative InPouch culture), a number of women tested positive for *T. vaginalis* infection 3-6 months later, despite reporting no sexual contact in the intervening time (Gatski & Kissinger, 2010).

Drug resistance to nitroimidazoles such as metronidazole and tinidazole has also been reported in 5-10% of clinical specimens (Upcroft & Upcroft, 2001). As there are currently no effective non-nitroimidazole treatments for trichomoniasis, drug resistant *T. vaginalis* must be treated by increasing medication dosages, which often leads to increased adverse effects. If these adverse reactions become severe enough to force cessation of therapy, trichomoniasis can become a chronic condition (Cudmore et al. 2004).

5.2 Other issues with treatment to control *T. vaginalis*

Sexually transmitted infections such as trichomoniasis are societal as well as medical problems. In order to successfully control the disease the personal, social, and cultural barriers associated with dealing with STI need to be addressed.

5.2.1 The education risk factor

Accurate and useful information on STI can be difficult to obtain. A study done with students (aged 13-16, male and female) in the United Kingdom showed that STI were recognized as a serious health problem. However, many of the teenagers were ill- or misinformed about the names of common STI, how to identify a possible infection, where to seek treatment, etc. (Garside et al., 2001). Lack of education has clearly been shown to be a risk factor for acquiring STI. Unfortunately education programs are not available in many areas where HIV and trichomoniasis are endemic due to reasons such as lack of finance and resources, geography, and cultural or personal discomfort about discussing sexuality and STI. As such, the importance of protecting those with little opportunity to access information about STI cannot be underestimated.

Lack of information and awareness regarding STI has been shown to lead to delays in seeking treatment for medical issues involving the genitals. Participants in a study in rural Zimbabwe had little awareness that having an STI could increase their risk of contracting HIV. Men were more aware of the link between STI and HIV (18% of men vs 5 % of women) and this knowledge was associated with seeking treatment more promptly upon noticing symptoms of genital disease. However many men (36%) and the majority of women (70%) ignored symptoms of urethral/vaginal discharge or discomfort, or lower abdominal pain for a week or more before seeking treatment (Gregson et al., 2001). Given the fact that trichomoniasis and other STI have been linked to sequelae such as infertility and adverse pregnancy outcomes, delays in seeking treatment puts reproductive health at risk.

Education about STI in the general population is not the only issue, part of the problem can stem from the lack of healthcare workers specialized in dealing with sexual issues and diseases. In many parts of the world specialist physicians are rare and general practitioners may not have sufficient background, or simply not be comfortable discussing "intimate" issues, especially with the opposite sex. Women are often more comfortable dealing with other women when discussing sexual issues, but a study in Bangladesh found that female healthcare workers were often uncomfortable discussing sexuality or performing genital exams (Gibney et al., 1999). Because of the embarrassment, social implications, etc. often attached to the subject of STI, an open discussion between a patient and healthcare provider can be difficult when medical personel are clearly uncomfortable with the subject. Patients may be less forthcoming about their symptoms and less likely to seek treatment if healthcare workers appear to be judgemental or reluctant to provide information and care.

5.2.2 Cultural barriers

There is a nearly universal stigma attached to having an STI. Sex and sexuality are generally considered to be very personal issues and seeking treatment for genital disease involves speaking about private matters. In addition reluctance to seek treatment can stem from fear of being associated with promiscuity and negative social behaviours, which are often linked with STI. A study of pregnant women in India showed that although the majority of women stated they were willing to be tested for HIV, they were also highly concerned about the reactions of their husbands, families, and community should it be found that they were seropositive. Additionally, not breastfeeding (recommended to prevent maternal-child HIV transmission) was widely believed to be a sign that a woman was a bad mother or had been unfaithful to her husband (Rogers et al., 2006).

Women in particular are often reluctant to speak about genital health issues, one study cites "shyness" as the single biggest barrier in seeking STI treatment (Gibney et al., 1999). A study of pregnant women in Nairobi found that over a quarter of women refused to answer portions of a health questionnaire related to vaginal discharge. Of the women who did respond, only 6% complained of discharge, but 51% were found were found to have abnormal vaginal discharge on clinical examination (Marx et al., 2010). Another study, also in pregnant women, found that although many of the women questioned recognized a variety of symptoms (including vaginal discharge/itching, dysuria, and genital ulcers or swelling) only 9% sought treatment (Blankhart et al., 1999). This statistic is particularly disturbing in view of the adverse outcomes associated with having an STI during pregnancy. Reluctance to seek STI treatment for fear of negative reactions from family and/or community is putting both child and maternal health at risk.

5.2.3 Sexual inequality and risk

Sexual risk behaviour in women has been found to significantly influence their likelihood of contracting trichomoniasis, but not HIV. Conversely high risk (male) partner behaviour significantly increased the female partner's risk of acquiring HIV, but was not associated with increased incidence of trichomoniasis (Mavedzenge et al., 2010). This issue of male sexual risk behaviour contributing to a female partner's risk of acquiring an STI, especially HIV, is important because many women do not have complete control of their sexual activities. A study of 481 pregnant young women in the Central African Republic showed that 72% reported voluntarily engaging in their first sexual intercourse, 18% were pressured their first intercourse, and 11% reported their first sexual intercourse was a rape. With respect to their pregnancies, 52% reported their pregnancy was planned and desired, 32% reported unplanned but accepted, and 16% reported that they did not desire the pregnancy (Blankhart et al., 1999).

A study on risk factors for HIV acquisition in Africa found that women's sexual choices are often limited or dictated by their male partners. Some women reported that they were forced into a sexual relationship as it was their only means to obtain food, shelter, or money for education. Others stated that they required their partner's permission to obtain medical care (including HIV testing) and to protect themselves (ie. use condoms). Marital standards are also unbalanced as while married women are expected to remain faithful to their husbands, men are not necessarily expected to maintain complete fidelity, especially if they are away from their wives (Chersich & Rees, 2008).

In many rural areas labourers must migrate to different locations or into cities to find work. This can result in significant periods of spousal separation and can result in one or both partners seeking extra-marital sexual intercourse. A study in Zimbabwe showed that while both partners may visit "beer halls" women are at statistically significant increased risk of HIV acquisition, while only a small non-significant increase in risk was seen for men (Gregson et al., 2001). In China, a study of migrant workers of both sexes found that they often engaged high risk sexual behaviours much more than the general population. In particular women were more likely to sell sex for money and men more likely to pay for sex. Interestingly, this increased involvement with the sex trade increased the prevalence of STI and HIV in women, but no statistically significant increase seen in men (Wang et al., 2007).

5.2.4 Marginalized populations

Female sex workers (FSW) are unsurprisingly at a high risk for STI. They can also act as a reservoir for STI that can be difficult to deal with using treatment alone as they can be sexually active on a daily basis. Additionally studies like one in Indonesia have shown that STI rates are highest in FSW in the lowest socioecomonic class, who charge the lowest prices per sex act and as such need to see more clients, increasing their risk for STI. These women are also more likely to have little ability to negotiate condom use, and have minimal money to spend on medical care and medication (Joesoef et al., 1997).

Even when healthcare initiatives aimed at FSW are in place, education and medical care are still not necessarily easily available to all. This is especially true for FSW who are non-residents or illegal immigrants in the country in which they are working. A study in Sydney, Australia showed an impressively low rate of STI amongst "local" FSW (women who were native Australian or had been in the country a significant period, and English-speaking) after partial legalization of the sex trade and an aggressive education campaign. However "international" FSW (women born outside of Australia whose first language was not English) showed high rates of STI. Language barriers, lack of access to the same medical programs as residents, and concerns about drawing attention to themselves by accessing medical care meant that these women remained at high risk despite there being a system in place to help protect them (O'Connor et al., 1996).

Sex trade workers are clearly an excellent target population for a vaccine that could provide long term, consistent protection from *T. vaginalis* infection and offer a reduced risk of HIV acquisition. They are part of a "core" group that acts as a reservoir for STI, and reducing the burden of infection in this population can be a community benefit.

5.3 Advantages of a vaccine for prevention of *T. vaginalis* infection

Trichomoniasis can be treated relatively easily and inexpensively, yet the disease is poorly controlled. Diverse factors lead to both a failure to recognize *T. vaginalis* infection and inability or unwillingness to seek or access treatment. A vaccine could provide long term protection eliminating the need for repeated doctor visits and treatments, the risk of misdiagnosis, and address the needs of high risk populations. In addition, given the link between trichomoniasis and other genital infection, especially HIV, a vaccine capable of preventing *T. vaginalis* infections has the potential to impact global STI burden.

6. *T. vaginalis* and HIV

6.1 Incidence and prevalence of trichomoniasis and HIV

It is estimated that approximately 33.3 million people are currently infected with HIV-1. About two-thirds of these (22.5 million) are living in sub-Saharan Africa and 4.1 million live in South and Southeast Asia (UN, 2009). Both these areas also have the highest rates of *T. vaginalis* infection, with about 32 million cases in sub-Saharan Africa and 76.5 million in South and Southeast Asia every year (WHO, 2001). Global rates of trichomoniasis and HIV tend to follow similar patterns in different areas of the world (ie. the higher the incidence of *T. vaginalis* infection, the higher the prevalence of HIV) with two exceptions. As stated above, sub-Saharan Africa has the highest prevalence of HIV and the second highest incidence of trichomoniasis, while the opposite is true for south and Southeast Asia. The other exception is North America, which has a fairly high prevalence of HIV (1.5 million cases) (UN, 2009) relative to a low incidence of *T. vaginalis* infection (8 million annually) (WHO, 2001).

Rates of co-infection with HIV and *T. vaginalis* in women have been reported to range from 16% to almost 30% (Allsworth et al., 2009; Gatski et al., 2010; Månsson et al., 2010; Marx et al., 2010). It is difficult to reliably estimate co-infection rates in men as trichomoniasis is generally asymptomatic and not usually considered a significant STI in males.

6.2 *T. vaginalis* and increased risk of HIV transmission

Trichomoniasis has been associated with a 1.52 to 2.05 times greater risk of seroconversion upon exposure to HIV (McClelland et al., 2007, Mavedzenge et al., 2010). A longitudinal study of almost 5000 women in South Africa and Zimbabwe showed that the link between HIV and *T. vaginalis* appears to be bi-directional. Compared to uninfected women, those with trichomoniasis were more likely to test positive for HIV at their next study visit, and HIV positive women were more likely to have acquired *T. vaginalis* infection by their following study visit (odds ratios were >2 for both cases, after adjusting for confounders such as age, other STIs, and sexual risk behaviours) (Mavedzenge et al., 2010). This leads to an increased risk of both *T. vaginalis* and HIV infection if both diseases are present in any combination between sexual partners.

6.2.1 Disruption of genital mucosa

As previously mentioned, *T. vaginalis* is capable of both contact dependent and contact independent disruption of cell layers (see section 2.5.2). This disruption can provide portals of entry that allow HIV access past the epithelium into tissue, can sometimes lead to the formation of punctuate mucosal hemorrhages (strawberry cervix) women.

Without co-factors such as STI co-infection or trauma to the genital mucosa, the odds of a woman acquiring HIV through sexual exposure are estimated to be 0.08%. The odds of female to male transmission are 0.04% per exposure. Healthy, intact genital mucosa is considered to be a significant barrier to HIV infection (Thurman & Doncel, 2011). Because trichomoniasis can disrupt the integrity of mucosal tissue this primary barrier against infection is breached and HIV transmission risk is increased.

The degree of epithelial disruption has been found in vitro to vary between different isolates of *T. vaginalis*. A study examining four different *T. vaginalis* clinical isolates (two from asymptomatic patients and two from symptomatic patients presenting with cervicitis and vaginal discharge) found that the symptomatic isolates rapidly disrupted cell monolayers, but the asymptomatic isolates had a much more limited effect on monolayer integrity. The potential impact of monolayer disruption on the ability of HIV to enter tissue was examined by adding HIV and *T. vaginalis* to the apical surface of stratified monolayers growing on transwell plates, then measuring the amount of virus present in the basolateral supernatant. The degree of monolayer disruption was found to correlate with the amount of HIV released into the basolateral supernatant. Symptomatic isolates (disrupted monolayers) caused a four- to five-fold increase in HIV released into supernatant, whereas asymptomatic isolates (intact monolayers) showed HIV supernatant levels similar to background (no trichomonads on monolayers) (Guenthner et al., 2005). Although only four isolates were used, this experiment suggests that not all isolates of *T. vaginalis* may have equal impact on the risk of acquiring HIV infection. This is an intriguing possibility that could potentially offer some explanation as to why the high incidence of trichomoniasis in South and Southeast Asia is not matched by an equally high prevalence of HIV.

6.2.2 Changes to vaginal flora

Both trichomoniasis and HIV transmission have been linked to disrupted or abnormal vaginal flora. A study examining the link between *T. vaginalis* infection and bacterial vaginosis (BV) showed that 61% of HIV positive women also had BV and 80% had abnormal vaginal flora (defined as Nugent scores of 7-10 and 4-10, respectively). In comparison HIV negative women with trichomoniasis showed 47.3% incidence of BV co-infection, and 58.9% had abnormal vaginal flora (Gatski et al., 2010). However, since co-infection with trichomoniasis and BV is relatively common, it is difficult to tell which, if either, infection acts as the primary risk factor.

Both trichomoniasis and BV are associated with an increase in vaginal pH and decreased or absent vaginal *Lactobacillus* species (Petrin et al., 1998 (trichomoniasis) and Sha et al., 2005 (BV)). Lactobacilli produce lactic acid which maintains the low pH of the (healthy) vagina. Lactic acid has been shown in vitro to inactivate HIV, as has H_2O_2 which is produced by some, but not all, lactobacilli (Klebanoff et al., 1991). Lactobacilli therefore contribute maintaining a vaginal milieu that is not permissive to infectious agents, and loss of *Lactobacillus* species can lead to increased chances of STI. Low vaginal pH and H_2O_2 can also inhibit activation and proliferation of vaginal lymphocytes, particularly CD4+ T cells (Hill & Anderson, 1992). This means that disruption of the vaginal environment by *T. vaginalis* can lead to greater risk of HIV infection due to an increase of activated CD4+ T cells that can be infected by the virus.

6.2.3 Inflammatory response

Infection with *T. vaginalis* leads to a local inflammatory response that includes chemoattractant (IL-8) and acute pro-inflammatory (TNF-α ,IL-1β, and IL-6) cytokines that are responsible for initiating immune response to infection and recruiting immune cells. Symptomatic infection is the result of a more vigorous immune response in which there is an increased amount of inflammation and cell recruitment. For example, in women vaginal discharge often contains neutrophils that respond to the presence of IL-8 (Thurman & Doncel, 2010). However immune response may fail to clear *T. vaginalis*, and does not provide long term immunological memory to prevent subsequent infections. Additionally immune response to trichomoniasis can attract lymphocytes that are the targets of HIV infection.

A powerful chemoattractant, IL-8 recruits immune cells to where they are needed to eliminate infection. However, it has also been shown that this cytokine can increase the susceptibility of monocytes, macrophages, and CD4+ T cells to HIV infection. IL-8 can also enhance HIV replication in infected immune cells (Narimatsu et al., 2005).

A study using cervicovaginal lavage samples from HIV positive women who were also infected with *T. vaginalis* showed elevated levels of IL-1β. Levels of IL-1β could be significantly different between visits, but clearly correlated with HIV viral load (Mitchell et al., 2011).

An in vitro study using HIV-infected peripheral blood mononuclear cells (PBMC) cultured with *T. vaginalis* resulted in increased replication of HIV compared to PBMCs alone. Unlike epithelial cell disruption, different isolates (symptomatic or asymptomatic) seemed to induce similar levels of increase in HIV replication. It was found that TNF-α levels were elevated in the supernatant of cultures containing *T. vaginalis* compared to controls and the addition of anti-TNF-α antibody could attenuate the increase in HIV replication (Guenthner et al., 2005).

The relationship between IL-6 and HIV is interesting in that they seem to be capable of upregulating each other in an apparent positive feedback loop. Examination of ectocervical tissue from HIV positive women found higher levels of IL-6 than in uninfected controls. Because the ectocervix was an area where high levels of HIV replication had been detected, recombinant IL-6 was applied to tissue explants and a greater than 300-fold increase in HIV transcription was seen (Asin et al., 2009). HIV appears to be capable of not only infecting immune cells, but of using immune response to its own advantage to enhance its replication.

6.2.4 Increased viral load

Inflammatory response to *T. vaginalis* infection leads to an influx of susceptible lymphocytes and the release of cytokines that can upregulate the rate of HIV replication. This in turn can increase HIV viral load and lead to a higher risk of spreading the infection to unprotected partners. A study looking at HIV positive men with genital ulcers found HIV RNA increased in ulcers caused by herpes simplex virus type 2 (HSV-2) only if HSV-2 was present in the ulcer. However, co-infection with *T. vaginalis* increased HIV viral load in ulcers regardless of the presence of HSV-2 indicating that trichomoniasis leads to increased shedding of HIV regardless of (or perhaps even in synergy with) other STI (Paz-Bailey et al., 2010).

While trichomoniasis does increase the amount of HIV viral shedding, elimination of *T. vaginalis* infection returns HIV RNA levels in the genitals to lower levels. A study in Africa of HIV positive women with trichomoniasis measured viral RNA at the time of trichomonal infection, and then 2 weeks later after treatment when infection had been resolved. There was a 4.2 fold decrease in the amount of HIV shed (Wang et al., 2001). Another study in New Orleans examined vaginal viral shedding in HIV positive women with and without trichomoniasis. Women with *T. vaginalis* infection were almost twice as likely as women without trichomoniasis to have detectable HIV RNA in their vaginal secretions at baseline (36.2% vs 19.6%). One month following successful treatment for trichomoniasis, the number of women shedding HIV was reduced (although it remained significantly higher than in women previously uninfected by *T. vaginalis*). At followup visits three months after initial interviews there was no significant difference in the number of women shedding vaginal HIV between the two groups (Kissinger et al., 2009), indicating that elimination of the parasite removes the enhanced HIV risks associated with trichomoniasis. As *T. vaginalis* clearly has a significant impact on HIV infection, reducing incidence of trichomoniasis has the potential to help control the incidence and prevalence of HIV.

6.3 Reducing *T. vaginalis* as a method of HIV prevention

Trichomoniasis is clearly associated with HIV risk, the question is can reducing *T. vaginalis* infections have an impact on the incidence of HIV? A study in Tanzania showed that a decrease in HIV prevalence in women was accompanied by a significant decrease in multiple STI, particularly trichomoniasis which dropped from 21.2% to 5% incidence over the 3-5 year cross-sectional study. This reduction in disease burden was attributed mainly to changes in sexual behaviour as a result of a multi-pronged sexual health awareness campaign. Interestingly very little change was seen in condom use or age of first sexual intercourse, but a dramatic decline was seen in women reporting having engaged in casual sex (Msuya et al., 2007). As a women's sexual risk behaviour is correlated with the risk of trichomonal infection, this study suggests that protecting women from *T. vaginalis* could contribute to protecting them from HIV. Since treatment has proved to be an ineffective method of reducing trichomoniasis, a vaccine could provide long term for protection to those who are both most at risk and least able to protect themselves.

A vaccine would also be helpful in targeting specific at risk populations. For example, black women have consistently been shown to have a higher incidence of trichomoniasis than women of other races (Shafir et al., 2009). This may be the result of sample bias, as many studies take place in inner-city clinics and in sub-Saharan Africa where other risk factors such as poverty and lack of education are also present. It could also be the result of certain common practices (eg. vaginal cleaning/douching), unknown biological factors, or a combination of factors that act synergistically to increase susceptibility to *T. vaginalis* infection. The availability of a vaccine could target protection to those with increased risk, while avoiding stigmatizing a specific population. As this population has also been found to have an increased risk of HIV infection, an single effective vaccine could potentially have a significant impact on the incidence of both diseases.

HIV and the spectrum of medical issues that arise from infection are complicated issues that are often not well understood by either the HIV positive or the HIV negative. For example, many people believe if an HIV-positive person has an undetectable viral load, that they cannot infect anyone else. However, it has been shown that up to 33% of women with undetectable serum viral load continue to shed the virus in cervicovaginal secretions (Neely et al., 2007). Due to high rates of co-infection with *T. vaginalis* it is likely that a number of these women have or will acquire trichomoniasis. A *T. vaginalis* vaccine could reduce the burden of disease in HIV positive individuals who are at high risk to acquire trichomoniasis, and protect their partners from the elevated risk associated with co-infection.

7. Conclusions

Current methods for reducing the incidence of HIV include education and public health programs (providing condoms and encouraging condom use, needle exchange, etc.) and antiretorviral therapy (ART) to reduce HIV viral titers and minimize the risk of transmission. However, HIV is endemic in developing countries where obtaining resources (financial, personal, etc.) and accessing (may need to travel from rural areas to cities) education and health programs can be difficult, potentially limiting positive impact. Providing ART also poses a problem in resource limited settings as it is an expensive multi-drug cocktail and therapy is often complicated by drug interactions and toxicity, and adverse patient reactions. Additionally, ART is usually prescribed based on CD4+ T cell count, and monitoring can be difficult if patients must travel to reach a medical facility capable of testing (WHO, 2006). Finding simple, inexpensive alternative methods to reduce the transmission of HIV could help reduce dependence on ART as a means of controlling HIV incidence.

Treatment of STI can be difficult for reasons beyond drug availability and efficacy and access to healthcare. Cultural barriers and personal beliefs can affect an individual's acceptance of their diagnosis and willingness to seek treatment. Limited control over one's sexual activity can lead to an inability to protect oneself and control sexual risk. In addition, some populations (eg. FSW) are at a persistently higher risk for STI and while treatment eliminates disease, it does not protect against subsequent infection thus will have minimal impact on STI incidence. The development of a *T. vaginalis* vaccine that could be offered as part of routine medical care for high risk groups could eliminate the need to seek treatment, reduce risk, and lower the incidence of trichomoniasis.

T. vaginalis infection has been shown to facilitate both transmission and acquisition of HIV through multiple mechanisms. Many of these mechanisms have been described in vitro, but their exact correlation to infection is not clearly defined. The existence of a mouse model of *T. vaginalis* infection provides a powerful and relatively inexpensive tool to elucidate the disease mechanisms of trichomoniasis in vivo. The model also allows for the evaluation of immune responses to *T. vaginalis* infection and vaccination as a part of an approach to rational vaccine design.

The actual increase in risk of acquiring HIV or infecting a sexual partner due to trichomoniasis is unknown. However, given that the high incidence of *T. vaginalis* infection (174 million cases annually), the fact that it is globally distributed in similar patterns to those of HIV, and that some populations have been found to have co-infection rates as high as almost 30% (Allsworth et al., 2009), even a small percentage of *T. vaginalis* infections leading to seroconversion could significantly impact the incidence of HIV. Vaccination against *T. vaginalis* offered to "core" groups that act as reservoirs of STI could have the potential to reduce community incidence of both trichomoniasis and HIV. Pregnant women are also often at increased risk of trichomoniasis due to hormonal changes. Vaccinating against *T. vaginalis* would not only prevent adverse birth outcomes associated with trichomoniasis, but could potentially protect against an HIV infection that could lead to maternal-child transmission of the virus. Thus, we suggest vaccination against *T. vaginalis* as an alternative approach to HIV control as well as for prevention of this highly prevalent STI.

8. References

Abraham MC, Desjardins M, Filion LG, Garber GE. Inducible immunity to Trichomonas vaginalis in a mouse model of vaginal infection. Infect Immun. 1996 Sep; 64 (9): 3571-5.

Alderete JF, Garza GE. Soluble Trichomonas vaginalis antigens in cell-free culture supernatants. Mol Biochem Parasitol. 1984 Oct; 13 (2): 147-58.

Alderete JF, Kasmala L, Metcalfe E, Garza GE. Phenotypic variation and diversity among Trichomonas vaginalis isolates and correlation of phenotype with trichomonal virulence determinants. Infect Immun. 1986 Aug; 53 (2): 285-93.

Alderete JF, Provenzano D, Lehker MW. Iron mediates Trichomonas vaginalis resistance to complement lysis. Microb Pathog. 1995 Aug; 19 (2): 93-103.

Allsworth JE, Ratner JA, Peipert JF. Trichomoniasis and other sexually transmitted infections: results from the 2001-2004 National Health and Nutrition Examination Surveys. Sex Transm Dis. 2009 Dec; 36 (12): 738-44.

Alvarez-Sánchez ME, Solano-González E, Yañez-Gómez C, Arroyo R. Negative iron regulation of the CP65 cysteine proteinase cytotoxicity in Trichomonas vaginalis. Microbes Infect. 2007 Nov-Dec; 9 (14-15): 1597-605.

Arroyo R, Engbring J, Alderete JF. Molecular basis of host epithelial cell recognition by Trichomonas vaginalis. Mol Microbiol. 1992 Apr; 6 (7): 853-62.

Asin SN, Eszterhas SK, Rollenhagen C, Heimberg AM, Howell AL. HIV type 1 infection in women: increased transcription of HIV type 1 in ectocervical tissue explants. J Infect Dis. 2009 Sep 15; 200 (6): 965-72.

Becker M, Stephen J, Moses S, Washington R, Maclean I, Cheang M, Isac S, Ramesh BM, Alary M, Blanchard J. Etiology and determinants of sexually transmitted infections in Karnataka state, south India. Sex Transm Dis. 2010 Mar; 37 (3): 159-64.

Blankhart D, Müller O, Gresenguet G, Weis P. Sexually transmitted infections in young pregnant women in Bangui, Central African Republic. Int J STD AIDS. 1999 Sep; 10 (9): 609-14.

Carlton JM, Hirt RP, Silva JC, Delcher AL, Schatz M, Zhao Q, Wortman JR, Bidwell SL, Alsmark UC, Besteiro S, Sicheritz-Ponten T, Noel CJ, Dacks JB, Foster PG, Simillion C, Van de Peer Y, Miranda-Saavedra D, Barton GJ, Westrop GD, Müller S, Dessi D, Fiori PL, Ren Q, Paulsen I, Zhang H, Bastida-Corcuera FD, Simoes-Barbosa A, Brown MT, Hayes RD, Mukherjee M, Okumura CY, Schneider R, Smith AJ, Vanacova S, Villalvazo M, Haas BJ, Pertea M, Feldblyum TV, Utterback TR, Shu CL, Osoegawa K, de Jong PJ, Hrdy I, Horvathova L, Zubacova Z, Dolezal P, Malik SB, Logsdon JM Jr, Henze K, Gupta A, Wang CC, Dunne RL, Upcroft JA, Upcroft P, White O, Salzberg SL, Tang P, Chiu CH, Lee YS, Embley TM, Coombs GH, Mottram JC, Tachezy J, Fraser-Liggett CM, Johnson PJ. Draft genome sequence of the sexually transmitted pathogen Trichomonas vaginalis. Science. 2007 Jan 12; 315 (5809): 207-12.

Centers for Disease Control and Prevention. Expedited partner therapy in the management of sexually transmitted diseases. Atlanta, GA: US Department of Health and Human Services. 2006.

Chang JH, Ryang YS, Morio T, Lee SK, Chang EJ. Trichomonas vaginalis inhibits proinflammatory cytokine production in macrophages by suppressing NF-kappaB activation. Mol Cells. 2004 Oct 31; 18 (2): 177-85.

Chersich MF, Rees HV. Vulnerability of women in southern Africa to infection with HIV: biological determinants and priority health sector interventions. AIDS. 2008 Dec; 22 Suppl 4:S27-40.

Corbeil LB. Use of an animal model of trichomoniasis as a basis for understanding this disease in women. Clin Infect Dis. 1995 Oct; 21 Suppl 2:S158-61.

Corbeil LB. Vaccination strategies against Tritrichomonas foetus. Parasitol Today. 1994 Mar; 10 (3): 103-6.

Cotch MF, Pastorek JG 2nd, Nugent RP, Hillier SL, Gibbs RS, Martin DH, Eschenbach DA, Edelman R, Carey JC, Regan JA, Krohn MA, Klebanoff MA, Rao AV, Rhoads GG. Trichomonas vaginalis associated with low birth weight and preterm delivery The Vaginal Infections and Prematurity Study Group. Sex Transm Dis. 1997 Jul; 24 (6): 353-60.

Crucitti T, Jespers V, Mulenga C, Khondowe S, Vandepitte J, Buvé A. Non-sexual transmission of Trichomonas vaginalis in adolescent girls attending school in Ndola, Zambia. PLoS One. 2011 Jan 31; 6 (1): e16310.

Crucitti T, Van Dyck E, Tehe A, Abdellati S, Vuylsteke B, Buve A, Laga M. Comparison of culture and different PCR assays for detection of Trichomonas vaginalis in self collected vaginal swab specimens. Sex Transm Infect. 2003 Oct; 79 (5): 393-8.

Cudmore SL, Delgaty KL, Hayward-McClelland SF, Petrin DP, Garber GE. Treatment of infections caused by metronidazole-resistant Trichomonas vaginalis. Clin Microbiol Rev. 2004 Oct; 17 (4): 783-93, table of contents.

de Miguel N, Lustig G, Twu O, Chattopadhyay A, Wohlschlegel JA, Johnson PJ. Proteome analysis of the surface of Trichomonas vaginalis reveals novel proteins and strain-dependent differential expression. Mol Cell Proteomics. 2010 Jul; 9 (7): 1554-66.

Domeika M, Zhurauskaya L, Savicheva A, Frigo N, Sokolovskiy E, Hallén A, Unemo M, Ballard RC, Eastern European Network for Sexual and Reproductive Health. Guidelines for the laboratory diagnosis of trichomoniasis in East European countries. J Eur Acad Dermatol Venereol. 2010 Oct; 24 (10): 1125-34.

Escario JA, Gómez Barrio A, Martínez Fernández AR. The relationship of experimental pathogenicity in vivo with in vitro cytoadherence and cytotoxicity of 6 different isolates of Trichomonas vaginalis. Int J Parasitol. 1995 Aug; 25 (8): 999-1000.

Fiori PL, Rappelli P, Addis MF, Sechi A, Cappuccinelli P. Trichomonas vaginalis haemolysis: pH regulates a contact-independent mechanism based on pore-forming proteins. Microb Pathog. 1996 Feb; 20 (2): 109-18.

Garber GE. The laboratory diagnosis of Trichomonas vaginalis. Can J Infect Dis Med Microbiol. 2005 Jan; 16 (1): 35-8.

Garber GE, Lemchuk-Favel LT. Association of production of cell-detaching factor with the clinical presentation of Trichomonas vaginalis. J Clin Microbiol. 1990 Nov; 28 (11): 2415-7.

Garber GE, Lemchuk-Favel LT, Rousseau G. Effect of beta-estradiol on production of the cell-detaching factor of Trichomonas vaginalis. J Clin Microbiol. 1991 Sep; 29 (9): 1847-9.

Garside R, Ayres R, Owen M, Pearson VA, Roizen J. "They never tell you about the consequences": young people's awareness of sexually transmitted infections. Int J STD AIDS. 2001 Sep; 12 (9): 582-8.

Gatski M, Kissinger P. Observation of probable persistent, undetected Trichomonas vaginalis infection among HIV-positive women. Clin Infect Dis. 2010 Jul 1; 51 (1): 114-5.

Gatski M, Mena L, Levison J, Clark RA, Henderson H, Schmidt N, Rosenthal SL, Martin DH, Kissinger P. Patient-delivered partner treatment and Trichomonas vaginalis repeat infection among human immunodeficiency virus-infected women. Sex Transm Dis. 2010 Aug; 37 (8): 502-5.

Gatski M, Martin DH, Clark RA, Harville E, Schmidt N, Kissinger P. Co-occurrence of Trichomonas vaginalis and bacterial vaginosis among HIV-positive women. Sex Transm Dis. 2011 Mar; 38 (3): 163-6.

Gibney L, Choudhury P, Khawaja Z, Sarker M, Islam N, Vermund SH. HIV/AIDS in Bangladesh: an assessment of biomedical risk factors for transmission. Int J STD AIDS. 1999 May; 10 (5): 338-46.

Gomez C, Esther Ramirez M, Calixto-Galvez M, Medel O, Rodríguez MA. Regulation of gene expression in protozoa parasites. J Biomed Biotechnol. 2010; 2010:726045.

Gregson S, Mason PR, Garnett GP, Zhuwau T, Nyamukapa CA, Anderson RM, Chandiwana SK. A rural HIV epidemic in Zimbabwe? Findings from a population-based survey. Int J STD AIDS. 2001 Mar; 12 (3): 189-96.

Guenthner PC, Secor WE, Dezzutti CS. Trichomonas vaginalis-induced epithelial monolayer disruption and human immunodeficiency virus type 1 (HIV-1) replication: implications for the sexual transmission of HIV-1. Infect Immun. 2005 Jul; 73 (7): 4155-60.

Hill JA, Anderson DJ. Human vaginal leukocytes and the effects of vaginal fluid on lymphocyte and macrophage defense functions. Am J Obstet Gynecol. 1992 Feb; 166 (2): 720-6.

Heine P, McGregor JA. Trichomonas vaginalis: a reemerging pathogen. Clin Obstet Gynecol. 1993 Mar; 36 (1): 137-44.

Huppert JS, Mortensen JE, Reed JL, Kahn JA, Rich KD, Miller WC, Hobbs MM. Rapid antigen testing compares favorably with transcription-mediated amplification assay for the detection of Trichomonas vaginalis in young women. Clin Infect Dis. 2007 Jul 15; 45 (2): 194-8.

Joesoef MR, Linnan M, Barakbah Y, Idajadi A, Kambodji A, Schulz K. Patterns of sexually transmitted diseases in female sex workers in Surabaya, Indonesia. Int J STD AIDS. 1997 Sep; 8 (9): 576-80.

Johnston VJ, Mabey DC. Global epidemiology and control of Trichomonas vaginalis. Curr Opin Infect Dis. 2008 Feb; 21 (1): 56-64.

Kissinger P, Amedee A, Clark RA, Dumestre J, Theall KP, Myers L, Hagensee ME, Farley TA, Martin DH. Trichomonas vaginalis treatment reduces vaginal HIV-1 shedding. Sex Transm Dis. 2009 Jan; 36 (1) :11-6.

Klebanoff SJ, Hillier SL, Eschenbach DA, Waltersdorph AM. Control of the microbial flora of the vagina by H2O2-generating lactobacilli. J Infect Dis. 1991 Jul; 164 (1): 94-100.

Krashin JW, Koumans EH, Bradshaw-Sydnor AC, Braxton JR, Evan Secor W, Sawyer MK, Markowitz LE. Trichomonas vaginalis prevalence, incidence, risk factors and antibiotic-resistance in an adolescent population. Sex Transm Dis. 2010 Jul; 37 (7): 440-4.

Kucknoor AS, Mundodi V, Alderete JF. Adherence to human vaginal epithelial cells signals for increased expression of Trichomonas vaginalis genes. Infect Immun. 2005 Oct; 73 (10): 6472-8.

Kummer S, Hayes GR, Gilbert RO, Beach DH, Lucas JJ, Singh BN. Induction of human host cell apoptosis by Trichomonas vaginalis cysteine proteases is modulated by parasite exposure to iron. Microb Pathog. 2008 Mar; 44 (3): 197-203.

Kvasnicka WG, Taylor RE, Huang JC, Hanks D, Tronstad RJ, Bosomworth A, Hall MR. Investigations of the incidence of bovine trichomoniasis in nevada and of the efficacy of immunizing cattle with vaccines containing Tritrichomonas foetus. Theriogenology. 1989 May; 31 (5): 963-71.

Lehker MW, Arroyo R, Alderete JF. The regulation by iron of the synthesis of adhesins and cytoadherence levels in the protozoan Trichomonas vaginalis. J Exp Med. 1991 Aug 1; 174 (2): 311-8.

Lehker MW, Alderete JF. Iron regulates growth of Trichomonas vaginalis and the expression of immunogenic trichomonad proteins. Mol Microbiol. 1992 Jan; 6 (1): 123-32.

Lossick JG (1990). Epidemiology of urogenital trichomoniasis. Therapy of urogenital trichomoniasis, In: *Trichomonads parasitic in humans*, BM Honigberg (ed.), pp. 324-341, Springer-Verlag, ISBN, New York, NY.

Lusk MJ, Naing Z, Rayner B, Rismanto N, McIver CJ, Cumming RG, McGeechan K, Rawlinson WD, Konecny P. Trichomonas vaginalis: underdiagnosis in urban Australia could facilitate re-emergence. Sex Transm Infect. 2010 Jun; 86 (3): 227-30.

Madhivanan P, Krupp K, Hardin J, Karat C, Klausner JD, Reingold AL. Simple and inexpensive point-of-care tests improve diagnosis of vaginal infections in resource constrained settings. Trop Med Int Health. 2009 Jun; 14 (6): 703-8

Malla N, Yadav M, Gupta I. Kinetics of serum and local cytokine profile in experimental intravaginal trichomoniasis induced with Trichomonas vaginalis isolates from symptomatic and asymptomatic women. Parasite Immunol. 2007 Feb; 29 (2): 101-5.

Marx G, John-Stewart G, Bosire R, Wamalwa D, Otieno P, Farquhar C. Diagnosis of sexually transmitted infections and bacterial vaginosis among HIV-1-infected pregnant women in Nairobi. Int J STD AIDS. 2010 Aug; 21 (8): 549-52.

Mavedzenge SN, Pol BV, Cheng H, Montgomery ET, Blanchard K, de Bruyn G, Ramjee G, Straten A.Epidemiological synergy of Trichomonas vaginalis and HIV in Zimbabwean and South African women. Sex Transm Dis. 2010 Jul; 37 (7): 460-6.

McClelland RS, Sangare L, Hassan WM, Lavreys L, Mandaliya K, Kiarie J, Ndinya-Achola J, Jaoko W, Baeten JM. Infection with Trichomonas vaginalis increases the risk of HIV-1 acquisition. J Infect Dis. 2007 Mar 1; 195 (5): 698-702.

McGrory T, Garber GE. Mouse intravaginal infection with Trichomonas vaginalis and role of Lactobacillus acidophilus in sustaining infection. Infect Immun. 1992 Jun; 60 (6): 2375-9. PubMed PMID:1587604;

Meysick KC, Garber GE. Interactions between Trichomonas vaginalis and vaginal flora in a mouse model. J Parasitol. 1992 Feb; 78 (1): 157-60.

Midlej V, Benchimol M. Trichomonas vaginalis kills and eats--evidence for phagocytic activity as a cytopathic effect. Parasitology. 2010 Jan; 137 (1): 65-76.

Mitchell C, Hitti J, Paul K, Agnew K, Cohn SE, Luque AE, Coombs R. Cervicovaginal shedding of HIV type 1 is related to genital tract inflammation independent of changes in vaginal microbiota. AIDS Res Hum Retroviruses. 2011 Jan; 27 (1): 35-9.

Moodley P, Wilkinson D, Connolly C, Moodley J, Sturm AW. Trichomonas vaginalis is associated with pelvic inflammatory disease in women infected with human immunodeficiency virus. Clin Infect Dis. 2002 Feb 15; 34 (4): 519-22.

Msuya SE, Mbizvo EM, Stray-Pedersen B, Uriyo J, Sam NE, Rusakaniko S, Hussain A. Decline in HIV prevalence among women of childbearing age in Moshi urban, Tanzania. Int J STD AIDS. 2007 Oct; 18 (10): 680-7.

Månsson F, Camara C, Biai A, Monteiro M, da Silva ZJ, Dias F, Alves A, Andersson S, Fenyö EM, Norrgren H, Unemo M. High prevalence of HIV-1, HIV-2 and other sexually transmitted infections among women attending two sexual health clinics in Bissau, Guinea-Bissau, West Africa. Int J STD AIDS. 2010 Sep; 21 (9): 631-5.

Narimatsu R, Wolday D, Patterson BK. IL-8 increases transmission of HIV type 1 in cervical explant tissue. AIDS Res Hum Retroviruses. 2005 Mar; 21 (3): 228-33.

Nye MB, Schwebke JR, Body BA. Comparison of APTIMA Trichomonas vaginalis transcription-mediated amplification to wet mount microscopy, culture, and polymerase chain reaction for diagnosis of trichomoniasis in men and women. Am J Obstet Gynecol. 2009 Feb; 200 (2): 188.e1-7. PubMed PMID:19185101.

Neely MN, Benning L, Xu J, Strickler HD, Greenblatt RM, Minkoff H, Young M, Bremer J, Levine AM, Kovacs A. Cervical shedding of HIV-1 RNA among women with low levels of viremia while receiving highly active antiretroviral therapy. J Acquir Immune Defic Syndr. 2007 Jan 1; 44 (1): 38-42.

O'Connor CC, Berry G, Rohrsheim R, Donovan B. Sexual health and use of condoms among local and international sex workers in Sydney. Genitourin Med. 1996 Feb; 72 (1): 47-51.

O'Hagan DT, De Gregorio E. The path to a successful vaccine adjuvant--'the long and winding road'. Drug Discov Today. 2009 Jun; 14 (11-12): 541-51.

Paintlia MK, Kaur S, Gupta I, Ganguly NK, Mahajan RC, Malla N. Specific IgA response, T-cell subtype and cytokine profile in experimental intravaginal trichomoniasis. Parasitol Res. 2002 Apr; 88 (4): 338-43.

Pastorek JG 2nd, Cotch MF, Martin DH, Eschenbach DA. Clinical and microbiological correlates of vaginal trichomoniasis during pregnancy The Vaginal Infections and Prematurity Study Group. Clin Infect Dis. 1996 Nov; 23 (5): 1075-80.

Paz-Bailey G, Sternberg M, Puren AJ, Steele L, Lewis DA. Determinants of HIV type 1 shedding from genital ulcers among men in South Africa. Clin Infect Dis. 2010 Apr 1; 50 (7): 1060-7.

Peterman TA, Tian LH, Metcalf CA, Satterwhite CL, Malotte CK, DeAugustine N, Paul SM, Cross H, Rietmeijer CA, Douglas JM Jr, RESPECT-2 Study Group. High incidence of new sexually transmitted infections in the year following a sexually transmitted infection: a case for rescreening. Ann Intern Med. 2006 Oct 17; 145 (8): 564-72.

Petrin D, Delgaty K, Bhatt R, Garber G. Clinical and microbiological aspects of Trichomonas vaginalis. Clin Microbiol Rev. 1998 Apr; 11 (2): 300-17.

Rogers A, Meundi A, Amma A, Rao A, Shetty P, Antony J, Sebastian D, Shetty P, Shetty AK. HIV-related knowledge, attitudes, perceived benefits, and risks of HIV testing among pregnant women in rural Southern India. AIDS Patient Care STDS. 2006 Nov; 20 (11): 803-11.

Roth AM, Williams JA, Ly R, Curd K, Brooks D, Arno J, Van Der Pol B. Changing Sexually Transmitted Infection Screening Protocol Will Result in Improved Case Finding for Trichomonas vaginalis Among High-Risk Female Populations. Sex Transm Dis. 2011 Jan 6; ahead of print.

Scott K, Manunta M, Germain C, Smith P, Jones M, Mitchell P, Dessi D, Branigan Bamford K, Lechler RI, Fiori PL, Foster GR, Lombardi G. Qualitatively distinct patterns of cytokines are released by human dendritic cells in response to different pathogens. Immunology. 2005 Oct; 116 (2): 245-54.

Seña AC, Miller WC, Hobbs MM, Schwebke JR, Leone PA, Swygard H, Atashili J, Cohen MS. Trichomonas vaginalis infection in male sexual partners: implications for diagnosis, treatment, and prevention. Clin Infect Dis. 2007 Jan 1; 44 (1): 13-22.

Sha BE, Zariffard MR, Wang QJ, Chen HY, Bremer J, Cohen MH, Spear GT. Female genital-tract HIV load correlates inversely with Lactobacillus species but positively with bacterial vaginosis and Mycoplasma hominis. J Infect Dis. 2005 Jan 1; 191 (1): 25-32.

Shafir SC, Sorvillo FJ, Smith L. Current issues and considerations regarding trichomoniasis and human immunodeficiency virus in African-Americans. Clin Microbiol Rev. 2009 Jan; 22 (1): 37-45.

Singh BN, Lucas JJ, Hayes GR, Kumar I, Beach DH, Frajblat M, Gilbert RO, Sommer U, Costello CE. Tritrichomonas foetus induces apoptotic cell death in bovine vaginal epithelial cells. Infect Immun. 2004 Jul; 72 (7): 4151-8.

Smith AJ, Chudnovsky L, Simoes-Barbosa A, Delgadillo-Correa MG, Jonsson ZO, Wohlschlegel JA, Johnson PJ. Novel Core Promoter Elements and a Cognate Transcription Factor in the Divergent Unicellular Eukaryote Trichomonas vaginalis. Mol Cell Biol. 2011 Apr; 31 (7): 1444-58.

Sutton M, Sternberg M, Koumans EH, McQuillan G, Berman S, Markowitz L. The prevalence of Trichomonas vaginalis infection among reproductive-age women in the United States, 2001-2004. Clin Infect Dis. 2007 Nov 15; 45 (10): 1319-26.

Thurman AR, Doncel GF. Innate immunity and inflammatory response to Trichomonas vaginalis and bacterial vaginosis: relationship to HIV acquisition. Am J Reprod Immunol. 2011 Feb; 65 (2): 89-98.

United Nations (UNAIDS) and World Health Organization. 2009 AIDS Epidemic Update. 2009.

Upcroft P, Upcroft JA. Drug targets and mechanisms of resistance in the anaerobic protozoa. Clin Microbiol Rev. 2001 Jan; 14 (1): 150-64.

Van Der Pol B, Williams JA, Orr DP, Batteiger BE, Fortenberry JD. Prevalence, incidence, natural history, and response to treatment of Trichomonas vaginalis infection among adolescent women. J Infect Dis. 2005 Dec 15; 192 (12): 2039-44.

Van Der Pol B, Kraft CS, Williams JA. Use of an adaptation of a commercially available PCR assay aimed at diagnosis of chlamydia and gonorrhea to detect Trichomonas vaginalis in urogenital specimens. J Clin Microbiol. 2006 Feb; 44 (2): 366-73.

Van der Pol B. Trichomonas vaginalis infection: the most prevalent nonviral sexually transmitted infection receives the least public health attention. Clin Infect Dis. 2007 Jan 1; 44 (1): 23-5.

Wang CC, McClelland RS, Reilly M, Overbaugh J, Emery SR, Mandaliya K, Chohan B, Ndinya- Achola J, Bwayo J, Kreiss JK. The effect of treatment of vaginal infections on shedding of human immunodeficiency virus type 1. J Infect Dis. 2001 Apr 1; 183 (7): 1017-22.

Wang B, Li X, Stanton B, Fang X, Liang G, Liu H, Lin D, Yang H. Gender differences in HIV-related perceptions, sexual risk behaviors, and history of sexually transmitted diseases among Chinese migrants visiting public sexually transmitted disease clinics. AIDS Patient Care STDS. 2007 Jan; 21 (1): 57-68.

Wendel KA, Erbelding EJ, Gaydos CA, Rompalo AM. Trichomonas vaginalis polymerase chain reaction compared with standard diagnostic and therapeutic protocols for detection and treatment of vaginal trichomoniasis. Clin Infect Dis. 2002 Sep 1; 35 (5): 576-80.

Wiesenfeld HC, Macio I. The infrequent use of office-based diagnostic tests for vaginitis. Am J Obstet Gynecol. 1999 Jul; 181 (1): 39-41.

Wira CR, Rossoll RM, Kaushic C. Antigen-presenting cells in the female reproductive tract: influence of estradiol on antigen presentation by vaginal cells. Endocrinology. 2000 Aug; 141 (8): 2877-85.

Wølner-Hanssen P, Krieger JN, Stevens CE, Kiviat NB, Koutsky L, Critchlow C, DeRouen T, Hillier S, Holmes KK. Clinical manifestations of vaginal trichomoniasis. JAMA. 1989 Jan 27; 261 (4): 571-6.

Workowski KA, Berman S, Centers for Disease Control and Prevention (CDC). Sexually transmitted diseases treatment guidelines, 2010. MMWR Recomm Rep. 2010 Dec 17; 59 (RR-12): 1-110.

World Health Organization. Global prevalence and incidence of selected curable sexually transmitted diseases: overview and estimates. Geneva, Switzerland: WHO. 2001.

World Health Organization. Guidelines for the management of sexually transmitted infections. Geneva, Switzerland: WHO. 2003.

World Health Organization. Antiretroviral therapy for HIV infection in adults and adolescents: recommendations for a public health approach. Geneva, Switzerland: WHO. 2006.

Yadav M, Gupta I, Malla N. Kinetics of immunoglobulin G, M, A and IgG subclass responses in experimental intravaginal trichomoniasis: prominence of IgG1 response. Parasite Immunol. 2005 Dec; 27 (12): 461-7.

Yin YP, Wu Z, Lin C, Guan J, Wen Y, Li L, Detels R, Rotheram-Borus MJ, NIMH Collaborative HIV/STD Prevention Trial Group. Syndromic and laboratory diagnosis of sexually transmitted infection: a comparative study in China. Int J STD AIDS. 2008 Jun; 19 (6): 381-4.

12

In Vitro and *In Vivo* Transactivation of HIV-1 by Human Herpesvirus 6

Ongrádi Joseph[1], Kövesdi Valéria[1], Nagy Károly[1], Matteoli Barbara[2], Ceccherini-Nelli Luca[2] and Ablashi Dharam[3]
[1]*Institute of Medical Microbiology, Semmelweis University, Budapest*
[2]*Virology Unit and Retrovirus Center, Department of Experimental Pathology, University of Pisa, Pisa*
[3]*HHV-6 Foundation, Santa Barbara, CA*
[1]*Hungary*
[2]*Italy*
[3]*USA*

1. Introduction

1.1 Latency and reactivation of HIV-1

Since the discovery of human immunodeficiency virus type 1 (HIV-1), there has been a great deal of interest in identifying cofactors that might accelerate the stages of development associated with acquired immunodeficiency syndrome (AIDS). Many environmental agents, namely inherent factors such as ethnicity and geographical location, were first implicated as risk factors in the study of HIV infection. However, speculation that infectious diseases may act as cofactors in HIV infection began to be studied soon thereafter. These speculations led to one of the early opinions that HIV plays a correlary role in AIDS, but not a causative role (Duesberg, 1989). AIDS patients have a history of both circumstantial serological and microbial evidence of increased exposure to a number of common and opportunistic infectious agents. It is difficult to ascertain, however, whether these various coinfections contribute anything to the progressive decline of the immune system (Pedersen et al., 1990). *In vivo,* infection with HIV-1 is followed by a long disease-free period, during which a low number of CD4+ mononuclear leukocytes (CCR5 coreceptor positive monocytes and CXCR4 coreceptor positive lymphocytes) containing transcriptionally silent integrated provirus can be found. HIV-1 replication can be demonstrated in only a small population of T cells without inducing clinical manifestations. This state of latency is partly due to low transcriptional activity of the integrated provirus in resting cells. Activation of CD4+ cells by antigens, mitogens (Tobiume et al., 1998) or superinfection by other viruses interacting with HIV-1 via viral and/or cellular transacting factors may terminate HIV-1 latency, leading to a productive HIV-1 infection. Transactivation of the HIV-1 long terminal repeat (LTR) in turn will induce gene expression, including the synthesis of the HIV-1 transactivator protein (TAT) (Arya et al., 1985). TAT will then independently amplify HIV-1 gene expression, ultimately leading to a high level of virus replication and death of infected cells. Onset and progression of AIDS correlates with augmented production of infectious virions parallel to a shift in their tropism from CCR5 towards the CXCR4 coreceptor. The number and ratio of infected cells, mainly CD4+ T lymphocytes, increases 100-1000-fold during this period (Ensoli et al., 1989).

Initiation and augmentation of transcription by HIV relies not only on the simultaneous binding of virus-encoded TAT polypeptide to TAR, but the normal cellular transcriptional factors (NF-κB, Sp1, and other regions of the 3′ HIV-1 mRNA start site) also anchor into specific binding sites of the proviral LTR. The production of such factors are augmented after mitogen treatment followed by signal transduction from cell surface receptors and through several parallel pathways including secondary messenger systems (Martin et al., 1991; Mosca et al., 1987a, 1987b; Nabel & Baltimore, 1987; Siekievitz et al., 1987). The basal level promoter activity does not require binding of NF-κB or other nuclear factors (Wang et al., 1994).

1.2 The role of heterologous viruses in HIV-1 activation

Two alternative ways exist for HIV transactivation by heterologous viruses. First, two (or more) viruses can simultaneously infect the same immune cell if the appropiate receptors are expressed on its surface. Several DNA viruses have been suggested as potential cofactors in AIDS due to their capability to transactivate *in vitro* the HIV-1 LTR-directed gene expression by a *tat*-independent mechanism. For example, herpes simplex virus type 1 (HSV-1) immediate early gene products ICP0 and ICP4 act via NF-κB and Sp1 (Mosca et al., 1987a, 1987b). Stimulating effects vary by cell type, indicating that the cellular environment plays an important role in viral transactivation (Albrecht et al.,1989). HSV-2 can coinfect, simultaneously replicate and transactivate HIV-1 (Kucera et al., 1990). Human cytomegalovirus (HCMV) IE genes activate via Sp1 and NF-κB sites (Davis et al., 1987; Ghazal & Nelson, 1993). HCMV also transactivates HIV-2 LTR (Duclos et al., 1989). Epstein-Barr virus (EBV) EBNA2, BRLF1 and LMP gene products act through NF-κB and Sp1 (Hammarskjöld et al., 1992; Kenney et al., 1988; Quinlivan et al., 1990). The IE protein of pseudorabies virus induces the overproduction of Sp1 (Yuan et al., 1989). Papovaviruses (JC, BK) transactivate through Sp1 (Gendelman et al., 1986), adenovirus (AdV) E1A 13S protein exerts activation on the TATA box and Sp1 sites (Nabel et al., 1988; Rice & Mathews, 1988). Vaccinia virus (Stellrecht et al., 1992), hepatitis B virus (HBV) X protein (Seto et al., 1988), and a retrovirus named human T lymphotropic virus type I (HTLV-I) *tax* polypeptide (Siekievitz et al., 1987) transactivate HIV-1. Lymphoid cells chronically infected with HTLV-I are more susceptible to infection *in vitro* with HIV-1, and coinfected cells produce higher levels of HIV-1 (De Rossi et al., 1986, Ongrádi et al., 2000b). It is likely that the activation of HIV-1 by heterologous viruses in dually infected cells results from the cumulative effects of various gene promoters. None of these viruses infects CD4+ T cells as their primary target. Their gene products do not bind directly to the HIV LTR sequences, and there is no apparent molecular link between these products and cellular transcriptional factors. Intracellular transactivation is mediated by those transcriptional factors that are upregulated upon external stimuli. They may act in a paracrine manner, whereby altering mediator production affects the producer cell or neighbouring cells. It has been established that tumor necrosis factor (TNF)-α via NF-κB activation acts in tandem with HSV-1 in augmenting HIV-1 in different CD4+ cells such as T lymphocytes, monocytes, and leukemic cell lines (Popik & Pitha, 1994). Thus, the relevance of these viruses to direct HIV-1 activation *in vivo* is still waiting for unequivocal confirmation. Simultaneous infection in a single cell is a relatively rare event, and as such the biological effects of an event of this nature could be minimal. On the contrary, cross-talk between immune cells carrying different viruses is more common, especially in lymph nodes where they are in the vicinity of one another. Heterologous viruses can infect many other types of cells which are not targets of HIV, but release several immunomodulating mediators. This transcellular transactivation can last a lifetime, and its intensity may vary on an individual basis, as well as on the synergistic or antagonistic effects of several factors including the heterologous viruses themselves. This category of interaction seems to have a more significant biological and clinical impact on HIV replication and AIDS progression. Expression of the early and/or immediate early genes of several heterologous viruses exert very strong modifying effects on the normal mediator pattern, which consequently alters HIV replication. HIV infected individuals carrying other viruses, therefore, may be at a greater risk for early onset and rapid progression of AIDS.

2. Human herpesvirus 6 as a broad-range virus transactivator

2.1 Characterization and genetic structure of HHV-6

Among heterologous viruses, human herpesvirus 6 (HHV-6, *Herpesviridae* family, *Betaherpesvirinae* subfamily, *Roseolovirus* genus) seems to be one of the most important HIV-1 transactivator. HHV-6 is predominantly a T cell tropic virus, and its unique immunomodulatory characteristics have made it a widely studied *in vitro* and *in vivo* model. HHV-6 has two variants, which differ on the basis of distinct genetic, immunological and biological characteristics.; Variant A (HHV-6A) was originally obtained from the peripheral blood mononuclear cells (PBMC's) of patients with HIV infection and other lymphoproliferative disorders (Salahuddin et al., 1986), while HHV-6B was originally obtained from the PBMC's of children suffering from exanthema subitum. Isolates were later grouped according to prototypes (e.g. GS and U1102 for HHV-6A, Z29 and HST for HHV-6B) (Ablashi et al., 1991). The viral genome is 160-162 kbp in size and is formed by a central unique (U) region (143-145 kbp) flanked at both ends by terminal direct repeats (DR, each 8-9 kbp long). The DR's contain a tandem repetitive sequence that is also present in human telomeres (Thomson et al., 1994a). The genome of HHV-6B contains 119 open reading frames (ORFs) encoded by 97 genes, 9 of which are absent in HHV-6A: DR4, DR5, DR8, U1, U61, U78, U88, U92, U93 (Dominguez et al., 1999; Gompels et al., 1995). Several conserved genes organized into 7 blocks are present in the genome of all herpesviruses. One additional block comprises 17 genes conserved in all Roseoloviruses (U20-21, U23-24, U26, U85, U100). Two genes are unique to HHV-6 and present in both variants: U83, which encodes chemokines (Dewin et al., 2006), and U94, which encodes for a homologue of the human adeno-associated virus type 2 (AAV-2) *rep* gene (Thomson et al., 1994b). The latter is transcribed in latently infected lymphocytes, suggesting it likely contributes to the maintenance of latency (Rotola et al., 1999). The overall nucleotide sequence identity between HHV-6A and -B variants is 90%, but the genes of DR, U86-U93, and U95-U100 show the highest degree of sequence divergence, reaching 72%. Increased divergence in consequent amino acid sequences explains the biological and pathogenic differences between variants A and B. Differences in the U100 gene products, designated gQ, determine differences in cell tropism between variants (Mori et al., 2003). The variants also differ in temporal regulation and splicing patterns of U91 transcripts in T cell lines (Mirandola et al., 1998). The products of U90 and U95 genes are hypothesized to play a role in the establishment of variant-specific niches within the host. The degree of heterogeneity between HHV-6 isolates within the same variant is less than 1% (Ablashi et al., 1991). In the isolates obtained from immunocompetent persons no genetic gradients and recombinants between HHV-6A and HHV-6B have been detected, making it clear that the two variants have independent biological niches and meet the criteria for classification into distinct species (Dominguez et al., 1999).

2.1.1 Molecular interactions between HHV-6 and the immune system

2.1.1.1 Modulation of surface receptor expression, cytokine and chemokine pattern

CD46 has been demonstrated as a cellular receptor for both HHV-6A and HHV-6B (Santoro et al., 1999). This glycoprotein is a complement regulator, and is expressed on the surface of all nucleated cells. Binding of HHV-6A gH structural polypeptides, but not HHV-6B gB structural polypeptides, to CD46 cell surface receptors induces the downregulation of IL-12 and CD46 with consequent disturbances in the complement system (Santoro et al., 1999), cell fusion, and CD4+ T lymphocyte depletion (Mori et al., 2002). Through CD46, HHV-6 has the ability to infect a wide variety of cell types including neuronal cells (references in De Bolle et al., 2005), but both variants express a non-naive phenotype and replicate most efficiently in CD4+ T lymphocytes (Ablashi et al., 1991; Grivel et al., 2003). This phenotype introduces a unique relationship to the immune system with profound implications on immunomodulation. They also infect monocyte/macrophages (Kondo et al., 1991) and dendritic cells (Kakimoto et al., 2002) to further establish their latent infection. HHV-6A efficiently infects CD8+ T cells (Lusso et al., 1991), γδ lymphocytes (Lusso et al., 1995), and natural killer (NK) cells (Lusso et al., 1993). This leads to the induction of CD4 expression on infected cells, which in turn potentially increases the range of cells susceptible to HIV infection. The genes responsible for transactivation of the CD4 promoter include U86 and U89 (Flamand et al., 1998). HHV-6A and HHV-6B viral envelope proteins inhibit T lymphocyte proliferation induced by phytohemagglutinin (PHA), IL-2 or antigens (Horvat et al., 1993). Not only do the infected cells experience programmed cell death (apoptosis), but adjacent healthy lymphocytes die as well due to high concentrations of both TNF-α and -β released from nearby infected cells (Inoue et al., 1997). Both variants inhibit the expression of CD3/T cell receptor (TCR) complex (Lusso et al., 1991), the lectin-like receptor DC-SIGN on dendritic cells (Niiya et al., 2004), CD14, CD64 and HLA-DR on antigen presenting cells (Janelle & Flamand, 2006).

HHV-6 profoundly modifies the bodily pattern of cytokine and chemokine production as well, which in turn significantly affects the functionality of effective immune responses. HHV-6A strongly inhibits IL-12 and IFN-γ production, consequently lowering the output of uninfected T lymphocytes (Arena et al., 1999). IL-12 production by macrophages (Smith et al., 2003), IL-2 production by CD4+ lymphocytes (Flamand et al., 1995), IL-2, IFN-γ production by HSB-2 cultures (Ongrádi et al., 1990), IL-10 and IL-14 production in SupT1 cultures is inhibited (Mayne et al., 2001). On the contrary, HHV-6A upregulates the production of IL-1β, IFN-α, TNF-α, IL-10 synthesis in PBMC's, TNF-α production in HSB-2 cultures, IL-10, IL-12 production in monocytes, and IL-15 production in both monocytes and NK cells (Arena et al., 1997, 1999, 2000; Flamand et al., 1990, 1991, 1996; Kikuta et al., 1990; Mayne et al., 2001; Li et al., 1997; Ongrádi et al., 1990). HHV-6A induces GM-CSF in the peripheral blood lymphocytes and the ensuing increase in macrophages consequently enhances differentiation of bone marrow progenitor cells, further sensitizing them to HIV infection (Furlini et al., 1996). All these changes result in a Th1 to Th2 shift in cytokine pattern, an impairment of cellular immunity and maintenance of persistent viral infections.

Similar to HHV-6A, HHV-6B increases expression of IL-18, IL-2 receptor and members of TNF-α superfamily receptors (Mayne et al., 2001). HHV-6B increases the production of IFN-α in PBMC's (Kikuta et al., 1990), IL-8 release from HepG2 human hepatoma cell lines without altering IL-1β expression (Inagi et al., 1996), and downregulates IL-12 production (Smith et al., 2001). Upon HHV-6B infection, the cytokine pattern produced by MOLT-3 CD4+ lymphoid cells drastically changes as compared to mock-infected cultures in synergism with IL-2, while the concentration of IL-3, IL-4, IL-10, IL-15, GM-CSF, TNF-α and -β decreases. These changes result in the suppression of innate, humoral and cellular immunity *in vivo* (Ongrádi et al., 2006).

It seems that the global effect of HHV-6 on human immune functionality differs by variant. HHV-6A targets the suppression of cellular immunity above all, while HHV-6B primarily weakens humoral immunity. The consequence of variant-specific immunomodulation is the onset of different clinical entities and provision of helper function for other viral diseases. These studies have suggested that HHV-6A induced chronic immune alterations contribute to HIV pathogenesis and AIDS progression as causative factors, while recurrent HHV-6B infection acts as a secondary contributor by aggravating and accentuating other immuncompromised conditions.

2.1.1.2 HHV-6 encoded chemokines and chemokine receptors

During co-evolution with animals, HHV-6 seems to have obtained genes from them via molecular piracy. The products of these genes may play important roles in pathogenesis and immune evasion. U83 of HHV-6B encodes for a functional β-chemokine (Zou et al., 1999). This protein is produced by infected cells, and as a highly active CCR2 agonist attracts CCR2-expressing cells such as monocytes/macrophages the virus establishes new infection, thus facilitating the spread of the virus. U83 of HHV-6A encodes for two different forms of β-chemokines. The full-length form acts as an agonist while the spliced form acts as an antagonist that interacts with other chemokine receptors, i.e. CCR1, CCR4, CCR5, CCR6 and CCR8, and is expressed on T cells, monocytes/macrophages, and dendritic cells (Dewin et al., 2006). Gene U22 also codes for yet another chemokine (French et al., 1999). Counterparts of U12 and U51 genes have been shown in the betaherpesviruses and they code for G-protein coupled receptor homologs: U12 protein of both variants acts as a β-chemokine (RANTES, macrophage inflammatory protein /MIP/-1α and -1β, monocyte chemoattractant protein /MCP/-1) binding receptor related to CCR1, CCR3, and CCR5. It is expressed at the late stage of infection of monocyte/macrophages and cord blood mononuclear cells. Its expression is activated by the above cytokines elicited on the effect of other factors, i.e. viruses, but not by the α-chemokine IL-8 (Isegawa et al., 1998, Kondo et al., 2002). While expressed on human epithelial cells, U51 protein specifically binds and down-regulates RANTES (Caruso et al., 2003; Milne et al., 2000) by mimicking receptors typically expressed on the surface of activated T cells (Menotti et al., 1999). Down-regulation of RANTES may consequentially compromise the ability of T-lymphocytes, monocytes and eosinophils to gather at sites of inflammation. The gene product of U51 may act as a positive regulator of viral replication, possibly promoting membrane fusion and facilitating cell-to-cell spread (Zhen et al., 2005).

The main task of the production of HHV-6 specific chemokines and chemokine receptors is to ensure the efficient dissemination of virus throughout the organism either by way of acute infection or latent carriage.

2.2 Clinical manifestations and transactivating potential of HHV-6A

The exact mode of transmission and pathomechanism of HHV-6A have not been established. In developed countries, HHV-6A does not or very rarely infects children, but from adolescence onward its prevalence increases. In several countries of the developing world, especially in Sub-Saharan and South Africa, as much as one quarter of children below the age of 18 months already carries this variant in both HIV-1 positive and negative groups. This suggests that early infections have a different exposure profile compared to North America and Europe (Kasolo et al., 1999). In a recent study of genotyping, variant A was identified in 85% of HHV-6 infections of asymptomatic African infants, and HHV-6B was largely detected as a co-infection alongside HHV-6A (Bates et al., 2009). In such cases, unusual recombinants between HHV-6A and HHV-6B were shown (Gompels & Kasolo, 2006; Kasolo et al., 1997). This is reminescent of the peculiar adenovirus recombinants found in the intestines of AIDS patients (Hierholzer et al., 1988). The molecular mechanisms are known in neither case, but each raise the idea of a common effect exerted by HIV-1. Saliva and breast milk contained neither HHV-6A virions nor viral DNA. It was found in 54% of the lungs of healthy adults (Cone et al., 1996). In the blood of children born to HIV seropositive mothers living in Africa, a high-quantity load of HHV-6A can be detected. HHV-6 DNA has been found in the semen of two thirds of healthy males, and although its variant specificity has not been established, epidemiological circumstances raise the possibility of sexual spread. Transmission is also suspected to occur from mother to child (Bates et al., 2009). The symptoms of acute infection are unknown, but in some well-documented cases febrile conditions in children were observed. Primary adult infections have been associated with severe inflammatory or neurological disease with increased neurotropism (Alvarez-Lafuente et al., 2007; Hall et al., 1998; Portolani et al., 2005). Persistent HHV-6A infection in the brain may also contribute to AIDS-associated dementia. Primary HHV-6A infection later in life may trigger the onset of multiple sclerosis (MS) (Akhyani et al., 2000; Alvarez-Lafuente et al., 2006; Ongrádi et al., 1999). HHV-6A also establishes life-long latency in CD4+ immune cells, and is usually reactivated in immunocompromised patients after bone marrow or organ transplantation along with HHV-6B, HHV-7 and HCMV (Griffiths et al., 1999). HHV-6A might be a cofactor in the progression of several tumors. The simultaneous detection of HHV-6A and human papilloma virus type 16 (HPV-16) in cervical carcinoma cells (Chen et al., 1994b) and the ability of HHV-6A U16 and U30 gene products to transactivate E6 and E7 of HPV-16 in cervical epithelial cells (Chen et al., 1994a) have prompted investigation of its role in the pathogenesis of cervical carcinoma. In a large clinical study, it was concluded that although HHV-6A is not the causative agent of cervical carcinoma, it can contribute to multistage carcinogenesis and the progression of cervical cancer (Di Paolo et al., 1994). It is of note that cervical cancer is one of the AIDS criteria. Furthermore, due to their high prevalence in the lymphoid tissues, HHV-6 and EBV are frequently detected simultaneously (Bertram et al., 1991). HHV-6A infection has been shown to activate EBV replication from latency by a mechanism of transactivation that targets a cyclic AMP response element with the EBV Zebra promoter (Flamand & Menezes, 1996) to increase expression of EBV early genes (Cuomo et al., 1995) and to enhance the transformative capacity of EBV (Cuomo et al., 1998). In return, the presence of EBV renders B cells susceptible to HHV-6 infection. EBV has been detected in all brain lymphomas and frequent detection occurs in other lymphomas of AIDS patients as well (Cuomo et al., 1995). HHV-6A has been shown to enhance the progression of lymphomagenesis. As mentioned earlier, the HHV-6A U94 gene product, known as the

RepH6 polypeptide, is able to complement replication of a *rep*-deficient AAV-2 genome (Thomson et al., 1994b). Contrary to HIV LTR activation by HHV-6, HHV-6 cannot transactivate latent infection by human T lymphotropic virus type I (HTLV-I) or subsequently affect the expression of its *tax* transactivator gene (Cao & Sullivan, 1992). Mediators released from actively replicating HHV-6A or carrier cells transactivate the human endogenous retrovirus (HERV) K18 and induce expression of HERV K18-encoded superantigen (Tai et al., 2009). HHV-6B also induces HERV K18-encoded superantigen expression (Turcanova et al., 2009).

In rare clinical manifestations of HHV-6A infection (e.g. hepatitis) or transmission by organ transplantation in Europe, North-America and Japan (Portolani et al., 2005; Potenza et al., 2008) where HHV-6B predominates, HHV-6A strains may be considered emergent infectious diseases. These cases will require careful genotyping as well as viral load and gene expression studies to further characterize the infection (Bates et al., 2009).

2.3 Epidemiology and biological effects of HHV-6B

Although both HHV-6 variants infect CD4+ immune cells, and despite their high molecular homology they profoundly differ in epidemiology and pathogenesis. Lack of reliable serological testing has hindered their differentiation in pathological conditions for several decades, but variant specific polymerase chain reaction (PCR) and other PCR based quantitative methods have yielded satisfactory data on their role played in acute and chronic diseases. The mode of transmission and pathomechanism of HHV-6B has sine been well-characterized, and evidence seems to indicate that humans are the only know reserviors of HHV-6B. The salivary gland serves as a reservoir for symptomless shedding, and the saliva of the caregivers of small children has been shown to transmit infection via droplets (Fox et al., 1990). By age 2, almost all children have become seropositive (references in Ongrádi et al., 1999d). The majority of infections are symptomless, but approximately 15% of infected children develop exanthema subitum (Yamanishi et al., 1988). Although HHV-6B DNA sequences were found in the genital tract of 20% of pregnant women, perinatal transmission is unlikely (Okuno et al., 1995). HHV-6B establishes life-long latency in CD4+ immune cells. HHV-6B is frequently reactivated in immunocompromised conditions, e.g. after transplantation of bone marrow, liver, kidney or pancreas. High fever, graft rejection and other lethal complications are not uncommon. HHV-6B reactivation is followed by HHV-7 and HCMV reactivation in a temporal pattern, aggravating clinical symptoms (Herbein et al., 1996). HHV-6B might also act as a cofactor in the pathogenesis of several chronic debilitating immunological or neurological diseases such as Hodgkin's lymphomas, multiple sclerosis, mesial temporal lobe epilepsy, chronic fatigue syndrome and drug induced hypersensitivity syndrome (references in Caselli & Di Luca 2007 and De Bolle et al., 2005). HHV-6B DNA is commonly detected in the brain of deceased AIDS patients and HHV-6B proteins are often located in the demyelinated areas, suggesting an active role in persistent infection and neurological complications in AIDS patients (Drobyski et al., 1994). No vaccination against HHV-6B exists, but for chemoprevention and treatment in severe conditions ganciclovir, valaciclovir, foscarnet and cidofovir have been used (references in Caselli & Di Luca, 2007 and De Bolle et al., 2005).

2.4 Chromosomally integrated HHV-6

It has recently been demonstrated that both variants of HHV-6 can integrate specifically into the telomeres of human chromosomes 1, 9, 10, 11, 17, 18, 19 and 22 of PBMC's *in vivo* and *in vitro* (Luppi et al., 1993; Morrisette & Flamand, 2010; Torelli et al., 1995). This behavior is unique among human herpesviruses. The presence of human telomeric-like repeat sequences at the HHV-6 genome termini (Gompels & Macaulay, 1995) and the HHV-6 U94 gene product (RepH6) might mediate the site-specific viral DNA integration within human cells (Surosky et al., 1997). Chromosomally integrated HHV-6 (CIHHV-6) can be passed through the germ line. Recent evidence from studies in the USA, UK, and Japan have shown that approximately 0.2-0.85% of infants experience vertical transmission of HHV-6 through the germ line, accounting for almost all HHV-6 congenital infections with no significant differences between distribution of variants (Hall et al., 2008; Tanaka-Taya et al., 1996; Ward et al., 2006). Cells containing CIHHV-6 copies do not have closed circular viral DNA (episomes), but produce a high viral load in the blood (10^6-10^7 copies per ml). A person with CIHHV-6 will never be negative by PCR in serum or whole blood (Ward et al., 206). While some individuals with CIHHV-6 are asymptomatic, the integrated virus appears to be capable of reactivating. Members of these families carry identical HHV-6 strains, and some of them suffer from severe neurological symptoms. It has been demonstrated that CIHHV-6 can be made to reactivate by chemically stimulating the integrated cells (Arbuckle et al., 2010). Several case reports have shown that CIHHV-6 patients with neurological problems responded to antivirals (Troy et al., 2008; Wittekind et al., 2010).

3. Transactivation of HIV by human herpesvirus 6 variant A and B

3.1 *In vitro* studies on the intracellular transactivation of HIV by HHV-6 variants

The fact that HHV-6 and HIV-1 infect overlapping subsets of CD4+ lymphocytes (Lusso & Gallo, 1995) and lytic HHV-6 infection may contribute to the decline of this cell population in HIV-infected individuals, has lead to the hypothesis that there is specific interaction between these viruses. To substantiate this claim, several arguments were initially raised based on *in vitro* data rather than on clinical observations. In the first logical investigation, freshly isolated and activated PBMC's containing CD4+ immune cells were simultaneously infected with HIV-1 and HHV-6A (GS). It was demonstrated that HHV-6A and HIV-1 could productively coinfect individual CD+ T cells, resulting in accelerated HIV-1 gene expression and enhanced cell death through apoptosis (Lusso et al., 1989). Infection of the ACH-2 leukemic T cells carrying latent HIV-1 with HHV-6A resulted in HIV-1 antigen co-expression with early-late HHV-6 products, suggesting that more IE gene products are involved in the activation of latent HIV-1 (Isegawa et al., 2007). Superinfection of U1 promonocytic cells latently carrying HIV-1 occurred by introducing HHV-6A (GS) and treating with TNF-α induced massive HIV-1 replication, whereas none of the clinical isolates of HHV-6B were able to break latency of HIV-1. It is of interest that HIV-1 upregulation elicited by HHV-6 was not inhibited by anti-TNF-α antibodies (Knox & Carrigan, 1996). Cloned fragments of HHV-6 and HIV-1 LTR were cotransfected into different cells, and the transactivating potential of HHV-6 infection on HIV-1 LTR was reported (Ensoli et al., 1989). Since then, transactivating functions have been assigned to an increasing number of individual HHV-6 genes. The protein encoded by HHV-6A (U1102) DR7 gene, expressed from 18h postinfection has been shown to transactivate HIV-1 LTR promoter and increase HIV-1 replication (Kashanchi et al., 1994, Thompson et al., 1994). Its oncogenic potential in NIH 3T3 fibroblast cells relates to its capacity for binding and intiating the tumor suppressor protein p53 (Kashanchi et al., 1997). The U3-encoded protein was found to transactivate the HIV-1 LTR promoter in money kidney CV-1 cells (Mori et al., 1998). The U16 to U19 genes encode transactivators that upregulate viral and cellular transcription. The immediate early (IE) expressed spliced gene products of U16/U17 and the IE U18- and U19-encoded proteins have all been shown to independently transactivate the HIV-1 LTR promoter *in vitro* (Flebbe-Rehwaldt et al., 2000; Geng et al., 1992; Nicholas & Martin, 1994). The DNA polymerase processing factor, encoded by the HHV-6 (U1102) U27 gene, was shown to transactivate the HIV-1 LTR in CV-1 cells. The presence of NF-κB binding sites was mandatory for the response to pU27 (Zhou et al., 1994). The HHV-6 IE-A locus encodes two proteins, IE1 and IE2, corresponding to the ORFs U89 and U86-87, respectively. Both are expressed from spliced mRNAs, and each contains an exon derived from the U90 gene (Nikolaou et al., 2003). IE1 of HHV-6A was shown capable of transactivating heterologous promoters. Compared to the IE1 protein of HHV-6A, the HHV-6B IE1 protein was found to exhibit much lower transactivating potential on HIV-1 LTR (Gravel et al., 2002). IE2 activates multiple promoters that have no regulatory element in common, such as the complex HIV-1 LTR promoter, or simple promoters containing zero or only one response element (NF-κB, CRE, or NF-AT (Gravel et al., 2003). It also transactivates the CD4 promoter (Flamand et al., 1998). HHV-6A (U1102) U94-encoded RepH6 acts as a transactivator by binding to a transcription factor, human TATA binding protein (Mori et al., 2000). RepH6 by itself possesses single-stranded DNA binding capacity, which is enhanced by cellular nuclear factors (Dhepakson et al., 2002), and is known to activate the HIV-1 LTR promoter in fibroblast cells (Thomson et al., 1994b).

HHV-6 encoded proteins with HIV-1 LTR transactivating potential not only stimulate HIV-1 expression (Ensoli et al., 1989; McCarthy et al., 1998), but these proteins (e.g. IE1) and the HIV-1 transactivating protein TAT have been shown to interact synergistically in this respect as early as 6.5 hours after HHV-6 infection (Di Luca et al., 1991, Garzino-Demo et al., 1996). HIV-1 TAT enhances HHV-6A titers and protein synthesis in cord blood lymphocytes and continuous CD4+ JJHAN T cells (Sieczkowski et al., 1995), but no activation was detected in Jurkat cells (Di Luca et al., 1991). More products of genes and cloned gene fragments of HHV-6A (U1102), namely *SalI* L, *EcoRI* (encoding p41) genomic fragments and HHV-6A (GS) pZVB70 and pZVB10 transactivate HIV-1 LTR at the NF-κB site, while pZVH14 acts through the Sp1 site in African green monkey kidney cells (CV-1) and human T cells (Geng et al., 1992), although in other experiments all three fragments have been shown to activate NF-κB. HHV-6A is able to activate HIV LTR in both stimulated and resting T lymphocytes, while HHV-6B (Z29) can carry out HIV LTR activation in T cells only (Horvat et al., 1991).

Patients and clinically normal individuals are frequently infected with multiple viruses. It is therefore important to understand the implications of simultaneous infection by multiple viruses. Coinfections with HIV, HHV-6A and hepatitis C virus (HCV) are frequently seen in the same individual. In a recent study, human lymphoid cells were simultaneously infected with all three viruses. Individual cells were able to support replication of all three viruses without dominance of one virus. All these viruses are highly cytolytic, and therefore triply-infected cells were short lived (Salahuddin et al., 2007).

There are several reports concerning the inhibitory effect of HHV-6 on HIV-1 in cell cultures. Peripheral blood lymphocytes, macrophages, and dendritic cells were coinfected. Unfortunately, in the majority of these studies, two different HHV-6 strains belonging to variant B were used: either strain Z29 (Asada et al., 1999; Carrigan & Knox, 1990; Spira et al., 1990) or SF (Levy et al., 1990b). Their further studies on cytokines produced by HHV-6 B infected cells showed inconclusive results, because virus infection was not synchronized. In this way, consecutive generations of viruses induced different cytokines at very different or overlapping time points.

3.2 *In vitro* studies on the transcellular transactivation of HIV by HHV-6 A and B

Next, to study the possible transcellular transactivation of HIV by HHV-6A, Ongrádi et al. infected HSB-2 CD4+ T lymphocytes with HHV-6A (GS). Supernatants of the infected cells contained a myriad of mediators and newly produced virions, similarly to the serum of patients. At regular time intervals, supernatant samples were removed and filtered until virus-free. Meanwhile CEM-ss cells were infected with HIV-1 (IIIB) at different multiplicities of infection (moi) and then mixed with HHV-6A-free supernatant samples. Next, HIV-1 production was quantitated by syncytia formation, reverse transcriptase (RT) activity and p24 antigen production. Supernatants obtained at 24 and 48 hours post-infection exerted the strongest HIV-1 activation. The smaller the HIV-1 inocula were, the higher activating effect was observed. This timing coincides with the expression of early HHV-6A genes. Elevated TNF-α, but suppressed IFN-γ production was exhibited, and IL-2 was found to have no role. Late supernatant samples obtained at the time of virion production showed slightly inhibited HIV production. Distinct cytokines and chemokines are produced in a sequential manner by the same cell. Their ratio continuously changes, and they furthermore exert pleiotropic effects. HIV-1 activation (and/or inhibition) via HHV-6 induced cytokine and chemokine production is the net effect of many soluble factors. This is the only known experiment in the literature describing that HHV-6 infected--but virus-free--media obtained from one type of CD4+ lymphoid culture modifies HIV-1 production in another lymphoid culture (Ongrádi et al., 1990, 1999c). Similarly, separated human peripheral blood monocytes were exposed to different viral antigens, and aliquots of the media of these monocytes were mixed to ACH-2 and U1 cells latently infected by HIV-1. Conditioned media obtained from HCMV and EBV antigen exposed monocyte cultures augmented HIV-1 replication, whereas others, such as HSV-1, HSV-2, VZV, HHV-6A failed to stimulate HIV-1 replication (Clouse et al., 1989). These suggest that HIV-1 is under several synergistic or antagonistic effects *in vivo*. Several studies have also shown that certain proinflammatory cytokines induced by HHV-6A infection--such as TNF-α, IL-1β and IL-6 enhance *in vitro* expression of HIV-1(Flamand et al.., 1991). The major mode of transcellular transactivation between HHV-6A (GS) infected and HIV-1 carrier lymphocytes is mediated by TNF-α and consequent NF-κB induction followed by its increased binding to LTR sequences. *In vivo,* HHV-6A induces the T helper cell profile to shift from Th1 to Th2 by upregulating IL-10 and downregulating IL-12 in infected PBMC's (Arena et al., 1999), which might act with the similar effects of HIV-1 to accelerate AIDS progression.

4. Epidemiological studies on the HIV transactivating and AIDS promoting potential of HHV-6

4.1 Cross sectional molecular studies

In vivo transactivation of HIV-1 by HHV-6 has been postulated on the basis of several *in vitro* experiments. Following the discovery of HHV-6A, it was frequently isolated from HIV-1 infected patients worldwide (Dowling et al., 1987; Levy et al.., 1990a; Lopez et al.., 1988; Tedder et al., 1987) although no opportunistic diseases had been associated with HHV-6A at that time. Concomitant infection by HHV-6A, HTLV-I and HIV-2 has also been described (Agout et al., 1988). Widespread HHV-6A infection was documented in patients with AIDS at post-mortem examination (Carrigan & Knox, 1994). HHV-6A infected cells--usually lung macrophages--were observed in all patients, whereas HHV-6A infected lymphocytes and epithelial cells were seen in approximately two thirds of patients. The kidneys and liver also showed wide-spread infection of lymphocytes in inflammatory infiltrates. In the lymph nodes, HHV-6A concentrated in lymphocytes in the medullary region. Lymphoid organs are important reservoirs of HIV infection, and progression from HIV-1 infection to AIDS is associated with the involution of these tissues. Cell destruction is synergistically enhanced leading to early disintegration of the lymphoid environment with higher viral load. HIV proviral viral load was higher in tissues taken at autopsy if the organ also harbored HHV-6, which could suggest upregulation of the former by the latter (Corbellino et al., 1993; Knox & Carrigan, 1994a, 1996). HHV-6B levels in the lymph nodes and in different organs of deceased patients also were found elevated alongside increased HIV-1 loads. It has been postulated that neighbouring cells exert mutual effects by altered cytokine milieu (Emery et al., 1999). Excretion of HHV-6B in the saliva of patients in successive stages of the disease was not significantly different (Gautheret et al.., 1995).

Ongrádi et al. also tested several groups of patients for double virus infection. In the first series of cross-sectional studies, patients in consecutive stages of HIV-1 infection with declining CD4+ cell number (symptomless, full blown and terminal AIDS, permanent HIV seronegative sexual partners, and control individuals) were screened for HHV-6A antibodies by immunofluorescence. As compared to controls, the mean level of IgM in the sexual partners raised 30-fold, that of IgG increased 10-fold, and 80% of individuals had low avidity IgG suggesting fresh HHV-6A infection. As compared to controls, the mean titer of IgM to HHV-6A remained elevated 10-fold in each group of HIV positive subjects. The highest level was found in the HIV seronegative partner group. The IgG level was 6-fold increased in asymptomatic HIV carriers, 4-fold in early and 5-fold in terminal AIDS patients. In the rapid progressors of AIDS patients HHV-6A IgG was higher, whereas in the subgroup of rapid progressors of terminal AIDS patients HHV-6A IgG was significantly lower compared to slow progressors. More than one quarter of AIDS patients had low avidity IgG to HHV-6A. These data suggest that, parallel to the decline of CD4+ T cell number and disease progression, HHV-6A maintains a chronic persistent infection in a significant number of HIV infected persons, and repeated HHV-6A infection furthermore occurs in the sexual partners of HIV-1 carriers. In the case of rapid progression, HHV-6A IgG production ceases (Maródi et al., 1998; Ongrádi et al., 1999b, 1999e), and as a result HHV-6A can become widely distributed by inflitrating the lymphocytes of several organs without specific tissue damaging effects (Knox & Carrigan, 1996).

Restricted expression of the same immediately early and early genes without the complete replication cycle, of several viruses can alter cellular machinery, resulting in malignant transformation and altering cytokine/chemokine production and subsequent HIV transactivation. The question then became whether simultaneous carriage of HIV-1 and HHV-6, or expression of viral genes reflecting active virus replication can influence depletion of CD4+ T cells and disease progression in different risk patients such as hemophiliacs and intravenous drug abusers (IVDA) compared to blood donors. DNA was extracted from plasma and peripheral blood lymphocytes (PBL's), while RNA was only extracted from PBL's. Carriage of both viruses was detected by PCR, and their expression by RT-PCR: PCR specific for HIV-1 *env* gene and nested PCR specific for HHV-6 ZVH14 fragment, was carried out. RT-PCR was carried out on complementer (c) DNA under the same conditions. The HHV-6 strain was characterised by endonuclease digestion fragments.

(Ceccherini-Nelli et al., Ongrádi et al. detected HHV-6A active replication more frequently in IVDA, 107/135, 79%), than in hemophiliacs (11/35, 31%, $p<0.001$) and blood donors (26/145, 18%, $p<0.001$). 81% of IVDA was positive by HIV-1 DNA PCR and, in spite of specific retroviral therapy, expressed HIV in 54% of cases. Furthermore, 43% (58/135) of these persons also expressed HHV-6 sequences evidently able to transactivate HIV-1. Expression of HHV-6 in HIV-1 seropositive patients is found to be 6.1 times more frequent than in HIV-1 seronegative counterparts. Simultaneous virus expression was shown to enhance CD4+ cell depletion. HHV-6 expression was found to enhance mortality of AIDS patients by approx. 35% in a two year period. These data prove that in the majority of patients HIV-1 expression is associated with active HHV-6A replication, but not with the latent state of HHV-6A. Among HIV-1 transactivating cofactors, HHV-6A seems to be relatively frequent. These data also suggest that the route of HHV-6A dispersal throughout the body is identical to that of HIV-1 (Ceccherini-Nelli et al., 1990; Ongrádi et al., 1994).

Patients	CD4+ cell counts	HIV-1 viral load (log Eq/ml)	HHV-6 DNA PCR 1µg 5µg	HHV-7 DNA PCR 1µg 5µg	Clinical stage (CDC 1993)
1	17	147.9	+ +	- -	C3
2	29	501.8	- -	- -	C3
3	59	32.66	- -	- -	B3
4	79	72.57	- +	- -	B3
5	97	190.06	+ +	- -	C3
6	139	388.4	+ +	- -	C3
7	197	10.9	- -	+ +	C3
8	217	117.46	- -	- -	A2
9	240	negative	- -	- +	A2
10	280	negative	- -	+ +	A2
11	321	18.9	- -	- -	A2
12	346	51.53	- -	+ +	A2
13	429	13.04	- +	+ +	A2
14	432	13.77	- +	+ +	C2
15	453	12.52	- -	- +	A2
16	504	11.48	+ +	+ +	A1
17	598	28.1	- -	- +	A1
18	735	negative	- +	+ +	A1

Table 1. Clinical, virological and immunological data of HIV-1 seropositive patients

As outlined in Section V, HHV-7 shows a marked reciprocal interference with HIV-1 *in vitro*. To investigate *in vivo* interactions of HHV-6, HHV-7 and HIV-1, another cross-sectional study comprising 18 HIV-1 seropositive patients and 33 blood donors has been recently described (Barsanti et al., submitted). Presence of HHV-6 was established as above, and nested PCR for HHV-7 on DNA extracted from PBLs was carried out using a set of specific primers and probe designed from the KHR strain of HHV-7 as described (Okuno et al., 1995). HIV-1 load was quantitated by branched DNA signal amplification. Although no significant difference in HHV-6 prevalence was found between patients and controls (22 and

33%, respectively), all 4 HHV-6 positive patients belonged to variant A, whereas among controls with HHV-6 DNA positivity had variant A and 4 had variant B, confirming that HHV-6A is predominantly associated with immunocompromised patients (Table 1). The percentage of HHV-7 positivity in HIV-1 seropositive patients (39%) is significantly lower than that of blood donors (82%, $p<0.01$, χ^2 test). HHV-7 positivity significantly correlated with a low level of HIV-1 ($p<0.01$, Mann-Whitney's test) as compared to HHV-7 negative HIV-1 positive patients. Interestingly, while the presence of HHV-6A was detected in patients with all consecutive stages of HIV-1 infection, distributed evenly, HHV-7 positivity was found more frequently in patients with earlier stages of HIV-1 infection: namely stages A1- 3/3, A2-5/7, C2-1/1, B3-0/2, and C3-1/3. Although the number of patients in each group is very small, the trend is clear: independent or synergistic destruction of CD4+ T cells by HHV-7 and HIV-1 lead to their rapid declination. Another possibility is that rapid declination of CD4+ cells by HIV-1 prevents the replication of HHV-7 in the later stages of HIV-1 infection, but the low level of HIV-1 load argues against this hypothesis. Irrespective of interpretation, these results raise the idea that HHV-7 may not be such a harmless virus in HIV-1 infected patients. Further *in vivo* studies on the interaction between HIV-1 and HHV-7 are warranted (Barsanti et al., submitted).

4.2 Longitudinal, serological and molecular studies

Follow-up studies could be done only in a limited number of double infected patients, and methodology was the same as described above. The first study of HHV-6 infection was carried out in two HIV-1 seropositive patients to provide *in vivo* evidence of HHV-6 reactivation. Concomitant with a significant rise of anti-HHV-6 IgG detected by IFA, a transient increase in HHV-6 viral load was shown in PBL's via PCR. During HHV-6 reactivation it was identified either as cell-free HHV-6 by PCR in plasma or by IgM antibody titers. HHV-6 reactivation was followed by a temporary decrease in CD4+ count and by a progressive dramatic loss of CD4+ cells during the 18 months post-reactivation. HHV-6 strain characterization by PCR demonstrated that the first patient (a woman with 232 CD4+ cell/mm^3 at the beginning, 34 CD4+/mm^3 with full-blown AIDS 16 months later) initially carried the B variant followed by reactivation and persistence of the A variant, while in the second patient (a man with 248 CD4+ at the beginning, then 14 CD4+/mm^3, *Pneumocystis carinii* pneumonia and esophageal candidiasis 13 months later) only the A variant was detected. The evidence of HHV-6A reactivation presented suggests its involvement in a mechanism of immunologic damage underlying the disease by either direct destruction of lymphoid cells or altering cytokine pattern (Iuliano et al., 1997). In another longitudinal follow-up of two AIDS patients from active HHV-6A infection evidence was demonstrated but the profile of infection in the two patients varied. One patient demonstrated the appearance and disappearance of HHV-6A indicating viral reactivation, whereas the other patient exhibited chronic or persistent HHV-6A infection (Ablashi et al., 1997). In another cohort, serum samples and PBMC's collected over a period of four years. IgG antibodies to HHV-6 gp110 late antigen did not differentiate between HIV-1 infected and control subjects, but IgG and IgM antibodies to p41/38 early antigens showed a significantly higher prevalence in HIV-1 infected individuals than in healthy donors, suggesting viral activation. HHV-6A was also shown in doubly infected PBL's of T lineage (CD2+, CD4+, CD38+) (Ablashi et al., 1998b). As Ceccherini-Nelli et al., Ongrádi et al. demonstrated, others have also shown that HHV-6A is frequently reactivated in early asymptomatic HIV-1 infected patients (Secchiero et al., 1995). AIDS progression is accelerated in infants with vertically

acquired HIV-1 and early acquisition of HHV-6A infection (Kositanont et al., 1999). Periodic reactivation or sustained persistence seem to be general phenomena among doubly infected persons. Additionally, high HHV-6 antibody titers were demonstrated in patients with consistently increasing HIV-1 load (Lenette et al., 2005).
HHV-6A upregulates CD4 expression, competitively inhibits binding of CCR5-trop HIV particles through RANTES overproduction, and ensures selective advantage of CXCR4-trop particles to infect T lymphocytes. HHV-6A persistence seems to sensitize the organism to HIV-1 infection. In the early phases of HIV infection, reactivated HHV-6A -especially in children- speeds up the disintegration of lymph nodes, as well as the onset and progression of AIDS in a vicious cycle. During the terminal phase of AIDS, a large amount of reactivated HHV-6A particles invade the whole body. In rapid AIDS progressors, both prevalence of HHV-6A virions and the titer of anti-HHV-6A antibodies are higher than in slow progressors. In AIDS-associated retinitis, HHV-6A proviral DNA, RNA and polypeptides are frequently shown beside HCMV (Qavi et al., 1989). In AIDS patients, HHV-6A might aggravate pneumonitis (Knox & Carrigan, 1994), Regarding the neuropathogenesis of HIV-1 infected children, HHV-6A is extensively disseminated in neural cells of the brain. It was reported that adult patients with AIDS had large areas of demyelination in their brain tissue at time of death (Knox & Carrigan, 1995).

5. Human herpesvirus 7 as a negative competitor of HIV infection

HHV-7 was isolated from the activated T lymphocytes of a healthy blood donor (Frenkel et al., 1990). HHV-6 and HHV-7 share similar genetic, biologic and immunologic features. HHV-7 also belongs to the *Roseolovirus* genus. The viral DNA is completely sequenced (Nicholas, 1996), it is formed by a unique segment of 133 kbp flanked by 6 to 10 kbp DR sequences, so that the genome length ranges between 145 and 153 kbp. Similar to HHV-6, the HHV-7 viral genome contains herpesvirus conserved genes arranged in 7 boxes. Nucleic acid sequence identity ranges from 20.7 to 75.7% in various genes, while amino acid sequence identity is between 41 and 75%. The coding ability of HHV-7 comprises 84 different ORFs (Megaw et al., 1998), only one gene (U55B) is HHV-7 specific, and there is no homologue to the HHV-6 U94 gene. It has been shown that HHV-7 gB attaches to CD4 molecules as a receptor (Lusso et al., 1994). It is likely that other molecules can act as receptors, and it is known that HHV-7 can infect cells that do not express CD4, e.g. lymphocytes, monocytes, epithelial cells, and fibroblasts. CD4 alone is not sufficient for a productive infection (Kempf et al., 1998). HHV-7 also establishes latent infection in CD4+ lymphocytes and macrophages, persistent infection occurs in salivary gland tissues as well, as shown by specific PCR (Sada et al., 1996). *In vitro*, only the CD4+ immature T cell line (SupT1) supports HHV-7 growth (Ablashi et al., 1998a). Due to CD4 affinity, HHV-7 competes for the shared receptor with HIV-1 (Lisco et al., 2007). Blockade of the CD4 molecule with anti-CD4 monoclonal antibodies (mAbs) or HIV-1 gp120 (which bind to CD4), inhibits HHV-7 infection of T cells. Exposure of terminally differentiated CD4+ macrophages derived from peripheral blood monocytes to intact or UV-inactivated HHV-7 prior to HIV-1 infection reduced the average level of HIV-1 p24 antigen production in cell culture supernatants by 91%, indicating that the mechanism of interference depends directly on the competition for CD4. It was suggested that this antagonistic effect be exploited to devise therapeutic approaches to AIDS. However, in prospective *in vivo* studies, HHV-7 was detected in only 3% of HIV-1 infected patients and 12% of controls. It was suggested that this low level of detection resulted from HIV-1 out-competing HHV-7 for infection of CD4+ cells. There was no association between HHV-7 viral load in PBL and progressson of HIV-1 disease (Crowley et al., 1996). HHV-7 has a strong down-regulation on CD4 mRNA and transcriptional activity in cord blood lymphocytes and SupT1 cell (Furukawa et al., 1994). The HHV-7 U21 open reading frame codes for an immunoevasin that inhibits the transport of class I MHC and CD4 molecules to the surface, thus infected cells are more difficulty recognizable by CD8+ cytotoxic T lymphocytes (Hudson et al., 2003). Expression of Kaposi's sarcoma herpesvirus (HHV-8), K5 protein (MIR2) (Paulson et al., 2001) and adenovirus E3/19K protein (Lippé et al., 1991) also restrict surface expression of MHC class I molecules. HIV Nef polypeptide down-regulates both MHC class I and CD4 molecules (Mangasarian et al., 1999). In patients carrying several viruses simultaneously, the concerted action of HIV Nef and immunoevasins of heterologous viruses dramatically diminishes cytotoxic immune cell activism, resulting in the survival of virus-producing cells and consequently increasing bodily viral load. HHV-7 down-modulates CXCR4 surface molecule independently of CD4 in infected cells (Secchiero et al., 1998), which inhibit HIV-1 spread through the body. Differently than HHV-6A, HHV-7 does not down-regulate CD3, and has no effect on CD1, CD2, CD44 and CD49 T cell adhesion molecules (Yasukawa et al., 1993). In addition, HHV-7 decreases CD38 levels, and slightly increases CD5 and CD57 on the surface of infected both SupT1 cells (Kirn et al., 1997). During the late stage of infection, HHV-7 increases the expression of CD46 at both the transcriptional and translational levels, as well as on the surface of SupT1 cells and primary CD4+ T cells. Together with CD59 overexpression, HHV-7 infected cells become more resistant to complement-dependent cytotoxicity than uninfected cells. CD46 overexpression facilitates infection of these immune cells by several heterologous viruses, among them HHV-6 and some adenovirus types, which are known to transactivate HIV-1 (Takemoto et al., 2007). Unlike with HHV-6, a generalized increase in host cell protein synthesis is observed in HHV-7 infected lymphocytes. Host genes whose expression is upregulated by HHV-7 infection include the lymphocyte specific G-protein coupled receptor EBI I, GADD45 (Kirn et al., 1997), GM-CSF and IL-15 (Atedzoé et al., 1997). Infection of PBMC's obtained from seronegative individuals (mimicking primary infection) increases the level of intracellular mRNA and secreted polypeptides of TNF-α, TGF-β, IFN-γ, but decreases the production of IL-2 from mitogen (bacterial endotoxin polysaccharide, LPS and OKT3 mAb) activated PBMC. On the other hand, HHV-7 does not affect IL-4 and IL-6 synthesis (Atedzoé et al., 1999). In PBMC's of seropositive persons (mimicking secondary infection), HHV-7 infection results in diminished IL-2 and IFN-γ production with or without mitogen activation. HHV-7 induces early IL-10 production, which is known to inhibit cytokine release from CD4+ helper lymphocytes. After a primary infection, HHV-7 causes significant inhibition of lymphocyte proliferation and overall the cellular immununity, but in repeated infections the overall effect of HHV-7 on cytokine production by infected cells is balanced.This might contribute to the moderate immunosuppression upon reactivation (Ongrádi et al., 1999a). HHV-7 also encodes two functional chemokine receptors, U12 and U51, which are counterparts of human CCR4 and CCR7. And whose natural ligands are CCL22 and CCL19, respectively. These receptors are expressed on T and B lymphocytes, and promote their translocation from the blood to the lymph nodes. Overexpression of these receptors facilitate the dissemination of infected lymphocytes throughout the body (Tadagaki et al., 2007).

HHV-7 is ubiquitous worldwide. Approximately 70% of children are infected and seroconvert before 4 years of age,usually following HHV-6B infection, but 30% of the population acquires infection later in life. In children, HHV-7 can induce exanthema subitum directly or, through activation of HHV-6B, may induce febrile convulsions or hepatitis. HHV-7 is reactivated in some patients 4 to 6 weeks after liver, kidney, bone marrow or stem cell transplantation, and may exacerbate human cytomegalovirus (HCMV) induced immunosuppression. HHV-7 can also reactivate HHV-6B *in vitro* (Katsafanas et al., 1996). In seronegative adults, HHV-7 can induce pityriasis rosea (PR) as presence of infective viruses, viral DNA and rising antibody as is indicated by increasing levels of IFN-α and -γ in the serum (Drago et al., 1997; Vág et al.., 2004a). Although rare, cases of PR have been described in patients with HIV-1 infection. Several types of papulosquamosus disorders might occur also in AIDS patients (Duvic et al., 1991). The lack of herald patch typical of genuine HHV-7 induced PR supports proper differential diagnosis. Due to some common immune pathways of HHV-7 and HIV-1 (e.g. alteration of cytokine pattern in the skin), PR might be mimicked in AIDS patients (Sadick et al., 1990). Interaction of HHV-6B or HHV-7 with human parvovirus B19 induces papular-purpuric gloves-and-socks syndrome (PPGSS, Ongrádi et al., 2000a; Vág et al., 2004b). HHV-7 is transmitted via saliva (Wyatt & Frenkel, 1992) and breast milk (Fujusaki et al., 1998). HHV-7 has been detected at the same ratio, more frequently, at higher viral loads, or in decreased quantitiy in saliva from HIV+ individuals with clinical symptoms of immunodeficiency than from controls by PCR in different studies (Di Luca et al., 1995; Lucht et al.., 1998; Gautheret-Dejean et al., 1997). There is no evidence for congenital infection, although 2.7% of cervical samples obtained from pregnant women during the third trimester are PCR positive (Hall et al., 2008). Viral DNA is sporadically detected in the urine of healthy individuals, and in 6.5% of the cellular fraction of urine samples from HIV-1 positive patients with low CD4+ cell count (Gautheret-Dejean et al., 1997), but no infectious virus has been obtained from cervical and urine samples simultaneously. The HHV-7 pp85 protein was detected in 9 of 32 HIV-associated cases, and in one of 7 classic sporadic Kaposi's sarcoma lesions, which was localized to the cytoplasm of CD4-CD68+ cells of the monocyte/macrophage lineage. Dually infected HHV-6B and HHV-7 CD4-CD68+ cells were detected in 9% of these lesions. The cytokine-rich environment of Kaposi's sarcoma might activate HHV-7 and subsequently HHV-6B (Kempf et al., 1997). These data suggest that HHV-7 also interacts with different viruses, among them HHV-6B, but does not activate HIV-1 directly and does not activate HIV-1 through HHV-6A activation. On the other hand, its immunomodulatory effects can be additive to immune suppression induced by HIV-1 *in vivo*.

6. Animal models to study transactivation by heterologous viruses

6.1 Simian AIDS model

A major hindrance to elucidating the *in vivo* role played by HHV-6A in AIDS has been the lack of a reliable animal model system (Lusso et al., 2007). Although simian (SIV) and feline (FIV) immunodeficiency viruses in their natural hosts provide appropriate models, the lack of known counterparts of *Roseolovirus* isolates from these animals impedes studies on the effect of simultaneous infection in AIDS progression. Peripheral blood lymphocytes of adult chimpanzees, pig-tailed macaques (*Macaca nemestrina*) and African green monkeys were found as susceptible to HHV-6A (Lusso et al., 1990, 1994) and HHV-6B (Levy et al., 1990) infections as were human PBL's. Although HHV-6A infected PBL cultures of chimpanzees exhibited CPE similar to that seen in human PBL and produced infectious virus (Lusso et al., 1990), this model is practically unavailable. The availability of pig-tailed macaques whose T cells are highly susceptible to HHV-6A infection is an ideal experimental model (Lusso et al., 1994). It has been established that *in vivo* coinfection with HHV-6A accelerates the course of SIV disease in pig-tailed macaques (Lusso et al., 2007). Three groups of young adult animals were infected by intravenous inoculation with either SIV_{smE660} alone, HHV-$6A_{GS}$ alone, or both SIV and HHV-6A. Dually infected animals were first inoculated with SIV and then superinfected with HHV-6A 14 days later. None of the animals had detectable antibodies to HHV-6A and SIV before inoculation. Animals were observed for 32 months. HHV-6A infected animals developed clinical manifestations of mild to moderate intensity such as fever, splenomegaly, and generalized lymphadenopathy. Anti-HHV-6A seroconversion appeared after a mean of 3±1.4 and 2.2±0.5 weeks in HHV-6A and dually infected animals, respectively. SIV infection resulted in plasma viremia, and $SIVp27_{Gag}$ antigenemia at two weeks post-inoculation in both groups. Clinical signs included fever, generalized lymphadenopathy and splenomegaly, while the fever was higher and longer in duration in animals coinfected with SIV and HHV-6A. A transient loss of circulating CD4+ T lymphocytes was detected in singly and coinfected macaques. During the follow-up, no long term clinical or hematological alterations were seen in animals singly infected with HHV-6A, and their CD4+ and CD8+ T cell counts remained stably with the normal range. By contrast, a progressive loss of circulating CD4+ and CD8+ T cells was seen in coinfected animals. SIV superinfection of animals carrying HHV-6B for 13 to 21 months resulted in a very rapid decline of CD4+ and CD8+ T cells, and these animals developed AIDS-related conditions after 69 and 15 weeks of SIV superinfection (Lusso et al., 2007). Interestingly, the longer the duration of HHV-6A latency was, the shorter of AIDS-related conditions developed. This means that even latent HHV-6A infection induces irreversible changes in the immune system. Unlike the immunological parameters, the levels of SIV plasma viremia and antigenemia during the follow up were not significantly different between singly or dually infected macaques. Interestingly, disease progression in dually infected animals was accompanied by frequent episodes of HHV-6A reactivation, suggesting that SIV infection exerted a boosting effect on HHV-6A replication. Dually infected animals also showed a significantly expedited decrease in anti-HHV-6A antibody reactivity over time demonstrating exhaustion of humoral immunity. Lymph node biopsy one month post-inoculation showed follicular hyperplasia in all animals. However, in macaques singly infected with SIV or HHV-6A the nodal architecture was conserved, whereas in dually infected monkeys it exhibited a florid follicular hyperplasia with confluent germinal centers. Coinfected lymph nodes showed higher levels of SIV RNA deposited on the surface of follicular dendritic cells and HHV-6A mRNA expression in the extrafollicular area. Thus, HHV-6A and SIV could simultaneously replicate in coinfected lymph nodes. In biopsies obtained 6 months after inoculation, lymph nodes of dually infected animals showed significant atrophy of germinal centers. During the 32 months of the study, AIDS-defining clinical conditions developed in all coinfected macaques, but in only one of 4 infected with SIV.

It was also shown that reisolated SIV obtained from HHV-6A coinfected macaques after one year of infection had acquired resistance to RANTES (regulated upon activation normal T cell expressed and secreted). RANTES is a CCR5 binding chemokine that blocks the entry of SIV into cells, since SIV depends on CCR5 for infection. As has been previously discussed, HHV-6A is a potent RANTES inducer in lymphoid tissue (Grivel et al., 2001). In HHV-6A coinfected macaques, SIV subsequently evolved toward RANTES resistance, most likely under the selective pressure of elevated RANTES levels. Resistance to RANTES is increasingly recognized as a key virulence factor in HIV infection (Grivel et al., 2003), which may allow the virus to replicate in the high-RANTES milieu. One of the possible mechanisms whereby HHV-6A may foster the progression to AIDS is by facilitating an early acquisition of RANTES resistance (Lusso et al., 2007). In a recent study, SIV were reisolated from singly and HHV-6A-coinfected macaques. Surgically removed human tonsils in the presence of RANTES and PBMC from randomly selected healthy donors or from a homozygous CCR5-Δ32 +/+ donor were infected with SIV reisolates. All SIV isolates were able to replicate in human lymphoid tissue. Inoculation of different cell lines expressing several coreceptors (CCR2b, CCR3, CCR4, CCR6, CCR8, CX_3CR1, and CXCR4) were not able to support SIV infection. The majority of SIV isolates from HHV-6A coinfected macaques were not able to replicate in CCR5-Δ32 +/+ PBMC's showing that SIV variants, despite maintaining exclusive CCR5 coreceptor sensitivity, become resistant to HHV-6A and RANTES receptor competition. Cytokine polypeptide production in PBMC's obtained from healthy donors was induced by infection using either SIV from singly infected animals or SIV from HHV-6 coinfected animals. IL-2 production was significantly down-regulated while IFN-γ production was significantly upregulated in cultures infected with SIV derived from coinfected macaques as compared to the cytokine-inducing ability of SIV obtained after a single infection. For other Th1 and Th2 cytokines (IL-1α and -β, IL-4, IL-7, IL-12, IL-15, IL-16, and TNF-α), chemokines (MIP-1α and –β), other mediators (GM-CSF, IP10, MIG, and SDF-1β) no significant differences between lymphoid tissue infected with the two groups of SIV isolates were recorded. These results also indicate that SIV isolates obtained from HHV-6A-coinfected animals undergo a biological evolution *in vivo*, with the emergence of viral strains containing a reduced sensitivity to RANTES-mediated inhibition, thus, bypassing an important mechanism of virus control. It has been learned from clinical studies, that progression toward full-blown AIDS is often associated with the evolution of HIV-1 toward increased virulence. HIV-1 acquires the ability to use CXCR4 as a coreceptor, becoming resistant to the inhibitory effects of endogenous CCR5-binding chemokines. This phenotypic switch is typically accompanied by an accelerated loss of CD4+ T cells and suppression of Th1 polarized responses that play an essential role in the clearance of viral infections. These results are conclusive *in vivo* evidence that HHV-6A accelerates the progression of SIV toward full-blown AIDS (Biancotto et al., 2009), and excellently support human clinical and experimental data on the interaction of HHV-6A and HIV-1.

6.2 Feline AIDS as an ideal small animal model to study the interaction between retroviruses and different heterologous viruses

Although SIV infection is very close to the human analog monkeys are not available for the majority of research groups due to short supply and ethical considerations. Specific pathogen-free populations are nonexistent. Feline immunodeficiency virus (FIV), another member of the family *Retroviridae* has a pathogenesis similar to that of HIV infection, and because cats are both plentiful and available in specific pathogen free (SPF) status, they might prove to be an ideal model for AIDS cofactor studies. FIV shares many genetic, structural and biological characteristics with HIV. Although FIV shows tropism for CD4+ cells, its receptor is CD134 (Shimojima et al., 2004), and it requires further interaction with chemokine coreceptors (CCR5 and CXCR4) for entry (de Parseval et al., 2006). RANTES inhibits FIV infection of feline PBMC's, while antibodies against CXCR4, CCR5 and CCR3 reduce FIV infection. CD4+ and CD8+ T cells monocytes/macrophages are the major targets of FIV, in which it might establish latent infection. Upon virus activation, cells die of apoptosis (references in Bendinelli et al., 1995 and Burkhard & Dean, 2003). FIV diverges from other lentiviruses throughout the genome. Beside *gag, pol, env* and other small ORFs encoding regulatory proteins, the provirus contains two LTR elements, one at each end, which accommodate multiple regulatory elements. FIV LTRs appear to be strong basal promoters and poorly active in transactivation (Sparger et al., 1992). Regulatory sequences include one or two TATA boxes, and a variety of enhancer or promoter protein-binding sites (AP-1, NF-κB, etc). FIV transactivation is significantly different than that seen for HIV because FIV lacks TAT and the transactivating response (TAR) element (Sparger et al., 1992). Instead, FIV contains Orf-2 (also designated as Orf-A), a *tat*-like gene encoding a viral transactivator necessary for productive FIV replication in primary T lymphocytes as well as feline T cell lines (de Parseval & Elder, 1999). Unlike other lentiviral transactivators, FIV Orf-2 requires additional LTR elements for transactivation (Chatterji et al., 2002). Infection with FIV is usually associated with direct inoculation of the virus into the body via bites, and there is a distinct transient initial stage of infection that follows exposure by several weeks. After recovery from this initial disease, afflicted cats enter into a long asymptomatic stage of the infection that lasts for months or years before other signs appear. CD4+ T lymphocyte decline and inversion of the CD4/CD8 ratio are hallmarks of FIV infection, especially in neonates (Diehl et al., 1996) due to apoptosis induced by TNF-α overproduction (Ohno et al., 1993). Serum levels of IL-1, IL-6 and TNF-α increase in parallel with viral replication (Kraus et al., 1996). After *in vitro* treatment of separated PBMC in experimentally infected cats CD4+ lymphocytes produce TNF-α, IFN-γ, IL-2, IL-4 and IL-8, while CD8+ T lymphocytes express TNF-α, IFN-γ, and IL-2. Monocytes/macrophages are the source of IL-1, IL-6, TNF-α, IL-10 and IL-12p40 (Ritchey et al., 2001). The terminal AIDS stage of FIV infection is associated with a number of chronic common and opportunistic-type infections. Like HIV infection of humans, other infectious diseases may interact with FIV infection in the field to cause a more severe disease syndrome.

Retroviruses and herpesviruses are associated with a variety of diseases in animals. It has been suspected for long time that their interaction may result in synergistic induction of diseases (Bacon et al., 1989). A possible interaction of feline herpesvirus type 1 (FHV-1, subfamily *Alphaherpesvirinae)* with FIV has been studied *in vivo* and *in vitro*. FHV-1 is a significant pathogen of family *Felidae*, causing an upper respiratory tract disease in cats. In dually infected animals it induces several immunological abnormalities (Reubel et al., 1992, 1994). FHV-1 also infects T lymphocytes. Productive coinfection of individual T lymphocytes has been detected (Kawaguchi et al., 1991). FHV-1 ICP4 was shown to modulate FIV LTR activity (Kawaguchi et al., 1994, 1995).

Among other AIDS-promoting DNA viruses, adenoviruses (AdV) are known to cause fatal enteritis among terminal AIDS patients. The only feline adenovirus isolate (FeAdV) was obtained (Ongrádi, 1999) from a PCR positive fecal sample (Lakatos et al., 1997) of a cat with unknown FIV status. In Europe, 10 to 20% of free roaming cats are seropositive (Lakatos et al., 1996, 2000). FeAdV DNA has been detected in fecal samples of a child and her cat in Japan (Phan et al., 2006), and in a Brazilian child with upper respiratory tract infection (Luiz et al., 2010). Sequences of its hexon (Pring-Akerblom & Ongrádi, GenBank Accession No.

AY512566) and fiber (Pring-Akerblom & Ongrádi, GenBank Accession No. AY518270) suggest that FeAdV is related to human AdV type 1. It would be ideal to explore its interrelationship with both HIV and FIV, especially with respect to the role of AdVs in the intestinal complications of AIDS.

Another common interaction in nature is between FIV infection and feline leukemia virus (FeLV). About 10 to 15% of the cats clinically ill with FIV infection are coinfected with FeLV worldwide (Hosie et al., 1989; Ishida et al., 1989; Yamamoto et al., 1989). FeLV can also induce immunodeficiency (Rojko & Olsen, 1984). In dually infected cats, the CD4+/CD8+ T lymphocyte ratio becomes rapidly inverted (Pedersen et al., 1990). FeLV induced tumors are a source of frequent and anticipated feline death (Shelton et al., 1990). This interrelationship is similar to what has been described for HIV and HTLV-I (Levy, 1993).

Besides viruses, other opportunistic infections can enhance the progression of feline AIDS. Both *Toxoplasma gondii* (Levy et al., 1998) and *Listeria monocytogenes* (Dean et al., 1998; Dean & Pedersen, 1998; Levy et al., 1998) disrupt the synergistic production of normal Th1 type cytokines, causing a loss of cellular immunity in FIV positive animals.

These different systems clearly show that the progression of feline AIDS is facilitated by a wide array of microbes. Further studies are warranted to better delineate the role of other putative cofactors among the Roseoloviruses in FIV infection as an ideal small animal model for human AIDS.

7. Importance of rapid viral diagnosis, treatment and prevention of HIV-1 and HHV-6 simultaneous infections

Several transactivating herpesviruses cause severe, long-lasting, and unusual opportunistic infections in HIV-1 infected and AIDS patients. Heterologous viruses frequently show unusual resistance to antiviral drugs. The potential to transactivate HIV and cause opportunistic infection shows an intimate mutual relationship between these viruses and their relationship within the immune system. Prevention and suppression of both phenomena ought to be a continuous clinical tasks while treating and improving the quality of life of these patients.

There are excellent laboratory methods available to diagnose HIV-1 and 2 antibodies, and to determine the actual viral load in the serum of patients. Determination of their resistance to antiviral drugs is also routinely analyzed during treatment. Unfortunately, no serological tests are routinelyavailable for the differential diagnosis of HHV-6 variants A and B. Immunfluorescent and ELISA methods determine the total quantity of anti-HHV-6 antibodies due to cross reactions, however the level of detectable serology can be insensitive when diagnosing immunocompromised populations. Several multiplex and real-time PCR assays are available for the simultaneous detection and quantification of HHV-6A, HHV-6B and HHV-7 specimens in patients (Safronetz et al., 2003). Recently, the success of highly active antiretroviral therapy (HAART) in controlling HIV-induced immunosuppression has resulted in the disappearance of HHV-6 opportunistic infections, according to the trend already described for HCMV (Martinez et al., 2007; Salzberger et al., 2005). HHV-6 variants are sensitive to ganciclovir, foscarnet, cidofovir, IFN-α and IFN-β, and all of them have already been used in a small number of patients with different immunocompromised conditions. Some HHV-6A strains can carry mutations in the U69 gene responsible for phosphotransferase activity, consequently displaying resistance to treatment with ganciclovir (De Clercq & Naesens, 2006).

8. Future dimensions

Future research efforts could be directed toward hot topics such as the following:
First, it has not been established that cytokines and other mediators excreted from HHV-6 infected cells are structurally normal or have altered chemical structure (e.g. glycosylation, phosphorylation). It is also conceivable that HHV-6 carrier cells produce one or more unique soluble mediators that strongly transactivate HIV-1. Such aspects ought to be explored.
Second, results strongly suggest that persistent HHV-6 gene expression and replication sensitizes to HIV infection and rapid progression. Rapid progressors might carry integrated HHV-6, or may be progressing due to other potential yet presently unknown genetic immunological defects. Available samples of former and recent patients ought to be retested with this goal in mind. More attention must also be payed to these HIV-1 infected, HHV-6 carrier patients concerning anti-HHV-6 therapy. Gene therapy to suppress HHV-6 expression would be ideal to treat patients carrying integrated HHV-6.
Finally, further studies on the *in vivo* interrelationship between FIV and feline roseolovirus are necessary to understand the clinical aspects of dual infections of this nature. A feline counterpart of HHV-6 ought to be discovered and characterized.

9. Conclusions

HIV-1 infection is followed by a long disease-free period due to low transcriptional activity of the integrated provirus in resting CD4+ immune cells. Activation of CD4+ cells by mitogens, altered cytokine/chemokine milieu, or superinfection by heterologous viruses upregulate cellular, nuclear transcriptional factors, which in turn upregulate HIV-1 LTR directed gene expression by a *tat*-independent mechanism leading to augmented HIV-1 production. HHV-6 variant A possesses several alternative ways to upregulate HIV-1 infection and promote AIDS progression. Co-infection of HIV-1 carrier CD4+ cells results in enhanced cell death through apoptosis *in vitro* and *in vivo*, especially in the lymph nodes. Infection of immune cells leads to a a shift in cytokine pattern from Th1 to Th2. Overproduction of TNF-α, IL-1 and IL-6 strongly transactivates HIV-1 via secondary messengers and the same nuclear transcriptional factors. Elevated levels of RANTES facilitate the change of CCR5-trop HIV-1 population towards the strongly cytopathic CXCR4 mutants. In the body, synergistic effects of immune evasion result in either a continuous or alternating presence of high level viremia, dissemination of the virus to all organs of the body which contributes to their failure and the consequentially premature death of AIDS patients. HHV-6A primarily damages cellular immunity, whereas HHV-6B predominantly suppresses the activity of humoral immune function. While HHV-6B infects CD+ immune cells, it hardly contributes to the activation of HIV-1, due to a differently modified cytokine/chemokine pattern. HHV-7 binds directly to CD4 molecules, therefore directly competing for this receptor with HIV-1. It is regarded as a harmless virus, but in successive stages of HIV-1 infection contributes to the gradual loss of CD4+ cells. There are molecular techniques for the simultaneous and rapid detection of these herpesviruses *in vivo*. Since the introduction of HAART, severe complications by HHV-6 have become rare, but if necessary ganciclovir and foscarnet can be used to inhibit these herpesviruses to improve the quality of life of HIV-1 infected patients.

10. Acknowledgement

We are thankful to Professor István Nász (Institute of Medical Microbiology, Semmelweis University, Budapest, Hungary) for his encouragement during preparation of the manuscript. The publication charge of the manuscript was partially defrayed by the Section of Medical Sciences, Hungarian Academy of Sciences. Kristin Loomis and Joshua Pritchett (HHV-6 Foundation, Santa Barbara, CA, USA) provided editorial assistance.

11. References

Ablashi, D.V., Balachandran, S .F., Josephs, C.L., Hung, C.L., Krueger, G.R., Kramarsky, B., Salahuddin, S.Z. & Gallo, R.C. (1991). Genomic Polymorphism, Growth Properties, and Immunologic Variations in Human Herpesvirus-6 Isolates. *Virology,* Vol.184, No.2, (October 1991), 545-552. ISSN 0042

Ablashi, D.V., Chatlynne, L.G. & Whitman, J.E Jr. (1997). Longitudinal follow-up of two AIDS patients for active human herpesvirus-6 (HHV-6) infection. *In vivo,* Vol.11, No.5, (September-October 1997), 383-386. ISSN 0189-6016S2005

Ablashi, D.V., Handy, M., Bernbaum, J., Chatlynne, L.G., Lapps, W., Kramarsky, B., Berneman, Z.N., Komaroff, A.L. & Whitman J.E. (1998a). Propagation and characterization of human herpesvirus-7 (HHV-7) isolates in a continuous T-lymphoblastoid cell line (SupT1). *Journal of Virologycal Methods,* Vol.73, No.2, (August 1998), 123-140. ISSN 0166-0934

Ablashi, D.V., Marsh, S., Kaplan, M., Whitman, J.E. Jr. & Pearson, GR.(1998b).HHV-6 infection in HIV-infected asymptomatic and AIDS patients. *Intervirology* Vol.41, No.1, (June 1997), 1-9. ISSN 0300-5526

Agut, H., Guetard, D., Collandre, H., Dauguet, C., Montagnie,r L., Miclea, J.M., Baurmann, H. & Gessain, A. (1988). Concomitant infection by human herpesvirus 6, HTLV-I, and HIV-2. *Lancet,* Vol.1, No.8587, (March 1998), 712. ISSN 0140-6736

Akhyani, N., Berti, R., Brennan, M.B., Soldan, S.S., Eaton, JM., McFarland, HF. & Jacobson S. (2000). Tissue distribution and variant characterization of human herpesvirus (HHV)-6: increased prevalence of HHV-6A in patients with multiple sclerosis. *Journal of Infectious Disease,* Vol.182, No.5, (November 2000), 1321-1325. ISSN 0934-9723

Albrecht, MA., DeLuca, NA., Byrn, RA., Schaffer, PA. & Hammer, SM. (1989). The herpes simplex virus immediate-early protein, ICP4, is required to potentiate replication of human immunodeficiency virus in CD4+ lymphocytes. *Journal of Virology,* Vol.63, No.5, (May 1989), 1861-1868. ISSN 0022-538x

Alvarez-Lafuente, R., García-Montojo, M., De las Heras, V., Bartolomé, M. & Arroyo, R. (2006). Clinical parameters and HHV-6 active replication in relapsing-remitting multiple sclerosis patients. *Journal of Clinical Virology,* Vol.37, No.1, (December 2006), 24-26. ISSN 1386-6532

Alvarez-Lafuente, R., de las Heras, V., García-Montojo, M., Bartolomé, M. & Arroyo, R. (2007). Human herpesvirus-6 and multiple sclerosis: relapsing-remitting versus secondary progressive. *Multiple Sclerosis,* Vol.13, No.5, (June 2007), 78-83. ISSN 1352-4585

Arbuckle, J.H., Medveczky, M.M., Luka, J., Luka, J., Hadley, S.H., Luegmayr, A., Ablashi, D., Lund, T.C., Tolar, J., De Meirleir, K., Montoya, J.G., Komaroff, A.L., Ambros, P.F. &

Medveczky, P.G. (2010). The latent human herpesvirus-6A genome specifically integrates in telomeres of human chromosomes in vivo and in vitro. *Proceedings of National Academy of Sciences of the United States of America*, Vol.107, No.12, (March 2010), 5563-5568. ISSN 0027-8424

Arena, A., Merendino, R.A., Bonina, L., Iannello, D., Stassi, G. & Mastroeni, P. (2000). Role of IL-15 on monocytic resistance to human herpesvirus 6 infection. *New Microbiologica* ,Vol.23, No.2, (April 200), 105-112. ISSN 1121-7138.

Arena, A., Liberto, M.C., Capozza, A.B. & Focà, A. (1997). Productive HHV-6 infection in differentiated U937 cells: role of TNF alpha in regulation of HHV-6. *New Microbiologica,* Vol.20, No.1, (January 1997), 13-20. ISSN 1121-7138.

Arena, A., Liberto, M.C., Iannello, D., Capozza, AB. & Focà, A. (1999). Altered cytokine production after human herpes virus type 6 infection. *New Microbiologica,* Vol.22, No.4, (October 1999), 293-300. ISSN 1121-7138.

Arya, S.K., Guo, C., Josephs, S.F. & Wong-Staal, F. (1985). Trans-activator gene of human T-lymphotropic virus type III (HTLV-III). *Science,* Vol.229, No.4708, (July 1985), 69-73. ISSN 0036-8075

Asada, H., Klaus-Kovtun.,V, Golding,H., Katz, SI. & Blauvelt, A. (1999). Human herpesvirus 6 infects dendritic cells and suppresses human immunodeficiency virus type 1 replication in coinfected cultures. *Journal of Virology*, Vol.73, No.5, (May 1999), 4019-4028. ISSN 0022-538x

Atedzoé, BN., Ahmad, A. & Menezes, J.(1977). Enhancement of natural killer cell cytotoxicity by the human herpesvirus-7 via IL-15 induction. *Journal of Immunology,* Vol.159, No.10, (November 1997), 4966-4972 ISSN 0022-1767

Atedzoé, B.N., Menezes, J., D'Addario, M., Xu, J., Ongrádi, J. & Ahmad, A. (1999). Modulatory effects of human herpesvirus-7 on cytokine synthesis and cell proliferation in human peripheral blood mononuclear cell cultures. *Journal of Leukocyte Biology,* Vol.66, No.5, (November 1999), 822-828, 1999. ISSN 0741-5400

Bacon, L.D., Witter, R.L. & Fadly, A.M. (1989). Augmentation of retrovirus-induced lymphoid leukosis by Marek's disease herpesviruses in White Leghorn chickens. *Journal of Virology,* Vol.63, No.2, (February 1989), 504-12. ISSN 0022-538x

Barsanti, L.A., Iuliano, R., Cannavò, E., Liuzzi, G., Brizzi, M., Mecocci, L., Mazzotta, F., Piazza, M. & Ceccherini-Nelli, L. (2011) HHV-6 and HHV-7 DNA PCR detection in HIV-1 seropositive individuals: correllation with CD4+ cell counts and HIV-1 RNA viral load. *Journal of Medical Virology,* submitted, ISSN 0146-6615

Bates, M., Monze, M,, Bima, H., Kapambwe, M., Clark, D., Kasolo, F,C. & Gompels, U.A. (2009). Predominant human herpesvirus 6 variant A infant infections in an HIV-1 endemic region of Sub-Saharan Africa. *Journal of Medical Virology,* Vol.8, No.5, (May 2009), 779-89. ISSN 0146-6615

Bendinelli, M., Pistello, M., Lombardi, S., Poli, A., Garzelli, C., Matteucci, D., Ceccherini-Nelli, L. & Malvaldi G, Tozzini. F. (1995). Feline immunodeficiency virus: an interesting model for AIDS studies and an important cat pathogen. *Clinical Microbiology Review,* Vol.8, No.1, (January 1995), 87-112. ISSN 0893-8512

Bertram, G., Dreiner,N., Krueger, G.R. , Ramon, A., Ablashi, D. V., Salahuddin, S.Z. & Balachandram, N. (1991). Frequent double infection with Epstein-Barr virus and human herpesvirus-6 in patients with acute infectious mononucleosis. *In vivo,* Vol.5, No.3, (May-June 1991), 271-279. ISSN 0189-6016S2005

Biancotto, A., Grivel, J.C., Lisco, A., Vanpouille, C., Markham, P.D., Gallo, R.C., Margolis, L.B. & Lusso, P. (2009). Evolution of SIV toward RANTES resistance in macaques rapidly progressing to AIDS upon coinfection with HHV-6A. *Retrovirology,* (July 2009), Vol.2, No.6, 61. ISSN 1742-4690

Burkhard M.J. & Dean, G.A. (2003). Transmission and immunopathogenesis of FIV in cats as a model for HIV. *Current HIV Research,* Vol.1, No.1, (January 2003), 15-29. ISSN 1570-162x

Cao, W. & Sullivan, C. (1992). Human herpesvirus 6 does not enhance human T cell lymphotropic virus type I (HTLV-I) expression in the HTLV-I-transformed cell line MT4. *Journal of Infectious Diseases,* Vol.166, No.2, (August 1992); 446-447.ISSN 0934-9723

Carrigan, D.R,. Knox, K.K. & Tapper, M.A. (1990). Suppression of human immunodeficiency virus type 1 replication by human herpesvirus-6. *Journal of Infectious Diseases.* Vol.162, No.4, (October 1990), 844-51 ISSN 0934-9723

Carrigan, D.R. & Knox, K.K. (1994). Human herpesvirus 6 (HHV-6) isolation from bone marrow: HHV-6-associated bone marrow suppression in bone marrow transplant patients. *Blood.* Vol.84, No.10, (November 1994), 3307-3310. ISSN 0006-4971

Caselli, E. & Di Luca, D. (2007). Molecular biology and clinical associations of Roseoloviruses human herpesvirus 6 and human herpesvirus 7. *New Microbiologica,* Vol.30, No.3, (July 2007), 173-87. ISSN 1121-7138

Caruso, A., Favilli, F., Rotola, A., Comar, M.,Horejsh, D., Alessandri, G.,Grassi, M., Di Luca, D. & Fiorentini, S. (2003). Human herpesvirus-6 modulates RANTES production in primary human endothelial cell cultures. *Journal of Medical Virology,* Vol.70, No.3, (July 2003), 451-458. ISSN 0146-6615

Ceccherini-Nelli, L., Rossi, L., Vanucchi, R., Barontini, L., Pistello, M., Ongrádi, J., Panicucci, F. & Bendinelli, M.HHV-6 seropositivity in HIV+ and HIV- hemophiliac patients. (1990). Annual Meeting of the Laboratory of Tumor Cell Biology, National Cancer Institute, Bethesda, MD, USA, 20-26 (August 1990). *AIDS Research and Human Retroviruses,* Vol.6, 151.

Chatterji, U., de Parseval, A. & Elder, J.H. (2002). Feline immunodeficiency virus OrfA is distinct from other lentivirus transactivators. *Journal of Virology,* Vol.76, No.19, (October 2002), 9624-9634. ISSN 0022-538x

Chen, M., Popescu, N., Woodworth, C., Berneman, Z., Corbellino, M., Lusso, P., Ablashi, D.V. & DiPaolo.J.A. (1994a). Human herpesvirus 6 infects cervical epithelial cells and transactivates human papillomavirus gene expression. *Journal of Virology,* Vol.68, No.2, (February 1994), 1173-1178. ISSN: 0022-538x.

Chen, M., Wang, H., Woodworth, C.D.,. Lusso, P., Berneman, Z., Kingma, D., Delgado, G. and DiPaolo, J.A. (1994b). Detection of human herpesvirus 6 and human papillomavirus 16 in cervical carcinoma. *American Journal of Pathology.* Vol.145, No.6, (December 1994), 1509-1516. ISSN 0002-9440

Clouse, K.A., Robbins, P.B., Fernie, B., Ostrove, J.M. & Fauci, A.S. (1989).Viral antigen stimulation of the production of human monokines capable of regulating HIV1 expression. *Journal of Immunology,* (July 1989) Vol.143, No.2, 470-475. ISSN 0022-1767

Cone, R.W., Huang, Meei-Li, W., Hackman RC. & Corey L. Coinfection with human herpesvirus 6 variants A and B in kung tissue. *Journal of Clinical Microbiology.* Vol.34, No.4, (April 1996), 877-881. ISSN 0095-1137

Corbellino, M., Lusso, P., Gallo, R,C,, Parravicini, C., Galli, M. & Moroni, M. (1993). Disseminated human herpesvirus 6 infection in AIDS. *Lancet*. Vol.342, No.8881, (November 1993), 1242. ISSN 0140-6736

Crowley, R.W., Secchiero, P., Zella, D., Cara, A., Gallo, R.C. & Lusso, P. (1996) Interference between human herpesvirus 7 and HIV-1 in mononuclear phagocytes. *Journal of Immunology*, Vol.156, No.5, (March 1996), 2004-2008. ISSN 0022-1767

Cuomo, L., Angeloni, A., Zompetta, C., Cirone, M., Calogero, A.,. Frati, L., Ragona, G. & Faggioni, A. (1995). Human herpesvirus 6 variant A, but not variant B, infects EBV-positive B lymphoid cells, activating the latent EBV genome through a BZLF-1-dependent mechanism. *AIDS Research and Human Retroviruses*, Vol.11, No.10, (October 1995), 1241-1245. ISSN 0889-2229

Cuomo, L., Trivedi, P., de Grazia, U., Calogero, A., D'Onofrio, M., Yan,g W., Frati, L., Faggioni, A., Rymo, L. & Ragona G. (1998). Upregulation of Epstein-Barr virus-encoded latent membrane protein by human herpesvirus 6 superinfection of EBV-carrying Burkitt lymphoma cells. *Journal of Medical Virology*, Vol.55, No.3, (July 1998), 219-226. ISSN 0146-6615

Davis, M.G., Kenney, S.C., Kamine, J., Pagano, J.S. & Huang, E.S. (1987). Immediate-early gene region of human cytomegalovirus trans-activates the promoter of human immunodeficiency virus. *Proceedings of National Academy of Sciences of the United States of America*, Vol.84, No.23, (December 1987), 8642-8646. ISSN 0027-8424

De Bolle, L., Naesens, L., De Clercq, E. (2005). Update on Human Herpesvirus 6 Biology, Clinical Features, and Therapy. *Clinical Microbiology Reviews*, Vol.18, No.1. (January 2005), 217-245. ISSN 0893-8512

De Clercq, E. & Naesens, L. (2006). In search of effective anti-HHV-6 agents. *Journal of Clinical Virology*. Vol.37, No.1, (December 2006), 82-86. ISSN 1386-6532

de Parseval, A. & Elder, J.H. (1999). Demonstration that orf2 encodes the feline immunodeficiency virus transactivating (Tat) protein and characterization of a unique gene product with partial rev activity. *Journal of Virology*, Vol.73, No.1, (January 1999), 608-617. ISSN 0022-538x

de Parseval, A., Grant, C.K., Sastry, K.J. & Elder, J.H. (2006). Sequential CD134-CXCR4 interactions in feline immunodeficiency virus (FIV): soluble CD134 activates FIV Env for CXCR4-dependent entry and reveals a cryptic neutralization epitope. *Journal of Virology*, Vol.80, No.6, (March 2006), 3088-91. ISSN 0022-538x

De Rossi, A., Franchini, G., Aldovini, A., Del Mistro, A., Chieco-Bianchi, L., Gallo, R.C. & Wong-Staal F. (1986). Differential response to the cytopathic effects of human T-cell lymphotropic virus type III (HTLV-III) superinfection in T4+ (helper) and T8+ (suppressor) T-cell clones transformed by HTLV-I. *Proceedings of National Academy of Sciences of the United States of America*, Vol.83, No.12, (June 1986), 4297-301. ISSN 0027-8424

Dean, G.A, Higgins, J., LaVoy, A., Fan, Z. & Pedersen, N.C. (1998). Measurement of feline cytokine gene expression by quantitative-competitive RT-PCR. *Veterinary Immunology and Immunpathology*, (May 1998) Vol.63, No.1-2, 73-82. ISSN 0921-4489

Dean, G.A. & Pedersen, N.C. (1998). Cytokine response in multiple lymphoid tissues during the primary phase of feline immunodeficiency virus infection. *Journal of Virology*, Vol.72, No.12, (December 1998), 9436-9440. ISSN 0022-538x

Dewin, D.R., Catusse, J. & Gompels, U.A. (2006) Identification and characterization of U83A viral chemokine, a broad and potent beta-chemokine agonist for human CCRs with unique selectivity and inhibition by spliced isoform. *Journal of Immunology,* Vol.176, No.1, (January 2006), 544-556. ISSN 0022-1767

Dhepakson, P., Mori, Y., Jiang, Y.B., Huang, H.L., Akkapaiboon, P., Okuno, T., and Yamanishi, K. (2002). Human herpesvirus-6 rep/U94 gene product has single-stranded DNA-binding activity. *Journal of General Virology,* Vol. 83, No.4, (April 2002), 847-854. ISSN 0022-1317

Di Luca, D., Secchiero, P., Bovenzi, P., Rotola, A., Caputo, A., Monini, P. & Cassai, E. (1991). Reciprocal in vitro interactions between human herpesvirus-6 and HIV-1 Tat. *AIDS,* Vol.5, No.9, (September 1991), 1095-1098. ISSN 0269-9370

Di Luca, D., Mirandola, P., Ravaioli, T., Dolcetti, R., Frigatti, A., Bovenzi, P., Sighinolfi, L., Monini, P. & Cassai. E. (1995). Human herpesviruses 6 and 7 in salivary glands and shedding in saliva of healthy and human immunodeficiency virus positive individuals. *Journal of Medical Virology,* Vol.45, No.4, (April 1995), 462-468. ISSN 0146-6615

Di Paolo, J.A., Popescu, N.C., Ablashi, D.V., Lusso, P., Zimonjic, D.B. & Woodworth C.D. (1994). Multistage carcinogenesis utilizing human genital cells and human papillomaviruses. Toxicology *Letters,* Vol.72, No.1-3, (June 1994), 7-11. ISSN 0378-4274.

Diehl, L.J., Mathiason-Dubard, C.K., O'Neil, L.L. & Hoover, EA. (1996). Plasma viral RNA load predicts disease progression in accelerated feline immunodeficiency virus infection. *Journal of Virology,* Vol.70. No.4, (April 1996), 2503-7. ISSN 0022-538x

Dominguez, G., Dambaugh, T.R., Stamey, F.R,, Dewhurst, S., Inoue, N. & Pellett, P.E. (1999). Human herpesvirus 6B genome sequence: coding content and comparison with human herpesvirus 6A. *Journal of Virology,* Vol.73. No.10, (October 1999), 8040-52. ISSN 0022-538x

Downing, R.G., Sewankambo, N., Serwadda, D., Honess, R., Crawford, D., Jarrett, R. & Griffin, B.E. (1987) Isolation of human lymphotropic herpesviruses from Uganda. *Lancet,* Vol. 2, No.8555, (August 1987), 390. ISSN 0140-6736

Drago, F., Ranieri, E., Malaguti, F., Battifoglio, M.L., Losi, E. & Rebora, A. (1997). Human herpesvirus 7 in patients with pityriasis rosea. Electron microscopy investigations and polymerase chain reaction in mononuclear cells, plasma and skin. *Dermatology,* Vol.195, No.4, (1997), 374-378. ISSN 1018-8665

Drobyski, W.R., Knox, K.K., Majewski, D. & Carrigan, D.R. (1994). Brief report: fatal encephalitis due to variant B human herpesvirus-6 infection in a bone marrow-transplant recipient. *New England Journal of Medicine,* Vol.330, No.19, (May 1994), 1356-1360. ISSN 0028-4793

Duclos, H., Elfassi, E., Michelson, S., Arenzana-Seisdedos, F., Hazan, U., Munier, A. & Virelizier JL.(1989). Cytomegalovirus infection and trans-activation of HIV-1 and HIV-2 LTRs in human astrocytoma cells. *AIDS Research and Human Retrovirusesroviruses,* (April 1989), Vol.5, No.2, 217-24. ISSN 0889-2229

Duesberg PH. (1989) Human immunodeficiency virus and acquired immunodeficiency syndrome: correlation but not causation. *Proceedings of National Academy of Sciences of the United States of America,* Vol.86, No.3, (February1989); 755–764. ISSN 0027-8424

Duvic M. (1991). Papulosquamous disorders associated with human immunodeficiency virus infection. *Clinical Dermatology,* Vol.9, No.3, (July1991), 523-550. ISSN 1075-6388.

Emery, V.C., Atkins, M.C., Bowen, E.F., Clark, D.A., Johnson, M.A., Kidd, I.M., McLaughlin, J.E., Phillips, A.N., Strappe, P.M. & Griffiths, P,D. (1999). Interactions between beta-herpesviruses and human immunodeficiency virus in vivo: evidence for increased human immunodeficiency viral load in the presence of human herpesvirus 6. *Journal of Medical Virology,* No.57, Vol.3, (March 1999), 278-282. ISSN 0146-6615

Ensoli, B., Lusso, P., Schachter, F., Josephs, S.F., Rappaport, J., Negro, F., Gallo, R.C. & Wong-Staal, F. Human herpes virus-6 increases HIV-1 expression in co-infected T cells via nuclear factors binding to the HIV-1 enhancer. *The European Molecular Biology Journal,* Vol.8, No.10, (October 1989), 3019-3027. ISSN 0261-4189

Flamand, L., Gosselin, J., D'Addario, M., Hiscott, J., Ablashi, D.V, Gallo, R.C. & Menezes, J. (1991). Human herpesvirus 6 induces interleukin-1 beta and tumor necrosis factor alpha, but not interleukin-6, in peripheral blood mononuclear cell cultures. *Journal of Virology,* Vol.65, No.9, (September 1991), 5105-5110. ISSN 0022-538x

Flamand, L., & Menezes, J. (1996). Cyclic AMP-responsive element-dependent activation of Epstein-Barr virus zebra promoter by human herpesvirus 6. *Journal of Virology,* Vol.70, No.3, (March 1996), 1784-1791. ISSN: 0022-538x.

Flamand, L., Romerio, F., Reitz, M.S. & Gallo R. C.. (1998). CD4 promoter transactivation by human herpesvirus 6. *Journal of Virology,* Vol.72, No.11, (November 1998), 8797-8805. ISSN: 0022-538x.

Flamand, L., Gosselin, J., Stefanescu, I., Ablashi, D. & Menezes, J. (1995). Immunosuppressive effect of human herpesvirus 6 on T-cell functions: suppression of interleukin-2 synthesis and cell proliferation. *Blood,* Vol.85, No.5, (March 1995), 1263-1271. ISSN 0006-4971

Flamand, L., Stefanescu, I. & Menezes, J. (1996). Human herpesvirus-6 enhances natural killer cell cytotoxicity via IL-15. *Journal of Clinical Investigation,* Vol.97, No.6, (March 1996), 1373-1381. ISSN 0021-9738

Flebbe-Rehwaldt, L.M., Wood, C. and Chandran, B. (2000). Characterization of transcripts expressed from human herpesvirus 6A strain GS immediate-early region B U16-U17 open reading frames. *Journal of Virology,* Vol.74, No.23, (December 2000) , 11040-11054. ISSN 0022-538X

Fox, J.D., Briggs, M., Ward, P.A. & Tedder, R.S. (1990) Human herpesvirus 6 in salivary glands. *Lancet,* Vol.336, No.8715, (September 1990) 590-593. ISSN 0140-6736

French, C., Menegazzi, P., Nicholson, L., Macaulay, H., Di Luca, D. & Gompels. U.A. (1999). Novel, nonconsensus cellular splicing regulates expression of a gene encoding a chemokine-like protein that shows high variation and is specific for human herpesvirus 6. *Virology,* Vol.262, No.1, (September 1999), 139-151 ISSN 0042-6822

Frenkel, N., Schirmer, E.C., Wyatt, L.S., Katsafanas, G., Roffman, E., Danovich, R.M. & June CH. (1990). *Proceedings of National Academy of Sciences of the United States of America,* Vol.87, No.2, 748-752. (January1990), Isolation of a new herpesvirus from human CD4+ T cells. Erratum in: *Proceedings of National Academy of Sciences of the United States of America,* Vol.87, No.19, (October 1990), 7797.

Fujisaki, H., Tanaka-Taya, K., Tanabe, H., Hara, T., Miyoshi, H., Okada, S. & Yamanishi, K. (1998). Detection of human herpesvirus 7 (HHV-7) DNA in breast milk by polymerase chain reaction and prevalence of HHV-7 antibody in breast-fed and bottle-fed children. *Journal of Medical Virology,* Vol.56, No.3, (November 1998), 275-279. ISSN 0146-6615

Furlini, G., Vignoli, M., Ramazzotti, E., Re, M.C., Visani, G. & La Placa. (1996). A concurrent human herpesvirus-6 infection renders two human hematopoietic progenitor (TF-1 and KG-1) cell lines susceptible to human immunodeficiency virus type-1. *Blood.* Vol.87, No.11, (June 1996), 4737-45. ISSN 0006-4971

Furukawa, M., Yasukawa, M., Yakushijin, Y. & Fujita, S. Distinct effects of human herpesvirus 6 and human herpesvirus 7 on surface molecule expression and function of CD4+ T cells. *Journal of Immunology.* Vol.152, No.12, (June 1994), 5768-5775. ISSN 0022-1767

Garzino-Demo, A., Chen, M., Lusso, P., Berneman, Z. & DiPaolo, J.A, (1996). Enhancement of TAT-induced transactivation of the HIV-1 LTR by two genomic fragments of HHV-6. *Journal of Medical Virology,* Vol.50, No.1, (September 1996), 20-24. ISSN 0146-6615

Gautheret, A., Aubin, J.T., Fauveau, V., Rozenbaum, W., Huraux, J,M. & Agut, H. (1995). Rate of detection of human herpesvirus-6 at different stages of HIV infection. *European Journal of Clinical Microbiology & Infectious Diseases,* Vol.14, No.9, (September 1995), 820-824. ISSN 0934-9723

Gautheret-Dejean A, Aubin JT, Poirel L, Huraux JM, Nicolas JC, Rozenbaum W, Agut H. (1997). Detection of human Betaherpesvirinae in saliva and urine from immunocompromised and immunocompetent subjects.*Journal of Clinical Microbiology,* Vol. 35, No.6, (June 1997), 1600-1603. ISSN 0095-1137

Gendelman, H.E., Phelps, W., Feigenbaum, L., Ostrove, J.M., Adachi, A., Howley, P.M., Khoury, G., Ginsberg, H.S. & Martin, M.A.(1986). Trans-activation of the human immunodeficiency virus long terminal repeat sequence by DNA viruses. *Proceedings of National Academy of Sciences of the United States of America,* Vol.83, No.24, (December 1986), 9759-9763. ISSN 0027-8424

Geng, Y.Q., Chandran, B., Josephs, S.F. & Wood, C. (1992). Identification and characterization of a human herpesvirus 6 gene segment that trans activates the human immunodeficiency virus type 1 promoter. *Journal of Virology* (March 1992), Vol.66, No.3, 1564-1570. ISSN 0022-538x

Ghazal, P. & Nelson, J.A. (1993). Interactions between cytomegalovirus immediate-early proteins and the long terminal repeat of human immunodeficiency virus. *Medical Virology,* Vol.3, No.1, (March 1993), 47-55. ISSN: 1052-9276

Gompels, U.A. & Kasolo, F.C. (2006). HHV-6 genome: Similar and different In: Kreuger AD, Ablashi D, editors. Human herpesvirus 6. 2nd edition. Oxford. UK: Elsevier. pp 23-46. ISSN 1132-6409

Gompels, U.A. & Macaulay, H.A. (1995). Characterization of human telomeric repeat sequences from human herpesvirus 6 and relationship to replication. *Journal of General Virology,* Vol.76, No.2, (February1995) 451-458. ISSN 0022-1317

Gompels, U.A., Nicholas, J., Lawrence, G., Jones, M., Thomson, B.J., Martin, M.E., Efstathiou, S., Craxton, M. & Macaulay, H.A. (1995). The DNA sequence of human herpesvirus-6: structure, coding content, and genome evolution. *Virology,* Vol.209, No.1, (May 1995), 29-51. ISSN 0042-6822

Gravel, A., Tomolu, A., Cloutier, N., Gosselin, J. & Flamand, L. (2003). Characterization of the immediate-early 2 protein of human herpesvirus 6, a promiscuous transcriptional activator. *Virology,* Vol.308, No.2, (April 2003) 340-353. ISSN 0042-6822

Gravel, A., Gosselin, J. & Flamand, L. (2002). Human herpesvirus 6 immediate-early 1 protein is a sumoylated nuclear phosphoprotein colocalizing with promyelocytic leukemia protein-associated nuclear bodies. *Journal of Biologcal Chemistry*, Vol.277, No.22, (May 2002), 19679-19687.ISSN 0021-9258

Griffiths, P.D., Ait-Khaled, M., Bearcroft, C.P., Clark, D. A., Quaglia, A,. Davies, S.E., Burroughs, A. K., Rolles, K., Kidd, I.M., Knight, S.N., Noibi, S.M., Cope, A.V., Phillips, A.N. & Emery, V.C. (1999). Human herpesviruses 6 and 7 as potential pathogens after liver transplant: prospective comparison with the effect of cytomegalovirus. *Journal of Medical Virology*, Vol.59, No.4, (December 1999), 496-501. ISSN 0146-6615

Grivel, J.C,. Ito, Y,. Faga, G,. Santoro, F,. Shaheen, F,. Malnati, M.S,. Fitzgerald, W,. Lusso, P. & Margolis, L. (2001). Suppression of CCR5- but not CXCR4-tropic HIV-1 in lymphoid tissue by human herpesvirus 6. *Nature Medicine*, Vol.7, No.11, (November 2001), 1232-1235. ISSN 1078-8956

Grivel, J.C,. Santoro, F,. Chen, S,. Faga, G,. Malnati, M.S,. Ito,Y,. Margolis, L. & Lusso, P. (2003). Pathogenic effects of human herpesvirus 6 in human lymphoid tissue ex vivo. *Journal of Virology*, Vol.77, No.15, (Augustus 2003), 8280-8289. ISSN 0022-538x

Hall, C.B,. Caserta, M.T,. Schnabel, K,. Shelley, L.M,. Marino, A.S,. Carnahan, J.A,. Yoo, C,. Lofthus, G.K. & McDermott, M.P. (2008). Chromosomal integration of human herpesvirus 6 is the major mode of congenital human herpesvirus 6 infection. *Pediatrics*, Vol,122, No.3, (September 2008), 513-520. ISSN 1098-4275

Hall, C.B., Caserta, M.T, Schnabel, K.C., Long, C., Epstein, L.G., Insel, R.A. & Dewhurst. S. (1998). Persistence of human herpesvirus 6 according to site and variant: possible greater neurotropism of variant A. *Clinical Infectious Diseases*, Vol.26, No.1, (January 1998), 132-137. ISSN 1058-4838

Hammarskjöld, M,L. & Simurda, M.C. Epstein-Barr virus latent membrane protein transactivates the human immunodeficiency virus type 1 long terminal repeat through induction of NF-kappa B activity. *Journal of Virology*, Vol.66, No.11, (November 1992), 6496-501. ISSN 0022-538x

Herbein, G., Strasswimmer, J., Altieri, M., Woehl-Jaegle, M.L., Wolf, P. & Obert, G. (1996). Longitudinal study of human herpesvirus 6 infection in organ transplant recipients. *Clinical Infectious Diseases*, Vol.22, No.1, (January 1996) 171-173. ISSN 1058-4838

Hierholzer, J.C., Wigand, R., Anderson, L.J., Adrian, T. & Gold, J.W. (1988). Adenoviruses from patients with AIDS: a plethora of serotypes and a description of five new serotypes of subgenus D (types 43-47). *Journal of Infectious Diseases*, Vol.158, No.4, (October 1988), 804-13. ISSN 0022-1899

Horvat, R.T., Parmely. M.J. & Chandran, B. (1993). Human herpesvirus 6 inhibits the proliferative responses of human peripheral blood mononuclear cells. Journal of Infectious Disease. Vol.167, No.6, (June 1993), 1274-1280. ISSN 0022-1899

Horvat, R.T., Wood, C., Josephs, S.F. & Balachandran, N. (1991). Transactivation of the human immunodeficiency virus promoter by human herpesvirus 6 (HHV-6) strains GS and Z-29 in primary human T lymphocytes and identification of transactivating HHV-6(GS) gene fragments. *Journal of Virology*, Vol.65, No.6, (June 1991), 2895-2902. ISSN 0022-538x

Hosie, M.J., Robertson, C. & Jarrett, O. (1989). Prevalence of feline leukaemia virus and antibodies to feline *Veterinary Records*, Vol.125, No.11, (September 1989), 293-297. ISSN 0042-4900

Hudson, A.W., Blom, D., Howley, P.M. & Ploegh, H.L. (2003), The ER-lumenal domain of the HHV-7 immunoevasin U21 directs class I MHC molecules to lysosomes. *Traffic,* No.4, Vol.12, (December 2003), 824-37. ISSN 1600-0854

Inagi, R., Guntapong, R., Nakao, M., Ishino, Y., Kawanishi, K., Isegawa, Y. & Yamanishi, K. (1996), Human herpesvirus 6 induces IL-8 gene expression in human hepatoma cell line, Hep G2. *Journal of Medical Virology,* Vol,49. No.1, (May 1996), 34-40. ISSN 0146-6615

Inoue, Y., Yasukawa, M. & Fujita, S. (1997). Induction of T-cell apoptosis by human herpesvirus 6. *Journal of Virology,* Vol.71, No.5, (May 1997), 3751-3759. ISSN: 0022-538x

Isegawa, Y., Katahira, J., Yamanishi, K. & Sugimoto, N. (2007). Reactivation of latent human immunodeficiency virus 1 by human herpesvirus 6 infection. *Acta Virologica* (2007), Vol.51, No.1, 13-20. ISSN 0001-723X

Isegawa, Y., Ping, Z., Nakano, K., Sugimoto, N. & Yamanishi, K. (1998). Human herpesvirus 6 open reading frame U12 encodes a functional beta-chemokine receptor. *Journal of Virology.* Vol.72, No.7, (July 1998), 6104-6112. ISSN: 0022-538x

Ishida, T., Washizu, T., Toriyabe, K., Motoyoshi, S., Tomoda, I. & Pedersen, N.C. (1989). Feline immunodeficiency virus infection in cats of Japan. *Journal of the American Veterinary Medical Axssociation,* Vol.194, No.2, (January 1989), 221-225. ISSN 0003-1488

Iuliano, R., Trovato, R., Lico, S., Luppi, M., Forastieri, G., Barsanti, L.A., Pizzigallo, A.M., Mecocci, L., Barozzi, P., Torelli, G., Mazzotta, F. & Ceccherini-Nelli L. (1997). Human herpesvirus-6 reactivation in a longitudinal study of two HIV-1 infected patients. *Journal of Medical Virology,* Vol.51, No.4, (April 1997), 259-264. ISSN 0146-6615

Janelle, M.E. & Flamand, L. Phenotypic alterations and survival of monocytes following infection by human herpesvirus-6. *Archieves of Virology,* Vol.151, No.8, (Augustus 2006), 1603-14. ISSN 034-8608

Kakimoto, M., Hasegawa, A., Fujita, S. & Yasukawa. M. (2002). Phenotypic and functional alterations of dendritic cells induced by human herpesvirus 6 infection. *Journal of Virology.* Vol.76, No.20, (October 2002), 10338-10345. ISSN: 0022-538x

Kashanchi, F., Araujo, J., Doniger, J., Muralidhar, S., Hoch, R., Khleif, S., Mendelson, E., Thompson, J., Azumi, N., Brady, J., N. Luppi, M., Torelli G. & Rosenthal. L. J. (1997). Human herpesvirus 6 (HHV-6) ORF-1 transactivating gene exhibits malignant transforming activity and its protein binds to p53. *Oncogene,* Vol.14, No.3, (January 1997), 359-367. ISSN 0950-9232

Kashanchi, F., Thompson, J. Sadaie, M. R. Doniger, J. Duvall, J. Brady, J. N. and Rosenthal. L. J. (1994). Transcriptional activation of minimal HIV-1 promoter by ORF-1 protein expressed from the SalI-L fragment of human herpesvirus 6. *Virology,* Vol.201, No.1, (May 1994), 95-106. ISSN 0042-6822

Kasolo, F.C., Monze, M., Obel, N., Anderson, R.A., French, C. & Gompels, U.A. (1998). Sequence analyses of human herpesvirus-8 strains from both African human immunodeficiency virus-negative and -positive childhood endemic Kaposi's sarcoma show a close relationship with strains identified in febrile children and high variation in the K1 glycoprotein. *Journal of General Virology,* (December 1998), Vol.79, No.12, 3055-3065. ISSN 0022-1317

Kasolo, F.C., Mpabalwani, E. & Gompels, U.A. (1997). Infection with AIDS-related herpesviruses in human immunodeficiency virus-negative infants and endemic childhood Kaposi's sarcoma in Africa. *Journal of General Virology*, Vol.78, No.Pt 4, (April 1997), 847-855. ISSN 0022-1317

Katsafanas, G.C., Schirmer, E.C., Wyatt, L.S. & Frenkel, N. (1996), In vitro activation of human herpesviruses 6 and 7 from latency. *Proceedings of National Academy of Sciences of the United States of America*, Vol.93, No.18, (September 1996), 9788-9792. ISSN 0027-8424

Kawaguchi, Y., Maeda, K., Miyazawa, T., Ono, M., Tsubota, K., Tomonaga, K. & Mikami, T. (1994). Inhibition of feline immunodeficiency virus gene expression and replication by alphaherpesvirus ICP4 homologues. *Journal of General Virology*, Vol. 75, No.10., (October 1994), 2783-2787. ISSN 0022-1317

Kawaguchi, Y., Maeda, K., Pecoraro, M.R., Inoshima, Y., Jang, H.K., Kohmoto, M. Iwatsuki, K., Ikeda, Y., Shimojima, M. & Tohya, Y., et al (1995). The feline herpesvirus type 1 ICP4 down-regulates feline immunodeficiency virus long terminal repeat (LTR)-directed gene expression via the C/EBP site in the LTR. *Journal of Veterinary Medical Science*. Vol.57, No.6, (December 1995), 1129-1131. ISSN 0916-7250

Kawaguchi, Y., Miyazawa, T., Horimoto, T., Itagaki, S., Fukasawa, M., Takahashi, E. & Mikami, T. (1991). Activation of feline immunodeficiency virus long terminal repeat by feline herpesvirus type 1. *Virology*, Vol.184, No.1, (September 1991), 449-454. ISSN 0916-7250. ISSN 0042-6822

Kempf, W., Adams, V., Mirandola, P., Menotti, L., Di Luca, D., Wey, N., Müller, B. & Campadelli-Fiume, G. (1998). Persistence of human herpesvirus 7 in normal tissues detected by expression of a structural antigen. *Journal of Infectious Diseases*. Vo.178, No.3, (September 1998), 841-845. ISSN 0934-9723

Kempf, W., Adams, V., Wey, N., Moos, R., Schmid, M., Avitabile, E. & Campadelli-Fiume, G. (1997). CD68+ cells of monocyte/macrophage lineage in the environment of AIDS-associated and classic-sporadic Kaposi sarcoma are singly or doubly infected with human herpesviruses 7 and 6B. *Proceedings of National Academy of Sciences of the United States of America*, Vol.94, No.14, (July 1997), 7600-7605. ISSN 0027-8424

Kenney, S., Kamine, J., Markovitz, D., Fenrick, R. & Pagano, J. (1988). An Epstein-Barr virus immediate-early gene product trans-activates gene expression from the human immunodeficiency virus long terminal repeat. *Proceedings of National Academy of Sciences of the United States of America*, Vol.85, No.5, (March 1988), 1652-1656. ISSN 0027-8424

Kikuta, H., Nakane, A., Lu, H., Taguchi, Y., Minagawa, T. & Matsumoto, S. (1990a). Interferon induction by human herpesvirus 6 in human mononuclear cells. *Journal of Infectious Diseases*, (July 1990), Vol.162, No.1, 35-38. ISSN 0022-1899

Kirn, E., Krueger, E., Boehmer, S., Klussmann, J.P. & Krueger. G.R. (1997). In vitro cytobiological effects of human herpesviruses 6 and 7: immunohistological monitoring of apoptosis, differentiation and cell proliferation. *Anticancer Research*, Vol.17, No.6, (November-December 1997), 4623-4632. ISSN 0250-7005

Knox, K.K. & Carrigan, D.R. (1995). Active human herpesvirus (HHV-6) infection of the central nervous system in patients with AIDS. *Journal of Acquired Immune Deficiency Syndromes and Human Retrovirology*, Vol.9, No.1, (May 1995), 69-73. ISSN 0003-4819

Knox, K.K. & Carrigan, D.R. (1996). Active HHV-6 infection in the lymph nodes of HIV-infected patients: in vitro evidence that HHV-6 can break HIV latency.*Journal of*

Acquired Immune Deficiency Syndromes and Human Retrovirology, Vol.11, No.4, (April 1996), 370-378. ISSN 0003-4819

Knox, K.K. & Carrigan, D.R. (1994). Disseminated active HHV-6 infections in patients with AIDS. *Lancet*. (March 1994), Vol.343, No.8897, 577-578. ISSN 0140-6736

Kondo, K., Kondo, T., Okuno, T., Takahashi, M. & Yamanishi. K. (1991). Latent human herpesvirus 6 infection of human monocytes/macrophages. *Journal of General Virology*, Vol.72, No.6, (June 1991), ISSN 1401-1408

Kondo, K., Shimada, K., Sashihara, J., Tanaka-Taya, K. and Yamanishi. K. 2002. Identification of human herpesvirus 6 latency-associated transcripts. *Journal of Virology*, Vol.76, No.8, (April 2002), 4145-4151. ISSN 0022-538x.

Kositanont, U., Wasi, C., Wanprapar, N., Bowonkiratikachorn, P., Chokephaibulkit, K., Chearskul, S., Chimabutra, K., Sutthent, R., Foongladda, S., Inagi, R., Kurata, T. & Yamanishi, K. (1999). Primary infection of human herpesvirus 6 in children with vertical infection of human immunodeficiency virus type 1. *Journal of Infectious Diseases*. Vol.180, No.1, (July 1999), 50-55. ISSN 0934-9723

Kraus, L.A., Bradley, W.G., Engelman, R.W., Brown, K.M., Good, R.A. & Day, N.K. (1996). Relationship between tumor necrosis factor alpha and feline immunodeficiency virus expressions. *Journal of Virology*, Vol.70, No.1, (January 1996), 566-569. ISSN 0022-538x

Kucera, L.S., Leake, E., Iyer, N., Raben, D. & Myrvik, Q.N. (1990). Human immunodeficiency virus type 1 (HIV-1) and herpes simplex virus type 2 (HSV-2) can coinfect and simultaneously replicate in the same human CD4+ cell: effect of coinfection on infectious HSV-2 and HIV-1 replication. *AIDS Research and Human Retroviruses*. Vol.6, No.5, (May 1990), 641-647. ISSN 0889-2229

Lakatos, B., Farkas, J., Ádám, É., Dobay, O., Jeney, Cs., Nász, I. & Ongrádi, J. (2000). Serological evidence of adenovirus infection in cats. *Archieves of Virology*, Vol.145, No.5, (2000), 1029-1033, ISSN 0304-8608

Lakatos, B., Farkas, J., Ádám, É., Jarrett, O., Egberink, H.F., Bendinelli, M., Nász, I. & Ongrádi, J. (1996). Data to the adenovirus infection of European cats. *Hungarian Veterinary Journal*, Vol.51, (1996), 543-545. ISSN 0025-004X

Lakatos, B., Farkas, J., Egberink, H.F., Vennema, H., Horzinek, M.C., van Vliet, A., Rossen, J., Benkő, M. & Ongrádi, J. (1997). PCR detection of adenovirus in a cat. *Hungarian Veterinary Journal*, Vol.119, (1997), 517-519. ISSN 0025-004x

Lennette, E.T., Busch, M.P., Hecht, F.M. & Levy, J.A. (2005). Potential herpesvirus interaction during HIV type 1 primary infection. *AIDS Research and Human Retroviruses*, Vol.21, No.10, (October 2005), 869-875. ISSN 0889-2229

Levy, J.A. Pathogenesis of human immunodeficiency virus infection. *Microbiol Reviews*, Vol.57, No.1, (March 1993), 183-289. ISSN 0983-8512

Levy, J.A., Ferro, F., Greenspan, D. & Lennette, E.T. (1990a). Frequent isolation of HHV-6 from saliva and high seroprevalence of the virus in the population. *Lancet*, Vol.335, No.8697, (May 1990), 1047-1050. ISSN 0140-6736

Levy, J.A., Hsueh, F., Blackbourn, D.J., Wara, D. & Weintrub, P.S. (1988). CD8 cell noncytotoxic antiviral activity in human immunodeficiency virus-infected and -uninfected children. *Journal of Infectious Diseases*, No.177, No.2, (February 1998), 470-472. ISSN 0934-9723

Levy, J.A., Landay, A. & Lennette, E.T. (1990b). Human herpesvirus 6 inhibits human immunodeficiency virus type 1 replication in cell culture. *Journal of Clinical Microbiology*, (October 1990), Vol.28, No.10, 2362-2364. ISSN 0095-1137

Li, C., Goodrich, J.M. & Yang, X. (1997). Interferon-gamma (IFN-gamma) regulates production of IL-10 and IL-12 in human herpesvirus-6 (HHV-6)-infected monocyte/macrophage lineage. *Clinical and Experimental Immunology*, Vol.109, No.3, (September 1997), 421-425 ISSN 0009-9104

Lippé, R., Luke, E., Kuah, Y.T., Lomas, C. & Jefferies, W.A. (1991). Adenovirus infection inhibits the phosphorylation of major histocompatibility complex class I proteins. *Journal of Experimental Medicine*, Vol.174, No.5, (November 1991), 1159-1166. ISSN 0022-1007

Lisco, A., Grivel, J.C., Biancotto, A., Vanpouille, C., Origgi, F., Malnati, M.S., Schols, D., Lusso, P. & Margolis, L.B. (2007). Viral interactions in human lymphoid tissue: Human herpesvirus 7 suppresses the replication of CCR5-tropic human immunodeficiency virus type 1 via CD4 modulation. *Journal of Virology*, Vol.81, No.2, (January 2007), 708-717. ISSN 0022-538x

Lopez, C., Pellett, P., Stewart, J., Goldsmith, C., Sanderlin, K., Black, J., Warfield, D. (1988). Feorino, P. Characteristics of human herpesvirus-6. *Journal of Infectious Diseases*, Vol.157, No.6, (June1988), 1271-1273. ISSN 0934-9723

Lucht, E., Brytting, M., Bjerregaard, L., Julander, I. & Linde A. (1998). Shedding of cytomegalovirus and herpesviruses 6, 7, and 8 in saliva of human immunodeficiency virus type 1-infected patients and healthy controls. *Clinical Infectious Diseases*, Vol.27, No.1, (July 1998), 137-141. ISSN 1058-4838

Luiz, L.N., Leite, J.P., Yokosawa, J., Carneiro, B.M., Pereira, Filho, E., Oliveira, T.F., Freitas, G.R., Costa, L.F., Paula, N.T., Silveira, H.L., Nepomuceno, J.C. & Queiróz, D.A. (2010). Molecular characterization of adenoviruses from children presenting with acute respiratory disease in Uberlândia, Minas Gerais, Brazil, and detection of an isolate genetically related to feline adenovirus. *Memórias do Instituto Oswaldo Cruz*, (Augustus 2010), Vol.105, No.5, 712-716. ISSN 0074-0276

Luppi, M., Marasca, R., Barozzi, P, Ferrari, S., Ceccherini-Nelli, L., Batoni, G., Merelli, E. & Torelli, G. (1993).Three cases of human herpesvirus-6 latent infection: integration of viral genome in peripheral blood mononuclear cell DNA. Journal of Medical Virology, Vol.40, No.1, (May 1993), 44-52. ISSN 0146-6615

Lusso, P., Crowley, R.W., Malnati, M.S., Di Serio, C., Ponzoni, M., Biancotto, A., Markham, P.D. & Gallo, R.C. (2007). Human herpesvirus 6A accelerates AIDS progression in macaques. *Proceedings of National Academy of Sciences of the United States of America* Vol.104, No.12, (March 2007), 5067-5072. ISSN 0027-8424

Lusso, P., De Maria, A., Malnati, M., Lori, F., DeRocco, S.E., Baseler, M., Gallo, R.C. (1991). Induction of CD4 and susceptibility to HIV-1 infection in human CD8+ T lymphocytes by human herpesvirus 6. *Nature*, Vol.349, No.6309, (February 1991), 533-535. ISSN 0028-0836

Lusso, P., Ensoli, B., Markham, P.D., Ablashi, D.V., Salahuddin, S.Z., Tschachler, E., Wong-Staal, F. & Gallo, R.C. Productive dual infection of human CD4+ T lymphocytes by HIV-1 and HHV-6. *Nature.* Vol.337, No.6205, (January 1989), 370-373. ISSN 0028-0836

Lusso, P. & Gallo, R.C. (1995). Human herpesvirus 6 in AIDS. *Immunology Today*, Vol.16, No.2, (February 1995), 67-71. ISSN 0167-5699

Lusso, P., Malnati, M.S., Garzino-Demo, A., Crowley, R.W., Long, E.O. & Gallo, R.C. (1993). Infection of natural killer cells by human herpesvirus 6. *Nature,* Vol.362, No.6419, (April 1993), 458-462. ISSN 0028-0836

Lusso, P., Markham, P.D., DeRocco, S.E. & Gallo, R.C. (1990). In vitro susceptibility of T lymphocytes from chimpanzees (Pan troglodytes) to human herpesvirus 6 (HHV-6): a potential animal model to study the interaction between HHV-6 and human immunodeficiency virus type 1 in vivo. *Journal of Virology,* Vol.64, No.6, (June 1990), 2751- 2758. ISSN 0022-538x

Lusso, P., Secchiero, P. & Crowley, R.W. (1994). In vitro susceptibility of Macaca nemestrina to human herpesvirus 6: a potential animal model of coinfection with primate immunodeficiency viruses. *AIDS Research and Human Retroviruses,* Vol.10, No.2, (February 1994), 181-187. ISSN 0889-2229

Mangasarian, A., Piguet, V., Wang, J.K., Chen, Y.L. & Trono, D. (1999). Nef-induced CD4 and major histocompatibility complex class I (MHC-I) down-regulation are governed by distinct determinants: N terminal alpha helix and proline repeat of Nef selectively regulate MHC-I trafficking. *Journal of Virology,* Vol.73, No.3, (March 1999),1964-1973. ISSN 0022-538x

Maródi, C.L., Csiszár, A., Sierra-Vazquez, B., Di Luca, D., Barabás, É., Nagy, K. & Ongrádi, J. (1998). Studies on the antibodies to human herpesvirus type 6 among Hungarian patients with asymptomatic HIV infection. *Pathology Oncology Research,* Vol.4, No.1, (1998), 56-61. ISSN 1219-4956

Martin, M.E., Nicholas, J., Thomson, B.J., Newman, C. & Honess, R.W. (1991). Identification of a transactivating function mapping to the putative immediate-early locus of human herpesvirus 6. *Journal of Virology,* Vol. 65, No.10, (October 1991), 5381-90. ISSN 0022-538x

Martínez, P.A., Díaz, R., González, D., Oropesa, L., González, R., Pérez, L., Viera, J. & Kourí, V. (2007). The effect of highly active antiretroviral therapy on outcome of central nervous system herpesviruses infection in Cuban human immunodeficiency virus-infected individuals. *Journal of Neurovirology,* Vol.13, No.5, 446-51. (October 2007), ISSN 1355-0248

Mayne, M., Cheadle, C., Soldan, S. S., Cermelli, C., Yamano, Y., Akhyani, N., Nagel, J.E., Taub, D.D., Becker, K.G. & Jacobson, S. (2001). Gene expression profile of herpesvirus-infected T cells obtained using immunomicroarrays: induction of proinflammatory mechanisms. *Journal of Virology,* Vol.75, No.23, (December 2001), 11641-11650. ISSN 0022-538x

McCarthy, M., Auger, D., He, J. & Wood, C. (1998). Cytomegalovirus and human herpesvirus-6 trans-activate the HIV-1 long terminal repeat via multiple response regions in human fetal astrocytes. *Journal of Neurovirology,* Vol.4, No.5, (October 1998), 495-511. ISSN 1355-0248

Megaw, A.G., Rapaport, D., Avidor, B., Frenkel, N. & Davison, A.J. (1998). The DNA sequence of the RK strain of human herpesvirus 7. *Virology,* Vol.244, No.1, (April 1998), 119-132. ISSN 0042-6822

Menotti, L., Mirandola, P., Locati, M. & Campadelli-Fiume, G. (1999). Trafficking to the plasma membrane of the seven-transmembrane protein encoded by human herpesvirus 6 U51 gene involves a cellspecific function present in T lymphocytes. *Journal of Virology,* Vol.73, No.1, (January 1999), 325-333. ISSN 0022-538x

Milne, R.S., Mattick, C., Nicholson, L., Devaraj, P., Alcami, A. & Gompels. U. A. (2000). RANTES binding and down-regulation by a novel human herpesvirus-6 beta chemokine receptor. *Journal of Immunology*, Vol.164, No.5, (March 2005), 2396-2404. ISSN 002-1767

Mirandola, P., Menegazzi, P., Merighi, S., Ravaioli, T., Cassai, E. & Di Luca D. (1998). Temporal mapping of transcripts in herpesvirus 6 variants. *Journal of Virology* Vol.72, No.5, (May 1995), 3837-3844. ISSN 0022-538x.

Mori, Y., Dhepakson, P., Shimamoto, T., Ueda, K., Gomi, Y., Tani, H., Matsuura, Y. & Yamanishi, K. (2000). Expression of human herpesvirus 6B within infected cells and binding of its gene product to the TATA-binding protein in vitro and in vivo. *Journal of Virology*, Vol.74, No.13, (July 2000), 6096-6104. ISSN 0022-538x.

Mori, Y., Seya, T., Huang, H.L., Akkapaiboon, P., Dhepakson, P. & Yamanishi K. (2002). Human herpesvirus 6 variant A but not variant B induces fusion from without in a variety of human cells through a human herpesvirus 6 entry receptor, CD46. *Journal of Virology*, Vol.76, No.13, (July 2002), 6750-6761. ISSN 0022-538x

Mori, Y., Yagi, H., Shimamoto, T., Isegawa, Y., Sunagawa, T., Inagi, R., Kondo, K., Tano, Y. & Yamanishi, K. (1998). Analysis of human herpesvirus 6 U3 gene, which is a positional homolog of human cytomegalovirus UL 24 gene. *Virology*, Vol.249, No.1, (September 1998), 129-139. ISSN 0042-6822

Mori, Y., Yang, X. Akkapaiboon, P. Okuno, T. & Yamanishi K. (2003). Human herpesvirus 6 variant A glycoprotein H- glycoprotein L-glycoprotein Q complex associates with human CD46. *Journal of Virology*, Vol.77, No.8, (April 2003), 4992-4999. ISSN 0022-538x.

Morissette, G., & Flamand, L. (2010). Herpesviruses and chromosomal integration. *Journal of Virology*, Vol.84, No.23, (December 2010), 12100-121009. ISSN 0022-538X

Mosca, J.D., Bednarik, D.P., Raj, N.B., Rosen, C.A., Sodroski, J.G., Haseltine, W.A., Hayward, G.S., Pitha, P.M. (1987a). Activation of human immunodeficiency virus by herpesvirus infection: identification of a region within the long terminal repeat that responds to a trans-acting factor encoded by herpes simplex virus 1. *Proceedings of National Academy of Sciences of the United States of America*, Vol.84, No.21, (November 1987), 7408-7412. ISSN 0027-8424

Mosca, J.D., Bednarik, D.P., Raj, N.B., Rosen, C.A., Sodroski, J.G., Haseltine, W.A. & Pitha, P.M. (1987b). Herpes simplex virus type-1 can reactivate transcription of latent human immunodeficiency virus. *Nature*, Vol.325, No.6099, (January 1987), 67-70. ISSN 0028-0836

Nabel, G. & Baltimore, D. (1987). An inducible transcription factor activates expression of human immunodeficiency virus in T cells. *Nature*. Vol.326, No.6114, (April 1987), 711-713. ISSN 0028-0836

Nabel, G.J., Rice, S.A., Knipe, D.M. & Baltimore, D. (1988). Alternative mechanisms for activation of human immunodeficiency virus enhancer in T cells. *Science*, Vol.239, No.4845, (March 1988), 1299-302. ISSN 0036-8075

Nicholas, J. (1996). Determination and analysis of the complete nucleotide sequence of human herpesvirus. *Journal of Virology*, Vol.70, No.9, (September 1996), 5975- 5989. ISSN 0022-538x

Nicholas, J. & Martin, M.E. (1994). Nucleotide sequence analysis of a 38.5-kilobase-pair region of the genome of human herpesvirus 6 encoding human cytomegalovirus immediate-early gene homologs and transactivating functions. *Journal of Virology*, Vol.68, No.2, (Februar 1994), 597-610. ISSN 0022-538x.

Niiya, H., Azuma, T., Jin, L., Uchida, N., Inoue, A., Hasegawa, H., Fujita, S., Tohyama, M., Hashimoto, K. & Yasukawa, M. (2004). Transcriptional downregulation of DC-SIGN in human herpesvirus 6-infected dendritic cells.*Journal of General Virology*, Vol.85, No.9, (September 2004), 2639-2642. ISSN 0022-1317

Nikolaou, K., Varinou, L., Inoue, N. & Arsenakis, M. (2003). Identification and characterization of gene products of ORF U90/89 of human herpesvirus 6. *Acta Virologica* Vol.47, No.1, (2003), 17-26. ISSN 0001-723X

Ohno, K., Nakano, T., Matsumoto, Y., Watari, T., Goitsuka, R., Nakayama, H., Tsujimoto, H. & Hasegawa, A. (1993). Apoptosis induced by tumor necrosis factor in cells chronically infected with feline immunodeficiency virus. *Journal of Virology*, Vol.67, No.5, (May 1993), 2429-2433. ISSN 0022-538x

Okuno, T., Oishi, H., Hayashi, K., Nonogaki, M., Tanaka, K. & Yamanishi, K. (1995). Human herpesviruses 6 and 7 in cervixes of pregnant women. *Journal of Clinical Microbiology*, Vol.33, No.7, (July1995), 1968-1970. ISSN 0095-1137

Ongrádi, J. (1999). Identification of a feline adenovirus isolate that replicates in monkey and human cells in vitro *American Journal of Veterinary Research.* Vol.60, No.12, 1463. (December 1999), ISSN 0002-9645.

Ongrádi, J., Ahmad, A. & Menezes, J. (1999a). In vitro cytokine induction by HHV-7 in leukocytes. *Hungarian Medical Journal*, Vol.140 (1999), 1935-1939. ISSN 1216- 8335

Ongrádi, J., Bánhegyi, D., Maródi,C.L., Nagy, K., Csiszár, A. & Horváth, A. (1999b). Antibody titres to HHV-6A at risk and during the course of HIV infection. *Hungarian Medical Journal*, Vol.140, 1881-1885. ISSN 1216-8335

Ongrádi, J., Becker, K., Horváth, A., Hidvégi, E. & Mezey, I. (2000a). Simultaneous infection by human herpesvirus 7 and human parvovirus B19 in papular-purpuric gloves-and-socks syndrome. *Archieves of Dermatology*, Vol.136, No.5, (May 2000), 672. ISSN 0003-987x

Ongrádi, J., Laird, H.M., Szilágyi, J.F., Horváth, A. & Bendinelli, M. (2000b). Unique morphological alterations of the HTLV-I transformed C8166 cells by infection with HIV-1. *Pathology Oncology Research*, Vol.6, No.1, (2000), 27-37. ISSN 1219-4956

Ongrádi, J., Ceccherini-Nelli, L., Matteucci, D., Bertók, L. & Bendinelli, M. (1999c). Human herpesvirus variant A enhances in vitro HIV-1 replication by soluble mediators, which effect is diminished by endotoxin. *Hungarian Medical Journal*, Vol.140, (1999), 2577-2579. ISSN 1216- 8335

Ongrádi, J., Ceccherini-Nelli, L., Soldaini, E., Bendinelli, M., Conaldi, P.G., Specter, S. & Friedman, H. (1990b). Endotoxin suppresses indirect activation of HIV-1 by human herpesvirus 6. In: Cellular and molecular aspects of endotoxin reactions. Eds: Nowotny, A., Spitzer, J.J. & Ziegler, E.J. Elsevier Science Publishers B.V., Amsterdam, (1990), p.387-394. ISBN 0-444-81365-9

Ongrádi, J., Csiszár, A., Maródi, C.L, Sólyom, J., Horváth, A. & Menezes J. (1999d). Onset of antibodies to human herpesvirus types 6 and 7 in Hungarian children. *Hungarian Medical Journal*, Vol.140, No.17, (1999), 935-940. ISSN 1216- 8335

Ongrádi, J., Iuliano, R., Rossi, M., Ceccherini-Nelli, L. (1994). Transcellular transactivation of HIV-1 by HHV-6Role of humoral factors in the progression of HIV disease, Sopron. *Acta Microbiologica et Immunologica Hungarica* Vol.52, (1994), 41. ISSN 1217-8950

Ongrádi, J., Laird, H.M., Szilágyi, J.F., Horváth, A. & Bendinelli,M. (2000b). Unique morphological alterations of the HTLV-I transformed C8166 cells by infection with HIV-1 *Pathology Oncology Research,* Vol.6, No.1, (2000), 27-37. ISSN 1219-4956

Ongrádi, J., Maródi, C.L., Nagy, K., Csiszár. A., Bánhegyi, D. & Horváth A. (1999e). Risk of HHV-6A primary infections at risk and recurrent infections during the course of AIDS. *Journal of Acquired Immune Deficiency Syndromes and Human Retrovirology.* Vol.22, No.3, (November 1999), 311-312, ISSN 0003-4819

Ongrádi, J., Pistello, M., Mazzetti, P., Zaccaro, L. & Bendinelli, M. (1996). Cytokines activate feline immunodeficiency virus (FIV) in macrophages. *Acta Microbiologica et Immunologica Hungarica,* Vol.43, (1996), 224. ISSN 1217-8950

Ongrádi, J., Rajda, C., Maródi, C.L., Csiszár, A. & Vécsei, L. (1999f). A pilot study on the antibodies to HHV-6 variants and HHV- 7 in CSF of MS patients. Journal of *Neurovirology,* Vol.5, No.5, (October 1999), 529-532. ISSN 1355- 0248

Ongrádi, J., Sonkoly, E., Kövesdi, V. & Széll, M. (2006). Cytokine pattern alterations in CD4 T lymphocytes by human herpesvirus 6B infection. 5th International Conference on HHV-6 and 7, Barcelona, Spain, April 30-May 3rd, 2006, Program Book, p. 45. *Journal of Clinical Virology,* 37, S106, 2006. ISSN1386-6532

Paulson. E., Tran, C., Collins, K. & Früh, K. (2001). KSHV-K5 inhibits phosphorylation of the major histocompatibility complex class I cytoplasmic tail. *Virology,* Vol.288, No.2, (September 2001), 369-378. ISSN 0042-6822

Pedersen, N.C., Torten, M., Rideout, B., Sparger, E., Tonachini, T., Luciw, P.A., Ackley, C., Levy, N. & Yamamoto J. (1990). Feline leukemia virus infection as a potentiating cofactor for the primary and secondary stages of experimentally induced feline immunodeficiency virus infection. *Journal of Virology,* Vol.64, No.2, (February 1990), 598-606. ISSN 0022-538x

Phan, T.G., Shimizu, H., Nishimura, S., Okitsu, S., Maneekarn, N. & Ushijima, H. (2006). Human adenovirus type 1 related to feline adenovirus: evidence of interspecies transmission. *Clinical Laboratory,* Vol.52, No.9-10, (2006), 515-518. ISSN 1433-6510

Popik, W. & Pitha, P.M.(1994). Differential effect of tumor necrosis factor-alpha and herpes simplex virus type 1 on the Tat-targeted inhibition of human immunodeficiency virus type 1 replication. *Virology,* Vol.202, No.2, (Augustus 1994), 521-529. ISSN 0042-6822

Portolani, M., Cermelli, C., Mirandola, P. & Di Luca, D. (1995). Isolation of human herpesvirus 7 from an infant with febrile syndrome. *Journal of Medical Virology,* Vol.45, No.3, (March 1995), 282-283. ISSN 0146-6615

Potenza, L., Luppi, M., Barozzi, P., Rossi, G., Cocchi, S., Codeluppi, M., Pecorari, M., Masetti, M., Di Benedetto, F., Gennari, W., Portolani, M., Gerunda, G.E., Lazzarotto, T., Landini, M.P., Schulz, T.F., Torelli, G. & Guaraldi, G. (2008). HHV-6A in syncytial giant-cell hepatitis. *New England Journal of Medicine,* Vol. 359, No.6, (Augustus 2008), 593-602. ISSN 0028-4793

Pring-Akerblom, P. & Ongrádi, J. Feline adenovirus hexon. GenBank Accession Number AY512566

Pring-Akerblom, P. & Ongrádi, J. Feline adenovirus fiber. GenBank Accession Number AY 518270

Qavi, H.B., Green, M.T., SeGall, G.K. & Font, R.L. (1989). Demonstration of HIV-1 and HHV-6 in AIDS-associated retinitis. Current Eye Research, (April 1989), Vol.8, No.4, 379-87. ISSN 0271-3683

Quinlivan, E.B., Holley-Guthrie, E., Mar, E.C., Smith, M,S. & Kenney, S. (1990).The Epstein-Barr virus BRLF1 immediate-early gene product transactivates the human immunodeficiency virus type 1 long terminal repeat by a mechanism which is enhancer independent. *Journal of Virology,* Vol.64, No.4, (April 1990), 1817-1820. ISSN 0022- 538x

Reubel, G.H., Dean, G.A., George, J.W., Barlough, J.E. & Pedersen, N.C. (1994). Effects of incidental infections and immune activation on disease progression in experimentally feline immunodeficiency virus-infected cats. *Journal of Acquired Immune Deficiency Syndromes,* Vol.7, No.10, (October 1994),1003-1015. ISSN 1525-4135

Reubel, G.H., George, J.W., Barlough, J.E., Higgins, J., Grant, C.K. & Pedersen, N.C. (1992). Interaction of acute feline herpesvirus-1 and chronic feline immunodeficiency virus infections in experimentally infected specific pathogen free cats. *Veterinary Immunology and Immunpathology,* Vol.35, No.1-2, (December 1992), 95-119. ISSN 0921-4489

Rice, A.P. & Mathews, M.B. (1998). Trans-activation of the human immunodeficiency virus long terminal repeat sequences, expressed in an adenovirus vector, by the adenovirus E1A 13S protein. *Proceedings of National Academy of Sciences of the United States of America,* Vol.85, No.12, (June 1988), 4200-4204. ISSN 0027-8424

Ritchey, J.W., Levy, J.K., Bliss, S.K., Tompkins, W.A. & Tompkins, M.B. (2001). Constitutive expression of types 1 and 2 cytokines by alveolar macrophages from feline immunodeficiency virus-infected cats.

Veterinary Immunology and Immunpathology, Vol.79, No.1-2, (May 2001), 83-100. ISSN 0921-4489

Rojko, J.L. & Olsen, R.G. (1994). The immunobiology of the feline leukemia virus. *Veterinary Immunology and Immunpathology,* Vol.6, No.1-2, (May 1984), 107-165. ISSN 0921-4489

Rotola, A., Cassai, E., Tola, M.R., Granieri, E. & Di Luca. D. (1999). Human herpesvirus 6 is latent in peripheral blood of patients with relapsing-remitting multiple sclerosis. *Journal of Neurology, Neurosurgery & Psychiatry,* Vol.67, No.4, (October 1999), 529-531. ISSN 0022-3050

Sada, E., Yasukawa, M., Ito, C., Takeda, A., Shiosaka, T., Tanioka, H. & Fujita, S. (1996). Detection of human herpesvirus 6 and human herpesvirus 7 in the submandibular gland, parotid gland, and lip salivary gland by PCR. *Journal of Clinical Microbiology,* Vol.34, No.9, (September 1996), 2320-2321. ISSN 0095-1137

Sadick, N.S., McNutt, N.S. & Kaplan, M.H. (1990). Papulosquamous dermatoses of AIDS. *Journal of the American Academy of Dermatology*, Vol.22, No.6, (June 1990), 1270-1277. ISSN 1097-6787

Safronetz, D., Humar, A. & Tipples, G.A. (2003). Differentiation and quantitation of human herpesviruses 6A, 6B and 7 by real-time PCR. *Journal of Virological Methods*, Vol.112, No.1-2, (September 2003), 99-105. ISSN 0166-0934

Salahuddin, S.Z., Ablashi, D.V., Markham, P.D., Josephs, S.F., Sturzenegger, S., Kaplan, M., Halligan, G., Biberfeld, P., Wong-Staal, F. & Kramarsky, B.(1986). Isolation of a new virus, HBLV, in patients with lymphoproliferative disorders. *Science,* Vol.234, No.4776, (October 1986), 596-601. ISSN 0036-8075

Salahuddin, S.Z., Snyder, K.A., Godwin, A., Grewal, R., Prichard, J.G., Kelley, A.S. & Revie, D. (2007). The simultaneous presence and expression of human hepatitis C virus (HCV), human herpesvirus-6 (HHV-6), and human immunodeficiency virus-1

(HIV-1) in a single human T-cell. *Virology Journal*. Vol.4, (October 2007), 106. ISSN 1743-422X

Salzberger, B., Hartmann, P., Hanses, F., Uyanik, B., Cornely, O.A., Wöhrmann, A. & Fätkenheuer, G. (2005). Incidence and prognosis of CMV disease in HIV-infected patients before and after introduction of combination antiretroviral therapy. *Infection*. Vol.33, No.5-6, (October 2005), 345-349. ISSN 0300-8126

Santoro, F., Kennedy, P.E., Locatelli, G., Malnati, M.S., Berger, E.A. & Lusso, P. (1999). CD46 is a cellular receptor for human herpesvirus 6. *Cell*, Vol.99, No.7, (December 1999), 817-827. ISSN 0092-8674

Secchiero, P., Carrigan, D.R., Asano, Y., Benedetti, L., Crowley, R.W., Komaroff, A.L., Gallo, R.C. & Lusso, P. (1995). Detection of human herpesvirus 6 in plasma of children with primary infection and immunosuppressed patients by polymerase chain reaction. *Journal of Infectious Diseases*, Vol.171, No.2, (February1995), 273-80. ISSN 0934-9723

Secchiero, P., Zella, D., Barabitskaja, O., Reitz, M.S., Capitani, S., Gallo, R.C. & Zauli, G.(1998). Progressive and persistent downregulation of surface CXCR4 in CD4(+) T cells infected with human herpesvirus 7. *Blood*, Vol.92, No.12, (December 1998), 4521-4528. ISSN 0006-4971

Seto, E., Yen, T.S., Peterlin, B.M. & Ou, J.H. (1988). Trans-activation of the human immunodeficiency virus long terminal repeat by the hepatitis B virus X protein. *Proceedings of National Academy of Sciences of the United States of America*, Vol,85. No.21. (November 1988), 8286-8290

Shelton, G.H., Grant, C.K., Cotter, S.M., Gardner, M.B., Hardy, W.D. Jr. & DiGiacomo, R.F. (1990). Feline immunodeficiency virus and feline leukemia virus infections and their relationships to lymphoid malignancies in cats: a retrospective study (1968-1988). *Journal of Acquired Immune Deficiency Syndromes*, No.3, No.6, (1990), 623-630. ISSN 1525-4135

Shimojima, M., Miyazawa, T., Ikeda, Y., McMonagle, E.L., Haining, H., Akashi, H., Takeuchi, Y., Hosie, M.J. & Willett, B.J. (2004). Use of CD134 as a primary receptor by the feline immunodeficiency virus. *Science*, Vol.303, No.5661, (February 2004), 1192-1195. ISSN 0036-8075.

Sieczkowski, L., Chandran, B. & Wood, C.(1995). The human immunodeficiency virus tat gene enhances replication of human herpesvirus-6. *Virology*, Vol.211, No.2, (Augustus 1995), 544-553. ISSN 0042-6822

Siekevitz, M., Josephs, S.F., Dukovich, M., Peffer, N., Wong-Staal, F. & Greene, W.C. Activation of the HIV-1 LTR by T cell mitogens and the trans-activator protein of HTLV-I. (1987) *Science*, Vol.238, No.4833, (December 1987), 1575-1578. ISSN 0036-8075

Smith, L.M., Bonafonte, M.T., Campbell, L.D. & Mead, J.R. (2001). Exogenous interleukin-12 (IL-12) exacerbates Cryptosporidium parvum infection in gamma interferon knockout mice. *Experimental Parasitology*, Vol.98, No.3, (July 2001), 123-133. ISSN 0014-4894

Smith, A., Santoro, F. Di Lullo, G. Dagna, L. Verani, A. & Lusso. P. (2003). Selective suppression of IL-12 production by human herpesvirus 6. *Blood*, Vol.102, No.8, (october 2003), 2877-2884. ISSN 0006-4971

Sparger, E.E., Shacklett, B.L., Renshaw-Gegg, L., Barry, P.A., Pedersen, N.C., Elder, J.H. & Luciw, P.A. (1992). Regulation of gene expression directed by the long terminal repeat of the feline immunodeficiency virus. *Virology,* Vol.87, No.1, (March 1992),165-177. ISSN 0042-6822

Spira, T.J., Bozeman, L.H., Sanderlin, K.C., Warfield, D.T., Feorino, P.M., Holman, R.C., Kaplan, J.E., Fishbein, D.B. & Lopez, C. (1990). Lack of correlation between human herpesvirus-6 infection and the course of human immunodeficiency virus infection. *Journal of Infectious Diseases,* Vol.161, No.3, (March 1990), 567-570. ISSN 0934-9723

Stellrecht, K.A., Sperber, K. & Pogo, B.G. (1992). Activation of the human immunodeficiency virus type 1 long terminal repeat by vaccinia virus. *Journal of Virology,* Vol.66, No.4, (April 1992), 2051-2056. ISSN 0022-538x

Surosky, R.T., Urabe, M., Godwin, S.G., McQuiston, S.A., Kurtzman, G.J., Ozawa, K. & Natsoulis. G. (1997). Adeno-associated virus Rep proteins target DNA sequences to a unique locus in the human genome. *Journal of Virology,* Vol.71, No.10, (October 1997), 7951-7959. ISSN: 0022-538x.

Tadagaki, K., Yamanishi, K. & Mori, Y. (2007). Reciprocal roles of cellular chemokine receptors and human herpesvirus 7-encoded chemokine receptors, U12 and U51. *Journal of General Virology,* Vol.88, No.5, (May 2007), 1423-1428. ISSN 0022-1317

Tai, A.K., Luka, J., Ablashi, D. & Huber, B.T. (2009). HHV-6A infection induces expression of HERV-K18-encoded superantigen. *Journal of Clinical Virology,* (September 2009), Vol.46, No.1, 47-48. ISSN1386-6532

Takemoto, M., Yamanishi, K. & Mori, Y. (2007). Human herpesvirus 7 infection increases the expression levels of CD46 and CD59 in target cells. *Journal of General Virology,* Vol.88, No.5, (May 2007), 1415-22. ISSN 0022-1317

Tanaka-Taya, K., Kondo, T., Mukai, T., Miyoshi, H., Yamamoto, Y., Okada, S. & Yamanishi. K. (1996). Seroepidemiological study of human herpesvirus-6 and -7 in children of different ages and detection of these two viruses in throat swabs by polymerase chain reaction. *Journal of Medical Virology,* Vol.48, No.1, (January 1996), 88-94. ISSN 0146-6615

Tedder, R.S., Briggs, M., Cameron, C.H., Honess, R., Robertson, D. & Whittle, H. (1987). A novel lymphotropic herpesvirus. *Lancet,* Vol.2, No.8555, (Augustus 1997), 390-392. ISSN 0140-6736

Thompson, J., Choudhury, S., Kashanchi, F., Doniger, J., Berneman, Z., Frenkel, N. & Rosenthal. L.J. (1994). A transforming fragment within the direct repeat region of human herpesvirus type 6 that transactivates HIV-1. *Oncogene,* Vol.9, No.4, (April 1994), 1167-1175. ISSN 0950-9232

Thomson, B.J., Dewhurst, S. & Gray. D. (1994a). Structure and heterogeneity of the a sequences of human herpesvirus 6 strain variants U1102 and Z29 and identification of human telomeric repeat sequences at the genomic termini. *Journal of Virology,* Vol.68, No.5. (May 1994), 3007-3014. ISSN: 0022-538x.

Thomson, B.J., Weindler, F.W., Gray, D., Schwaab, V. & Heilbronn. R. (1994). Human herpesvirus 6 (HHV-6) is a helper virus for adeno-associated virus type 2 (AAV-2) and the AAV-2 rep gene homologue in HHV-6 can mediate AAV-2 DNA replication and regulate gene expression. *Virology,* Vol.204, No.1, (October 1994), 304-311. ISSN 0042-6822

Tobiume, M., Fujinaga, K., Kameoka, M., Kimura, T., Nakaya, T., Yamada, T. & Ikuta, K. (1998). Dependence on host cell cycle for activation of human immunodeficiency virus type 1 gene expression from latency. *Journal of General Virology.* Vol.79, No.6, (June 1998), 1363-1371. ISSN 0022-1317

Torelli, G., Barozzi, P., Marasca, R., Cocconcelli, P., Merelli, E., Ceccherini-Nelli, L., Ferrari, S. & Luppi M. (1995). Targeted integration of human herpesvirus 6 in the p arm of chromosome 17 of human peripheral blood mononuclear cells in vivo. Journal of Medical *Virology*, Vol.46, No.3, (July 1995), 178-188. ISSN 0146-6615

Troy, S.B., Blackburn, B.G., Yeom, K., Caulfield, A.K., Bhangoo, M.S. & Montoya, J.G. (2008). Severe encephalomyelitis in an Immunocompetent Adult with chromosomally integrated human herpesvirus 6 and clinical response to treatment with foscarnet plus ganciclovir. *Clinical Infectious Diseases,* Vol47, No.12, (December 2008), 93-96. ISSN 1058-4838

Turcanova, V. L., Bundgaard, B., Höllsberg, P. (2009). Human herpesvirus-6B induces expression of the human endogenous retrovirus K18-encoded superantigen. *Journal of Clinical Virology,* Vol.46, No.1, (September 2009), 15-19. ISSN 1386-6532

Vág, T., Sonkoly, E., Kárpáti, S., Kemény, B. & Ongrádi, J. (2004). Avidity of antibodies to human herpesvirus 7 suggests primary infection in young adults with pityriasis rosea. *Journal of the European Academy of Dermatology and Venereology,* Vol.18, No.6, (November 2004), 738-740, 2004. ISSN 0926-9959

Vág, T., Sonkoly, E., Kemény, B., Kárpáti, S., Horváth, A. & Ongrádi, J. (2004). Familial occurence of papular-purpuric "gloves-and-socks" syndrome with human herpesvirus-7 and human parvovirus B19 infection. *Journal of the European Academy of Dermatology and Venereology,* Vol.18, No.5, 639-641, (September 2004), ISSN 0926-9959

Wang, J., Jones, C., Norcross, M., Bohnlein, E. & Razzaque, A. (1994). Identification and characterization of a human herpesvirus 6 gene segment capable of transactivating the human immunodeficiency virus type 1 long terminal repeat in an Sp1 binding site-dependent manner. *Journal of Virology,* Vol.68, No.3, (March, 1994), 1706-13. ISSN 0022-538x

Ward, K.N., Leong, H.N., Nacheva, E..P, Howard, J., Atkinson, C.E., Davies, N.W., Griffiths, P.D. & Clark, D.A. (2006). Human herpesvirus 6 chromosomal integration in immunocompetent patients results in high levels of viral DNA in blood, sera, and hair follicles. *Journal of Clinical Microbiology,* Vol.44, No.4, (April 2006), 1571-1574. ISSN 0095-1137

Wittekindt, B., Berger, A., Porto, L., Vlaho, S., Grüttner, H.P., Becker, M. & Lehrnbecher, T. (2009). Human herpes virus-6 DNA in cerebrospinal fluid of children undergoing therapy for acute leukaemia. *British Journal of Haematology,* Vol.145, No.4, (May 2009), 542-545. ISSN 0007-1048

Wyatt, L.S. & Frenkel, N. (1992). Human herpesvirus 7 is a constitutive inhabitant of adult human saliva. *Journal of Virology,* Vol.66, No.5, (May 1992), 3206-3209. ISSN 0022-538x

Yamamoto, J.K., Hansen, H., Ho, E.W., Morishita, T.Y., Okuda, T., Sawa, T.R., Nakamura, R.M. & Pedersen, N.C. (1989). pidemiologic and clinical aspects of feline immunodeficiency virus infection in cats from the continental United States and Canada and possible mode of transmission. *Journal of American Veterinary Medical Association*, Vol.194, No.2, (January 1989), 213-210. ISSN 0003-1488

Yamanishi, K., Okuno, T., Shiraki, K., Takahashi, M., Kondo, T., Asano Y. & Kurata, T. (1988). Identification of human herpesvirus-6 as a causal agent for exanthem subitum. *Lancet*, Vol.1, No.8594, (May 1988), 1065-1067. ISSN 0140-6736

Yasukawa, M., Yakushijin, Y., Furukawa, M. & Fujita, S. (1993). Specificity analysis of human CD4+ T-cell clones directed against human herpesvirus 6 (HHV-6), HHV-7, and human cytomegalovirus. *Journal of Virology,* Vol.67, No.10. (October 1993), 6259-6264. ISSN 0022-538x

Yuan, R., Bohan, C., Shiao, F.C., Robinson, R., Kaplan, H.J. & Srinivasan, A. (1989). Activation of HIV LTR-directed expression: analysis with pseudorabies virus immediate early gene. *Virology,* Vol.172, No.1, 92-99 (September 1989), ISSN 0042-6822

Zhen, Z., Bradel-Tretheway, B., Sumagin, S., Bidlack, J.M. & Dewhurst, S. (2005). The human herpesvirus 6 G protein-coupled receptor homolog U51 positively regulates virus replication and enhances cell-cell fusion in vitro. *Journal of Virology,* Vol.79, No.18, (September 2005), 11914-24. ISSN 0022-538x

Zhou, Y., Chang, CK., Qian, G., Chandran, B. & Wood, C. (1994). Trans-activation of the HIV promoter by a cDNA and its genomic clones of human herpesvirus-6. *Virology,* Vol.199, No.2, (March 1994), 311-322. ISSN 0042-6822

Zou, P., Isegawa, Y. Nakano, K. Haque, M. Horiguchi, Y. & Yamanishi. K. (1999). Human herpesvirus 6 open reading frame U83 encodes a functional chemokine. *Journal of Virology,* Vol.73, No.7, (July 1999), 5926-5933. ISSN: 0022- 538x.

Part 5

Animal Model

13

The Quest for a Small Animal Model for HIV Infection and Disease

Jorge C.G. Blanco[1], Lioubov M. Pletneva[1],
Lorraine E. Earle[2] and William I. Frels[2]
[1]*Sigmovir Biosystems Inc.*
[2]*Virion Systems Inc., Rockville, Maryland*
U.S.A

1. Introduction

Development of a small animal model to study human immunodeficiency virus type-1 (HIV-1) infection began with the discovery of the disease itself. Such a model would significantly facilitate studies of disease pathogenesis, vaccine and anti-viral drug development and testing. However, HIV-1 replication is subject to a number of species-specific restrictions at the level of cellular entry and/or post-entry. Although many attempts to develop a model that can overcome these cellular restrictions have been attempted, no satisfactory small animal model for HIV-1 infection has been identified to date.

The cotton rat has been a superb model for human infectious diseases. This "new world" wild rodent, that is now highly inbred, was shown to be susceptible to an extraordinary spectrum of human pathogens, particularly viruses. Importantly, it was shown by two different laboratories that cotton rats can be infected with the Human Immunodeficiency Virus (HIV-1), and that virus can be detected long after infection and antibodies are generated against viral proteins. In more recent studies, cotton rat cells were made permissive to HIV infection by engineering the expression of human co-receptors for HIV-1, supporting HIV-1 infection, DNA integration, and more importantly, production of infective HIV particles.

Importantly, the cotton rat is susceptible to other two pathogens that are extraordinarily associated with HIV-AIDS, *Mycobacterium tuberculosis* (TB) and herpes simplex virus (HSV). We will review previous attempts to develop a small animal model for HIV infection and explore the scientific and commercial significance of developing such a model. We will describe the cotton rat model of HIV, TB, HSV as they stand today. Finally, we will describe recent advances in the production of transgenic cotton rats that express HIV receptor molecules.

2. Animal models for HIV-1

The total number of Human Immunodeficiency Virus (HIV)-infected people worldwide is estimated at 40 million (and 600 new infections per hour). Preventive vaccine and prophylactic therapies against HIV infection and more efficient drugs for AIDS are not only urgently needed, but also, scientifically possible. However, one of the major obstacles in translational HIV research rests in the absence of inexpensive and efficient pre-clinical trial models.

Several animal models for HIV-1 infection have been useful, adding complementary information for specific aspects of HIV-1 disease in humans. Limitations of the current models include the limited availability and high cost (non-human primates), absence of or delay in an acquired immunodeficiency syndrome (AIDS), lack of viremia, and permissiveness only to related retroviruses. These models include human HIV-1 in chimpanzees, macaques, mice, rats, rabbits, and Simian HIV in several species of monkeys (Cohen, 2001; Nath, Schumann, and Boyer, 2000; van Maanen and Sutton, 2003).

HIV-1 replication is subject to a series of species-specific restrictions in cells of non-primate species. Binding of HIV-1 envelope protein (*Env*) to both CD4 and the appropriate member of the seven-transmembrane G-protein-coupled receptor superfamily are necessary for efficient entry of HIV-1 (Berger, Murphy, and Farber, 1999; Deng et al., 1996). Several different chemokine receptors (CCR2b, CCR3, CCR5, or CXCR4) or orphan chemokine receptor-like molecules (STRL33, GPR1, GPR15, V28, APJ) may participate in HIV-1 entry, but hCXCR4 and hCCR5 are the principal co-receptors for X4 (T-cell line-tropic) or R5 (macrophage-tropic) isolates, respectively. Blocking and down-regulation of these two cytokine receptors are ways by which their physiological ligands or modified analogues can reduce HIV-1 entry (Stantchev and Broder, 2001).

One approach for developing animal models in laboratory rodents has been to identify and then overcome specie-specific barriers that HIV encounters during its replication. The ultimate goal is to use the knowledge to develop an immunocompetent transgenic small animal model that is fully permissive to HIV replication. The barriers that stall replication in mouse and rat cells have been studied. Mice that express hCD4 and hCCR5 or hCXCR4 were first developed (Browning et al., 1997; Sawada et al., 1998). Preliminary results with these mice were initially exciting because the expression of the transgenes promoted viral entry, but were ultimately disappointing because the mice did not support viral replication (Browning et al., 1997). These results were partly explained by differences between the human and the mouse cyclin T1 (CycT1), which is an important cellular component of the p-TEFb transcription factor complex that is responsible for transcription from the viral long terminal repeat (HIV-LTR) (Garber et al., 1998; Wei et al., 1998). Recent studies indicate additional restrictions in mouse cells. Transgenic mice expressing human cyclin T1, human CD4, and the human chemokine receptor failed to produce high levels of HIV (Garber et al., 1998; Mariani et al., 2001) and other downstream elements like the maturation of the *gag* protein to produce p24 were also shown to be compromised in mouse cells (Mariani et al., 2001). These post-transcriptional defects result in a dramatically reduced yield of infectious virus (up to 10,000-fold) in a single cycle of HIV replication, as compared to human cells (Bieniasz and Cullen, 2000).

In 2001, Goldsmith and co-workers made improvements in the rat model for HIV. They first demonstrated that rat cells are more efficient for replication of HIV than mouse cells (Keppler et al., 2001), producing substantial levels of viral $p24^{gag}$. Based on these results, they engineered rats transgenic for the hCD4 and the hCCR5 that expressed the genes in CD4+ T lymphocytes, macrophages, and microglia (Keppler et al., 2002). They found that these cells could be productively infected by various recombinant and primary R5 strains of HIV-1 *ex vivo*, although the animals do not support viremia during infection.

The laboratory rabbit appears to be susceptible to HIV, but requires large inocula and viral replication does not spread (Dunn et al., 1995; Filice, Cereda, and Varnier, 1988). Rabbit cell lines expressing hCD4 and hCCR5 demonstrated an increase in infection and replication of CCR5 dependent strain of HIV (JR-CSF and YU-2)(Speck et al., 1998). Recently, new studies support the previous evidence for the susceptibility of rabbit cells, especially T cells, to HIV infection and suggest that in addition to the receptor complex transgenesis, modifications in *gag* and possibly *vif* of the HIV-1 might render the rabbit model fully permissive to infection by HIV-1 (Tervo and Keppler, 2010).

Recently, a small animal model of HIV transmission was developed by transplanting human bone marrow, liver, and thymus (BLT) into severe combined immunodeficient mice (Melkus et al., 2006). Consequently, human APCs and lymphocytes populate the mucosal surfaces, and the model can be used to assess some strategies to prevent vaginal HIV transmission (Denton et al., 2008). Further, once infected, the BLT mice generate humoral and cellular HIV-specific immune responses (Brainard et al., 2009). Some of these models allow transmission of HIV via the vaginal and rectal mucosa and display high-level viremia and CD4 T cell depletion. Unfortunately, these models are technically challenging, time-consuming, and not amenable to widespread use. Moreover, HIV-1 infected, xenotransplant mice mount low or dysfunctional adaptive immune responses to HIV infection, limiting these studies of natural immune control and vaccine testing.

3. The cotton rat

The cotton rat is a common New World rodent ranging in distribution from the southern United States through Mexico, Central America, Colombia and Venezuela. Eight species are recognized, with a karyotype ranging from 22 to 52 chromosomes. The most recent classification is to the Subfamily *Sigmodentinae* of the family *Cricetidae*, which includes New World mice, rats, voles, lemmings and muskrat. *Sigmodon hispidus* is the most commonly used cotton rat in biomedical research, but some investigators have also utilized laboratory-bred *S. fulviventer* (Piazza et al., 1992; Porter et al., 1991).

In the 1930's, it was discovered that inoculation of the cotton rat with poliovirus induced a paralytic disease, while other laboratory rodents did not develop disease (Armstrong, 1939). For over a decade, *S. hispidus* remained the prime animal model for polio until supplanted by monkeys and mice, with mice requiring extensive adaptation of virus. Since then, the cotton rat has been extensively used as a model to study different aspects of infection by respiratory syncytial virus (Li et al., 2000; Malley et al., 1998; Prince et al., 2001; Prince et al., 1978; Prince et al., 1999; Rodriguez et al., 1997; Tang et al., 2001), influenza A and B (Sadowski et al., 1987), parainfluenza viruses types 1, 2, and 3 (Ottolini et al., 2000; Porter et al., 1991; Prince et al., 2001; Sadowski et al., 1987), herpes simplex virus type 1 (HSV-1) (Lewandowski et al., 2002), HSV-2 (Yim et al., 2005), measles virus (Niewiesk, 2001; Niewiesk et al., 1997; Wyde et al., 1999), as well as several serotypes of adenovirus (Brunori et al., 2001; Ginsberg et al., 1989; Ginsberg, Moldawer, and Prince, 1999; Rojas-Martinez et al., 1998; Tsubota et al., 1998; Wildner and Morris, 2002). Finally, cotton rats are also natural reservoirs of several viruses of importance as emerging human pathogens. These include Venezuelan equine encephalitis (Wang et al., 2001), Guaranito and Pirital viruses (Fulhorst et al., 1999); and several species of hantavirus (Fulhorst et al., 1997; Glass et al., 1998; Hutchinson, Rollin, and Peters, 1998; Mantooth et al., 2001).

S. hispidus and *S. fulviventer* are fully inbred and both species are available from the Sigmovir Biosystems Inc. colony, a USDA licensed dealer for cotton rats.

4. HIV infection in cotton rat

Infection by HIV is defined as the replication of detectable virus in the host and the development of antibodies against HIV-1 proteins. Previously, one laboratory in the U.S. (Langley, Prince, and Ginsberg, 1998) and another in Russia (Rytik et al., 1995; Rytik et al., 2004) demonstrated that HIV-1 was detected in tissues of cotton rats previously infected with HIV-1. In the U.S. study (Langley, Prince, and Ginsberg, 1998), cotton rats were infected with HIV-1 and proviral DNA was detected in peripheral blood mononuclear cells (PBMCs) and tissues including spleen, thymus, and bone marrow from infected animals. Virus stimulated a strong, specific, and long-lasting immune response (in some animals included neutralizing antibodies and antibodies recognizing major HIV antigens) that was maintained up to 1 year post-infection. Although not demonstrable by direct culture of PBMCs or tissues from infected animals, infectious virus replicated at a low level in PBMCs of these animal because its presence was detected in animals that received three serial passages of blood from the original infected cotton rats.
In addition, Rytik and collaborators have also described the permissiveness of the cotton rat to HIV-1 infection by detection of viral DNA in spleen and brain (100% of the animals after 6 month), increase in mortality (17%), and morphological changes in cells of the central nervous system (CNS). These data strongly indicate that non-transgenic cotton rats are semi-permissive to HIV-1 replication. These findings imply that a productive infection may occur in cotton rats. The cotton rat offers several advantages for the development of an animal model, including small size, convenience of breeding, and the increasing availability of reagents to study the immunological and pathological aspects of HIV-1 disease (R&D Systems Inc).

4.1 Cotton rat primary macrophages support HIV-1 gene expression

Recently, the ability of cotton rat cells to support HIV-1 transcription was assessed by our laboratory using macrophages from two different cotton rat species (*S. hispidus and S. fulviventer*), from BALB/c mice, and from humans. Macrophages were transfected with a luciferase reporter gene encoding pNL4 env-R+, which provides a quantitative marker of HIV-1 gene expression. Macrophages from *S. hispidus* and *S. fulviventer* supported transcription of the HIV-1 derived backbone as indicated by enhanced luciferase activity compared with that of cells transfected with the control promotor-less luciferase construct (Fig. 1). The levels of transcription found in cotton rat macrophages were comparable to that measured in human macrophages, and all were significantly greater in comparison to mouse macrophages transfected with the HIV-1 reporter plasmid. Interestingly, the levels of transcription in macrophages of *S. hispidus* was at least 10 folds higher than the activity recorded in macrophages of humans or *S. fulviventer*. Although the nature of this high transcription efficiency of the LTR in *S. hispidus* is unknown, it could be related to the lift of a particular blockage or to an increase RNA/protein stability of luciferase. Transfection efficiencies measured by the expression of a CMV promoter-driven β-galactosidase activity were equivalent in cells of all species. These data indicate that cotton rat macrophages support transcription from the HIV-1-LTR and apparently lack the transcriptional blocks found in mouse cells.

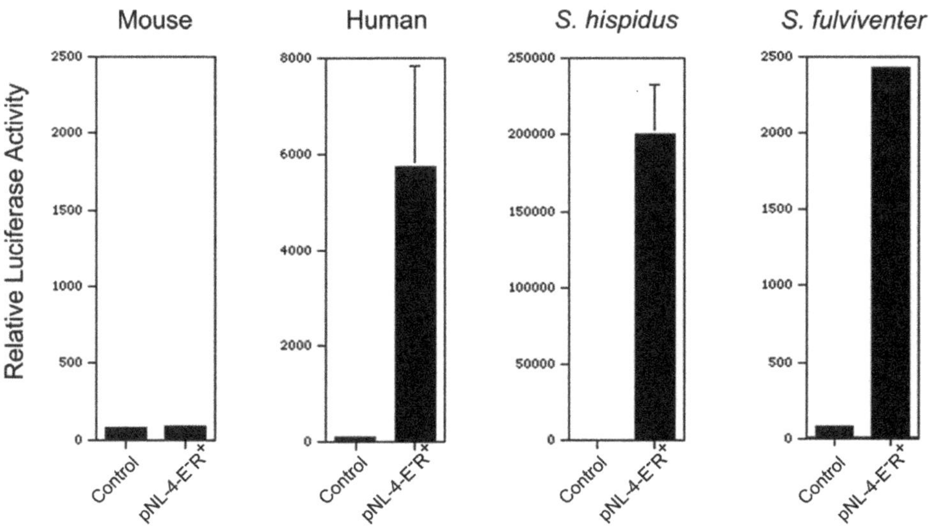

Fig. 1. Macrophages from *S. hispidus* and *S. fulviventer* supported transcription of the HIV-1 derived backbone. Mouse, human, *S.hispidus* and *S. fulviventer* macrophages were transfected with a control plasmid (pGL3-basic, Promega) or a plasmid containing a HIV-1 NL-4-E-R$^+$. Human macrophages were prepared by differentiating elutriated monocytes (from the NIH Blood Bank) for 14 days in high-cell density cultures of D-MEM media supplemented with 10% human AB serum, 2 mM L-glutamine and antibiotics in 100 mm square Petri. Cotton rat peritoneal macrophages from *S. hispidus* and *S. fulviventer* were prepared by injecting 3-month-old rats intraperitoneally with 8 ml of thioglycollate broth. Mouse macrophages were obtained in similar fashion injecting 3 ml of thioglycollate broth into the peritoneal cavity of Balb/c mice. Four days post injection, animals were sacrificed by CO_2 inhalation and the peritoneal cavity was washed twice with cold saline solution. Cells obtained were seeded in culture plates as indicated for human macrophages. For transfection of human, mouse, and cotton rat macrophages the ratio of transfection reagent in µl (FuGENE 6, Roche Molecular Biochemical) to NL4-3 derived backbone plasmid in µg was 4 to 1, where the total of 4.5 µg of plasmid DNA were used for each 10^6 macrophages. Transfection was carried out overnight at 37°C and the next day macrophages were washed and incubated for an additional 48 h before lysis and quantification of luciferase activity. The results represent luciferase activity obtained from transfected cells in triplicate wells from a representative experiment.

4.2 Cotton rat cell lines expressing the HIV-1 receptor complex are susceptible to HIV-1 infection

Two different cotton rat cells lines, CCRT (an osteosarcoma) and VCRT (an undifferentiated spindle cell sarcoma), that were selected for expression of hCD4/hCXCR4 and hCD4/hCCR5, were tested for infection with three well characterized isolates of HIV-1 virus: the MN isolate (a T-tropic HIV isolate that infects T cell lines and peripheral T cells, but not monocytes, and uses hCXCR4 as co-receptor), and the BAL and US1 isolates (M-tropic HIV isolates that infect monocytes and use hCCR5 as co-receptor). In all cases, the levels of $p24^{gag}$ in the supernatant of cotton rat cells expressing the HIV receptor complex were significantly higher than in control, untransfected cell cultures, with a peak of $p24^{gag}$ production evidenced on day 6 post-infection (Blanco et al., 2009). Fully mature, infectious HIV-1 particles were efficiently synthesized and assembled in HIV-1-infected cotton rat cells since PHA-activated PBMCs (pool of human PBMC from negative donors) or H9 cells incubated with the derived supernatants from cotton rat cells produced detectable amounts of $p24^{gag}$ (~200pg/ml) as early as day 3 post-transfer of all cotton rat-derived stocks. Furthermore, proviral DNA was detected in infected cotton rat cells, and subsequent direct cloning demonstrated that HIV-1 DNA integrates into the genome of infected cells (Blanco et al., 2009). The sequence of one of the integrated fragments (~ 1.6 kb) revealed the presence of 650 bp corresponding to sequence of the 5′ LTR of HIV-MN attached to 950 bp of a cotton rat genomic DNA sequence (GenBank acc# AY703985), and further demonstrates that cotton rat cells are able to support integration of viral DNA in their genome (Blanco et al., 2009).

5. The cotton rat model of tuberculosis

HIV fuels the TB epidemic in many ways. HIV promotes progression to active TB in both categories, that is, people with recently acquired TB and those with latent *Mycobacterium tuberculosis* infection (LTBI). HIV is the most powerful known risk factor for reactivation of LTBI to active disease. HIV also appears to increase the risk of pediatric TB, which is itself difficult to diagnose. A small animal model that is susceptible to infection with both pathogens could lead to development of treatments and vaccines that can target more efficiently this unparalleled problem for the population of third world countries.

The natural history of TB infection in *S. hispidus and S. fulviventer* has been studied (Elwood et al., 2007). The relatively short life span of the cotton rat (12-18 months) makes it possible to study TB infections throughout the entire life span of the animal. The studies demonstrated that young cotton rats experience a primary tuberculous pulmonary infection characterized by typical granuloma formation. There were differences in response to infection between the two species, with *S. fulviventer* demonstrating greater mortality than *S. hispidus*. Gross inspection of TB-infected cotton rat lungs show whitish nodular lesions and large numbers of TB (1 X 10^{5-7} cfu) were cultured from granulomas, spleen, and occasionally in smaller numbers from liver and bone marrow. Tuberculous lesions may also be seen in the adrenal glands (other organs remain to be examined) (Elwood et al., 2007). Established granulomas in some cases underwent central necrosis and calcification and cytokine genes are more highly expressed in the granuloma than in the unaffected areas of the lung. A minority of animals, about 20-30% with primary infection, develop serious progressive TB pulmonary disease, wasting, and succumb to infection. The remaining animals control or clear their infection by two to four months after challenged. Later, about half of these otherwise well appearing animals continue to have small numbers of TB recovered from lungs (1 X 10^{2-3} cfu) despite no microscopic evidence of inflammation or clinical disease. However, 50% of immunocompetent animals surviving past 9 months demonstrated positive lung tissue cultures for TB without histological evidence of disease. These findings are consistent with the development of LTBI. Furthermore, reactivation of disease occurs in the surviving animals after immunosuppression with cyclophosphamide (Elwood et al., 2009), indicating that a model of HIV-1 infection in the cotton rat more likely will parallel the course of TB disease seen in co-infected individual.

6. The cotton rat model of HSV infection

Genital herpes is one of the most prevalent sexually transmitted diseases (STD) worldwide and is the most common cause of genital ulcers. In the US, 17% of the population is seropositive for herpes simplex virus type 2 (HSV-2) and 58% for HSV-1, which is emerging as a major cause of genital herpes infections in developed countries (Roberts, 2005; Roberts, Pfister, and Spear, 2003; Xu et al., 2006). The HSV-2 seroprevalence rates are much higher in some populations, reaching 90-95% among HIV-infected subjects and female sex workers in developing countries where HSV-2 remains the dominant cause of genital ulcerative disease (Nagot et al., 2007). Implications of genital herpes infection include the risk of transmission to sexual partners and offspring as well as an increased risk of acquiring and transmitting HIV. Epidemiological studies consistently demonstrate that mucosal HIV-1 shedding is more frequent and in greater amounts during mucosal and subclinical reactivations (Corey et al., 2004; Nagot et al., 2007; Watson-Jones et al., 2008). HSV-2 can be detected in swabs obtained from the cervix from seropositive subjects by culture on 3% of days and by sensitive DNA PCR on about 20% of days, illustrating the high frequency of asymptomatic shedding (Wald et al., 2000). Being sero-positive for HSV-2 is associated with a 3- to 10-fold increased risk of HIV-1 acquisition in women, based on longitudinal cohort studies showing HSV-2 infection preceding HIV-1 acquisition and adjusted for sexual behavior (Celum et al., 2004; Celum, 2004; Freeman et al., 2006). In sub-Saharan Africa, more than a quarter of incident HIV infections may be attributed directly to HSV-2 (Abu-Raddad et al., 2008). A recently completed Phase IIb study, CAPRISA 004, found that 1% Tenofovir (TFV) vaginal gel was effective in reducing HIV transmission to high risk, seronegative, sexually active women (Abdool Karim et al., 2010). An unanticipated finding in these trials was that TFV gel provided 51% protection against HSV-2 (Q. Abdool Karim, unpublished data). Together, these results highlight the importance of the development of a preclinical model for testing combined therapies against HIV and HSV.

Female cotton rats (***S. hispidus***) are susceptible to genital HSV infection and do not require hormonal treatment to become infected (Yim et al., 2005). After HSV inoculation, animals develop lesions by day 12, without mortality. This contrasts significantly with the murine model, where medroxyprogesterone treatment is required for consistent infection, a higher inoculum is typically required, and mice develop hind limb paralysis and must be euthanized (Parr et al., 1994; Parr and Parr, 2003). In humans, primary genital herpes infections may be associated with constitutional symptoms, aseptic meningitis, and clinically asymptomatic spread of the virus to liver, lungs, and kidneys. In cotton rats, viral DNA was readily detected in vaginal swabs on days 3, 5, and 7 post-infection and could also be detected in the liver, lung, kidney, lumbosacral cord, and brain on the same days. Viral DNA was detected 100 days post-infection in lumbosacral cord, but not the brain, suggesting a state of latency in cotton rat dorsal root ganglia. Following healing of the primary lesions, 15-20% of female cotton rats display clinical signs of spontaneous reactivation with lesion formation at any given time (Yim et al., 2005). The lesions associated with reactivation are generally smaller than primary lesions, similar to human disease. Spontaneous recurrences are often preceded by virus being detected in vaginal swabs by PCR or culture, again similar to the human situation. Reactivation can be enhanced experimentally by dexamethasone treatment, increasing the rate to two- to three-fold higher than the rate of spontaneous reactivation.

Clinically silent reactivation of HSV is much more common than previously recognized and may play an important role in fueling both the HSV and HIV epidemic. For example, in a study of shedding in HSV-2 seropositive subjects who self-collected swabs 4 times daily for 60 days, HSV-2 was detected by PCR on 19% of days with a median duration of 13 h (Mark et al., 2008). Intermittent spontaneous viral shedding was observed in the absence of clinical lesions and was also detected by PCR and culture prior to the onset of clinical recurrences (Yim et al., 2005); these findings are consistent with those observed with human HSV infection and set up a potential valuable model of HSV and HIV co-infection and treatment.

7. Progress toward the development of a cotton rat model of HIV infection

Mammalian transgenic experiments have contributed tremendously to our understanding of numerous complex biological processes. While other laboratory animals have been used to produce transgenic lines, genetic manipulation has never been attempted in cotton rats. Development of transgenic cotton rat that is permissive to infection with HIV-1 was considered a project of sufficient importance to justify the development of the transgenic technique in this relatively new animal model. Since cotton rat stem cells are not available, pronuclear microinjection of DNA and subsequent embryonic transfer is required. To do that, an entire characterization of the reproductive habits of the cotton rat *S. hispidus* (52 chromosomes, inbred for more than 70 generations) including understanding the anatomy of its reproductive system, mating, and mothering habits, hormone stimulation, and fertilized egg recovery was required to optimize specific parameters for the production of transgenic cotton rats.

Female cotton rats maintained in 12-hour light-dark cycle (lights off from 6 PM to 6 AM) ovulate approximately every 9 days. Superovulation by hormone injection has been used in mice and rats to increase the number of one-celled fertilized eggs to use for microinjection. This is achieved by a course of treatment with pregnant mare serum gonadotrophin (PMS), followed by human chorionic gonadotrophin (HCG). The optimal age for hormone treatment of female cotton rats was 12 weeks, with the treatment consisting of 30 IU of PMS, followed with the same amount of HCG, 4 days later. Following these pretreatment conditions, matings were successful 65% of the time (*i.e.*, 65% of females exhibit a copulatory plug) producing an average of 6 fertilized eggs per female (Fig. 2).

Two hours after coitus, fertilized eggs can be retrieved from the oviduct (Fig. 3A). The shape and size of the cotton rat fertilized eggs resemble those of mice (Fig. 3B) with a distinguishable male and female pronucleus (FIG. 3C). Microinjection is performed using standard procedures by injecting 1 pl of purified and linearized DNA into the male pronucleus (Fig. 3D). Pseudopregnant recipients are used as surrogate mothers to nurture microinjected eggs to birth. These are young female cotton rats that are set for mating with vasectomized males. First, young female cotton rats at the peak of oestrus are identified and placed with vasectomized males at the beginning of the dark cycle. The mating rate of the young females with the vasectomized males is ~30%.

There is a very different anatomy of the cotton rat female reproductive system when compared to the mouse or laboratory rats, *e.g.*, the mouse and the rat have an evident ampulla where the fertilized eggs are located and where the transfer of embryos take place through the infundibulum. However, we could not find any evidence of the existence of an ampulla in the cotton rat. The infundibulum, however, is located inside the bursal sac as in the mouse. In contrast to the mouse that has the infundibulum free and accessible into the bursa to transfer the eggs, the cotton rat infundibulum is associated with the wall of the bursal sac. Eggs are implanted in the part of the oviduct that is proximal to the bursal sac (were the ampulla is anatomically located), and where the eggs are located at 20 hr post-coitum in the superovulated females (Fig. 3A).

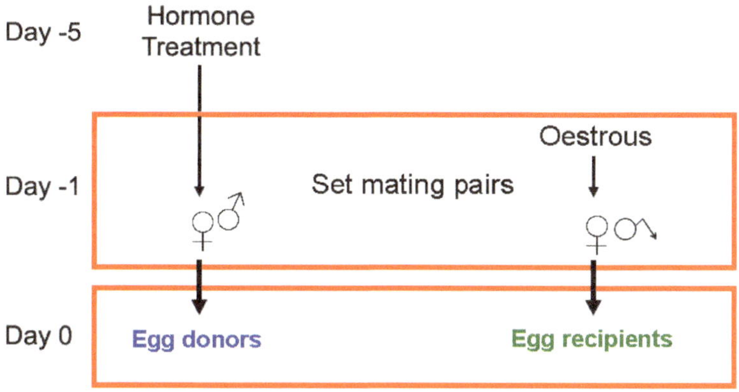

Fig. 2. Schematized protocol for the isolation of cotton rat fertilized eggs (egg donors, left side), and for the preparation of recipient pseudo-pregnant females (egg recipients, right side). Super-ovulation of female cotton rats is achieved by course of treatment of PMS followed by HCG before caging them with males for mating. In addition, female cotton rats in estrous are identified and set in mating pairs with vacectomized males. On day 0, females that have copulatory plugs are identified; eggs are isolated from oviducts of super-ovulated females, microinjected with DNA, and transferred to oviducts of pseudo-pregnant recipient females.

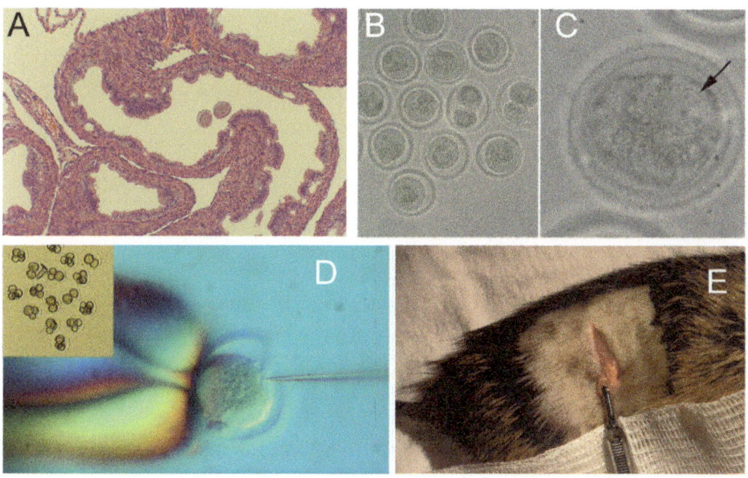

Fig. 3. Development of the transgenic technique in cotton rats. (A) H&E staining of cotton rat oviduct showing the location of the eggs. (B).Cotton rat fertilized eggs isolated from a super-ovulated cotton rat. (C) Fertilized cotton rat egg in which the male pro-nucleus, where DNA microinjection takes place, is depicted. (D) Microinjection of DNA in a fertilized egg. Insert shows viable eggs in culture after DNA microinjection. (E).Exposure of the oviduct of a pseudopregnant female cotton rat for embryo transfer.

8. Generation of transgenic cotton rats

The original genomic constructs for human CD4, CCR5 and CycT1 that were previously used in the mouse and rats (Keppler et al., 2002; Sawada et al., 1998), and that expressed their products in a tissue-specific manner (kindly provided by Dr. Dan R. Littman, M.D., Ph.D., Director of the Molecular Pathogenesis at Skirball Institute of Biomolecular Medicine) were purified to homogeneity for pronuclear microinjections. In the first set of microinjections and embryo transfer experiments, a set of three founders (2 females and one male) were obtained. After crossing, the F1 generation was genotyped for human CD4 and CCR5. Several animals in the F1 generation were positive by PCR and Southern blot genotyping for hCD4 and CCR5, indicating the production of transgenic cotton rats (Fig. 4). None of the animal genotyped were found to be transgenic for both transgenes. We are currently in process of determining expression of these genes in the transgenic cotton rats in order to produce double transgenics and subsequently initiate infection experiments to determine the degree of susceptibility to HIV-1 infection achieved.

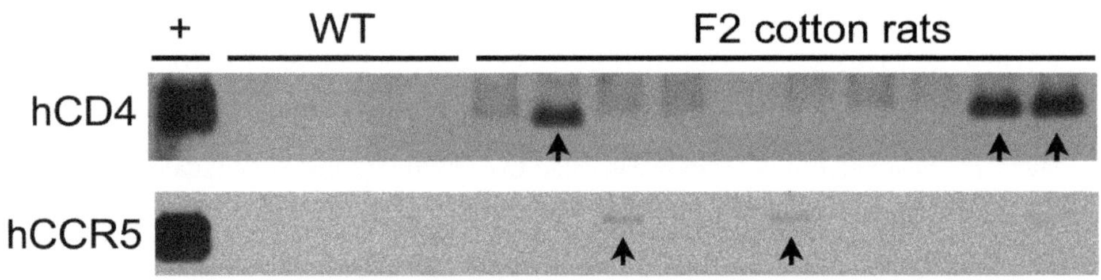

Fig. 4. Genotyping the F2 generation of cotton rats harboring transgenic hCD4 (upper panel) and transgenic hCCR5 (lower panel) by RT-PCR followed by Southern blot. PCR amplifications using DNA from the original transgenic constructs (+), and from wild-type cotton rats (wt) are depicted as controls.

9. Acknowledgment

The authors will like to acknowledge Drs Gregory A. Prince, Val Hemming, Vicky Polonis, Christopher Broader, Tsanko Stantchev for participating in this work during the years. Part of this work has been supported by NIH grant R44 AI054297 to JCGB.

10. References

Abdool Karim, Q., Abdool Karim, S. S., Frohlich, J. A., Grobler, A. C., Baxter, C., Mansoor, L. E., Kharsany, A. B., Sibeko, S., Mlisana, K. P., Omar, Z., Gengiah, T. N., Maarschalk, S., Arulappan, N., Mlotshwa, M., Morris, L., and Taylor, D. (2010). Effectiveness and safety of tenofovir gel, an antiretroviral microbicide, for the prevention of HIV infection in women. *Science* 329(5996), 1168-74.

Abu-Raddad, L. J., Magaret, A. S., Celum, C., Wald, A., Longini, I. M., Jr., Self, S. G., and Corey, L. (2008). Genital herpes has played a more important role than any other sexually transmitted infection in driving HIV prevalence in Africa. *PLoS ONE* 3(5), e2230.

Armstrong, C. (1939). The experimental transmission of poliomyelitis to the eastern cotton rat, *Sigmodon hispidus jispidus*. *Public Health Reports, Wash DC* 54, 1719-1721.

Berger, E. A., Murphy, P. M., and Farber, J. M. (1999). Chemokine receptors as HIV-1 coreceptors: roles in viral entry, tropism, and disease. *Annu Rev Immunol* 17, 657-700.

Bieniasz, P. D., and Cullen, B. R. (2000). Multiple blocks to human immunodeficiency virus type 1 replication in rodent cells. *J Virol* 74(21), 9868-77.

Blanco, J. C., Pletneva, L. M., Wieczorek, L., Khetawat, D., Stantchev, T. S., Broder, C. C., Polonis, V. R., and Prince, G. A. (2009). Expression of Human CD4 and chemokine receptors in cotton rat cells confers permissiveness for productive HIV infection. *Virol J* 6(1), 57.

Brainard, D. M., Seung, E., Frahm, N., Cariappa, A., Bailey, C. C., Hart, W. K., Shin, H. S., Brooks, S. F., Knight, H. L., Eichbaum, Q., Yang, Y. G., Sykes, M., Walker, B. D., Freeman, G. J., Pillai, S., Westmoreland, S. V., Brander, C., Luster, A. D., and Tager, A. M. (2009). Induction of robust cellular and humoral virus-specific adaptive immune responses in human immunodeficiency virus-infected humanized BLT mice. *J Virol* 83(14), 7305-21.

Browning, J., Horner, J. W., Pettoello-Mantovani, M., Raker, C., Yurasov, S., DePinho, R. A., and Goldstein, H. (1997). Mice transgenic for human CD4 and CCR5 are susceptible to HIV infection. *Proc Natl Acad Sci U S A* 94(26), 14637-41.

Brunori, M., Malerba, M., Kashiwazaki, H., and Iggo, R. (2001). Replicating adenoviruses that target tumors with constitutive activation of the wnt signaling pathway. *J Virol* 75(6), 2857-65.

Celum, C., Levine, R., Weaver, M., and Wald, A. (2004). Genital herpes and human immunodeficiency virus: double trouble. *Bull World Health Organ* 82(6), 447-53.

Celum, C. L. (2004). The interaction between herpes simplex virus and human immunodeficiency virus. *Herpes* 11 Suppl 1, 36A-45A.

Cohen, J. (2001). Building a small-animal model for AIDS, block by block. *Science* 293(5532), 1034-6.

Corey, L., Wald, A., Patel, R., Sacks, S. L., Tyring, S. K., Warren, T., Douglas, J. M., Jr., Paavonen, J., Morrow, R. A., Beutner, K. R., Stratchounsky, L. S., Mertz, G., Keene, O. N., Watson, H. A., Tait, D., and Vargas-Cortes, M. (2004). Once-daily valacyclovir to reduce the risk of transmission of genital herpes. *N Engl J Med* 350(1), 11-20.

Deng, H., Liu, R., Ellmeier, W., Choe, S., Unutmaz, D., Burkhart, M., Di Marzio, P., Marmon, S., Sutton, R. E., Hill, C. M., Davis, C. B., Peiper, S. C., Schall, T. J., Littman, D. R., and Landau, N. R. (1996). Identification of a major co-receptor for primary isolates of HIV-1. *Nature* 381(6584), 661-6.

Denton, P. W., Estes, J. D., Sun, Z., Othieno, F. A., Wei, B. L., Wege, A. K., Powell, D. A., Payne, D., Haase, A. T., and Garcia, J. V. (2008). Antiretroviral pre-exposure prophylaxis prevents vaginal transmission of HIV-1 in humanized BLT mice. *PLoS Med* 5(1), e16.

Dunn, C. S., Mehtali, M., Houdebine, L. M., Gut, J. P., Kirn, A., and Aubertin, A. M. (1995). Human immunodeficiency virus type 1 infection of human CD4-transgenic rabbits. *J Gen Virol* 76 (Pt 6), 1327-36.

Elwood, R. L., Rajnik, M., Wilson, S., Yim, K., Blanco, J. C., Nikonenko, B., and Hemming, V. G. (2009). Characterization of late tuberculosis infection in Sigmodon hispidus. *Tuberculosis (Edinb)* 89(2), 183-8.

Elwood, R. L., Wilson, S., Blanco, J. C., Yim, K., Pletneva, L., Nikonenko, B., Samala, R., Joshi, S., Hemming, V. G., and Trucksis, M. (2007). The American cotton rat: a novel model for pulmonary tuberculosis. *Tuberculosis (Edinb)* 87(2), 145-54.

Filice, G., Cereda, P. M., and Varnier, O. E. (1988). Infection of rabbits with human immunodeficiency virus. *Nature* 335(6188), 366-9.

Freeman, E. E., Weiss, H. A., Glynn, J. R., Cross, P. L., Whitworth, J. A., and Hayes, R. J. (2006). Herpes simplex virus 2 infection increases HIV acquisition in men and women: systematic review and meta-analysis of longitudinal studies. *Aids* 20(1), 73-83.

Fulhorst, C. F., Bowen, M. D., Salas, R. A., Duno, G., Utrera, A., Ksiazek, T. G., De Manzione, N. M., De Miller, E., Vasquez, C., Peters, C. J., and Tesh, R. B. (1999). Natural rodent host associations of Guanarito and pirital viruses (Family Arenaviridae) in central Venezuela. *Am J Trop Med Hyg* 61(2), 325-30.

Fulhorst, C. F., Monroe, M. C., Salas, R. A., Duno, G., Utrera, A., Ksiazek, T. G., Nichol, S. T., de Manzione, N. M., Tovar, D., and Tesh, R. B. (1997). Isolation, characterization and geographic distribution of Caño Delgadito virus, a newly discovered South American hantavirus (family Bunyaviridae). *Virus Res* 51(2), 159-71.

Garber, M. E., Wei, P., KewalRamani, V. N., Mayall, T. P., Herrmann, C. H., Rice, A. P., Littman, D. R., and Jones, K. A. (1998). The interaction between HIV-1 Tat and human cyclin T1 requires zinc and a critical cysteine residue that is not conserved in the murine CycT1 protein. *Genes Dev* 12(22), 3512-27.

Ginsberg, H. S., Lundholm-Beauchamp, U., Horswood, R. L., Pernis, B., Wold, W. S., Chanock, R. M., and Prince, G. A. (1989). Role of early region 3 (E3) in pathogenesis of adenovirus disease. *Proc Natl Acad Sci U S A* 86(10), 3823-7.

Ginsberg, H. S., Moldawer, L. L., and Prince, G. A. (1999). Role of the type 5 adenovirus gene encoding the early region 1B 55-kDa protein in pulmonary pathogenesis. *Proc Natl Acad Sci U S A* 96(18), 10409-11.

Glass, G. E., Livingstone, W., Mills, J. N., Hlady, W. G., Fine, J. B., Biggler, W., Coke, T., Frazier, D., Atherley, S., Rollin, P. E., Ksiazek, T. G., Peters, C. J., and Childs, J. E. (1998). Black Creek Canal Virus infection in Sigmodon hispidus in southern Florida. *Am J Trop Med Hyg* 59(5), 699-703.

Hutchinson, K. L., Rollin, P. E., and Peters, C. J. (1998). Pathogenesis of a North American hantavirus, Black Creek Canal virus, in experimentally infected Sigmodon hispidus. *Am J Trop Med Hyg* 59(1), 58-65.

Keppler, O. T., Welte, F. J., Ngo, T. A., Chin, P. S., Patton, K. S., Tsou, C. L., Abbey, N. W., Sharkey, M. E., Grant, R. M., You, Y., Scarborough, J. D., Ellmeier, W., Littman, D. R., Stevenson, M., Charo, I. F., Herndier, B. G., Speck, R. F., and Goldsmith, M. A. (2002). Progress toward a human CD4/CCR5 transgenic rat model for de novo infection by human immunodeficiency virus type 1. *J Exp Med* 195(6), 719-36.

Keppler, O. T., Yonemoto, W., Welte, F. J., Patton, K. S., Iacovides, D., Atchison, R. E., Ngo, T., Hirschberg, D. L., Speck, R. F., and Goldsmith, M. A. (2001). Susceptibility of rat-derived cells to replication by human immunodeficiency virus type 1. *J Virol* 75(17), 8063-73.

Langley, R. J., Prince, G. A., and Ginsberg, H. S. (1998). HIV type-1 infection of the cotton rat (Sigmodon fulviventer and S. hispidus). *Proc Natl Acad Sci U S A* 95(24), 14355-60.

Lewandowski, G., Zimmerman, M. N., Denk, L. L., Porter, D. D., and Prince, G. A. (2002). Herpes simplex type 1 infects and establishes latency in the brain and trigeminal ganglia during primary infection of the lip in cotton rats and mice. *Arch Virol* 147(1), 167-79.

Li, X., Sambhara, S., Li, C. X., Ettorre, L., Switzer, I., Cates, G., James, O., Parrington, M., Oomen, R., Du, R. P., and Klein, M. (2000). Plasmid DNA encoding the respiratory syncytial virus G protein is a promising vaccine candidate. *Virology* 269(1), 54-65.

Malley, R., DeVincenzo, J., Ramilo, O., Dennehy, P. H., Meissner, H. C., Gruber, W. C., Sanchez, P. J., Jafri, H., Balsley, J., Carlin, D., Buckingham, S., Vernacchio, L., and Ambrosino, D. M. (1998). Reduction of respiratory syncytial virus (RSV) in tracheal aspirates in intubated infants by use of humanized monoclonal antibody to RSV F protein. *J Infect Dis* 178(6), 1555-61.

Mantooth, S. J., Milazzo, M. L., Bradley, R. D., Hice, C. L., Ceballos, G., Tesh, R. B., and Fulhorst, C. F. (2001). Geographical distribution of rodent-associated hantaviruses in Texas. *J Vector Ecol* 26(1), 7-14.

Mariani, R., Rasala, B. A., Rutter, G., Wiegers, K., Brandt, S. M., Krausslich, H. G., and Landau, N. R. (2001). Mouse-human heterokaryons support efficient human immunodeficiency virus type 1 assembly. *J Virol* 75(7), 3141-51.

Mark, K. E., Wald, A., Magaret, A. S., Selke, S., Olin, L., Huang, M. L., and Corey, L. (2008). Rapidly cleared episodes of herpes simplex virus reactivation in immunocompetent adults. *J Infect Dis* 198(8), 1141-9.

Melkus, M. W., Estes, J. D., Padgett-Thomas, A., Gatlin, J., Denton, P. W., Othieno, F. A., Wege, A. K., Haase, A. T., and Garcia, J. V. (2006). Humanized mice mount specific adaptive and innate immune responses to EBV and TSST-1. *Nat Med* 12(11), 1316-22.

Nagot, N., Ouedraogo, A., Foulongne, V., Konate, I., Weiss, H. A., Vergne, L., Defer, M. C., Djagbare, D., Sanon, A., Andonaba, J. B., Becquart, P., Segondy, M., Vallo, R., Sawadogo, A., Van de Perre, P., and Mayaud, P. (2007). Reduction of HIV-1 RNA levels with therapy to suppress herpes simplex virus. *N Engl J Med* 356(8), 790-9.

Nath, B. M., Schumann, K. E., and Boyer, J. D. (2000). The chimpanzee and other non-human-primate models in HIV-1 vaccine research. *Trends Microbiol* 8(9), 426-31.

Niewiesk, S. (2001). Studying experimental measles virus vaccines in the presence of maternal antibodies in the cotton rat model (Sigmodon hispidus). *Vaccine* 19(17-19), 2250-3.

Niewiesk, S., Eisenhuth, I., Fooks, A., Clegg, J. C., Schnorr, J. J., Schneider-Schaulies, S., and ter Meulen, V. (1997). Measles virus-induced immune suppression in the cotton rat (Sigmodon hispidus) model depends on viral glycoproteins. *J Virol* 71(10), 7214-9.

Ottolini, M. G., Porter, D. D., Hemming, V. G., and Prince, G. A. (2000). Enhanced pulmonary pathology in cotton rats upon challenge after immunization with inactivated parainfluenza virus 3 vaccines. *Viral Immunol* 13(2), 231-6.

Parr, M. B., Kepple, L., McDermott, M. R., Drew, M. D., Bozzola, J. J., and Parr, E. L. (1994). A mouse model for studies of mucosal immunity to vaginal infection by herpes simplex virus type 2. *Lab Invest* 70(3), 369-80.

Parr, M. B., and Parr, E. L. (2003). Intravaginal administration of herpes simplex virus type 2 to mice leads to infection of several neural and extraneural sites. *J Neurovirol* 9(6), 594-602.

Piazza, F. M., Johnson, S. A., Ottolini, M. G., Schmidt, H. J., Darnell, M. E., Hemming, V. G., and Prince, G. A. (1992). Immunotherapy of respiratory syncytial virus infection in cotton rats (Sigmodon fulviventer) using IgG in a small-particle aerosol. *J Infect Dis* 166(6), 1422-4.

Porter, D. D., Prince, G. A., Hemming, V. G., and Porter, H. G. (1991). Pathogenesis of human parainfluenza virus 3 infection in two species of cotton rats: Sigmodon hispidus develops bronchiolitis, while Sigmodon fulviventer develops interstitial pneumonia. *J Virol* 65(1), 103-11.

Prince, G. A., Curtis, S. J., Yim, K. C., and Porter, D. D. (2001). Vaccine-enhanced respiratory syncytial virus disease in cotton rats following immunization with Lot 100 or a newly prepared reference vaccine. *J Gen Virol* 82(Pt 12), 2881-8.

Prince, G. A., Jenson, A. B., Horswood, R. L., Camargo, E., and Chanock, R. M. (1978). The pathogenesis of respiratory syncytial virus infection in cotton rats. *Am J Pathol* 93(3), 771-91.

Prince, G. A., Prieels, J. P., Slaoui, M., and Porter, D. D. (1999). Pulmonary lesions in primary respiratory syncytial virus infection, reinfection, and vaccine-enhanced disease in the cotton rat (Sigmodon hispidus). *Lab Invest* 79(11), 1385-92.

Roberts, C. (2005). Genital herpes in young adults: changing sexual behaviours, epidemiology and management. *Herpes* 12(1), 10-4.

Roberts, C. M., Pfister, J. R., and Spear, S. J. (2003). Increasing proportion of herpes simplex virus type 1 as a cause of genital herpes infection in college students. *Sex Transm Dis* 30(10), 797-800.

Rodriguez, W. J., Gruber, W. C., Groothuis, J. R., Simoes, E. A., Rosas, A. J., Lepow, M., Kramer, A., and Hemming, V. (1997). Respiratory syncytial virus immune globulin treatment of RSV lower respiratory tract infection in previously healthy children. *Pediatrics* 100(6), 937-42.

Rojas-Martinez, A., Wyde, P. R., Montgomery, C. A., Chen, S. H., Woo, S. L., and Aguilar-Cordova, E. (1998). Distribution, persistency, toxicity, and lack of replication of an E1A-deficient adenoviral vector after intracardiac delivery in the cotton rat. *Cancer Gene Ther* 5(6), 365-70.

Rytik, P. G., Il'kevich Iu, G., Poleshchuk, N. N., Miuller, V., Kucherov, I. A., Duboiskaia, G. P., Podol'skaia, I. A., Novikova, I. E., and Kvacheva, Z. B. (1995). [Morphological characteristics of the course of HIV infection in laboratory animals]. *Vestn Ross Akad Med Nauk*(6), 37-41.

Rytik, P. G., Kutcherov, II, Muller, W. E., Poleschuk, N. N., Duboiskaya, G. P., Kruzo, M., and Podolskaya, I. A. (2004). Small animal model of HIV-1 infection. *J Clin Virol* 31 Suppl 1, S83-7.

Sadowski, W., Semkow, R., Wilczynski, J., Krus, S., and Kantoch, M. (1987). [The cotton rat (Sigmodon hispidus) as an experimental model for studying viruses in human respiratory tract infections. I. Para-influenza virus type 1, 2 and 3, adenovirus type 5 and RS virus]. *Med Dosw Mikrobiol* 39(1), 33-42.

Sawada, S., Gowrishankar, K., Kitamura, R., Suzuki, M., Suzuki, G., Tahara, S., and Koito, A. (1998). Disturbed CD4+ T cell homeostasis and in vitro HIV-1 susceptibility in transgenic mice expressing T cell line-tropic HIV-1 receptors. *J Exp Med* 187(9), 1439-49.

Speck, R. F., Penn, M. L., Wimmer, J., Esser, U., Hague, B. F., Kindt, T. J., Atchison, R. E., and Goldsmith, M. A. (1998). Rabbit cells expressing human CD4 and human CCR5 are highly permissive for human immunodeficiency virus type 1 infection. *J Virol* 72(7), 5728-34.

Stantchev, T. S., and Broder, C. C. (2001). Human immunodeficiency virus type-1 and chemokines: beyond competition for common cellular receptors. *Cytokine Growth Factor Rev* 12(2-3), 219-43.

Tang, R. S., Nguyen, N., Cheng, X., and Jin, H. (2001). Requirement of cysteines and length of the human respiratory syncytial virus M2-1 protein for protein function and virus viability. *J Virol* 75(23), 11328-35.

Tervo, H. M., and Keppler, O. T. High natural permissivity of primary rabbit cells for HIV-1, with a virion infectivity defect in macrophages as the final replication barrier. *J Virol* 84(23), 12300-14.

Tsubota, K., Inoue, H., Ando, K., Ono, M., Yoshino, K., and Saito, I. (1998). Adenovirus-mediated gene transfer to the ocular surface epithelium. *Exp Eye Res* 67(5), 531-8.

van Maanen, M., and Sutton, R. E. (2003). Rodent models for HIV-1 infection and disease. *Curr HIV Res* 1(1), 121-30.

Wald, A., Zeh, J., Selke, S., Warren, T., Ryncarz, A. J., Ashley, R., Krieger, J. N., and Corey, L. (2000). Reactivation of genital herpes simplex virus type 2 infection in asymptomatic seropositive persons. *N Engl J Med* 342(12), 844-50.

Wang, E., Bowen, R. A., Medina, G., Powers, A. M., Kang, W., Chandler, L. M., Shope, R. E., and Weaver, S. C. (2001). Virulence and viremia characteristics of 1992 epizootic subtype IC Venezuelan equine encephalitis viruses and closely related enzootic subtype ID strains. *Am J Trop Med Hyg* 65(1), 64-9.

Watson-Jones, D., Weiss, H. A., Rusizoka, M., Changalucha, J., Baisley, K., Mugeye, K., Tanton, C., Ross, D., Everett, D., Clayton, T., Balira, R., Knight, L., Hambleton, I., Le Goff, J., Belec, L., and Hayes, R. (2008). Effect of herpes simplex suppression on incidence of HIV among women in Tanzania. *N Engl J Med* 358(15), 1560-71.

Wei, P., Garber, M. E., Fang, S. M., Fischer, W. H., and Jones, K. A. (1998). A novel CDK9-associated C-type cyclin interacts directly with HIV-1 Tat and mediates its high-affinity, loop-specific binding to TAR RNA. *Cell* 92(4), 451-62.

Wildner, O., and Morris, J. C. (2002). Subcutaneous Administration of a Replication-Competent Adenovirus Expressing HSV-tk to Cotton Rats: Dissemination, Persistence, Shedding, and Pathogenicity. *Hum Gene Ther* 13(1), 101-12.

Wyde, P. R., Moore-Poveda, D. K., Daley, N. J., and Oshitani, H. (1999). Replication of clinical measles virus strains in hispid cotton rats. *Proc Soc Exp Biol Med* 221(1), 53-62.

Xu, F., Sternberg, M. R., Kottiri, B. J., McQuillan, G. M., Lee, F. K., Nahmias, A. J., Berman, S. M., and Markowitz, L. E. (2006). Trends in herpes simplex virus type 1 and type 2 seroprevalence in the United States. *Jama* 296(8), 964-73.

Yim, K. C., Carroll, C. J., Tuyama, A., Cheshenko, N., Carlucci, M. J., Porter, D. D., Prince, G. A., and Herold, B. C. (2005). The cotton rat provides a novel model to study genital herpes infection and to evaluate preventive strategies. *J Virol* 79(23), 14632-9.

14

Macaque-Tropic HIV-1 Derivatives: A Novel Experimental Approach to Understand Viral Replication and Evolution In Vivo

Masako Nomaguchi, Naoya Doi, Sachi Fujiwara and Akio Adachi
The University of Tokushima Graduate School
Japan

1. Introduction

The use of animal models in the study of human diseases is obviously important. Fundamental properties of the disease can be investigated analytically and thoroughly by this approach, contributing much to the progress of basic science as well as clinical medicine (Nomaguchi & Adachi, 2010). Researchers in various specialties, therefore, have made every effort to establish animal models for human diseases including those caused by infectious agents. Acquired immunodeficiency syndrome (AIDS) of humans has long been one of the major targets for the model study in appropriate animals. However, human immunodeficiency virus type 1 (HIV-1) itself, the predominant causative virus of human AIDS, can not be used due to its very narrow host range. Because HIV-1 has adapted itself dexterously from the ancestral virus to replicate, persist and spread strictly in humans, it is very unique among various primate immunodeficiency viruses and no good counterparts are available in nature (Desrosiers, 2007; Kirchhoff, 2009; Sauter et al., 2009). Therefore, it can be concluded that practical and meaningful animal systems of non-alternative nature for HIV-1 study do not exist at all to date, although there are pre-existing animal models of some significance.

HIV-1 does not replicate in animal species except for chimpanzees and humans (Nomaguchi et al., 2008a). Animals frequently used for our experiments on virology, such as rodents and nonhuman primates, are not exceptions to this barrier. However, if we are to search for, develop and establish a fruitful animal model system for HIV-1 research, nonhuman primates are considered to be most suited, for HIV-1 is best fitted with humans and some apes. Ever since the discovery of HIV-1 (Barre-Sinoussi et al., 1983), many prominent researchers keen on understanding its biology and molecular biology have done investigations extensively to elucidate the bases underlying the species-specificity unique to HIV-1. These studies have highlighted the presence of potent anti-HIV-1 factors in nonhuman cells that efficiently restrict or even abolish the replication of HIV-1 and successfully raised an epoch-making notion of the intrinsic immunity (Andrew & Strebel, 2010; Arhel & Kirchhoff, 2010; Ayinde et al., 2010; Bergamaschi & Pancino, 2010; Douglas et al., 2010; Fujita et al., 2010; Huthoff & Towers, 2008; Kirchhoff, 2010; Luban, 2007; Malim & Emerman, 2008; Nakayama & Shioda, 2010; Nomaguchi et al., 2008a, 2008b; Planelles & Barker, 2010; Sauter et al., 2010; Strebel et al., 2009; Towers, 2007). Cellular factors shoulder this intrinsic immunity known to date are cyclophilin A (CypA) (Franke et al., 1994; Thali et al., 1994), apolipoprotein B mRNA-editing enzyme-catalytic polypeptide-like 3G (APOBEC3G)/APOBEC3F (Sheehy et al., 2002), tripartite motif protein 5α (TRIM5α) (Stremlau et al., 2004), TRIMCyp (Nisole et al., 2004; Sayah et al., 2004), and tetherin (alternatively called BST-2) (Neil et al., 2008; Van Damme et al., 2008). Because HIV-1 can indeed counteract human orthologs of these restriction factors effectively, it is well anticipated that HIV-1 in turn can be genetically engineered to replicate efficiently in nonhuman primates such as macaques. Nonetheless, most likely due to the lack of extensive and appropriate biological studies, we are still forced to use macaque-derived simian immunodeficiency virus (SIVmac) or SIVmac chimeric with a small portion of HIV-1 (SHIV) as an input virus for in vivo model studies in macaques. SIVmac and SHIV are genetically and biologically distinct from HIV-1 in a number of critical points, albeit they are quite similar to HIV-1 in the genome organization and pathogenic potentials (Desrosiers, 2007; Freed & Martin, 2007). They might not be used for future model studies aimed at understanding the biology of HIV-1 as a highly replicable/mutable, persistent, and pathogenic virus. We must go behind the outward form to grasp the inner meaning of the phenomenon, i.e., the species-specificity.

On the collective basis of molecular and biochemical studies performed by us and others so far, we recently have constructed a series of HIV-1 derivative clones tropic for macaque cells and/or macaques (Hatcho et al., 2008; Igarashi et al., 2007; Kamada et al., 2006, 2009; Kuroishi et al., 2009; Nomaguchi et al., 2008a; Saito et al., 2011; Yamashita et al., 2008), and are currently further modifying them for in vivo studies (our unpublished results). The viruses we have generated carry a minimal sequence of SIVmac, and overcome at least some species barriers. Importantly, these viruses are regarded to be genetically HIV-1, since they have less than 10% SIVmac genetic content (Igarashi et al., 2007). While we firmly believe that HIV-1 derivative viruses already constructed in our laboratory are useful for a variety of studies on HIV-1 infection in individuals, further improvement of the viruses by deliberating the evolutional process of SIV/HIV would surely add more scientific significance to basic and applied research fields. Needless to say, our goal is to generate a macaque-tropic HIV-1 (HIV-1mt) that replicates efficiently and is pathogenic for macaques as a standard pathogenic SIVmac clone such as SIVmac239 (Kestler et al., 1990). Through construction and biochemical/biological characterization of the ideal HIV-1mt clone with ability to induce AIDS at least in some species of macaques, we would be able to clarify the detailed molecular mechanisms for the narrow host range (species-tropism) of HIV-1. Viral Gag-capsid (CA) and accessory proteins (Vif, Vpx, Vpr, Vpu and Nef) are targets for those studies as a matter of course. Moreover, by using this persistent and pathogenic HIV-1mt clone as a seed virus for macaque infection experiments, we can trace and analyze its mutation, adaptation, evolutional direction to generate viral quasi-species, and finally pathogenesis in the context of immunological interaction. In addition, we can evaluate and develop the anti-HIV-1 drugs/vaccines by this HIV-1mt/macaque system.

In this chapter, we first outline the early and current studies on HIV-1, SIVmac and SHIV to emphasize and address the unique characteristics of HIV-1 and scientific issues to resolve. We then describe viral and cellular factors that are responsible for or potentially associated with restriction of viral replication. We finally focus on our recent studies on the strategies to obtain HIV-1mt clones and on the biology/molecular biology of HIV-1mt clones. Main parts of this chapter consist of: (i) Overview of the biology and molecular biology of HIV-1, SIVmac and SHIV; (ii) Determinants for HIV-1 species-tropism; (iii) Generation and characterization of various HIV-1mt clones. The primary mission of we basic virologists is to understand viral replication and viral pathogenesis in vivo by multilateral approaches (Nomaguchi & Adachi, 2010). We then take over our new important findings to functional parties in related fields, thus promoting further progress in virology.

2. Overview of the biology and molecular biology of HIV-1, SIVmac and SHIV

Numerous immunodeficiency viruses of distinct groups have been isolated from humans and a wide variety of African nonhuman primates (Desrosiers, 2007; Freed & Martin, 2007). These viruses infect the immune system of primates, kill cells that are critical for effective immune responses, and eventually cause AIDS in some hosts (Desrosiers, 2007; Kuritzkes & Walker, 2007). Soon after the discovery in 1983 (Barre-Sinoussi et al., 1983; Barre-Sinoussi, 2010; Montagnier, 2010), HIV-1 was demonstrated to belong to a lentiviral genus of the retrovirus family, and expected to exhibit the properties characteristic of the family (Goff, 2007). In 1986, another human immunodeficiency virus was identified and designated HIV-2 (Clavel et al., 1986; Montagnier, 2010). Among these primate lentiviruses, HIV-1, HIV-2 and its close relative SIVmac are most well-studied through biological, biochemical and medical approaches, and many findings crucial for the biological and medical sciences have been generated (Ho & Bieniasz, 2008).

Basically, HIV/SIV exhibit a virological phenotype common to the retroviruses. Viral proteins are synthesized from viral DNA genome integrated into host chromosomal DNA, and progeny viral particles (virions) are produced from cells in a typical manner. However, HIV/SIV are unique, as primate lentiviruses, in the genome and virion composition among the retroviruses (Fig. 1). They all have additional genes relative to a standard retrovirus. Importantly, these extra genes encode, in addition to structural Gag, Pol and Env proteins common to all retroviruses, viral regulatory (Tat and Rev) and accessory proteins that are essential for the specific and unique characteristics of HIV/SIV. HIV/SIV virions, therefore, contain some viral proteins not found in the other retroviral virions. The common and unique properties are also applicable to their replication cycle. HIV/SIV replicate in their target cells essentially in the same way with the other retroviruses. Retroviral replication cycle consists of early and late phases. The early phase (Fig. 2) begins with the virion entry step into cells, and proceeds to the reverse transcription of viral RNA genome, uncoating, nuclear import of viral DNA genome, and integration of viral DNA genome into host DNA to generate proviral DNA. The late phase (Fig. 3) then starts with the proviral transcription, and proceeds to the viral RNA export to cytoplasm, translation into viral proteins, assembly of the viral RNA/proteins at cell surface, budding/release from cells, and maturation into infectious virions.

Of viral proteins unique to HIV/SIV, Tat and Rev are essential for virus replication as is the case for structural proteins Gag, Pol, and Env, and act as regulators for expression of the other viral proteins (Freed & Martin, 2007). Tat is a potent trans-activator of transcription, and is the primary switch of viral gene expression. Rev is responsible for the viral RNA export process, and required for expression of viral structural proteins and most of the accessory proteins except for Nef. Thus, Rev can be considered to be the second expression switch. In contrast to the two regulatory proteins, accessory proteins are not always necessary for viral replication in cells (Freed & Martin, 2007). Early studies indicated that these proteins are unnecessary or dispensable for virus replication in the established cell lines. However, it was soon noticed that, in the primary natural target cells such as CD4-positive T-lymphocytes and macrophages, or in some specific cell lines, the accessory proteins are essential or important for virus replication. These findings have led to the identification of innate anti-viral factors APOBEC proteins (Sheehy et al., 2002) and tetherin as described above (Neil et al., 2008; Van Damme et al., 2008), and to the search for an anti-viral macrophage factor(s) (Fujita et al., 2010). Although some aspects of the accessory proteins are becoming more organized and much clearer than before as summarized in Table 1, detailed mechanisms for their activity remain to be elucidated. In particular, much is still unknown about structurally related Vpr and Vpx proteins. Moreover, functional studies in animals on HIV-1 and HIV-2 accessory proteins have not yet been performed.

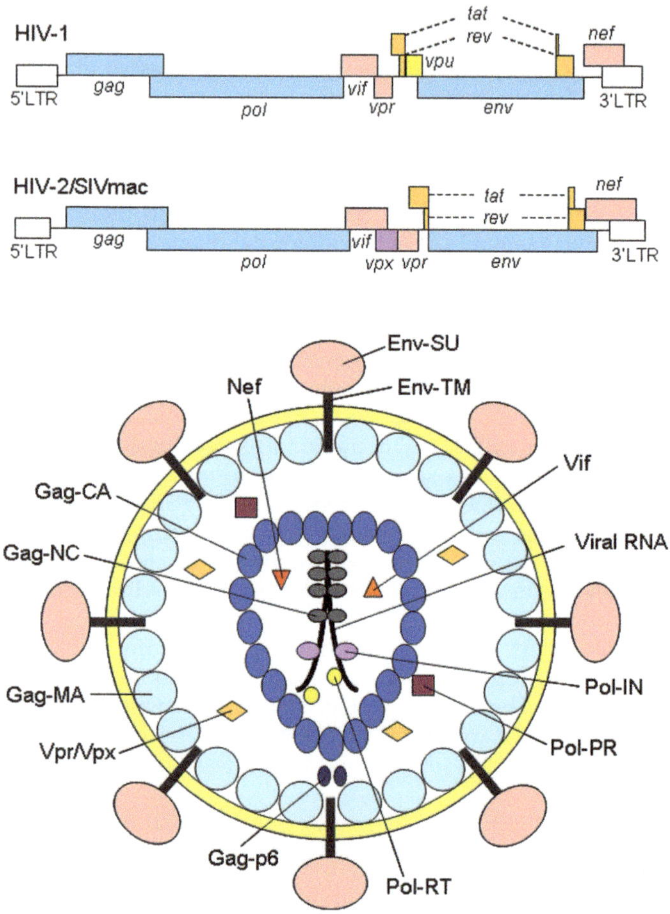

Fig. 1. Genome and virion characteristics of HIV/SIV. Upper: Proviral genome structure is schematically shown. Blue, orange, pink areas (boxes) indicate the structural, regulatory and accessory genes, respectively. Accessory genes unique to HIV-1 (*vpu*) and HIV-2/SIVmac (*vpx*) are indicated by yellow and purple, respectively. LTR, long terminal repeat. Lower: A schema of viral particle (virion). Viral proteins reported to be present in virion are illustrated. CA, capsid; IN, integrase; MA, matrix; NC, nucleocapsid; PR, protease; RT, reverse transcriptase; SU, surface; TM, transmembrane.

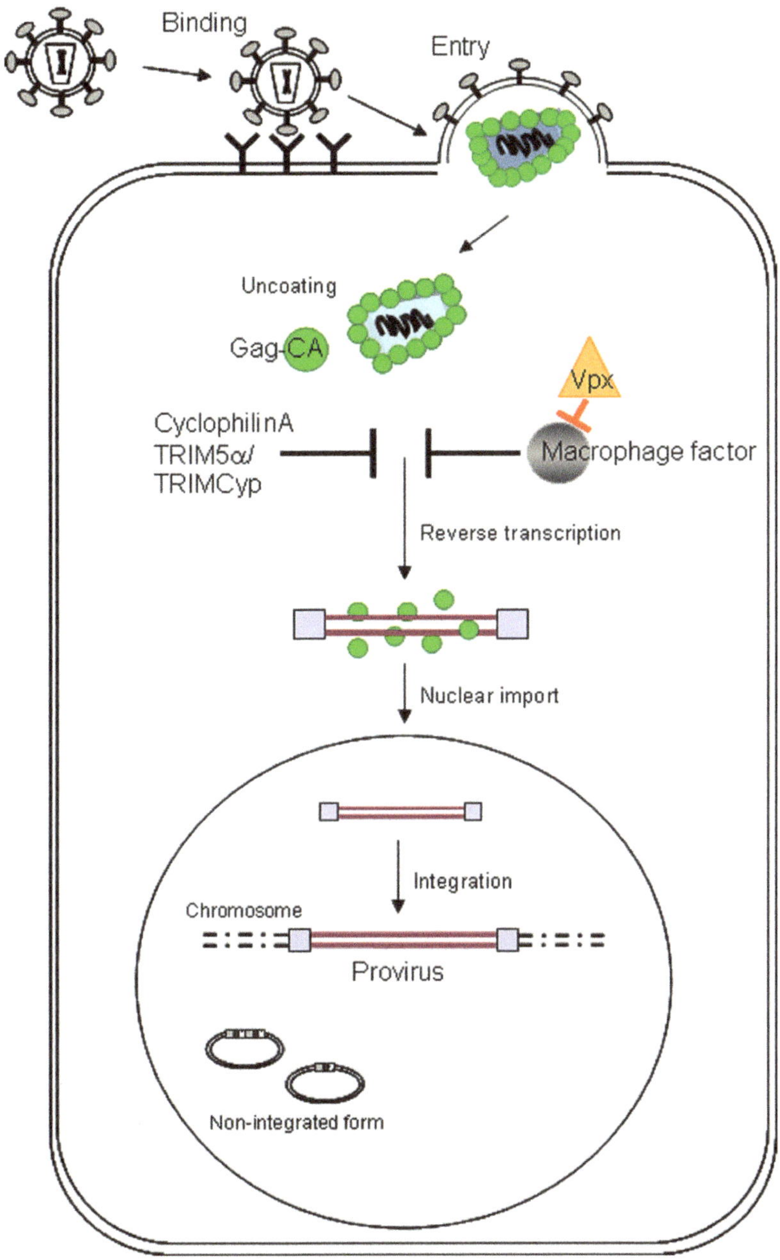

Fig. 2. The early phase of HIV/SIV replication cycle in target cells. Viral replication steps from the binding to generation of provirus are shown. Viral and cellular proteins particularly important in this chapter are highlighted. For details, see the reference (Freed & Martin, 2007).

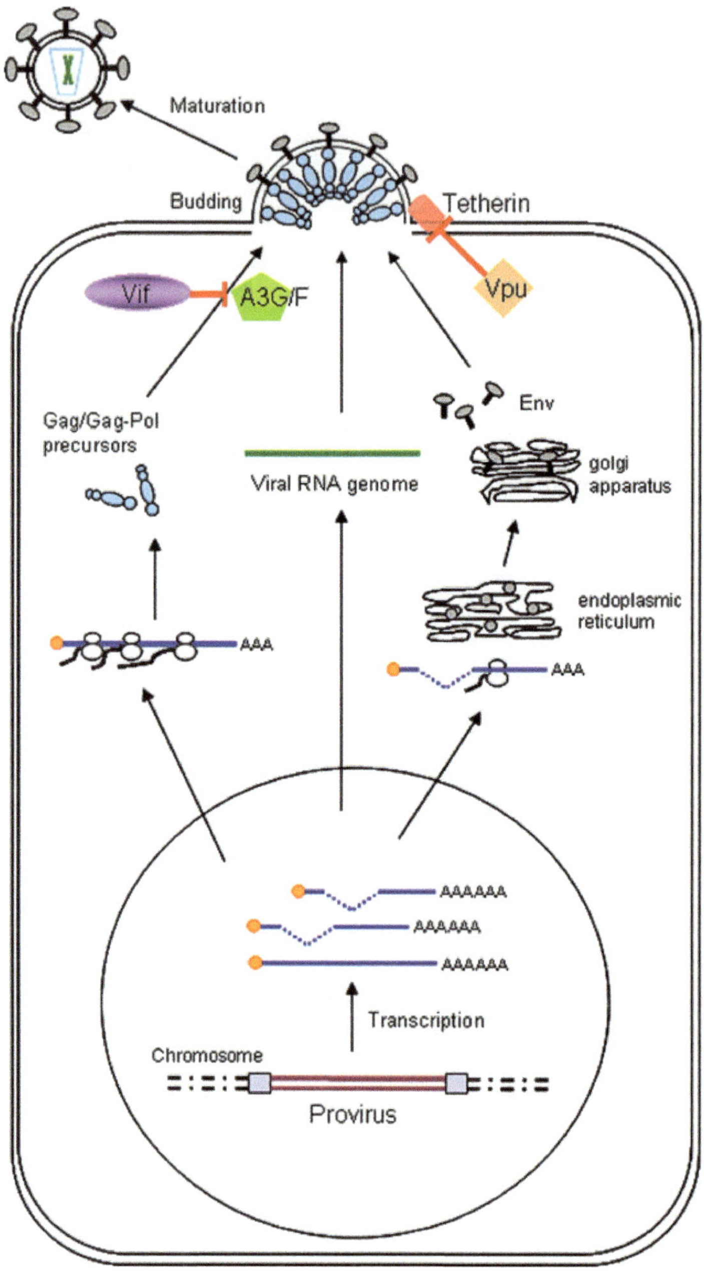

Fig. 3. The late phase of HIV/SIV replication cycle in target cells. Viral replication steps from the transcription of proviral genome to maturation are shown. Viral and cellular proteins particularly important in this chapter are highlighted. For details, see the reference (Freed & Martin, 2007).

Accessory proteins	Activities	References
Vif	Neutralization of antiviral activities of APOBEC3G/F Induction of G2 cell cycle arrest	Holmes et al., 2007 Huthoff & Towers, 2008 Izumi et al., 2010
Vpx	Inactivation of macrophage factor	Fujita et al., 2010
Vpr	Induction of G2 cell cycle arrest Trans-activation of transcription Promotion of nuclear import of pre-integration complex	Le rouzic & Benichou, 2005 Andersen et al., 2008 Ayinde et al., 2010 Fujita et al., 2010
Vpu	Degradation of tetherin Degradation of newly synthesized CD4 in ER	Bour & Strebel, 2003 Nomaguchi et al., 2008b Tokarev et al., 2009
Nef	Down-regulation of cell surface molecules (CD4, MHC-I etc.) Enhancement of viral infectivity	Kirchhoff et al., 2008 Kirchhoff, 2009 Jere et al., 2009

Table 1. Multi-functional activity of HIV/SIVmac accessory proteins. Major functions or activities are listed. For details, refer to the articles shown. ER, endoplasmic reticulum; MHC, major histocompatibility complex.

One of the most outstanding biological properties of HIV-1 is its especially narrow host range. It was recognized soon after the virus isolation that HIV-1 can not infect macaque cells and macaques, animals frequently used for experimental infection. We, therefore, pioneered the work to determine viral determinants for this species-tropism by construction and characterization of chimeric viruses between SIVmac and HIV-1 (Nomaguchi et al., 2008; Sakuragi et al., 1992; Shibata et al., 1991, 1995; Shibata & Adachi, 1992). SIVmac has a wider host range relative to HIV-1, and can efficiently replicate both in macaque and human cells. The chimeric viruses (Fig. 4), later called SHIV, were useful to localize the viral genetic area responsible for the tropism. Among NM-1, NM-3, and NM-8 in Fig.4, only NM-3 was shown to display infectivity to macaque cells. In addition, Gag-CA region was suggested to be important for the tropism by a similar analysis of chimeric viruses (Dorfman & Gottlinger, 1996). Totally, these SHIV studies revealed that Gag-CA plus some viral protein(s) encoded by the central viral genomic region may determine the HIV-1 species-tropism.

As for input viruses of model infection studies in macaques, SIVmac and SHIVs have been widely and frequently used (Ambrose et al., 2007; Nomaguchi et al., 2008). SIVmac is thought to emerge by a cross-species infection of rhesus macaques with SIVsmm naturally occurring in African sooty mangabeys (Fultz et al., 1986; Murphey-Corb et al., 1986). It targets CD4-positive cells such as T-lymphocytes and macrophages, persists, and finally cause AIDS in rhesus macaques. Pathogenic SHIVs have been obtained from the original prototype SHIV by serial animal passages, and were used for infection experiments in rhesus macaques. An SIVmac derivative that has reverse transcriptase (RT) of HIV-1 (RT-SHIV) (Fig. 4) was also constructed to test the effect of anti-RT drugs on virus replication (Uberla et al., 1995). Although these viruses did contribute much to HIV-1 model studies including the assessment of immune response, evaluation of anti-viral drugs, analysis of drug-resistance, and establishing the strategy for vaccine development, there are some intrinsic differences among important virological properties of HIV-1, SIVmac and SHIVs as summalized in Table 2. These should be seriously considered for the future model studies. To underscore the essential need for the suitable primate model research to answer basic questions about HIV-1 in vivo, we wish to mention here, as an example, that the trials to develop anti-viral vaccines have been unsuccessful due to the lack of appropriate models (Hayden, 2008; Watkins et al., 2008).

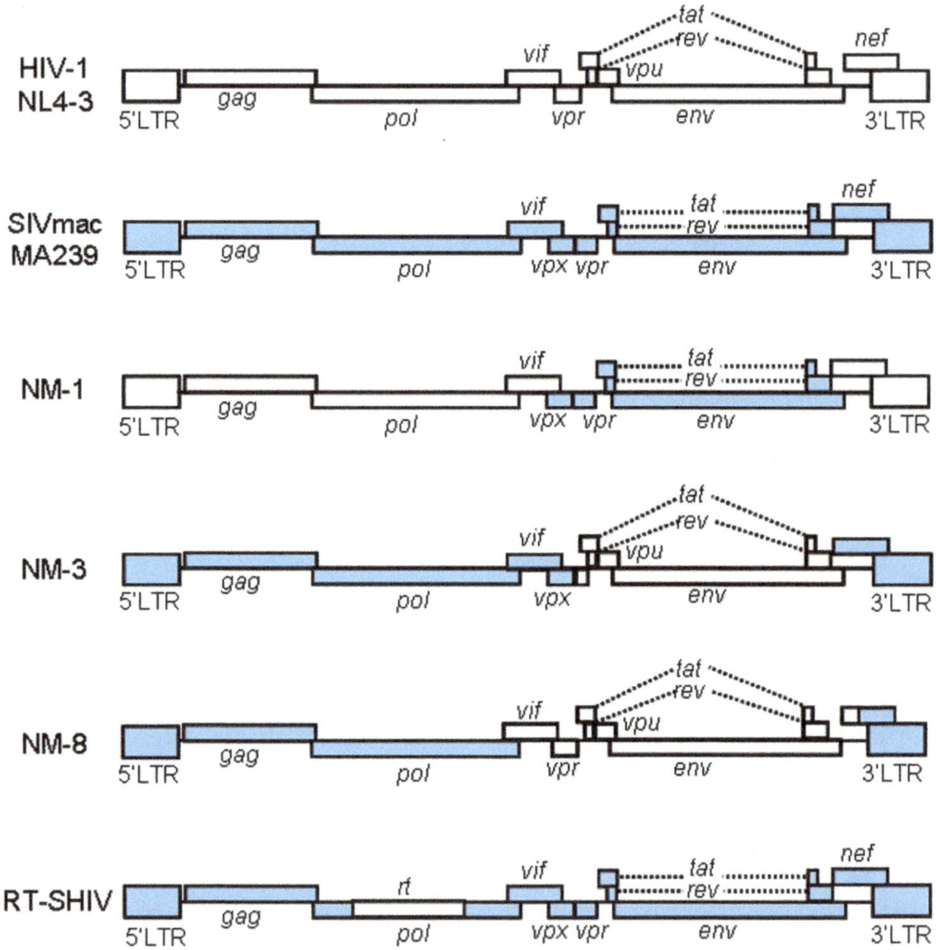

Fig. 4. Genome organization of HIV/SIV and representative SHIVs. Proviral genome structure is schematically shown. White and blue areas (boxes) indicate the genes and LTR of HIV-1 NL4-3 (Adachi et al., 1986) and SIVmac MA239 (Shibata et al., 1991), respectively. Areas without gene names indicate that the genes there are inactivated by genetic manipulations.

	HIV-1/human	SIVmac/rhesus	SHIV/rhesus	References
Outcomes in individuals				
Response to vaccines			Easily vaccinated	Ambrose et al., 2007 Freed & Martin, 2007
Response to drugs		Not always inhibited by anti-HIV-1 drugs	Not always inhibited by anti-HIV-1 drugs	Ambrose et al., 2007 Uberla et al., 1995
Median disease course	Approximately 10 years	One to three years	Rapid	Brown et al., 2007 Freed & Martin, 2007
Emergence of X4-tropic isolates	Frequent (Subtype B)	Rare		Brown et al., 2007
Accessory proteins in cells				
Vpx	Not present	Inactivate an unidentified anti-viral factor in macro-phages		Fujita et al., 2008 Sharova et al., 2008
Vpr	Influence viral replication in macrophages	Act on viral replication nothing in macrophages		Fujita et al., 2010
Vpu	Antagonize tetherin	Not present		Neil et al., 2008
Nef	Not antagonize tetherin Not down-regulate CD3	Antagonize tetherin Down-regulate CD3		Zhang et al., 2009 Kirchhoff, 2009

Table 2. Biology of HIV-1, SIVmac, and SHIV in infected hosts. For details, see the main references shown.

3. Determinants for HIV-1 species-tropism

Our early studies on systematic analysis of HIV-1 proviral mutants by site-directed mutagenesis have clearly demonstrated the cell-dependent functionality of some viral proteins (Gag-CA, Vif, Vpu, and Vpx) and the cell-dependent viral replication (Adachi et al., 1999; Kawamura et al., 1994b, 1998; Sakai et al., 1993, 1995; Sakuragi et al., 1995). These results have strongly suggested the presence of specific intracellular factors, other than receptor molecules for viruses, responsible for viral cellular tropism. Importantly, restriction factors against HIV-1 (APOBEC3/Vif, TRIM5α/Gag-CA, and tetherin/Vpu) have been recently identified and molecularly cloned (Neil et al., 2008; Sheehy et al., 2002; Stremlau et al., 2004; Van Damme et al., 2008). Furthermore, a new restriction factor functional in macrophages and antagonized by Vpx has been proposed (Fujita et al., 2008; Fujita et al., 2010; Sharova et al., 2008; Srivastava et al., 2008). Taken altogether, these findings have prompted active researchers to examine whether these cellular proteins are associated with the HIV-1 species-tropism. As results of a series of comparative biological and biochemical studies on the interaction between HIV/SIV and human/monkey restriction factors, it has been revealed that various species-specific cellular proteins in Table 3 determine or modulate the species-tropism of HIV-1. As can be understood in Table 3, viral accessory proteins Vif, Vpu, Vpx (and/or Vpr), and Nef (in the case of some SIVs) play significant roles (Tables 1 and 2) against the restriction factors present in host cells (Malim & Emerman,

Host restriction factors	Viral proteins	Antiviral effects
APOBEC3G/F	Vif	Induction of lethal mutations in the viral genome
CypA and TRIM5α/TRIMCyp	Gag-CA	Block of post-entry replication steps
Tetherin/BST-2	Vpu	Inhibition of virion release
Macrophage factor?	Vpx/Vpr?	Suppression of uncoating / reverse transcription?

Table 3. Restriction factors against HIV-1. Cellular anti-HIV-1 factors identified and one of potential anti-viral factors are listed. As for the details of restriction factors of these two categories, see the text.

2008). It is well-predicted that primate immunodeficiency viruses now have evolved by acquiring the appropriate accessory genes through numerous mutations and recombinations (Kirchhoff, 2009, 2010; Sauter et al., 2009, 2010). Among viral structural proteins, only Gag-CA, which constitutes a major virion component, appears to be deeply involved in the species-tropism of HIV-1. By adapting Gag-CA and accessory proteins to the hostile environment, HIV/SIV could spread, persist, and survive. In this regard, HIV-1 has developed its specific characteristics from the progenitor form, and may be still uniquely altering its virological property through multiple rounds of the infection cycle in human populations.

3.1 Vif and APOBEC3G/F

Accessory protein Vif (Table 1) is essential for HIV/SIV replication in certain cell types such as natural target cells (T-lymphocytes and macrophages) that express APOBEC3G/APOBEC3F. APOBEC3G/F are members of a polynucleotide cytidine deaminase family that displays diverse functions (Holmes et al., 2007), and are potent inhibitors of viral replication counteracted by Vif. Vif degrades APOBEC3G/F via the ubiquitin-proteasome pathway (Table 1 and Fig. 3). In the absence of Vif, APOBEC3G/F are incorporated into virions, and cause lethal mutations in viral genome during the reverse transcription process in a new infection cycle (Table 3). There are two functional domains in Vif, that is, N-terminal binding region to APOBEC proteins and C-terminal region for degradation (Strebel et al., 2009). Noteworthy, HIV-1 Vif does not degrade APOBEC3Gs of the rhesus macaque and African green monkey probably due to its inability to binding to them. In contrast, SIVmac Vif can inactivate both human and simian APOBEC3Gs. Thus, the interaction of Vif and APOBEC3G/F is critically important for the unique species-tropism of HIV-1. In our experience, APOBEC3G/F is the strongest determinant for this tropism among the restriction factors listed in Table 3. Whether another activity of Vif to induce G2 cell cycle arrest (Izumi, T., 2010) (Table 1) is involved in the species-tropism is presently unknown.

3.2 Gag-CA and its interacting cellular proteins (CypA, TRIM5α and TRIMCyp)

Early studies have already indicated that Gag-CA is responsible for the HIV-1 species-tropism as described above (Shibata et al., 1991; Dorfman & Gottlinger, 1996). Recent works have focused on the interaction of Gag-CA and its counterpart (CypA, TRIM5α and a TRIM5α/CypA fusion protein, TRIMCyp). It is well-established now that CypA, TRIM5α and TRIMCyp act as an inhibitor of HIV-1 replication in a species-specific manner (Lim et al., 2010; Luban, 2007; Nakayama & Shioda, 2010; Price et al., 2009; Towers, 2007; Ylinen, 2010). These cellular proteins exert their anti-viral powers on the incoming virion core in a poorly defined way (Table 3 and Fig. 2). Of note, CypA positively and negatively regulates HIV-1 replication in human and macaque cells, respectively. Importantly, rhesus TRIM5α, cynomolgus TRIM5α and cynomolgus TRIMCyp effectively inhibit HIV-1 replication, but not rhesus TRIMCyp. Therefore, CypA, TRIM5α and TRIMCyp can determine the unique species-tropism of HIV-1. We estimate that Gag-CA is the second strongest determinant for the tropism. It should be stressed here that the polymorphism observed in TRIM5 alleles affects the sensitivity of hosts to virus infection.

3.3 Vpu and tetherin

Accessory protein Vpu (Table 1) is required for optimal replication of HIV-1 in certain cell types that express tetherin. Tetherin specifically inhibits the virion release from cells (Table 3) and is countered by Vpu (Nomaguchi et al. 2008b; Strebel et al., 2009). Vpu degrades cellular tetherin and CD4 effectively. It is generally accepted that Vpu enhances virion release from the cell surface by down-regulation of tetherin (Table1, Table 2 and Fig.3), and thereby promote viral replication. However, Vpu proteins of HIV-1 and some SIVs can not efficiently antagonize simian tetherin molecules relative to those of SIVs with a high ability (Sauter et al, 2009). In fact, HIV-1 NL4-3 scarcely suppressed the anti-viral activity of the rhesus tetherin. Based on this finding, it can be concluded that tetherin is associated with the species-tropism of HIV-1. However, in our experience, the positive effect of Vpu on viral replication is much smaller than those of Vif and Gag-CA. Moreover, another functional activity of Vpu to degrade cellular CD4 is considered to be irrelevant to the HIV-1 species-tropism. Whether Vpu is associated with the HIV-1 pathogenesis is an important question to address. Interestingly and importantly, Env of some HIV-2 isolates and Nef of some SIVs have the Vpu-like ability to enhance virion release (Strebel et al., 2009; Zhang et al., 2009).

3.4 Potential determinants for HIV-1 species-tropism

It has been recently reported that HIV-2/SIVmac Vpx is necessary for the post-entry step of viral replication, such as uncoating/reverse transcription, in monocyte-derived dendritic cells and macrophages (Fujita et al., 2008; Goujon et al., 2007; Srivastava et al., 2008). Vpx is supposed to counter an unidentified anti-retroviral factor(s) present in cells of this lineage (Tables 1-3 and Fig. 2). Because Vpx can also up-regulate the HIV-1 replication, the unidentified macrophage factor appears to be commonly important for HIV/SIV replication. To substantiate the macrophage entity as a restriction factor against HIV/SIV and/or the other retroviruses, its identification is urgently required.

During a systemic characterization of HIV-1mt CA mutants, we have noticed a TRIM5α-independent enhancement of viral infectivity in macaque cells (Nomaguchi et al., manuscript in preparation). This result suggests the presence of unknown anti-viral factor that interact with HIV-1 Gag-CA. We also have found a mutation in the Env-SU region that confers the mutant a significant affinity to macaque CD4, considerably promoting virus replication (Nomaguchi et al., manuscript in preparation). These observations may be relevant to the HIV-1 species-tropism.

4. Generation and characterization of various HIV-1mt clones

To obtain a novel class of HIV-1 that infects, replicates and finally causes AIDS in macaques, we and a research group in USA have independently initiated the work on HIV-1mt and have done macaque model studies (Hatcho et al., 2008; Hatziioannou, 2006, 2009; Igarashi et al., 2007; Kamada et al., 2006, 2009; Kuroishi et al., 2009; Nomaguchi et al., 2008a; Saito et al., 2011; Yamashita et al., 2008). Another group has published a report on HIV-1mt derivatives very recently (Thippeshappa et al., 2011). We now are actively and thoroughly amending the HIV-1mt genome by computer-assisted and structure-guided mutagenesis.

Our prototype HIV-1mt designated NL-DT5R (Kamada et al., 2006) contains a 21-nucleotide SIVmac Gag-CA element (corresponding to the HIV-1 CypA-binding loop) and the entire SIVmac *vif* gene inserted into the genetic background of HIV-1 NL4-3 (Adachi et al., 1986). From this clone, we have systemically generated a series of HIV-1mt clones as shown in Fig. 5. Because CCR5-tropic (R5) viruses of HIV-1 are thought to be clinically more important than CXCR4-tropic (X4) viruses, we have constructed two sets of HIV-1mt clones. Our strategy for generation of HIV-1mt clones pathogenic for macaques are as follows: (i) Adaptation of viruses in macaque cells. Targets for infection are cynomolgus and rhesus macaque lymphocyte cell lines immortalized by Herpesvirus saimiri (HVS) (Table 4).; (ii) In vitro mutagenesis of the clones based on bioinformatics. With the aid of the computational sciences, new viral genome sequences are designed.; (iii) Selection of appropriate clones by their replication kinetics in macaque lymphocyte cell lines in Table 4. Viruses which replicates similarly with or more robustly than SIVmac239 in cynomolgus and rhesus peripheral blood mononuclear cells are then chosen. On the basis of this strategy, we have successfully obtained a number of new generations with increasing ability to replicate from the original prototype NL-DT5R (see below). However, so far, none of the HIV-1mt clones tested are pathogenic for macaques (pig-tailed and cynomolgus) (Igarashi et al., 2007; Nomaguchi et al., manuscript in preparation; Saito et al., 2011), although they all can replicate in the monkeys. The newest clones in Fig. 5 (MN4Rh-3V and MN5Rh-3V), which replicate best in macaque cells among our HIV-1mt clones, have not yet been examined for their pathogenicity. It should be mentioned here that the replication potentials of the HIV-1mt clones in cell lines parallel with those in individuals.

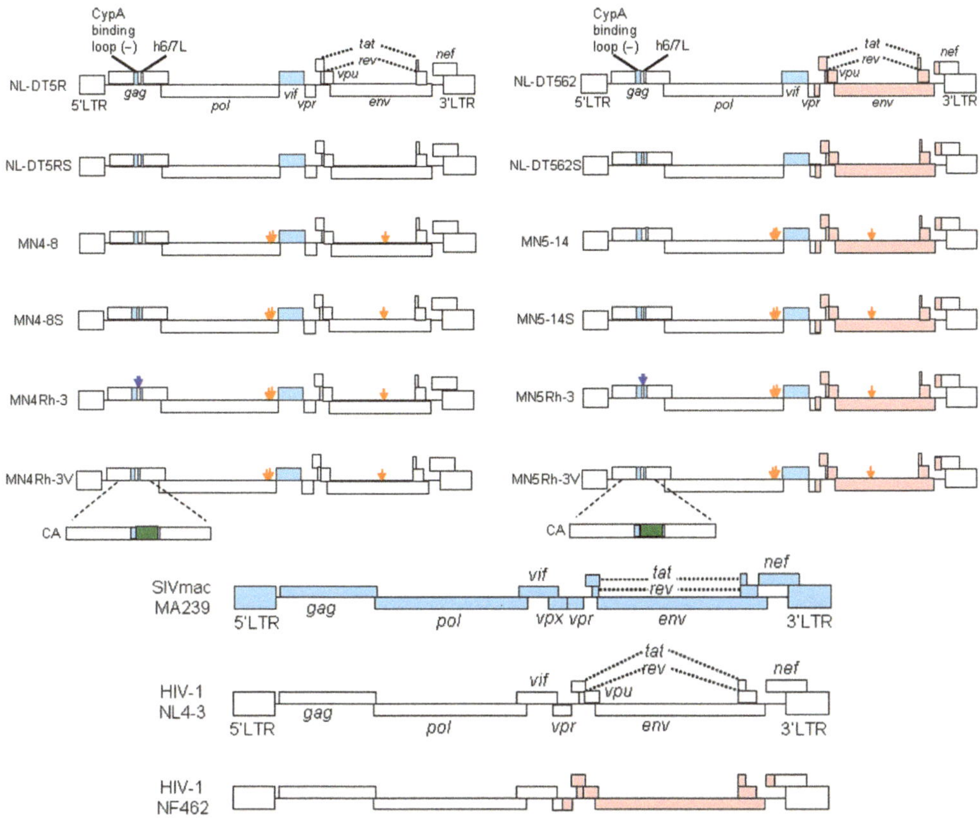

Fig. 5. Genome organization of HIV/SIV and various clones of HIV-1mt. Proviral genome structure is schematically shown. Blue, white and pink areas (boxes) indicate the genes and LTR of SIVmac MA239 (Shibata et al., 1991), X4-tropic HIV-1 NL4-3 (Adachi et al., 1986) and R5-tropic HIV-1 NF462 (Kawamura et al., 1994a), respectively. HIV-1mt clones on the left and right are X4 and R5 viruses, respectively. Arrows indicate the site of each single/double nucleotide-mutation introduced (Nomaguchi et al., manuscripts in preparation). There are several single-nucleotide mutations in the green area of Gag-CA (Nomaguchi et al., unpublished). h6/7L, Loop between helices 6 and 7.

In parallel with the generation and characterization of a series of HIV-1 mt clones, we have searched for and established macaque cell lines suitable for our projects. Table 4 lists the cell lines we routinely use now. Since the lymphocyte cell lines immortalized by HVS do not lose their original characteristics as primary lymphocytes in most cases and are readily maintained for experiments, to biologically characterize viruses like HIV-1, it is quite important for laboratory researchers to have HVS-immortalized cell lines. In our laboratory, cynomolgus HSC-F (Akari et al., 1996; Fujita et al., 2003) and rhesus M1.3S (Doi et al., 2011) cell lines are chosen as targets for virus infection, and frequently used. HSC-F cells are very sensitive to HIV-1mt and SIVmac clones, and produce a large amount of progeny viruses after infection. M1.3S cells are quite resistant to HIV-1mt and SIVmac clones, and are appropriate for selection of highly replicable and potentially pathogenic viruses. Because we are interested in analyzing the species-tropism of HIV-1, we need to have various target cell lines of human and simian origins with a unique property. Monolayer cell lines of cynomolgus MK.P3 (F) and rhesus LLC-MK2 are easily used for transfection experiments and for monitoring the single-cycle viral infectivity assays. In fact, we have differentially and successfully used the cell lines in Table 4 depending on the purpose of each project.

Macaques	Cell lines	Origins	TRIM5 alleles
Cynomolgus	HSC-F	lymphocyte	TRIM5α and TRIMCyp
	MK.P3 (F)	kidney	TRIM5α and TRIMCyp
Rhesus	HSR1.4	lymphocyte	Mamu-3 and Mamu-4
	HSR5.4	lymphocyte	Mamu-7
	M1.3S	lymphocyte	Mamu-1 and Mamu-3
	LLC-MK2	kidney	Mamu-1 and Mamu-7

Table 4. Cell lines for virological evaluation of HIV-1mt. TRIM5 alleles of the cell lines listed have been determined in our laboratory (Doi et al., 2010; our unpublished results). For the polymorphism of TRIM5 alleles, see the references (Newman et al., 2006; Virgen et al., 2008; Wilson et al., 2008).

We have repeatedly examined the replication kinetics of HIV-1mt clones in various macaque cell lines. Fig. 6 shows the typical kinetics (a schema) based on the results from our numerous infection experiments. In highly sensitive HSC-F cells, all the viruses do replicate to distinct extents. As is clear, MN4Rh-3V and MN5Rh-3V replicate most robustly among HIV-1mt clones. In relatively resistant M1.3S cells, three clones do replicate but the others do not. In both cell lines, SIVmac239 (MA239N) (Doi et al., 2010) displays the best potential to replicate. These results indicate that we still need to improve MN4Rh-3V and MN5Rh-3V to obtain the ideal clone, the pathogenic HIV-1mt. In this situation, there are two directions. These are the selection of host macaques susceptible to the currently available clones and the further efforts to obtain the desired clones. First, pig-tailed and/or the other macaque species sensitive to the viruses can be selected by their TRIM5 alleles (Newman et al., 2006; Virgen et al., 2008; Wilson et al., 2008), and used for infection. Indeed, American research groups have adopted this strategy using the pig-tailed macaques/variants of simian-tropic (st) HIV-1 with a *vif*-substitution only (Hatziioannou et al., 2009; Thippeshappa et al., 2011). However, we very much prefer to take the second possibility. Through this approach, we would be able to better understand the molecular mechanism underlying various events between the pathogen and host. Furthermore, if one is interested in the studies to analyze the mutations, adaptations, and evolution of the pathogen, the pressure-giving environment (Malim & Emerman, 2008), i.e., natural hosts having a wide variety of restriction factors, would be much better. Of a particular note, pig-tailed monkeys infected with various st HIV-1s have not yet develop AIDS (Igarashi et al., 2007; Hatziioannou et al., 2009; Thippeshappa et al., 2011).

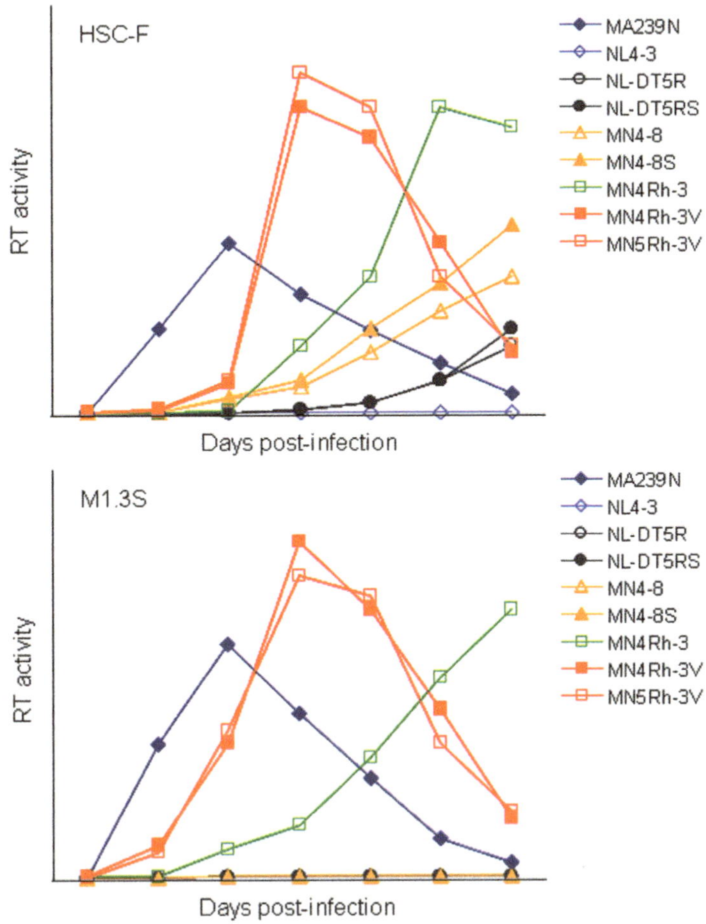

Fig. 6. Schematic representation of replication kinetics of various viral clones. A schema of replication kinetics is illustrated. Molecular proviral clones for study are shown on the right. Routinely, cell-free virus samples are prepared by transfection of proviral clones into 293T cells (Kamada et al., 2006), and viruses produced in cells of equal RT units are inoculated into HSC-F and M1.3S cells (Table 4). After infection, viral replication is monitored at intervals by RT activity in the culture supernatants.

5. Conclusion

We have described the generation of CXCR4-tropic and CCR5-tropic HIV-1 clones with macaque cell-tropism (HIV-1mt) in this chapter. The best X4 and R5 viruses we have now replicate comparably with a standard SIVmac clone in macaque cells, although their pathogenicity for macaques needs to be determined. The genomes of these HIV-1 mt clones contain the entire *vif* gene of SIVmac, some nucleotide substitutions in the *gag* gene to give a small number of mutated amino acids, two adaptive mutations in the *pol* gene, and one adaptive mutation in the *env* gene (Fig. 5).

For the moment, our goal is to have the HIV-1mt clones pathogenic for cynomolgus and/or rhesus macaques with the aid of computational sciences. The clones are expected to have the HIV-1-derived or closely related accessory genes except for the *vif* gene. With these ideal HIV-1mt clones, we would be able to authentically investigate the HIV-1/host interaction including: (i) viral replication in individuals; (ii) viral pathogenesis; (iii) viral mutations/adaptations/evolution. Once these clones are available, a wide variety of basic and clinical studies would be initiated otherwise impossible.

6. Acknowledgment

We thank Mrs. Kazuko Yoshida of our laboratory (Institute of Health Biosciences, The University of Tokushima Graduate School) for excellent editorial assistance. This work was supported in part by a Grant-in-Aid for Scientific Research (B) from the Japan Society for the Promotion of Science (ID no. 21390141).

Our recent studies described in this chapter have been done in collaboration with the following researchers: Akatsuki Saito and Hirofumi Akari (Primate Research Institute, Kyoto University, Japan); Ken Kono, Emi E. Nakayama and Tatsuo Shioda (Research Institute for Microbial Diseases, Osaka University, Japan); Masaru Yokoyama and Hironori Sato (Center for Pathogen Genomics, National Institute of Infectious Diseases, Japan). We are indebted to these scientists for their critical contribution to our work. We also thank all staffs in our department and the other institutions who have supported our work.

Many original articles reporting the scientifically new and important findings could not be cited due to the tremendous numbers of publications and the space limitations. We express our sincere regret over these omissions based on rather subjective considerations.

7. References

Adachi, A.; Gendelman, H.E.; Koenig, S.; Folks, T.; Willey, R.; Rabson, A. & Martin, M.A. (1986). Production of acquired immunodeficiency syndrome-associated retrovirus in human and nonhuman cells transfected with an infectious molecular clone. *Journal of Virology*, Vol.59, No.2, (August 1986), pp. 284-291, ISSN 0022-538X

Adachi, A.; Tamaki, M.; Shimano, R.; Inubushi, R.; Naito, T.; Yoshida, K.; Oshima, Y.; Kawamura, M.; Koyama, A.H. (1999). Cell-dependent replication potentials of HIV-1 gag mutants. *Microbes and Infection*, Vol.1, No.9, (July 1999), pp. 671-676, ISSN 1286-4579

Akari, H.; Mori, K.; Terao, K.; Otani, I.; Fukasawa, M.; Mukai, R. & Yoshikawa, Y. (1996). In vitro immortalization of Old World monkey T lymphocytes with Herpesvirus saimiri: its susceptibility to infection with simian immunodeficiency viruses. *Virology*, Vol.218, No.2, (April 1996), pp. 382-388, ISSN 0042-6822

Ambrose, Z.; KewalRamani, V.N.; Bieniasz, P.D. and Hatziioannou, T. (2007). HIV/AIDS: in search of an animal model. *Trends in Biotechnology*, Vol.25, No.8, (August 2007), pp. 333-337, ISSN 0167-7799

Andersen, J.L.; Le Rouzic, E. & Planelles, V. (2008). HIV-1 Vpr: mechanism of G2 arrest and apoptosis. *Experimental and Molecular Pathology*, Vol.85, No.1, (August 2008), pp. 2-10, ISSN 0014-4800

Andrew, A. & Strebel K. (2010). HIV-1 Vpu targets cell surface markers CD4 and BST-2 through distinct mechanisms. *Molecular Aspects of Medicine*, Vol.31, No.5, (October 2010), pp. 407-417, ISSN 0098-2997

Arhel, N. & Kirchhoff, F. (2010). Host proteins involved in HIV infection: new therapeutic targets. *Biochimica et Biophysica Acta–Molecular Basis of Disease*, Vol.1802, No.3, (March 2010), pp. 313-321, ISSN 0925-4439

Ayinde, A.; Maudet, C.; Transy, C. & Margottin-Goguet, F. (2010). Limelight on two HIV/SIV accessory proteins in macrophage infection: is Vpx overshadowing Vpr? *Retrovirology*, Vol.7, (April 2010), 35, ISSN 1742-4690

Barre-Sinoussi, F.; Chermann, J.C.; Rey, F.; Nugeyre, M.T.; Chamaret, S.; Gruest, J.; Dauguet, C.; Axler-Blin, C.; Vezinet-Brun, F.; Rouzioux, C.; Rosenbaum, W. & Montagnier, L. (1983). Isolation of a T-lymphotropic retrovirus from a patient at risk for acquired immune deficiency syndrome (AIDS). *Science*, Vol.220, No.4599, (May 1983), pp. 868-871, ISSN 0036-8075

Barre-Sinoussi, F. (2010). HIV: a discovery opening the road to novel scientific knowledge and global health improvement. *Virology*, Vol.397, No.2, (February 2010), pp. 255-259, ISSN 0042-6822

Bergamaschi, A. & Pancino G. (2010). Host hindrance to HIV-1 replication in monocytes and macrophages. *Retrovirology*, Vol.7, (April 2010), 31, ISSN 1742-4690

Bour, S. & Strebel K. (2003). The HIV-1 Vpu protein: a multifunctional enhancer of viral particle release. *Microbes and Infection*, Vol.5, No,11, (September 2003), pp. 1029-1039, ISSN 1286-4579

Brown, C.R.; Czapiga, M.; Kabat, J.; Dang, Q.; Ourmanov, I.; Nishimura, Y.; Martin, M.A. & Hirsch, V.M. (2007). Unique pathology in simian immunodeficiency virus-infected rapid progressor macaques is consisitent with a pathogenesis distinct from that of classical AIDS. *Journal of Virology*, Vol.81, No.11, (June 2007), pp. 5594-5606, ISSN 0022-538X

Clavel, F.; Guetard, D.; Brun-Vezinet, F.; Chamaret, S.; Rey, M.A.; Santos-Ferreira, M.O.; Laurent, A.G.; Dauguet, C.; Katlama, C.; Rouzioux, C.; Klatzmann, D.; Champalimaud, J.L. & Montagnier, L. (1986). Isolation of a new human retrovirus from West African patients with AIDS. *Science*, Vol.233, No.4761, (July 1986), pp. 343-346, ISSN 0036-8075

Desrosiers, R.C. (2007). Nonhuman lentiviruses, In : *Fields Virology 5th edition*, D.M. Knipe, P.M. Howley, D.E. Griffin, R.A. Lamb, M.A. Martin, B. Roizman & S.E. Straus, (Eds.), 2215-2243, Lippencott Williams & Wilkins, ISBN 978-0-7817-6060-7, Philadelphia, USA.

Doi, N.; Fujiwara, S.; Adachi, A. & Nomaguchi, M. (2010). Growth ability in various macaque cell lines of HIV-1 with simian cell-tropism. *Journal of Medical Investigation*, Vol.57, No.3/4, (August 2010), pp. 284-292, ISSN 1343-1420

Doi, N.; Fujiwara, S.; Adachi, A. & Nomaguchi, M. (2011). Rhesus M1.3S cells suitable for biological evaluation of macaque-tropic HIV/SIV clones. *Frontiers in Microbiology*, Vol.2, (May 2011), 115, ISSN 1664-302X

Dorfman, T. & Gottlinger H.G. (1996). The human immunodeficiency virus type 1 capsid p2 domain confers sensitivity to the cyclophilin-binding drug SDZ NIM 811. *Journal of Virology*, Vol.70, No.9, (September 1996), pp. 5751-5757, ISSN 0022-538X

Douglas, J.L.; Gustin, J.K.; Viswanathan, K.; Mansouri, M.; Moses, A.V. & Fruh, K. (2010). The great escape: viral strategies to counter BST-2/tetherin. *PLoS Pathogens*, Vol.6, No.5, (May 2010), e1000913, ISSN 1553-7366

Franke, E.K.; Yuan, H.E. & Luban, J. (1994). Specific incorporation of cyclophilin A into HIV-1 virions. *Nature*, Vol.372, No.6504, (November 1994), pp. 359-362, ISSN 0028-0836

Freed, E.O. & Martin, M.A. (2007). HIVs and their replication, In : *Fields Virology 5th edition*, D.M. Knipe, P.M. Howley, D.E. Griffin, R.A. Lamb, M.A. Martin, B. Roizman & S.E. Straus, (Eds.), 2107-2185, Lippencott Williams & Wilkins, ISBN 978-0-7817-6060-7, Philadelphia, USA.

Fujita, M.; Yoshida, A.; Sakurai, A.; Tatsuki, J.; Ueno, F.; Akari, H. & Adachi, A. (2003). Susceptibility of HVS-immortalized lymphocytic HSC-F cells to various strains and mutants of HIV/SIV. *International Journal of Molecular Medicine*, Vol. 11, No.5, (2003), pp. 641-644, ISSN 1107-3756

Fujita, M.; Otsuka, M.; Miyoshi, M.; Khamsri, B.; Nomaguchi, M. & Adachi, A. (2008). Vpx is critical for reverse transcription of the human immunodeficiency virus type 2 genome in macrophages. *Journal of Virology*, Vol.82, No.15, (August 2008), pp. 7752-7756, ISSN 0022-538X

Fujita, M.; Otsuka, M.; Nomaguchi, M. & Adachi, A. (2010). Multifaceted activity of HIV Vpr/Vpx proteins: the current view of their virological functions. *Reviews in Medical Virology*, Vol.20, No.2, (March 2010), pp. 68-76, ISSN 1099-1654

Fultz, P.N.; McClure, H.M.; Anderson, D.C.; Swenson, R.B.; Anand, R. & Srinivasan, A. (1986). Isolation of a T-lymphotropic retrovirus from naturally infected sooty mangabey monkeys (Cercocebus atys). *Proceedings of the National Academy of Sciences of the United States of America*, Vol.83, No.14, (July 1986), pp. 5286-5290, ISSN 0027-8424

Goff, S.P. (2007). The retroviruses and their replication, In : *Fields Virology 5th edition*, D.M. Knipe, P.M. Howley, D.E. Griffin, R.A. Lamb, M.A. Martin, B. Roizman & S.E. Straus, (Eds.), 1999-2069, Lippencott Williams & Wilkins, ISBN 978-0-7817-6060-7, Philadelphia, USA.

Goujon, C.; Riviere, L.; Jarrosson-Wuilleme, L.; Bernaud, J.; Rigal, D.; Darlix, J.L. & Cimarelli, A. (2007). SIV_{SM}/HIV-2 Vpx proteins promote retroviral escape from a proteasome-dependent restriction pathway present in human dendritic cells. *Retrovirology*, Vol.4, (January 2007), 2, ISSN 1742-4690

Hayden, E.C. (2008). US plans more primate research. *Nature*, Vol.453, No.7194, (May 2008), p.439, ISSN 0028-0836

Hatcho, K.; Kamada, K.; Yamashita, T.; Adachi, A. & Nomaguchi, M. (2008). Replication potentials of *vif* variant viruses generated from monkey cell-tropic HIV-1 derivative clones NL-DT5/NL-DT5R. *Microbes and Infection*, Vol.10, No.10/11, (August/September 2008), pp. 1218-1222, ISSN 1286-4579

Hatziioannou, T.; Princiotta, M.; Piatak, M. Jr.; Yuan, F.; Zhang, F.; Lifson, J.D. & Bieniasz, P.D. (2006). Generation of simian-tropic HIV-1 by restriction factor evasion. *Science*, Vol.314, No.5796, (October 2006), p. 95, ISSN 0036-8075

Hatziioannou, T.; Ambrose, Z.; Chung, N.P.Y.; Piatak, M. Jr.; Yuan, F.; Trubey, C.M.; Coalter, V.; Kiser, R.; Schneider, D.; Smedley, J.; Pung, R.; Gathuka, M.; Estes, J.D.; Veazey, R.S.; KewalRamani, V.N.; Lifson, J.D. & Bieniasz, P.D. (2009). A macaque model of HIV-1 infection. *Proceedings of the National Academy of Sciences of the United States of America*, Vol.106, No.11, (March 2009), pp. 4425-4429, ISSN 0027-8424

Ho, D.D. & Bieniasz, P.D. (2008). HIV-1 at 25. *Cell*, Vol.133, No.4, (May 2008), pp. 561-565, ISSN ISSN 0092-8674

Holmes, R.K.; Malim, M.H. & Bishop, K.N. (2007). APOBEC-mediated viral restriction: not simply editing? *Trends in Biochemical Sciences*, Vol.32, No.3, (March 2007), pp. 118-128, ISSN 0968-0004

Hutoff, H & Towers, G.J. (2008). Restriction of retroviral replication by APOBEC3G/F and TRIM5alpha. *Trends in Microbiology*, Vol.16, No.12, (December 2008), pp. 612-619, ISSN 0966-842X

Igarashi, T.; Iyengar, R.; Byrum, R.A.; Buckler-White, A.; Dewar, R.L.; Buckler, C.E.; Lane, H.C.; Kamada, K.; Adachi, A. & Martin, M.A. (2007). Human immunodeficiency virus type 1 derivative with 7% simian immunodeficiency virus genetic content is able to establish infections in pig-tailed macaques. *Journal of Virology*, Vol.81, No.20, (October 2007), pp. 11549-11552, ISSN 0022-538X

Izumi, T.; Io, K.; Matsui, M.; Shirakawa, K.; Shinohara, M.; Nagai, Y.; Kawahara, M.; kobayashi, M.; Kondoh, H.; Misawa, N.; Koyanagi, Y.; Uchiyama, T. & Takaori-Kondo A. (2010). HIV-1 viral infectivity factor interacts with TP53 to induce G2 cell cycle arrest and positively regulate viral replication. *Proceedings of the National Academy of Sciences of the United States of America*, Vol.107, No.48, (November 2010), pp. 20798-20803, ISSN 0027-8424

Jere, A.; Fujita, M.; Adachi, A. & Nomaguchi, M. (2010). Role of HIV-1 Nef protein for virus replication in vitro. *Microbes and Infection*, Vol.12, No.1, (January 2010), pp. 65-70, ISSN 1286-4579

Kamada, K.; Igarashi, T.; Martin, M.A.; Khamsri, B.; Hatcho, K.; Yamashita, T.; Fujita, M.; Uchiyama, T. & Adachi, A. (2006). Generation of HIV-1 derivatives that productively infect macaque monkey lymphoid cells. *Proceedings of the National Academy of Sciences of the United States of America*, Vol.103, No.45, (November 2007), pp. 16959-16964, ISSN 0027-8424

Kamada, K.; Yamashita, T.; Hatcho, K.; Adachi, A. & Nomaguchi, M. (2009). Evasion from CypA- and APOBEC-mediated restrictions is insufficient for HIV-1 to efficiently grow in simian cells. *Microbes and Infection*, Vol.11, No.2, (February 2009), pp. 164-171, ISSN 1286-4579

Kawamura, M.; Ishizaki, T.; Ishimoto, A., Shioda, T.; Kitamura, T. & Adachi, A. (1994a). Growth ability of human immunodeficiency virus type 1 auxiliary gene mutants in primary blood macrophage cultures. *Journal of General Virology*, Vol.75, No.9, (September 1994), pp. 2427-2431, ISSN 0022-1317

Kawamura, M.; Sakai, H. & Adachi, A. (1994b). Human immunodeficiency virus Vpx is required for the early phase of replication in peripheral blood mononuclear cells. *Microbiology and Immunology*, Vol. 38, No.11, (November 1994), pp. 871-878, ISSN 0385-5600

Kawamura, M.; Shimano, R.; Inubushi, R.; Akari, H. & Adachi, A. (1998). Early function of Gag proteins is cell-dependent. *Biochemical and Biophysical Research Communications*, Vol.248, No.3, (July 1998), pp. 899-903, ISSN 0006-291X

Kestler, H.; Kodama, T.; Ringler, D.; Marthas, M.; Pedersen, N.; Lackner, A.; Regier, D.; Sehgal, P.; Daniel, M.; King, N. & Desrosiers, R. (1990). Induction of AIDS in rhesus monkeys by molecularly cloned simian immunodeficiency virus. *Science*, Vol.248, No.4959, (June 1990). pp. 1109-1112, ISSN 0036-8075

Kirchhoff, F. (2009). Is the high virulence of HIV-1 an unfortunate coincidence of primate lentiviral evolution? *Nature Reviews Microbiology*, Vol.7, No.6, (June 2009), pp. 467-476, ISSN 1740-1526

Kirchhoff, F. (2010). Immune evasion and counteraction of restriction factors by HIV-1 and other primate lentiviruses. *Cell Host & Microbe*, Vol.8, No.1, (July 2010), pp. 55-67, ISSN 1931-3128

Kirchhoff, F.; Schindler, M.; Specht, A.; Arhel, N. & Munch, J. (2008). Role of Nef in primate lentiviral immunopathogenesis. *Cellular and Molecular Life Sciences*, Vol.65, No.17, (September 2008), pp. 2621-2636, ISSN 1420-682X

Kuritzkes, D.R. & Walker, B.D. (2007). HIV-1 pathogenesis, clinical manifestations and treatment, In : *Fields Virology 5th edition*, D.M. Knipe, P.M. Howley, D.E. Griffin, R.A. Lamb, M.A. Martin, B. Roizman & S.E. Straus, (Eds.), 2187-2214, Lippencott Williams & Wilkins, ISBN 978-0-7817-6060-7, Philadelphia, USA.

Kuroishi, A.; Saito, A.; Shingai, Y.; Shioda, T.; Nomaguchi, M.; Adachi, A.; Akari, H. & Nakayama, E.E. (2009). Modification of a loop sequence between alpha-helices 6 and 7 of virus capsid (CA) protein in a human immunodeficiency virus type 1 (HIV-1) derivative that has simian immunodeficiency virus (SIVmac239) vif and CA alpha-helices 4 and 5 loop improves replication in cynomolgus monkey cells. *Retrovirology*, Vol. 6, (August 2009), 70, ISSN 1742-4690

Le Rouzic, E. & Benichou, S. (2005). The Vpr protein from HIV-1: distinct roles along the viral life cycle. *Retrovirology*, Vol.2, (February 2005), 11, ISSN 1742-4690

Lim, S.-Y.; Rogers, T.; Chan, T.; Whitney, J.B.; Kim, J.; Sodroski, J. & Letvin, N.L. (2010). TRIM5α modulates immunodeficiency virus control in rhesus monkeys. *PLoS Pathogens*, Vol.6, No.1, (January 2010), e1000738, ISSN 1553-7366

Luban, J. (2007). Cyclophilin A, TRIM5, and resistance to human immunodeficiency virus type 1 infection. *Journal of Virology*, Vol.81, No.3, (February 2007), pp. 1054-1061, ISSN 0022-538X

Malim, M.H. & Emerman, M. (2008). HIV-1 accessory proteins-ensuring viral survival in a hostile environment. *Cell Host & Microbe*, Vol.3, No.6, (June 2008), pp. 388-398, ISSN 1931-3128

Montagnier, L. (2010). 25 years after HIV discovery: prospects for cure and vaccine. *Virology*, Vol.397, No.2, (February 2010), pp. 248-254, ISSN 0042-6822

Murphey-Corb, M.; Martin, L.N.; Rangan, S.R.; Baskin, G.B.; Gormus, B.J.; Wolf, R.H.; Andes, W.A.; West, M. & Montelaro, R.C. (1986). Isolation of an HTLV-III-related retrovirus from macaques with simian AIDS and its possible origin in asymptomatic mangabeys. *Nature*, Vol.321, No.6068, (May 1986), pp. 435-437, ISSN 0028-0836

Nakayama, E.E. & Shioda, T. (2010). Anti-retroviral activity of TRIM5 alpha. *Reviews in Medical Virology*, Vol.20, No.2, (March 2010), pp. 77-92, ISSN 1099-1654

Neil, S.J.; Zang, T. & Bieniasz, P.D. (2008). Tetherin inhibits retrovirus release and is antagonized by HIV-1 Vpu. *Nature*, Vol.451, No.7177, (January 2008), pp. 425-430, ISSN 0028-0836

Newman, R.M.; Hall, L.; Connole, M.; Chen, G.-L.; Sato, S.; Yuste, E.; Diehl, W.; Hunter, E.; Kaur, A.; Miller, G.M. & Johnson, W.E. (2006). Balancing selection and the evolution of functional polymorphism in Old World monkey TRIM5α. *Proceedings of the National Academy of Sciences of the United States of America*, Vol.103, No.50, (December 2006), pp. 19134-19139, ISSN 0027-8424

Nisole, S., Lynch, C., Stoye, J.P. & Yap, M.W. (2004). A trim5-cyclophilin A fusion protein found in owl monkey kidney cells can restrict HIV-1. *Proceedings of the National Academy of Sciences of the United States of America*, Vol.101, No.36, (September 2004), pp. 13324-13328, ISSN 0027-8424

Nomaguchi, M.; Doi, N.; Kamada, K. & Adachi, A. (2008a). Species barrier of HIV-1 and its jumping by virus engineering. *Reviews in Medical Virology*, Vol.18, No.4, (July/August 2008), pp. 261-275, ISSN 1099-1654

Nomaguchi, M.; Fujita, M. & Adachi, A. (2008b). Role of Vpu protein for virus spread and pathogenesis. *Microbes and Infection*, Vol.10, No.9, (July 2008), pp. 960-967, ISSN 1286-4579

Nomaguchi, M. & Adachi, A. (2010). Virology as biosystematics: towards understanding the viral infection biology. *Frontiers in Microbiology*, Vol.1, (July 2010), 2, ISSN 1664-302X

Planelles, V. & Barker, E. (2010). Roles of Vpr and Vpx in modulating the virus-host cell relationship. *Molecular Aspects of Medicine*, Vol.31, No.5, (October 2010), pp. 398-406, ISSN 0098-2997

Price, A.J.; Marzetta, F.; Lammers, M.; Ylinen, L.M.J.; Schaller, T.; Wilson, S.J.; Towers, G.J. & James, L.C. (2009). Active site remodeling switches HIV specificity of antiretroviral TRIMCyp. *Nature Structural & Molecular Biology*, Vol.16, No.10, (October 2009), pp. 1036-1042, ISSN 1545-9993

Saito, A.; Nomaguchi, M.; Iijima, S.; Kuroishi, A.; Yoshida, T.; Lee, Y.J.; Hayakawa, T.; Kono, K.; Nakayama, E.E.; Shioda, T.; Yasutomo, Y.; Adachi, A.; Matano, T. & Akari, H. (2011). Improved capacity of a monkey-tropic HIV-1 derivative to replicate in cynomolgus monkeys with minimal modifications. *Microbes and Infection*, Vol.13, No.1, (January 2011), pp. 58-64, ISSN 1286-4579

Sakai, H.; Shibata, R.; Sakuragi, J.; Sakuragi, S.; Kawamura, M. & Adachi, A. (1993). Cell-dependent requirement of human immunodeficiency virus type 1 Vif protein for maturation of virus particles. *Journal of Virology*, Vol.67, No.3, (March 1993), pp. 1663-1666, ISSN 0022-538X

Sakai, H.; Tokunaga, K.; Kawamura, M. & Adachi, A. (1995). Function of human immunodeficiency virus type 1 Vpu protein in various cell types. *Journal of General Virology*, Vol.76, No.11, (November 1995), pp. 2717-2722, ISSN 0022-1317

Sakuragi, J.; Sakai, H.; Kawamura, M.; Tokunaga, K.; Ueda, S. & Adachi, A. (1995). Generation and characterization of a host cell-dependent gag gene mutant of human immunodeficiency viruis type 1. *Virology*, Vol.212, No.1, (September 1995), pp. 251-254, ISSN 0042-6822

Sakuragi, S.; Shibata, R.; Mikai, R.; Komatsu, T.; Fukasawa, M.; Sakai, H.; Sakuragi, J.; Kawamura, M.; Ibuki, K.; Hayami, M. & Adachi, A. (1992). Infection of macaque monkeys with a chimeric human and simian immunodeficiency virus. *Journal of General Virology*, Vol.73, No.11, (November 1992), pp. 2983-2987, ISSN 0022-1317

Sauter, D.; Schindler, M.; Specht, A.; Landford, W.N.; Munch, J.; Kim, K.-A.; Votteler J.; Schubert, U.; Bibollet-Ruche, F.; Keele, B.F.; Takehisa, J.; Ogando, Y.; Ochsenbauer, C.; Kappes, J.C.; Ayouba, A.; Peeters, M.; Learn, G.H.; Shaw, G.; Sharp, P.M.; Bieniasz, P.; Hahn, B.H.; Hatziioannou, T. & Kirchhoff, F. (2009). Tetherin-driven adaptation of Vpu and Nef function and the evolution of pandemic and nonpandemic HIV-1 strains. *Cell Host & Microbe*, Vol.6, No.5, (November 2009), pp. 409-421, ISSN 1931-3128

Sauter, D.; Specht, A. & Kirchhoff, F. (2010). Tetherin: holding on and letting go. *Cell*, Vol.141, No.3, (April 2010), pp. 392-398, ISSN 0092-8674

Sayah, D.M.; Sokolskaja, E.; Berthoux, L. & Luban, J. (2004). Cyclophilin A retrotransposition into TRIM5 explains owl monkey resistance to HIV-1. *Nature*, Vol.430, No.6999, (July 2004), pp. 569-573, ISSN 0028-0836

Sharova, N.; Wu, Y.; Zhu, X.; Stranska, R.; Kaushik, R.; Sharkey, M. & Stevenson, M. (2008). Primate lentiviral Vpx commanders DDB1 to counteract a macrophage restriction. *PLoS Pathogens*, Vol.4, No.5, (May 2008), e1000057, ISSN 1553-7366

Sheehy, A.M.; Gaddis, N.C.; Choi, J.D. & Malim, M.H. (2002). Isolation of a human gene that inhibits HIV-1 infection and is suppressed by the viral Vif protein. *Nature*, Vol.418, No.6898, (August 2002), pp. 646-650, ISSN 0028-0836

Shibata, R.; Kawamura, M.; Sakai, H.; Hayami, M.; Ishimoto, A. & Adachi, A. (1991). Generation of a chimeric human and simian immunodeficiency virus infectious to monkey peripheral blood mononuclear cells. *Journal of Virology*, Vol.65, No.7, (July 1991), pp. 3514-3520, ISSN 0022-538X

Shibata, R. & Adachi A. (1992). SIV/HIV recombinants and their use in studying biological properties. *AIDS Research and Human Retroviruses*, Vol.8, No.3, (March 1992), pp. 403-409, ISSN 0889-2229

Shibata, R.; Sakai, H.; Kawamura, M.; Tokunaga, K. & Adachi, A. (1995). Early replication block of human immunodeficiency virus type 1 in monkey cells. *Journal of General Virology*, Vol.76, No.11, (November 1995), pp. 2723-2730, ISSN 0022-1317

Srivastava, S.; Swanson, S.K.; Manel, N.; Florens, L.; Washburn, M.P. & Skowronski, J. (2008). Lentiviral Vpx accessory factor targets VprBP/DCAF1 substrate adaptor for cullin 4 E3 ubiquitin ligase to enable macrophage infection. *PLoS Pathogens*, Vol.4, No.5, (May 2008), e1000059, ISSN 1553-7366

Strebel, K.; Luban, J. & Jeang, K.-T. (2009). Human cellular restriction factors that target HIV-1 replication. *BMC Medicine*, Vol.7, (September 2009), 48, ISSN 1741-7015

Stremlau, M.; Owens, C.M.; Perron, M.J.; Kiessling, M.; Autissier, P. & Sodroski, J. (2004). The cytoplasmic body component TRIM5α restricts HIV-1 infection in Old Word monkeys. *Nature*, Vol.427, No.6977, (February 2004), pp. 848-853, ISSN 0028-0836

Thali, M.; Buskovsky, A.; Kondo, E.; Rosenwirth, B.; Walsh, C.T.; Sodroski, J. & Gottlinger, H.G. (1994). Functional association of cyclophilin A with HIV-1 virions. *Nature*, Vol.372, No.6504, (November 1994), pp. 363-365, ISSN 0028-0836

Thippeshappa, R.; Polacino, P.; Kimata, M.T.Y.; Siwak, E.B.; Anderson, D.; Wang, W.; Sherwood, L.; Arora, R.; Wen, M.; Zhou, P.; Hu, S.-L. & Kimata, J.T. (2011). Vif substitution enables persistent infection of pig-tailed macaques by human immunodeficiency virus type 1. *Journal of Virology*, Vol.85, No.8, (April 2011), pp. 3767-3779, ISSN 0022-538X

Tokarev, A.; Skasko, M.; Fitzpatrick, K. & Guatelli, J. (2009). Antiviral activity of the interferon-induced cellular protein BST-2/tetherin. *AIDS Research and Human Retroviruses*, Vol.25, No.12, ISSN 0889-2229

Towers, G.J. (2007). The control of viral infection tripartite motif proteins and cyclophilin A. *Retrovirology*, Vol.4, (June 2007), 40, ISSN 1742-4690

Uberla, K.; Stahl-Hennig, C.; Bottiger, D.; Matz-Rensing, K.; Kaup, F.J.; Li, J.; Haseltine, W.A.; Fleckenstein, B.; Hunsmann, G.; Oberg, B. & Sodroski, J. (1995). Animal model for the therapy of acquired immunodeficiency syndrome with reverse transcriptase inhibitors. *Proceedings of the National Academy of Sciences of the United States of America*, Vol.92, No.18, (August 1995), pp. 8210-8214, ISSN 0027-8424

Van Damme, N.; Goff, D.; Katsura, C.; Jorgenson, R.L.; Mitchell, R.; Johnson, M.C.; Stephens, E.B. & Guatelli, J. (2008). The interferon-induced protein BST-2 restricts HIV-1 release and is downregulated from the cell surface by the viral Vpu protein. *Cell Host & Microbe*, Vol.3, No.4, (April 2008), pp. 245-252, ISSN 1931-3128

Virgen, C.A.; Kratovac, Z.; Bieniasz, P.D. & Hatziioannou, T. (2008). Independent genesis of chimeric TRM-cyclophilin proteins in two primate species. *Proceedings of the National Academy of Sciences of the United States of America*, Vol.105, No.9, (March 2008), pp. 3563-3568, ISSN 0027-8424

Watkins, D.I.; Burton, D.R.; Kallas, E.G. ; Moore, J.P. & Koff, W.C. (2008). Nonhuman primate models and the failure of the Merck HIV-1 vaccine in humans. *Nature Medicine*, Vol.14, No.6, (June 2008), pp. 617-621, ISSN 1078-8956

Wilson, S.J.; Webb, B.L.; Ylinen, L.M.; Verschoor, E.; Heeney, J.L. & Towers, G.J. (2008). Independent evolution of an antiviral TRIMCyp in rhesus macaques. *Proceedings of the National Academy of Sciences of the United States of America*, Vol.105, No.9, (March 2008), pp. 3557-3562, ISSN 0027-8424

Yamashita, T.; Doi, N.; Adachi, A. & Nomaguchi, M. (2008). Growth ability in simian cells of monkey cell-tropic HIV-1 is greatly affected by downstream region of the *vif* gene. *Journal of Medical Investigation*, Vol.55, No.3/4, (August 2008), pp. 236-240, ISSN 1343-1420

Ylinen, L.M.; Price, A.J.; Rasaiyaah, J.; Hue, S.; Rose, N.J.; Marzetta, F.; james, L.C. & Towers, G.J. (2010). Conformational adaptation of Asian macaque TRIMCyp directs lineage specific antiviral activity. *PLoS Pathogens*, Vol.6, No.8, (August 2010), e1001062, ISSN 1553-7366

Zhang, F.; Wilson, S.J.; Landford, W.C.; Virgen, B.; Gregory, D.; Johnson, M.C.; Munch, J.; Kirchhoff, F.; Bieniasz, P.D. & Hatziioannou, T. (2009). Nef proteins from simian immunodeficiency viruses are tetherin antagonists. *Cell Host & Microbe*, Vol.6, No.1, (July 2009), pp. 54-67, ISSN 1931-3128

Permissions

The contributors of this book come from diverse backgrounds, making this book a truly international effort. This book will bring forth new frontiers with its revolutionizing research information and detailed analysis of the nascent developments around the world.

We would like to thank Dr. Theresa L. Chang, for lending her expertise to make the book truly unique. She has played a crucial role in the development of this book. Without her invaluable contribution this book wouldn't have been possible. She has made vital efforts to compile up to date information on the varied aspects of this subject to make this book a valuable addition to the collection of many professionals and students.

This book was conceptualized with the vision of imparting up-to-date information and advanced data in this field. To ensure the same, a matchless editorial board was set up. Every individual on the board went through rigorous rounds of assessment to prove their worth. After which they invested a large part of their time researching and compiling the most relevant data for our readers. Conferences and sessions were held from time to time between the editorial board and the contributing authors to present the data in the most comprehensible form. The editorial team has worked tirelessly to provide valuable and valid information to help people across the globe.

Every chapter published in this book has been scrutinized by our experts. Their significance has been extensively debated. The topics covered herein carry significant findings which will fuel the growth of the discipline. They may even be implemented as practical applications or may be referred to as a beginning point for another development. Chapters in this book were first published by InTech; hereby published with permission under the Creative Commons Attribution License or equivalent.

The editorial board has been involved in producing this book since its inception. They have spent rigorous hours researching and exploring the diverse topics which have resulted in the successful publishing of this book. They have passed on their knowledge of decades through this book. To expedite this challenging task, the publisher supported the team at every step. A small team of assistant editors was also appointed to further simplify the editing procedure and attain best results for the readers.

Our editorial team has been hand-picked from every corner of the world. Their multi-ethnicity adds dynamic inputs to the discussions which result in innovative outcomes. These outcomes are then further discussed with the researchers and contributors who give their valuable feedback and opinion regarding the same. The feedback is then collaborated with the researches and they are edited in a comprehensive manner to aid the understanding of the subject.

Apart from the editorial board, the designing team has also invested a significant amount of their time in understanding the subject and creating the most relevant covers. They scrutinized every image to scout for the most suitable representation of the subject and create an appropriate cover for the book.

The publishing team has been involved in this book since its early stages. They were actively engaged in every process, be it collecting the data, connecting with the contributors or procuring relevant information. The team has been an ardent support to the editorial, designing and production team. Their endless efforts to recruit the best for this project, has resulted in the accomplishment of this book. They are a veteran in the field of academics and their pool of knowledge is as vast as their experience in printing. Their expertise and guidance has proved useful at every step. Their uncompromising quality standards have made this book an exceptional effort. Their encouragement from time to time has been an inspiration for everyone.

The publisher and the editorial board hope that this book will prove to be a valuable piece of knowledge for researchers, students, practitioners and scholars across the globe.

List of Contributors

Yasutsugu Suzuki
Yong Loo Lin School of Medicine, National University of Singapore, Singapore
Graduate School of Biostudies, Kyoto University, Japan

Youichi Suzuki and Naoki Yamamoto
Yong Loo Lin School of Medicine, National University of Singapore, Singapore

Ben Haij N., Planès R., Mzoughi O. and Bahraoui E.
Université Paul Sabatier, Unité mixte INSERM/CNRS/UPS 1043, Toulouse, France

Daniëlle Hoogmoed, Marion Cornelissen and Antoinette van der Kuyl
University of Amsterdam, The Netherlands

Giovanna Romeo
Department of Infectious, Parasitic and Immune-Mediated Diseases, Istituto Superiore di Sanità, Rome, Italy
Department of Medical-Surgical Sciences and Biotechnologies, Sapienza University of Rome, Rome, Italy

Zulema A. Percario, Valentina Gallo and Elisabetta Affabris
Department of Biology, University Roma Tre, Rome, Italy

Maria Vincenza Chiantore
Department of Infectious, Parasitic and Immune-Mediated Diseases, Istituto Superiore di Sanità, Rome, Italy

Gianna Fiorucci
Department of Infectious, Parasitic and Immune-Mediated Diseases, Istituto Superiore di Sanità, Rome, Italy
Institute of Molecular Biology and Pathology, Consiglio Nazionale delle Ricerche, Rome, Italy

Giorgio Mangino
Department of Biology, University Roma Tre, Rome, Italy
Department of Medical-Surgical Sciences and Biotechnologies, Sapienza University of Rome, Rome, Italy

Rachna Shah and Theresa L. Chang
Public Health Research Institute and Department of Microbiology and Molecular Genetics, University of Medicine and Dentistry of New Jersey-New Jersey Medical School, United States

Wilfried Posch, Cornelia Lass-Flörl and Doris Wilflingseder
Innsbruck Medical University, Division of Hygiene and Medical Microbiology, Austria

Marta Epeldegui and Christel H. Uittenbogaart
UCLA AIDS Institute, David E. Geffen School of Medicine, University of California, Department of Microbiology, Immunology & Molecular Genetics, Los Angeles, CA , USA

Bianca Blom
Academic Medical Center, University of Amsterdam, Dept. Of Cell Biology & Histology, Amsterdam, The Netherlands

Daniel Pérez-Núñez
Centro de Biología Molecular Severo Ochoa (CSIC-UAM), Madrid, Spain

Narcisa Martínez-Quiles
Department of Microbiology, Facultad de Farmacia, Universidad Complutense de Madrid, Spain

Christina Guzzo, Nor Fazila Che Mat, Xiubo Zhang and Katrina Gee
Department of Biomedical and Molecular Sciences, Queen's University, Kingston, ON, Canada

Zoltan Beck
Division of Retrovirology, U.S. Military HIV Research Program, Walter Reed Army Institute of Research, Silver Spring, MD, USA
Henry M. Jackson Foundation for the Advancement of Military Medicine, Rockville, MD, USA

Carl R. Alving
Division of Retrovirology, U.S. Military HIV Research Program, Walter Reed Army Institute of Research, Silver Spring, MD, USA

Sarah Cudmore, Jeffrey Smith and Gary Garber
University of Ottawa, Canada

Ongrádi Joseph, Kövesdi Valéria and Nagy Károly
Institute of Medical Microbiology, Semmelweis University, Budapest, Hungary

Ablashi Dharam
HHV-6 Foundation, Santa Barbara, CA, USA

Matteoli Barbara and Ceccherini-Nelli Luca
Virology Unit and Retrovirus Center, Department of Experimental Pathology, University of Pisa, Pisa, Italy

Jorge C.G. Blanco and Lioubov M. Pletneva
Sigmovir Biosystems Inc., USA

Lorraine E. Earle and William I. Frels
Virion Systems Inc., Rockville, Maryland, USA

Masako Nomaguchi, Naoya Doi, Sachi Fujiwara and Akio Adachi
The University of Tokushima Graduate School, Japan